CANCER AND OCCUPATIONAL THERAPY

ENABLING
PERFORMANCE
AND PARTICIPATION
ACROSS THE
LIFESPAN

Edited by
Brent Braveman, OTR, PhD, FAOTA
Robin Newman, OTD, OT, OTR, CLT, FAOTA

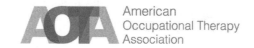

American
Occupational Therapy
Association

AOTA Vision 2025
Occupational therapy maximizes health, well-being, and quality of life for all people, populations, and communities through effective solutions that facilitate participation in everyday living.

Mission Statement
The American Occupational Therapy Association advances occupational therapy practice, education, and research through standard-setting and advocacy on behalf of its members, the profession, and the public.

AOTA Staff
Sherry Keramidas, *Executive Director*
Matthew Clark, *Chief Officer, Innovation & Engagement*

Elizabeth Dooley, *Vice President, Strategic Marketing & Communications*
Laura Collins, *Director of Communications*
Caroline Polk, *Digital Manager and AJOT Managing Editor*
Ashley Hofmann, *Development/Acquisitions Editor*
Barbara Dickson, *Production Editor*

Rebecca Rutberg, *Director, Marketing*
Amanda Goldman, *Marketing Manager*
Jennifer Folden, *Marketing Specialist*

American Occupational Therapy Association, Inc.
6116 Executive Boulevard, Suite 200
North Bethesda, MD 20852-4929
Phone: 301-652-AOTA (2682)
Fax: 301-652-7711
www.aota.org
To order: 1-877-404-AOTA or store.aota.org

Disclaimers
This publication is designed to provide accurate and authoritative information in regard to the subject matter covered. It is sold or distributed with the understanding that the publisher is not engaged in rendering legal, accounting, or other professional service. If legal advice or other expert assistance is required, the services of a competent professional person should be sought.
—*From the Declaration of Principles jointly adopted by the American Bar Association and a Committee of Publishers and Associations*

It is the objective of the American Occupational Therapy Association to be a forum for free expression and interchange of ideas. The opinions expressed by the contributors to this work are their own and not necessarily those of the American Occupational Therapy Association.

ISBN: 978-1-56900-410-4
Ebook ISBN: 978-1-56900-602-3
Library of Congress Control Number: 2020938494

Cover design by Debra Naylor, Naylor Design, Inc., Washington, DC
Composition by Manila Typesetting Company, Philippines
Printed by P.A. Hutchison, Lancaster, PA

Suggested Citation
Braveman, B., & Newman, R. (Eds.). (2020). *Cancer and occupational therapy: Enabling performance and participation across the lifespan*. North Bethesda, MD: AOTA Press.

Dedication

We dedicate this book to the many cancer survivors and caregivers who have taught us invaluable lessons about living life to the fullest. We also dedicate this book to the occupational therapy practitioners and members of the cancer rehabilitation team who continually strive to improve the quality of life of cancer survivors across the life span through their dedication, compassion and care.
—Brent & Robin

I dedicate this book to my loving parents, Shirley C. Braveman and William D. Braveman, and my life partner, Michael Paul Appleman, whose love and support has provided me the confidence and courage to constantly strive to live a life worth living.
—Brent

I dedicate this book to my husband, Peter, and my children, Ryan and Laela. Thank you for always encouraging me to reach for the stars and follow my dreams.
—Robin

Contents

Part I. Understanding Cancer and Cancer Rehabilitation   1

Part II. Impact of Common Forms of Cancer Across the Lifespan   41

Part III. Cancer Care Continuum and Cancer Rehabilitation   101

List of Appendixes, Case Examples, Exhibits, Figures, and Tables

Figures

Tables

About the Editors

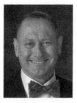 **Brent Braveman, OTR, PhD, FAOTA,** is the Director of the Department of Rehabilitation Services at the University of Texas MD Anderson Cancer Center. The department employs more than 100 occupational therapy and physical therapy practitioners, treats 25,000 patients each year, and had a gross revenue of more than $34 million in fiscal year 2019.

Dr. Braveman earned his Bachelor of Science in Occupational Therapy in 1984 from the University of New Hampshire, a Master of Arts in Education and Human Development from the George Washington University in 1992, and a Doctor of Philosophy in Public Health from the University of Illinois at Chicago in 2002. He has been an author on 44 refereed journal articles and book chapters, has presented at numerous national and international conferences, and is author of two occupational therapy textbooks, *Leading and Managing Occupational Therapy Services: An Evidence-Based Approach* and *Work: Occupational Therapy Intervention to Promote Participation and Productivity.*

Dr. Braveman has served on multiple national expert panels providing consultation on issues related to work disability and employment, HIV/AIDS, and oncology rehabilitation, including for the American Cancer Society, the National Quality Forum, the Institute of Medicine, and the National Institutes of Health. He has been a Co-Investigator on $1.2 million of federally funded research grants. He has a long history of volunteer service in state and national association activities, including serving as a State Association President, a member of AOTA's Roster of Accreditation Evaluators, the Chairperson of AOTA's Administration and Management Special Interest Section, the AOTA Special Interest Section Council Chairperson, Speaker of the AOTA Representative Assembly, and Secretary of AOTA.

Dr. Braveman has a passion for occupational therapy, leadership development, and social justice and is committed to the promotion of the profession and to helping occupational therapy practitioners to meet society's occupational needs.

 Robin Newman, OTD, OT, OTR, CLT, FAOTA, is a Clinical Assistant Professor in the Department of Occupational Therapy at Boston University College of Health and Rehabilitation Sciences: Sargent College. She has worked with survivors of cancer since 2000. Her clinical and research interests include developing self-management interventions for cancer survivors, with a particular focus on the late effects of cancer treatments and their impact on occupational performance and participation in meaningful life roles.

Dr. Newman earned her Bachelor of Science in History of Science with a Biomedical Focus in 1995 from the University of Wisconsin–Madison, a Master of Arts in 2000 from New York University, and a Post-Professional Doctor of Occupational Therapy in 2011 from Boston University. She received her certification in Manual Lymph Drainage and Complete Decongestive Therapy from Klose Norton Training and Consulting in 2002.

Dr. Newman has authored many articles in reviewed journals and has presented at conferences, both nationally and internationally, on topics related to occupational therapy and cancer rehabilitation. She served as an AOTA Special Interest Section Oncology Forum Moderator, AOTA Media Expert in Cancer Rehabilitation and Lymphedema, Planning Committee Member of an American Occupational Therapy Foundation Grant Planning Collective entitled "Catalyzing Research to Optimize Participation in Work & Life Roles of Cancer Survivors," and as a national expert on a transdisciplinary panel at the National Cancer Institute on issues related to work disability and cancer rehabilitation. She is active in the American Congress of Rehabilitation Medicine Cancer Rehabilitation Network Group (ACRM), serving as Co-Chair of the ACRM Oncology Cognitive Rehabilitation Task Force, and serving as a Member of the ACRM Oncology Rehabilitation Research and Outcomes Task Force.

Dr. Newman has a passion for mentoring occupational therapy students and occupational therapy practitioners in topics related to cancer rehabilitation. She was added to the American Occupational Therapy Roster of Fellows in 2020 for her commitment to optimizing occupational performance and participation of cancer survivors.

Contributors

Latoya Adekoya, OTR, MOT
Senior Occupational Therapist
MD Anderson Cancer Center
Houston

Megan Bailey, OTD, OTR/L
Department of Occupational Therapy
College of Health and Rehabilitation Sciences: Sargent
    College
Boston University

Brent Braveman, OTR, PhD, FAOTA
Director of the Department of Rehabilitation Services
MD Anderson Cancer Center
Houston

Claudine Campbell, OTD, OTR/L, CLT
Lead Occupational Therapist
Memorial Sloan Kettering Cancer Center
New York

Christine Connelly, MSOT, OTR/L
Occupational Therapy Supervisor
Memorial Sloan Kettering Cancer Center
New York

Anissa E. Hill, OTR, MOT
Senior Occupational Therapist
MD Anderson Cancer Center
Houston

Elizabeth G. Hunter, PhD, OTR/L
Assistant Professor
The Graduate Center for Gerontology
College of Public Health
University of Kentucky
Lexington

Mack Ivy, OTR, PhD
Senior Occupational Therapist
MD Anderson Cancer Center
Houston

Chrysanne Karnick, MOT, OTR/L, CAPS, CLT
Advanced Clinician Occupational Therapist
Memorial Sloan Kettering Cancer Center
New York

Donna Kelly, OTR, MED, CLT
Senior Occupational Therapist and Clinical Point Person
MD Anderson Cancer Center
Houston

Courtland Lee, OTR, MOT
Senior Occupational Therapist
MD Anderson Cancer Center
Houston

Caitlyn Lombardo, MSOT, OTR/L, CLT
Advanced Clinician Occupational Therapist
Memorial Sloan Kettering Cancer Center
New York

Kathleen Lyons, ScD, OTR/L
Senior Scientist
Norris Cotton Cancer Center at Dartmouth–Hitchcock
    Medical Center
Lebanon, NH

Assistant Professor of Psychiatry
Geisel School of Medicine at Dartmouth
Hanover, NH

Asfia Mohammed, OTR, MOT
Senior Occupational Therapist
MD Anderson Cancer Center
Houston

Brianne Morris, MOT, OTR/L
Advanced Clinician Occupational Therapist
Memorial Sloan Kettering Cancer Center
New York

Robin Newman, OTD, OT, OTR, CLT, FAOTA
Clinical Assistant Professor
Department of Occupational Therapy
College of Health and Rehabilitation Sciences:
    Sargent College
Boston University
Boston

Vi Nguyen, OTR, BSRC, MOT
Inpatient Supervisor
Department of Rehabilitation Services
MD Anderson Cancer Center
Houston

Jennifer Nicholson, OTR, MOT
Senior Occupational Therapist
MD Anderson Cancer Center
Houston

Mackenzi Pergolotti, PhD, OTR/L
Director of Research
ReVital Cancer Rehabilitation, Select Medical, Inc.
Mechanicsburg, PA

Assistant Professor
Colorado State University
Fort Collins

Katie M. Polo, DHS, OTR, CLT–LANA
Associate Professor
School of Occupational Therapy
University of Indianapolis
Indianapolis

Mary Vining Radomski, PhD, OTR/L, FAOTA
Senior Scientific Adviser
Courage Kenny Research Center
Minneapolis, MN

Joshua Skuller, PhD, OTR/L, BCP, ATP
Associate Professor
Auerbach School of Occupational Therapy
Spalding University
Louisville, KY

Alix G. Sleight, PhD, OTD, MPH, OTR/L
Cancer Prevention Fellow
National Cancer Institute
Bethesda, MD

Jessica Sparrow, OTD, OTR/L, BCP
Lead Occupational Therapist
St. Jude Children's Research Hospital
Memphis, TN

Laura Stimler, OTD, OTR/L, BCP, C/NDT
Assistant Professor
Auerbach School of Occupational Therapy
Spalding University
Louisville, KY

Shelby Ubrich, OTR, MOT
Senior Occupational Therapist
MD Anderson Cancer Center
Houston

Amanda Wheeler, MOT, OTR/L
Compliance and Education Manager, Rehabilitation Service
Memorial Sloan Kettering Cancer Center
New York

Tish Williams, OTR
Senior Occupational Therapist
MD Anderson Cancer Center

Suzänne (Taylor) Zeta, PhD, MBA, OTR/L
Vice President of Operations, VBHRC Virginia Catalyst
Affiliate Researcher, Massey Cancer Center
Richmond, VA

Preface

Brent Braveman, OTR, PhD, FAOTA, and Robin Newman, OTD, OT, OTR, CLT, FAOTA

There is a compelling need to help the growing number of cancer survivors participate in meaningful occupations across the lifespan and treatment continuum. Further, cancer and its treatments provide challenges and obstacles to full participation in life roles and life situations. The number of incident cases of cancer and the number of cancer survivors is growing, with an estimated 1,762,450 new cases in the United States and an expected 20.3 million survivors by 2026 (American Cancer Society, 2019; National Cancer Institute, 2018).

The burgeoning population of cancer survivors across the lifespan presents an immediate challenge and opportunity for occupational therapy practitioners to provide occupation-focused and evidence-based interventions to support occupational performance and participation in society across the lifespan. The American Occupational Therapy Association (2015) asserts that occupational therapy's distinct value is "to improve health and quality of life through facilitating participation and engagement in occupations, the meaningful, necessary, and familiar activities of everyday life" (para. 6). In the case of cancer, the meaningful, necessary, and familiar activities of everyday life such as self-care, IADLs, work and educational participation, and leisure and social participation may be disrupted by cancer, cancer treatment, and the sequelae of treatment. Occupational therapy's distinct value in cancer rehabilitation is to help survivors participate fully in such occupations at all points in the cancer experience, from diagnosis through treatment and survivorship or end of life.

Though many cancer survivors do not receive the intensity of rehabilitation services necessary to promote optimal engagement in meaningful occupations, the availability of occupational therapy and other rehabilitation services are increasing. As a result, occupational therapy practitioners need to be ready to meet the needs of cancer survivors along the cancer care continuum. This book seeks to fill a gap in available evidence-based and occupation-focused resources for occupational therapy practitioners working with survivors of cancer.

As you read this text, note that the terms *client, patient,* and *cancer survivor* may all be used to refer to a person with cancer; we have chosen to use the term *cancer survivor* whenever appropriate. The term *cancer survivor* can be used to refer more generally to any person with cancer at any point in their cancer journey. In 1986, the founders of National Coalition for Cancer Survivorship (NCCS) sought to "replace the words 'cancer victim' with 'cancer survivor' and bring about a different notion of the cancer experience" (NCCS, 2018, para. 2). The term *survivor* is defined as "from the time of diagnosis and for the balance of life" and is used in this text to represent that view of the person with cancer (NCCS, 2018, para. 1). We use the terms *patient* or *client* only in direct quotations or when referencing resources or cases. Similarly, we are intentional about the use of the terms *occupational therapy practitioner, occupational therapist,* and *occupational therapy assistant.* We use the term *occupational therapy practitioner* whenever it applies to services appropriate for either an occupational therapist or occupational therapy assistant.

The goal of this text is to support occupational therapy practitioners and occupational therapy students to expand their knowledge and readiness to confidently practice in cancer rehabilitation settings, whether it be an academic medical center, community-based rehabilitation setting, elementary school, worksite, or the home. This text can also be a valuable resource for those designing cancer rehabilitation programs along the cancer care continuum, beginning with primary and secondary prevention, through acute and medically complex settings to survivorship or end-of-life care. It is our hope that the focus on occupation throughout the book will empower occupational therapy practitioners to address the occupational performance needs of survivors across the life span, in addition to addressing the sequelae of cancer and cancer treatment.

This text seeks to provide occupational therapy practitioners with practical, up-to-date evidence that will prepare them to design comprehensive cancer rehabilitation interventions and to understand when additional advanced information and training on specific techniques is necessary.

HOW THIS TEXT IS ORGANIZED

This book is organized in five sections.

Section I: Understanding Cancer and Cancer Rehabilitation

Chapters 1, 2, and 3 review cancer demographics and trends in cancer across the lifespan, treatment approaches aimed at curing cancer, and applying the occupational therapy domain and process to cancer survivors.

Section II: Impact of Common Forms of Cancer Across the Lifespan

Chapters 4 through 7 discuss special considerations for working with cancer survivors across the lifespan. This section is organized in four chapters that address special considerations with children, adolescents and young adults, adults, and older adults.

Section III: Cancer Care Continuum and Cancer Rehabilitation

Chapters 8 through 14 explore occupational therapy intervention with cancer survivors in different practice contexts, including primary and secondary prevention, acute and medically complex settings, prehabilitation, acute inpatient rehabilitation, survivorship, palliative care and hospice, and home health and the community.

Section IV: Sequelae of Cancer and Interventions Across the Lifespan

Chapters 15 through 20 address occupational therapy intervention for the primary consequences of cancer and its treatments, including cancer-related fatigue, pain, cancer-related cognitive impairment, lymphedema, chemotherapy-induced peripheral neuropathy, and psychosocial issues.

Section V: Cancer and Participation in Occupations Across the Lifspan

Chapters 21 through 27 review occupational therapy intervention to address primary areas of occupation, including ADLs and IADLs, rest and sleep, play and leisure, education, work, social participation, and caregiving.

We hope that this book proves to be a valuable contribution toward improving the quality of life, occupational performance, and participation of cancer survivors. We also hope that it proves to be a valuable resource to occupational therapy students and practitioners as occupational therapy becomes more widely recognized for its contributions to comprehensive cancer rehabilitation.

REFERENCES

American Cancer Society. (2019). *Cancer facts and figures 2019.* Retrieved from https://www.cancer.org/content/dam/cancer-org/research/cancer-facts-and-statistics/annual-cancer-facts-and-figures/2019/cancer-facts-and-figures-2019.pdf

American Occupational Therapy Association. (2015). *Articulating the distinct value of occupational therapy.* Retrieved from https://www.aota.org/Publications-News/AOTANews/2015/distinct-value-of-occupational-therapy.aspx

National Cancer Institute. (2018). *Cancer statistics.* Retrieved from https://www.cancer.gov/about-cancer/understanding/statistics

National Coalition for Cancer Survivorship. (2018). *The National Coalition for Cancer Survivorship.* Retrieved from https://www.canceradvocacy.org/about-us/our-history/

PART I.

Understanding Cancer
and Cancer Rehabilitation

Cancer Demographics and Trends Across the Lifespan

1

Brent Braveman, OTR, PhD, FAOTA

LEARNING OBJECTIVES

After completing this chapter, readers should be able to
- Identify and describe demographic trends in cancer across the lifespan, including the most common forms of cancer and trends in cancer deaths and survivorship;
- Identify key factors to be considered in the prevention of cancer and describe relevant trends in cancer prevention; and
- Explain the pros and cons related to recommendations for approaches to screening for cancer.

KEY TERMS AND CONCEPTS

- Active surveillance
- Burden of disease
- Cancer
- Cancer screening
- Late effects
- Social determinants of health
- Staging
- Watchful waiting

INTRODUCTION

This chapter aims to provide a general introduction to cancer and demographics and trends in cancer prevention, screening and early diagnosis, treatment, and survivorship across the lifespan. Summarizing demographics and trends in cancer can present a challenge because statistics are constantly being updated, and any static statement such as the projected number of incident cases of cancer or estimated cancer deaths quickly becomes outdated. For this reason, the numbers and statistics in this chapter are best viewed as a snapshot of the current time period. Excellent resources that are frequently updated include the American Cancer Society (ACS; www.cancer.org) and the National Cancer Institute (NCI; www.cancer.gov). These sources are cited liberally throughout this chapter, and it is recommended that you use these resources and others to obtain the most current statistics and information.

Many of the topics broadly discussed in this chapter are explored in more depth in later chapters.

CANCER BASICS

Cancer is a group of diseases that can begin anywhere in the body, rather than one single disease. All cancers have abnormal cell growth in common, which can impede on the normal function of body structures and systems as cancer cells affect normal cells. Some cancers grow or spread quickly; some cancers progress slowly enough that the patient may choose to not intervene with treatment and instead pursue active surveillance or watchful waiting. This choice may be made because the negative effects of the treatment may be worse than the cancer, especially in people with shorter expected lifespans at the time of diagnosis (MD Anderson Cancer Center, 2017; Heidenreich et al., 2014). NCI (2019b) defines *active surveillance* as

A treatment plan that involves closely watching a patient's condition but not giving any treatment unless there are changes in test results that show the condition is getting worse. Active surveillance may be used to avoid or delay the need for treatments such as radiation therapy or surgery, which can cause side effects or other problems. During active surveillance, certain exams and tests are done on a regular schedule. It may be used in the treatment of certain types of cancer, such as prostate cancer, urethral cancer, and intraocular (eye) melanoma. (n.p.)

Watchful waiting is

Closely watching a patient's condition but not giving treatment unless symptoms appear or change. Watchful waiting is sometimes used in conditions that progress slowly. It is also used when the risks of treatment are greater than the possible benefits. During watchful waiting, patients may be given certain tests and exams. Watchful waiting is sometimes used in prostate cancer. (NCI, 2019b)

Some cancers form tumors that are solid masses of cancer cells. Other cancers such as blood cancers (e.g.,

---

leukemia, lymphoma) do not form solid tumors; they are described as "liquid tumors." Cancers are identified and named based on where they originate even if they spread (metastasize) to other parts of the body. Lung cancer is called lung cancer if it started in the lungs but is first found in the brain or the bones (American Cancer Society, 2015). In fact, more than 100 types of cancer have been identified. The most common forms are

- Carcinoma (skin or tissue lining the organs),
- Sarcoma (connective tissue),
- Leukemia (bone marrow or blood-forming organs),
- Lymphoma (immune system),
- Multiple myeloma (plasma cells and bone marrow),
- Melanoma (skin), and
- Central nervous system (brain and spine; NCI, 2015c).

The severity of a cancer diagnosis is often indicated by its stage, which conveys the extent of cancer (NCI, 2015b). A common system for **staging** is the TNM system:

- *T* represents the size and extent of a tumor.
- *N* represents the number of nearby lymph nodes that are positive for cancer cells.
- *M* represents whether the cancer has metastasized.

Another common method of staging is to designate the cancer as Stage 0 to Stage IV:

- In *Stage 0,* abnormal cells are present but have not spread to nearby tissue.
- In *Stage I, Stage II,* and *Stage III,* cancer cells are present, and the cancer tumor's size and how much the cancer has spread are greater in each progressive stage.
- In *Stage IV,* the cancer has metastasized to distant parts of the body.

TRENDS IN CANCER SURVIVORSHIP

The number of cancer survivors around the globe is growing substantially. By 2024, it is estimated that there will be 22 million cancer survivors in the United States (ACS, 2019b). In 2019, it was estimated that there would be more than 1.7 million new cases of cancer in the United States and more than 600,000 cancer deaths. Worldwide, about 1 in every 7 deaths can be attributed to cancer (ACS, 2019a). By 2040, there will be an estimated total of 27.5 million new cancer cases worldwide and 6.3 million cancer deaths annually because of increased population growth and aging populations (ACS, 2018b). National expenditures for cancer care in the United States totaled nearly $147.3 billion in 2017 and were estimated to reach $156 billion in 2020 (NCI, 2019b).

The 3 most common forms of new cancer in men are prostate (20%), lung and bronchus (13%), and colon and rectum (9%); in women they are breast (30%), lung and bronchus (13%), and colon and rectum (7%). These same cancers are also the leading causes of cancer death in men and women. Lung and bronchial cancers are the leading cause of cancer death in both genders, followed by colon and rectum and prostate in men, and breast and colon and rectum in women (ACS, 2019b). Men and women have a 1-in-3 lifetime risk of developing cancer (ACS, 2019b).

Five-year survivorship has improved in many cancers because of improvements in cancer prevention, cancer screening, and early detection, and in advances in treatments (DeSantis et al., 2014; Miller et al., 2016). In addition, cancer is, to a large extent, a disease of aging. According to the NCI (2015a), the most important risk factor for developing cancer is getting older. The NCI's Surveillance, Epidemiology, and End Results Program reports that the average age of a cancer diagnosis is 66 years, and 25% of cancer is diagnosed in people between the ages of 65 and 74.

CANCER DEMOGRAPHICS

Long-term trends in cancer incidence rates have been influenced by associated trends in health behaviors that contribute to the development of cancer and changes in practices, such as improved screening and early detection (Siegel et al., 2017). The overall cancer rate in men has declined about 2% per year since the mid 1990s, when there was a spike in incidence rates because of the significant increase in the diagnosis of asymptomatic prostate cancer. There have also been large declines in lung and colorectal cancers. The overall cancer rate in women has remained relatively stable since 1987, with decreases in lung and colorectal cancer and increases in breast and thyroid cancer and melanomas. As with other cancers, an increase in screening procedures such as colonoscopies is responsible for the decreases seen in colorectal cancers.

In the past 30 years, the 5-year survival rate for all cancers has increased 20 percentage points among Whites and 24 percentage points among Blacks (Siegel et al., 2017). When comparing survival rates for the most common cancers in patients 50–64 years with patients 65 and older, the younger group shows higher rates. It can also be that older adults die with, not from, cancer. This result is likely because treatments are less effective for older adults or new therapies are used less often in the elderly population.

During much of the 20th century, the cancer death rate increased as a result of tobacco use, but it has declined by around 1.5% per year since the early 1990s. Still, smoking continues to be the world's most preventable cause of death (ACS, 2018c). Smoking causes an estimated 480,000 premature deaths, including 42,000 deaths related to secondhand smoke exposure. Although cigarette smoking has decreased, the use of other tobacco products, including e-cigarettes and pipe tobacco, has increased.

DEMOGRAPHICS AND TRENDS ACCORDING TO AGE

There is some variation to how cancers are grouped according to age. For example, the NCI's (2019c) Surveillance, Epidemiology, and End Results Program groups age according to less than 20, 20–49, 50–64, 65–74, and 75 and older. Elsewhere on the NCI site, children are described as ages 0–14, adolescents are described as 15–24, and young adults as 25–39. Certainly there is great variation in the treatment and other therapeutic considerations for a child who is 1 or 2 years old and a child (or adolescent) who is 12 or 13.

Although you must be aware of age groupings when considering statistical or epidemiological data to ensure you are comparing apples to apples, the specific start and endpoints used to define an age cohort are probably less important for rehabilitation professionals than functional considerations related to age-related developmental milestones. Whether you refer to a 13-year-old as a child or an adolescent, most 13-year-olds face similar developmental challenges and events. The following sections use age groupings pulled from the NCI general website.

Demographics and Trends in Cancer in Children (Ages 0–14 Years)

A primary difference between cancer that develops in children and cancer that occurs in adults is that childhood cancers are not strongly linked to preventable lifestyle or modifiable environmental risks (ACS, 2017). Childhood cancers are more often related to changes in DNA, although the causes of most childhood cancers are not known (NCI, 2017a). Childhood cancers make up a tiny percentage of all cancers diagnosed each year (less than 1%). It is estimated that a little more than 10,000 children in the United States were diagnosed in 2017. The 5-year survival rate for children is greater than 80%. Cancer is the second leading cause of death in children ages 0–14 years with accidents being number one. The most common forms of cancer in children are leukemia, brain and central nervous system cancers, and lymphomas (ACS, 2017).

According to the NCI (2017a),

> Survivors of childhood cancer need follow-up care and enhanced medical surveillance for the rest of their lives because of the risk of complications that can occur many years after they complete treatment for their cancer. Health problems that develop months or years after treatment has ended are known as late effects. *Late effects* [emphasis added] can include second cancers, joint replacements, hearing loss, and congestive heart failure. (para. 30)

Rehabilitative and therapeutic concerns with children with cancer focus on helping children cope with the physical, emotional, social, and psychological effects of cancer and promoting societal participation, typical role development, and occupational performance. Cancer and its treatments can cause significant interruptions in children's roles, routines, and habits and can pose significant challenges to typical age-related developmental events.

Demographics and Trends in Cancer in Adolescents and Young Adults (Ages 15–39 Years)

According to the NCI (2017b),

> About 70,000 young people (ages 15–39) are diagnosed with cancer each year in the United States—accounting for about 5% of cancer diagnoses in the United States. This is about 6 times the number of cancers diagnosed in children ages 0–14. (para. 1)

The most common forms of cancer in adolescents are leukemia, brain and central nervous system cancer, and Hodgkin lymphoma (ACS, 2019b). Hodgkin lymphoma, melanoma, testicular cancer, thyroid cancer, and sarcomas are more likely to be seen in young adults than in children or older adults. Leukemia, lymphoma, testicular cancer, and thyroid cancer are the most common cancers among 15- to 24-year-olds. Among 25- to 39-year-olds, breast cancer and melanoma are the most common cancers (NCI, 2017b). Cancer is the leading cause of disease-related death in the adolescent and young adult population, and only accidents, suicide, and homicide were responsible for more deaths in this age group in 2011 (NCI, 2017b).

Some special considerations for young adults with cancer include fertility preservation, lack of health insurance, financial concerns, age-related social and emotional concerns, and the fact that cancers are often found later in young adults than in other age groups. Although concerns over body image may occur at any age, they may be particularly heightened in adolescents and young adults with cancer who are faced with forging personal relationships as well as relationships in school or in the workplace. Cancer and its treatments can result in a wide range of changes in physical presentation, including hair loss, skin coloring, and scars. Young adults can be caught between physicians and programs that specialize in treating of children with cancer and those that specialize in treating adults and older adults, resulting in confusion over recommendations for intervention.

Adolescents and young adults can also face the risk of late effects of cancer treatments, including chemotherapy and radiation. Late effects can range from mild to severe, and they can affect more than one part of the body or organ system. Late effects in adolescents and young adults can include things like

- Impaired fertility (ability to have children) in both women and men;
- Increased risk of developing another cancer later in life;
- Heart or lung problems (from certain chemo drugs or radiation to the chest);
- Hearing or vision problems (from certain chemo drugs or radiation to the head);
- Problems with other organs, such as the kidneys, or bones;
- Pain or swelling in parts of the body; and
- Hormone deficiencies (ACI, 2018d).

Demographics and Trends in Cancer in Adults (Ages 40–64 Years)

Approximately 43% of all cancers occur in adults ages 35–64 years (NCI, 2015a). Adults have just over a 40% chance of being diagnosed with cancer and approximately a 21% chance of dying from cancer (White et al., 2014).

Midlife is seen as a time of increased vulnerability for cancer for several reasons. Health status and health behaviors at midlife establish the foundation for health and function in older adulthood. Midlife is also the time when some significant and modifiable risk factors for cancer and other diseases begin to take a toll on the body. These factors include tobacco use, lack of physical activity, poor nutrition, excessive alcohol consumption, drug use and certain chronic infections. Several preventable chronic conditions and diseases (e.g., obesity, Type 2 diabetes) increase during midlife, and some of these conditions have been associated with increased cancer risk and reduced cancer survival (Ott et al., 2010; Prasad et al., 2012).

For most people, adulthood is a time of independence and productivity in several key occupational roles, including worker, spouse or family member, parent, leisure participant or hobbyist, and community participant. Cancer and its treatments can have a substantial negative effect on occupational performance and interrupt role performance. Cancer and its treatments can create a burden for the adult and their family and support system. Robert Havighurst, a noted developmental theorist, lists seven major developmental tasks in the middle years, each of which may be affected by cancer (Havighurst, 1963; University of Wyoming, 2018):

1. Accepting and adjusting to physiological changes, such as menopause,
2. Reaching and maintaining satisfaction in one's occupation,
3. Adjusting to and possibly caring for aging parents,
4. Helping teenage children become responsible adults,
5. Achieving adult social and civic responsibility,
6. Relating to one's spouse as a person, and
7. Developing leisure-time activities.

Occupational therapy practitioners can play critical roles in aiding the adult with cancer to successfully accomplish each of these tasks.

Demographics and Trends in Cancer in Older Adults (Ages 65 or Over)

A substantial number of people will live their lives without ever experiencing cancer. But as noted earlier, age is a contributing risk to developing cancer. In 2009, just over half of all cancers occurred in adults older than 64. As baby boomers age, the number of cancers in this population will increase. The number of diagnoses in older adults is projected to increase by 45% between 2010 and 2030, and by 2030, an estimated 70% of cancer cases will occur in those older than 64 (White et al., 2014).

Health and function vary a great deal among older adults. Some older adults exhibit characteristics of the frail elderly in their sixties, and others live vibrant and active lives into their nineties and beyond. A challenge to occupational performance in older adults with cancer includes the compounding effects of age, function, mobility, strength, and endurance. Limited social and family support are also challenges to some older adults, as are limited financial resources.

GLOBAL DEMOGRAPHICS AND TRENDS IN CANCER

Global Trends in Cancer Screening

Cancer screening involves examination of the body by a medical professional or by a person examining their own body (e.g., self-examination) to detect early symptoms of cancer. Screening can vary from simple self-examination of the breast using the hands or of the skin using a mirror, to medical tests that are provided on an outpatient basis using various medical technologies. Exhibit 1.1 lists various types of cancer screening approaches and provides a brief explanation of each.

For many years, there was an emphasis on increasing the prevalence of cancer screening, and increased screening and early detection have generally been credited with lower rates of cancer mortality. According to the NCI (2018b), estimates of the premature deaths that could have been prevented through screening vary from 3% to 35%, depending on a variety of assumptions. Beyond the potential for avoiding death, screening may reduce cancer morbidity because treatment of earlier-stage cancers is often less aggressive than for more advanced-stage cancers.

However, the most recent trend has to been to recommend less screening, not more (NCI, 2018a). These recommendations are

> based on an emerging—if counterintuitive—understanding that more screening does not necessarily translate into fewer cancer deaths and that some screening may actually do more harm than good. Much of the confusion surrounding the benefits of screening comes from interpreting the statistics that are often used to describe the results of screening studies. An improvement in survival—how long a person lives after a cancer diagnosis—among people who have undergone a cancer screening test is often taken to imply that the test saves lives. (ACS, 2018b, para. 1)

There is no doubt that, when properly used, cancer screenings save lives, but we have come to understand that cancer screenings also include risks. NCI (2018a) identified some of these risks:

- Some screening tests can cause serious problems such as bleeding.
- False-positive test results are possible.
- False-negative test results are possible.
- Finding the cancer may not improve a person's health or extend the length of their life.
- In teenagers and adults, there is an increased risk of suicide in the year following cancer diagnosis, and cancer treatments have significant side effects.

It is understandable that one might ask, "Does screening for cancer result in early detection and save lives, or does it cause problems and carry risks that are not worth it?" Fortunately, recommendations for when cancer screening should occur are readily available from reliable sources such as NCI, ACS, and leading institutions such as MD Anderson Cancer Center and Memorial Sloan Kettering Cancer Center (American Cancer Society, 2018a; American Society of Clinical Oncology, 2019; MD Anderson Cancer Center, 2018; Memorial Sloan Kettering Cancer Center, 2018; NCI, 2018a).

Smith et al. (2015) summarized data on screening prevalence for colorectal, breast, and cervical cancer between 2005 and 2015 collected through the National Health Information Survey (NHIS). During this time, screening for colorectal cancer increased by 19.5% because of the increased use of colonoscopies. Cervical cancer screening declined by 3.8%, and there has been little change in breast cancer screening since 2005. Prostate cancer screening rates were stable between 2005 and 2010 but declined by 18% between 2010 and 2013, and the proportion of men reporting undergoing a prostate-specific antigen test in the past year for routine reasons declined from 37.8% to 30.8%, according to NHIS data. The authors also addressed disparities in cancer screening, noting the following variations in screening according to race and health insurance status:

- When it comes to colorectal screening, 49.4% of Asians get screened, 49.9% of Hispanics do, and 65.4% of non-Hispanic Whites do. For adults ages 50–64, more

EXHIBIT 1.1.	Types of Cancer Screening

BREAST CANCER

- Mammography is a type of X ray designed to view the breast and identify tumors or irregularities of breast tissue. The images are called *mammograms.*
- Clinical breast examinations performed by a medical professional can detect changes in breast size, shape, and skin.
- Breast self-examination is an exam in which a woman looks and feels for changes in her own breast.
- MRIs may be used instead of mammography in women who are at high risk or have dense breast tissue, or if a lump is found.

CERVICAL CANCER

- HPV testing can identify strains of HPV that are strongly linked to cervical cancer.
- Pap tests use cells from the outside of the cervix to identify precancerous cells.

COLORECTAL CANCER

- *Colonoscopy* is the use of a flexible lighted tube inserted into the rectum to allow visual inspection of the entire colon for polyps or cancer.
- *Sigmoidoscopy* is the use of a flexible lighted tube to check the lower part of the colon for polyps or cancer.
- Fecal occult blood tests may find blood in the feces or stool, which may indicate polyps or cancer.
- Barium enemas provide for x-ray examination of the colon and rectum.

HEAD AND NECK CANCERS

- General exams by physicians and dentists involve a check for abnormalities in the nose, mouth, throat, and neck.

LUNG CANCER

- Low-dose CT scans create three-dimensional pictures of the body to identify abnormalities or tumors.

PROSTATE CANCER

- Digital rectal examinations involve a doctor inserting their gloved and lubricated finger into a man's rectum to feel for irregularities in the prostate's surface.
- PSA tests measure the level of PSA in the blood, which may indicate cancer.

SKIN CANCER

- Physicians can perform a complete skin examination for signs of skin cancer.
- Individuals can perform a skin self-examination of the entire body using a mirror to check for signs of skin cancer.
- *Dermascopy* is the use of a handheld device by a physician to evaluate the size, shape, and pigmentation patterns of lesions for the early detection of melanoma.

Note. CT = computed tomography; HPV = human papillomavirus; MRI = magnetic resonance imaging; PSA = prostate-specific antigen.

than twice as many (59.6%) insured adults get screened compared with uninsured adults (25.1%).

- When it comes to getting mammograms, 45.7% of Hispanic women get screened for breast cancer compared with 55.4% of non-Hispanic Black women. For women ages 50–64, screening rates were 2.5 times higher (52.5%) for insured women compared with uninsured women (20.9%).
- When it comes to screening for cervical cancer, 73.3% of Asian women get screened while 84.4% of non Hispanic White women do. Screening rates were one-third higher (84.4%) for insured women than for uninsured women (60.8%).

General Trends in Cancer Prevention and Early Diagnosis

The ***burden of disease*** refers to the full impact of the disease on a population. It goes beyond incidence and mortality and includes functional limitations and disability and non-health well-being (e.g., financial effects). Quantifying risk factors known to be associated with specific diseases is also part of the measurement of burden of disease (Lopez et al., 2006). Increases in the global burden of cancer have been documented, although cancer mortality rates in countries of all income levels are decreasing. As noted earlier, cancer might be considered a disease of aging. Because cancer risk increases with age, a 20%–43% increase in cases from 1990 to 2013 is attributed to the aging population. With greater life expectancy worldwide, the future burden of cancer will also likely increase (Fitzmaurice et al., 2015).

The burdens associated with cancer are most significant in low- and middle-income countries and may be exacerbated by the trends in these nations to adopt unhealthy behaviors and lifestyles associated with rapid income growth (e.g., smoking, poor diet, physical inactivity), and changes in reproductive patterns (e.g., fewer children, later age at first childbirth; Torre et al., 2015). The incidence rates of specific types of cancer vary widely from country to country. For example, prostate cancer is the most commonly diagnosed cancer among men in nearly 90 countries, especially in North and South America and all European countries outside of Eastern Europe. Men in Eastern Europe are diagnosed with lung cancer more than any other cancer (Torre et al., 2015).

According to Hashim et al. (2016), disparities in age-standardized cancer mortality rates among countries are shaped by three main determinants in addition to population demographic characteristics: (1) prevalence of risk factors; (2) early diagnostic protocols, including screening; and (3) access to treatment. Such disparities are influenced by a country's economic and industrial development. As explained by Fidler et al. (2018), "As a country transitions socially, economically and behaviorally with increasing human development, the cancer profile also transitions with decreases in infection-related cancers offset by increases in industrialization-related cancers" (p. 29).

Cancer Disparities

Disparities in the early detection and treatment of cancer across members of racial and ethnic minorities and people with lower socioeconomic status (SES) are widely reported, as is decreased access to health insurance and health care. The incidence of cancer deaths is higher among people with lower SES, regardless of demographic factors such as race or ethnicity. For example,

> cancer mortality rates among both black and non-Hispanic white men with 12 or fewer years of education are almost 3 times higher than those of college graduates for all cancers combined. This is partly because incidence rates are higher in people with lower SES for many cancers because many factors that increase cancer risk are more prevalent. (ACS, 2019a, p. 52)

Multiple influences, including social, economic, cultural, environmental, and health system factors, contribute to these disparities and interact in complex ways. The term *social determinants of health* is commonly used to describe the "conditions in the environments in which people are born, live, learn, work, play, worship, and age that affect a wide range of health, functioning, and quality-of-life outcomes and risks" (Office of Disease Prevention and Health Promotion, 2018, para. 5).

Disparities mostly arise from "inequities in work, wealth, education, housing, and overall standard of living, as well as social barriers to high-quality cancer prevention, early detection, and treatment services" (ACS, 2019a, p. 52). Occupational therapy practitioners treating cancer patients should be aware of disparities in treatment and understand that treatment received may differ from patient to patient or from location to location. Moreover, the American Occupational Therapy Association (2013) stated in its societal statement on health disparities,

> Occupational therapy practitioners have the responsibility to intervene with individuals and communities to limit the effects of inequities that result in health disparities. Practitioners have knowledge and skills in evaluating and intervening with individuals and groups who face physical, social, emotional, or cultural challenges to participation. (p. S7)

Trends in Cancer Prevention

NCI's (2019a) *Cancer Trends Progress Report* provides a comprehensive summary of trends in U.S. cancer control measures. The report organizes information on trends

EXHIBIT 1.2.	Major Categories of Risk Factors for Cancer

BEHAVIORAL FACTORS

- Tobacco use
- Smoking cessation
- Diet, physical activity, and weight
- Ultraviolet exposure and sun protective principles

TOBACCO POLICY/REGULATORY FACTORS

- Advertising and promotion of tobacco products
- Provision of smoking cessation under Medicaid

ENVIRONMENTAL FACTORS

- Secondhand smoke
- Chemical and environmental exposures (arsenic, benzene, cadmium, nitrate, radon)

in three major groups of risk factors: (1) behavioral, (2) environmental, and (3) policy or regulatory. Exhibit 1.2 shows the individual risk factors in each of these major groups. All data reported in the summaries of prevention trends in the following sections are from the NCI *Cancer Trends Progress Report.*

Smoking and tobacco use initiation

Smoking often begins in adolescence, with approximately 90% of smokers starting by age 18 years and 98% starting by age 26 years. In addition to cigarettes, tobacco use includes cigars and smokeless tobacco (i.e., tobacco that is chewed or snuffed). Decreases in smoking initiation and other uses of tobacco products have been achieved among children and adolescents ages 12–17 years, decreasing from 7.8% to 5.5% between 2008 and 2014. During the same time period, smoking decreased in those ages 18–25 years from 10.9% to 9.3%. Significant decreases have been noted in the percentage of adults who smoke cigarettes over the time period 1991–2016 (from 29.6% to 15.7%), but decreases of less than 1% were noted among cigar smokers and users of smokeless tobacco.

Recently there has been an increase in the use of e-cigarettes or "vaping." The use of vape pens can be traced back to ancient times, but the first e-cigarette was produced by a Chinese firm in the mid-2000s. Research on the effects of vaporizers is still evolving. Stephens (2017) noted that e-cigarette device settings, liquid formulation, and vaping behavior generally emit significantly less carcinogenic potency than tobacco smoke, but the cancer risks of e-cigarettes can sometimes greatly escalate. When the causes of the cancer risk escalation are known (e.g., smoking initiation), their circumstances are often avoidable.

Smoking cessation

Quitting smoking has major and immediate health benefits and dramatically reduces the risk of lung and other cancers, coronary heart disease, stroke, and chronic lung disease. For example, the risk of lung cancer can decrease by between one-third to one-half within 10 years after quitting. Between 1998 and 2016, 53.4% of adult smokers ages 18 years and older attempted to stop smoking for at least

1 day. Few people are successful in totally abstaining from smoking on their first attempt.

Advertising and promotion of tobacco products

The advertising and promotion of tobacco products has been associated with tobacco use, and cigarettes are highly promoted. In 1970, U.S. tobacco companies spent $1.72 billion (adjusted to 2014 dollars) on advertising. This increased to an all-time high of $19 billion in 2003. However, efforts via federal legislation to limit advertising and promotion have been effective, and in 2014 total expenditures decreased to $8.49 billion (Courtney, 2015).

Medicaid coverage of tobacco dependence treatments

The rate of smoking prevalence is higher among people who receive Medicaid than the general population. However, smoking cessation funding for Medicaid enrollees is limited. All state Medicaid programs must provide tobacco cessation services (both counseling and pharmacotherapy) for pregnant women under the Patient Protection and Affordable Care Act (ACA; P. L. 111-148), and state Medicaid programs cannot exclude coverage for cessation medications approved by the U.S. Food and Drug Administration. However, coverage still varies widely by state. As of June 2015, only 9 states covered 9 evidence-based cessation treatments (7 medications, individual counseling, and group counseling) for all Medicaid enrollees. As of September 2017, only 11 states provided comprehensive coverage of all 9 evidence-based cessation treatments for all Medicaid enrollees.

Secondhand smoke

Secondhand smoke can cause premature death and disease in those who do not smoke but are exposed. Exposure to secondhand smoke has decreased from 83.6% of nonsmokers ages 3 and older in 1988 to 28.5% in 2012. The dramatic decrease in exposure is the result of widespread public education and the prevalence of smoke-free laws and policies in workplaces and public locations.

Diet, physical activity, and weight

Up to one-third of cancer cases in the United States are related to poor nutrition, physical inactivity, or excess body weight or obesity. Dietary factors that can prevent cancer include regular consumption of fruits and vegetables; limiting consumption of red meat, fat, and alcohol; maintaining physical activity, including weekly moderate-intensity aerobic activity; and maintaining a healthy weight (e.g., a body mass index between 18.5 and 24.9).

Ultraviolet exposure and sun-protective practices

The risk of melanoma skin cancer can be decreased by moderating sunburns and high-intensity sun exposure. Sun-protective behaviors include using a broad-spectrum sunscreen (i.e., protection against both UVA and UVB rays) and wearing sunglasses and sun-protective clothing. In 2015,

it was estimated that only 70.8% of adults ages 18 years or older were taking steps to protect themselves from the sun most of the time or always. Fewer than 34% of adults protected themselves by using sunscreen with a protective factor of 15 or higher most of the time or always. Fortunately, there has been a decrease in the percentage of adolescents and adults who use an indoor tanning device. In adolescents, males decreased their use from 6.7% to 4.0% and females decreased their use from 25.4% to 10.6%. Use by adults is lower, with a decrease among adult males from 2.2% to 1.7% and among adult females from 8.9% to 5.6%.

Chemical and environmental exposure

Chemical and environmental exposure to cancer-causing agents that exist as pollutants in our air, food, water, and soil also influence the incidence of cancer. Most exposure to toxic substances and hazardous wastes results from human activities, particularly through agricultural and industrial production. Exposure to chemicals including arsenic, benzene, cadmium, nitrate, and radon at levels that could cause cancer is typically limited, and some level of exposure to these compounds is common. Higher-than-normal levels of exposure may occur during the use of and exposure to fertilizers, mining or smelting activities, or plastics production, among other occupational activities. However, radon, which is the second leading cause of lung cancer, can be present in people's homes, and radon levels can be measured and mitigated.

SUMMARY

Cancer is a group of diseases that can begin anywhere in the body. All cancers have abnormal cell growth in common, which can impede the normal function of body structures and systems as cancer cells affect normal cells. The most common forms of cancer occur in the skin or tissue lining the organs (carcinoma), the connective tissue (sarcoma), the bone marrow or blood-forming organs (leukemia), the immune system (lymphoma), cells that become melanocytes (melanoma), and the central nervous system (brain and spine). Cancers are staged according to the extent of the cancer and if it has spread (metastasized).

The number of cancer survivors is growing substantially around the globe, with just over half of cancers affecting people over the age of 65. Screening for cancer varies from simple self-examination to complex medical imaging, and it is estimated that as many as 35% of cancer-related deaths could be prevented by effective screening and early detection. Cancer prevention targets three major groups of risk factors: behavioral, environmental, and policy/regulatory.

Smoking is the world's most preventable cause of cancer, and 98% of smokers begin smoking by age 26 years. Other foci of cancer prevention include improvements in diet, increased physical activity and better weight control, decreased ultraviolet exposure and increased use of sun protection, limited advertising and promotion of tobacco products, increased Medicaid funding for smoking cessation, limited secondhand smoke exposure, and reduced chemical and environmental exposure.

Occupational therapy practitioners play a critical role in the rehabilitation of cancer survivors. Practitioners may encounter cancer survivors in a wide range of practice settings, including hospitals, skilled nursing facilities, in the community, and when providing home health services. Understanding demographic trends in cancer across the lifespan, including the most common forms of cancer and trends in cancer deaths and survivorship, will help practitioners to develop appropriate and effective occupational therapy services.

REFERENCES

American Cancer Society. (2015). *Cancer basics.* Retrieved from https://www.cancer.org/cancer/cancer-basics/what-is-cancer.html

American Cancer Society. (2017). *What are the differences between cancers in adults and children?* Retrieved from https://www.cancer.org/cancer/cancer-in-children/differences-adults-children.html

American Cancer Society. (2018a). *American Cancer Society guidelines on the early detection of cancer.* Retrieved from https://www.cancer.org/healthy/find-cancer-early/cancer-screening-guidelines/american-cancer-society-guidelines-for-the-early-detection-of-cancer.html

American Cancer Society. (2018b). *Crunching numbers: What cancer screening statistics really tell us.* Retrieved from https://www.cancer.gov/about-cancer/screening/research/what-screening-statistics-mean

American Cancer Society. (2018c). *How smoking tobacco affects your cancer risk.* Retrieved from https://www.cancer.org/cancer/cancer-causes/tobacco-and-cancer/health-risks-of-smoking-tobacco.html

American Cancer Society. (2018d). *Late and long-term effects of cancer treatment in young adults.* Retrieved from https://www.cancer.org/cancer/cancer-in-young-adults/late-effects.html

American Cancer Society. (2019a). *Cancer facts and figures 2019.* Retrieved from https://www.cancer.org/content/dam/cancer-org/research/cancer-facts-and-statistics/annual-cancer-facts-and-figures/2019/cancer-facts-and-figures-2019.pdf

American Cancer Society. (2019b). *Cancer statistics 2019: A presentation from the American Cancer Society.* Retrieved from https://www.cancer.org/research/cancer-facts-statistics/all-cancer-facts-figures/cancer-facts-figures-2019.html

American Occupational Therapy Association. (2013). AOTA's societal statement on health disparities. *American Journal of Occupational Therapy, 67,* S7–S8. https://doi.org/10.5014/ajot.2013.67S7

American Society of Clinical Oncology. (2019). *Cancer screening.* Retrieved from https://www.cancer.net/navigating-cancer-care/prevention-and-healthy-living/cancer-screening

Courtney, R. (2015). *The health consequences of smoking—50 years of progress: A report of the Surgeon General, 2014 U.S. Department of Health and Human Services.* Atlanta: Department of Health and Human Services, Centers for Disease Control and Prevention, National Center for Chronic Disease Prevention and Health Promotion, Office on Smoking and Health. *Drug and Alcohol Review, 34*(6), 694–695. Available at http://www.surgeongeneral.gov/library/reports/50-years-of-progress.

DeSantis, C. E., Lin, C. C., Mariotto, A. B., Siegel, R. L., Stein, K. D., Kramer, J. L., . . . Jemal, A. (2014). Cancer treatment and survivorship statistics, 2014. *CA: A Cancer Journal for Clinicians, 64,* 252–271. https://doi.org/10.3322/caac.21235

Fidler, M. M., Bray, F., & Soerjomataram, I. (2018). The global cancer burden and human development: A review. *Scandinavian Journal of Public Health, 46,* 27–36. https://doi.org/10.1177/1403494817715400

Fitzmaurice, C., Dicker, D., Pain, A., Hamavid, H., Moradi-Lakeh, M., MacIntyre, M. F., . . . Naghavi, M.; Global Burden of Disease Cancer Collaboration. (2015). The global burden of cancer 2013. *JAMA Oncology, 1,* 505–527. https://doi.org/10.1001/jamaoncol.2015.0735

Hashim, D., Boffetta, P., La Vecchia, C., Rota, M., Bertuccio, P., Malvezzi, M., & Negri, E. (2016). The global decrease in cancer mortality: Trends and disparities. *Annals of Oncology: Official Journal of the European Society for Medical Oncology, 27,* 926–933. https://doi.org/10.1093/annonc/mdw027

Havighurst, R. J. (1963). Successful aging. *Processes of Aging: Social and Psychological Perspectives, 1,* 299–320.

Heidenreich, A., Bastian, P. J., Bellmunt, J., Bolla, M., Joniau, S., van der Kwast, T., . . . Mottet, N.; European Association of Urology. (2014). EAU guidelines on prostate cancer. Part 1: Screening, diagnosis, and local treatment with curative intent-update 2013. *European Urology, 65,* 124–137. https://doi.org/10.1016/j.eururo.2013.09.046

Lopez, A. D., Mathers, C. D., Ezzati, M., Jamison, D. T., & Murray, C. J. L. (2006). *Global burden of disease and risk factors.* New York: Oxford University Press.

MD Anderson Cancer Center. (2017). *Active surveillance for prostate cancer.* Retrieved from https://www.mdanderson.org/publications/oncolog/july-2017/active-surveillance-for-prostate-cancer.html

MD Anderson Cancer Center. (2018). *Cancer screenings.* Retrieved from https://www.mdanderson.org/prevention-screening/get-screened.html

Memorial Sloan Kettering Cancer Center. (2018). *Screening guidelines.* Retrieved from https://www.mskcc.org/cancer-care/risk-assessment-screening/screening-guidelines

Miller, K. D., Siegel, R. L., Lin, C. C., Mariotto, A. B., Kramer, J. L., Rowland, J. H., . . . Jemal, A. (2016). Cancer treatment and survivorship statistics, 2016. *CA: A Cancer Journal for Clinicians, 66,* 271–289. https://doi.org/10.3322/caac.21349

National Cancer Institute. (2015a). *Age and cancer risk.* Retrieved from https://www.cancer.gov/about-cancer/causes-prevention/risk/age

National Cancer Institute. (2015b). *Diagnosis and staging.* Retrieved from http://www.cancer.gov/about-cancer/diagnosis-staging/staging

National Cancer Institute. (2015c). *What is cancer?* Retrieved from http://www.cancer.gov/about-cancer/what-is-cancer

National Cancer Institute. (2017a). *Adolescents and young adults with cancer.* Retrieved from https://www.cancer.gov/types/aya

National Cancer Institute. (2017b). *Cancer in children and adolescents.* Retrieved from https://www.cancer.gov/types/childhood-cancers/child-adolescent-cancers-fact-sheet

National Cancer Institute. (2018a). *Cancer Screening Overview (PDQ®)–Health Professional Version.* Retrieved from https://www.cancer.gov/about-cancer/screening/hp-screening-overview-pdq#link

National Cancer Institute. (2018b) *Cancer statistics.* Retrieved from https://www.cancer.gov/about-cancer/understanding/statistics

National Cancer Institute. (2019a). *Cancer trends progress report: Prevention.* Retrieved from https://progressreport.cancer.gov/prevention.

National Cancer Institute. (2019b). *NCI dictionary of cancer terms*. Retrieved from https://www.cancer.gov/publications/dictionaries/cancer-terms

National Cancer Institute. (2019c). *Surveillance, Epidemiology, and End Results Program fast stats*. Retrieved from https://seer.cancer.gov/faststats/selections.php?series=age

Office of Disease Prevention and Health Promotion. (2018). *Social determinants of health*. Retrieved from https://www.healthypeople.gov/2020/topics-objectives/topic/social-determinants-of-health

Ott, J. J., Ullrich, A., Mascarenhas, M., & Stevens, G. A. (2010). Global cancer incidence and mortality caused by behavior and infection. *Journal of Public Health, 33,* 223–233. https://doi.org/10.1093/pubmed/fdq076

Patient Protection and Affordable Care Act, Pub. L. 111-148, 42 U.S.C. §§ 18001–18121 (2010).

Prasad, S., Sung, B., & Aggarwal, B. B. (2012). Age-associated chronic diseases require age-old medicine: Role of chronic inflammation. *Preventative Medicine, 54*(Suppl.), S29–S37. https://doi.org/10.1016/j.ypmed.2011.11.011

Siegel, R. L., Miller, K. D., & Jemal, A. (2017). Cancer statistics, 2017. *CA: A Cancer Journal for Clinicians, 67,* 7–30. https://doi.org/10.3322/caac.21387

Smith, R. A., Manassaram-Baptiste, D., Brooks, D., Doroshenk, M., Fedewa, S., Saslow, D., . . . Wender, R. (2015). Cancer screening in the United States, 2015: A review of current American Cancer Society guidelines and current issues in cancer screening. *CA: A Cancer Journal for Clinicians, 65,* 30–54. https://doi.org/10.3322/caac.21261

Stephens, W. E. (2017). Comparing the cancer potencies of emissions from vapourised nicotine products including e-cigarettes with those of tobacco smoke. *Tobacco Control, 27,* 10–17. https://doi.org/10.1136/tobaccocontrol-2017-053808

Torre, L. A., Siegel, R. L., Ward, E. M., & Jemal, A. (2015). Global cancer incidence and mortality rates and trends—An update. *Cancer Epidemiology, Biomarkers & Prevention, 25,* 16–27. https://doi.org/10.1158/1055-9965.EPI-15-0578

University of Wyoming. (2018). *Learning theories for educators: Robert Havinghurst: Developmental states and tasks of the adult*. Retrieved from http://www.uwyo.edu/aded5050/5050unit4/havighurst.asp

White, M. C., Holman, D. M., Boehm, J. E., Peipins, L. A., Grossman, M., & Henley, S. J. (2014). Age and cancer risk: A potentially modifiable relationship. *American Journal of Preventive Medicine, 46*(Suppl. 1), S7–S15. https://doi.org/10.1016/j.amepre.2013.10.029

Cancer Treatment Approaches Across the Lifespan

2

Brent Braveman, OTR, PhD, FAOTA

LEARNING OBJECTIVES

After completing this chapter, readers should be able to
- Name and briefly describe the major approaches to treating cancer;
- Identify the risks and side effects of common approaches to treating cancer;
- Identify opportunities for occupational therapy practitioners to intervene to improve participation in roles and life situations, occupational performance, and quality of life for cancer survivors undergoing treatment for cancer; and
- Identify the members of the interprofessional cancer care and cancer rehabilitation teams and describe their role in caring for the cancer survivor.

KEY TERMS AND CONCEPTS

- Ablation therapy
- Adoptive cell therapy
- Allogeneic stem cell transplant
- Autologous stem cell transplant
- Cancer rehabilitation team
- Case managers
- Cellular therapy
- Chaplains
- Chemotherapy
- Child life specialists
- Clinical dietitians
- Clinical psychologists
- Complementary medicine
- Conventional medicine
- Cryoablation
- End-of-life care
- General immunotherapies
- Graft-versus-host disease
- High-intensity focused ultrasound
- Hospice
- Integrative medicine
- Monoclonal antibodies
- Nurses
- Occupational therapists
- Occupational therapy assistants
- Oncologists
- Palliative care
- Pencil-beam scanning
- Pharmacists
- Physiatrists
- Physical therapist assistants
- Physical therapists
- Proton therapy
- Radiation therapy
- Radiofrequency ablation
- Small molecule drugs
- Social workers
- Stem cell transplant
- Surgery
- Targeted immunotherapies
- Targeted therapy

INTRODUCTION

As noted in Chapter 1, "Cancer Demographics and Trends Across the Lifespan," cancer is a group of diseases, not a single disease, and all cancers have abnormal cell growth in common. Just as there are a variety of cancers that each brings different challenges to the body, there are various treatments for cancer, and each treatment brings different challenges and negative side effects. This chapter reviews the various types of cancer treatments and their effects. Opportunities for occupational therapy practitioners to improve participation in roles and life situations, occupational performance, and quality of life (QoL) in cancer survivors undergoing treatment are highlighted. In addition, members of the cancer rehabilitation teams are introduced.

APPROACHES TO TREATING CANCER

When treating cancer, a variety of approaches may be used in isolation or in combination depending on the type of cancer and its stage (see Chapter 1, "Cancer Demographics and Trends Across the Lifespan," for information on staging cancer). Each treatment presents benefits and possible risks and side effects. Occupational therapy practitioners working with cancer survivors should have a clear understanding of the treatment that each survivor is receiving, the signs and symptoms of complications from treatment, and how treatments or their side effects can affect occupational performance. Although the focus of occupational therapy intervention may vary across the course of treatment, the promotion of increased participation in life roles and improved occupational performance for a cancer survivor's valued occupations are always the primary focus of intervention.

Surgery

Surgery is a common cancer treatment and may be performed as the sole treatment or in combination with other interventions, such as chemotherapy and radiation. Surgery involves cutting, abrading, suturing, or otherwise physically changing body tissues and organs (MedicineNet.com, 2019). About 60% of patients undergo some type of surgery to treat their cancer (MD Anderson Cancer Center, 2019h). Several types of cancer surgery are presented in Table 2.1.

Surgery for cancer can include such side effects and complications as bleeding, blood clots, damage to nearby tissue, drug reactions (e.g., anesthesia reactions, allergies to antibiotics), damage to other organs, pain, infections, negative effects on body functions, and post-surgical complications, such as lymphedema (American Cancer Society [ACS], 2018).

Occupational therapy practitioners can help cancer survivors overcome the negative effects of surgery and its complications and promote occupational performance in various ways. These include strategies to address the negative effects of surgery (e.g., compression bandages for edema) and the use of occupation to promote performance in ADLs and in roles important to the cancer survivor, such as return to school, work, or parenting. Strategies to help manage post-surgical pain and to promote early mobility are also commonly used.

Some surgeries for cancer can be disfiguring and may cause significant disruption to body image. Occupational therapy practitioners can assist cancer survivors in exploring and implementing strategies to become more comfortable with their altered physical presentation (e.g., practicing answering questions about limb loss or scars). These strategies are explored in later chapters of this book.

Ablation Therapy

Ablation therapy is a minimally invasive procedure in which special probes are used to deliver heat or cold to destroy, or ablate, cancer tumors without the need for more invasive surgery. Ablation therapy has several advantages. It causes less pain and has a shorter recovery time than surgery or radiation therapy, can often be done as an outpatient procedure, and can be used in conjunction with other cancer treatments (Mayo Clinic, 2019).

Cryoablation is also known as cryotherapy or cryosurgery (RadiologyInfo.org, 2018). During cryoablation, extreme cold with temperatures well below freezing is used to kill cancer by inserting a probe into the tumor. A ball of ice forms at the tip of the probe, and the ice freezes and destroys the cancerous tissue. Cryotherapy is used to treat bone, cervical, eye, kidney, liver, lung, and prostate cancer. Cryotherapy can sometimes be performed as an outpatient procedure because it is not as invasive as surgery. Side effects of cryotherapy include loss of erectile function in men being treated for prostate surgery.

Radiofrequency ablation (RFA) uses heat to destroy cancer tissue by inserting a needle-thin probe and delivering radiofrequency waves directly to the tumor. RFA is best for smaller, localized tumors. It can be used to treat a variety of cancers, including bone, liver, lung, and kidney. The risks of RFA are low, but side effects can include weakness or numbness in the legs or other parts of the body if the spine is involved, and swelling and bruising at the incision site. Activity may have to be limited for 24–48 hours after the procedure (Cleveland Clinic, 2019).

High-intensity focused ultrasound (HIFU) is a nonsurgical treatment that uses a nonionizing physical agent to treat prostate cancer

> Focused ultrasound applied to tissue produces mechanical, thermal, and cavitation effects; all of which induce irreversible tissue damage. Despite these effects, there is no maximum dose for HIFU, nor is there any diffusion to other organs outside of the targeted volume. High-intensity focused ultrasound can also be used with external beam radiotherapy (before or after HIFU) and it can be repeated. HIFU treatment is performed under real time monitoring with ultrasound. (Gelet et al., 2017, p. 251)

Some forms of ablation therapy may have a minimal effect on occupational performance, and cancer survivors may return to normal activity quickly. For more invasive

---

TABLE 2.1.   Common Types of Cancer Surgeries

TYPE OF SURGERY	DESCRIPTION
Curative	Involves removal of a cancerous tumor and is most effective on localized cancers that haven't spread to other parts of the body. Curative surgery is often followed by radiation therapy or chemotherapy.
Preventive	Used to stop cancer before it occurs (e.g., colon cancer can be prevented by removing precancerous polyps before they become malignant). Some women may choose preventive breast removal if they are at high risk for breast cancer because of family history or genetic mutations.
Reconstructive	Seeks to restore normal or near-normal appearance or function after other cancer treatment. Examples include breast reconstruction after mastectomy or facial reconstruction.
Staging	Performed to determine the stage and extent of cancer and can sometimes be done via endoscopy.
Supportive	Performed to aid cancer treatments, such as placing a chemotherapy port under the skin.
Palliative	Used to improve a patient's QoL by easing pain or other symptoms caused by advanced or untreatable cancer.

Note. QoL = quality of life.
Source. Adapted from MD Anderson Cancer Center (2019g).

ablation therapy, including ablation surgery, risks include those of any invasive procedure or surgery. The use of heat or cold near vital organs such as the kidneys or the lungs may affect the organ's function. Other risks include nerve damage and resulting weakness or numbness or impotence if the therapy is used to treat the prostate. Occupational therapy may address negative effects of ablation therapy on occupational performance through strategies to limit the impact of nerve damage or other side effects as well as use of those strategies previously described for surgical interventions.

Radiation Therapy

Radiation therapy kills cancer cells through the use of focused, high-energy photon beams (MD Anderson Cancer Center, 2019d). The use of radiation therapy is common: more than 50% of cancer patients receive some sort of radiation therapy. It can be used as a stand-alone treatment or in combination with other therapies, such as chemotherapy. Radiation may shrink tumors before surgery or chemotherapy and can be used to kill any remaining cancer cells after other treatments.

One dose of radiation is called a *fraction,* and most radiation treatments require several fractions. A standard radiation treatment plan calls for 5 fractions a week for 4–6 weeks. Radiation therapy must be carefully planned to focus on the tumor and minimize the impact on surrounding healthy tissues (MD Anderson Cancer Center, 2019d). Before the patient undergoes treatment, doctors simulate treatment; computed tomography scanners are used to test various beam fields and various immobilization devices, which prevent the patient from moving during treatment. Doctors use the data from the simulators to calculate the appropriate dose of radiation before the patient's treatment begins. Table 2.2 provides information on how radiation therapy is often used on the basis of the disease site and treatment guideline (Barton et al., 2014).

Radiation therapy may produce several side effects, including fatigue, nausea and vomiting, skin changes, reduced range of motion (ROM), headache, hair loss, edema, skin tenderness, cough, shortness of breath, difficulty swallowing, sexual dysfunction, fertility problems, and difficulty with urination (National Cancer Institute [NCI], 2018d). Many of these side effects also occur with other treatments

for cancer, and occupational therapy practitioners can intervene to guide cancer survivors in minimizing the impact on occupational performance. Comprehensive programs to manage cancer-related fatigue (CRF) and the use of energy conservation and work simplification may lessen the impact of side effects (see Chapter 15, "Cancer-Related Fatigue," for more information on CRF). At times, intervention may focus on improving ROM, which may be limited because of surgery or previous cancer treatments, before radiation so a survivor can be positioned appropriately.

Proton Therapy

Proton therapy is similar to traditional radiation therapy, but it uses a different type of energy and is much more accurate for targeting tumors (Medical News Today, 2018). Standard radiation therapy may result in side effects from damage to nearby healthy tissues or organs because of the use of x-ray beams. To minimize side effects, the radiation dose delivered to the tumor must be limited. Alternatively, proton therapy uses protons, which are positively charged atomic particles, to deliver a targeted and more precise dose of radiation. For this reason, higher doses may be used, resulting in less damage to surrounding tissues and organs. Moreover, proton beams enter the body with a low dose of radiation that increases as it approaches the tumor before stopping. There is no "exit dose" beyond the tumor (American Society of Clinical Oncology, 2018a).

Pencil-beam scanning, also known as *spot scanning,* is a proton therapy technique used to treat complex tumors. The technology allows proton therapy to be delivered in a single, narrow proton beam that is about 4–5 millimeters in diameter. Pencil-beam scanning deposits the radiation dose layer-by-layer like a painter's brush strokes. It forms to the specific shape of a tumor and can be adjusted for intensity to achieve the desired dose distribution (Scripps, 2014). Pencil-beam scanning is used to treat cancers of the prostate, brain, base of the skull, and eye.

Drug Therapy (Chemotherapy)

Chemotherapy involves the use of pharmaceuticals to limit the growth of cancer cells, destroy them, or relieve pain

TABLE 2.2. Radiotherapy Use for Cancer Survivors, by Disease Site	
DISEASE SITE	**DESCRIPTION OF USE OF RADIOTHERAPY**
Breast	Postoperative treatment to some patients after cancer treated by surgery improves survival. These survivors may also be treated with hormonal therapy and chemotherapy.
Lung	The 5-year survival rate for nonoperable lung cancer is very low (approximately 5%), but tumor control may be improved in early disease with high-dose hypofractionated radiotherapy.
Cervix	Radiotherapy is used in combination with chemotherapy for more advanced cancer, and control varies from 70% in Stage 1 to 7% in Stage IV.
Head and neck	Radiotherapy is used with surgery in early disease and with surgery and chemotherapy in more advanced disease.
Lymphoma	Radiotherapy controls approximately 80%–90% of early stage Hodgkin lymphoma, but chemotherapy can result in lower doses of radiotherapy.
Bladder	There is wide variation in treatment success based on disease stage. Radiotherapy may be an alternative to surgery in early disease, and 5-year survival rates exceed 50% whether surgery or radiotherapy is used.

symptoms. This type of treatment can be used alone or in combination with other cancer treatments. Chemotherapy may be classified as *adjuvant*, which is focused on eliminating cancer cells after other treatments have been performed, or as *neoadjuvant*, which is focused on shrinking tumors before surgery or radiation (neoadjuvant therapy).

Chemotherapy is administered in several ways:

- *Intravenous (IV):* IV administration is the most common method of delivering chemotherapy. IV administration is performed by inserting a needle, which is attached to a plastic bag containing the chemotherapy drug, into the patient's vein. For patients requiring repeated administrations (doses), a catheter may be inserted into one of the large veins and left in place until treatment is concluded. A metal or plastic port is implanted under the skin as an IV connection device.
- *Oral chemotherapy:* Chemotherapy drugs are taken by mouth either in pill or liquid form.
- *Injections:* Injections are administered into the muscle, under the skin, or directly into a cancer lesion, depending on the type or location of the cancer.
- *Isolated limb perfusion:* Isolated limb perfusion is used to treat advanced or metastatic melanoma and some sarcomas. This approach targets tumors in the arm or leg by administering heated chemotherapy directly to the tumor. The blood supply of the affected limb is isolated from the rest of the body, and the chemotherapy drugs are pumped into the treatment area through tubes inserted into tiny incisions.
- *Hepatic arterial infusion:* Used to treat liver cancer, hepatic arterial infusion requires a tiny pump to be surgically inserted under the skin and connected to the hepatic artery, which supplies blood to the liver. Drugs are administered through the pump over a period of about 2 weeks.

The side effects of chemotherapy depend on the type of chemotherapy drugs used. The side effects will vary in length and severity in each patient; most side effects are temporary and disappear after treatment is complete (MD Anderson Cancer Center, 2019a). Noninvasive complementary therapies and medications can be administered to alleviate the severest symptoms.

The most common side effects of chemotherapy include (Pearce et al., 2017)

- Temporary hair loss,
- Fatigue,
- Nausea or vomiting,
- Diarrhea,
- Pain,
- Chest pain,
- Increased risk of infection,
- Depression,
- Mucositis,
- Rash,
- Anemia,
- Increased sun sensitivity,
- Numbness or weakness in the hands and feet (peripheral neuropathy), and
- Chemobrain (i.e., cognitive dysfunction due to chemotherapy) or cognitive issues that include memory problems, trouble concentrating, and other mental

symptoms. Strategies for addressing cognitive dysfunction due to chemotherapy and other causes are included in Chapter 17, "Cancer-Related Cognitive Impairment."

Various strategies can be used to reduce the negative impact of chemotherapy side effects, some of which are appropriate for use by occupational therapy practitioners. These preparatory activities include biofeedback and relaxation training, systematic desensitization, hypnosis, acupuncture or acupressure, and positive thinking (Kamen et al., 2014). CRF is one of the most common symptoms of chemotherapy and ranges from mild to severe. Strategies for addressing CRF are included in Chapter 15, "Cancer-Related Fatigue."

Targeted Therapy

Targeted therapy, sometimes also called *precision medicine,* is "a type of treatment that uses drugs or other substances to identify and attack specific types of cancer cells with less harm to normal cells" (NCI, 2018b, para. 1). Targeted therapies can be given in pill form or through an infusion and are often combined with chemotherapy or radiation.

The genes that cause cancer often produce protein molecules that cause the cancer to grow and spread. Targeted therapies are designed to interfere with, or *target*, these molecules or the cancer-causing genes that create them. Some targeted therapies work by attaching to the molecule and stopping it from doing its job. Other targeted therapies use chemotherapy drugs that block the molecule from the place it normally goes or deliver toxic substances to the cancer cells (NCI, 2018c).

There are two main types of targeted therapies drugs (MD Anderson Cancer Center, 2019i):

1. *Small molecule drugs* target molecules that are inside cancer cells. Because of their small size, they can easily enter the cells and interfere with the molecules.
2. *Monoclonal antibodies* are larger and work outside of cancer cells. They target molecules on the surface of the cancer cells or nearby. These are made using cloned cells that produce antibodies that interfere with the targeted molecule. Monoclonal antibodies also can be used to deliver a toxic molecule directly into a cancer cell.

Targeted therapies can only be effective if enough molecules that can be affected by a chemotherapy drug are present. To determine this, blood or DNA tests are used to see if and how many of a particular type of molecule are present in the patient's body. Drugs will be administered only if enough molecules of a specific type are present. Targeted therapies may fail because cancers can find other ways of progressing; if this happens, the targeted therapy will be discontinued.

Although targeted therapies generally have fewer side effects than chemotherapy, the side effects can be serious and depend on the targeted therapy drug a patient is taking. Common side effects include (ACS, 2019)

- Skin problems, including hives and intense itching;
- Allergic-like reactions, including trouble breathing, tightness in the chest or throat, dizziness, and swelling in the lips or tongue;
- Elevated liver enzymes;
- Diarrhea or constipation;

- Fatigue;
- Nausea and vomiting;
- Low blood cell counts;
- Poor blood clotting and wound healing; and
- High blood pressure.

By this point, readers should realize that different treatments for cancer can result in many of the same side effects. The interventions to promote participation and occupational performance are also similar across different types of cancer. Although some symptoms and side effects (e.g., impotence, nerve damage, edema) are more common with some types of cancer than others, occupational therapy practitioners assess each survivor in the context of their occupational profile to customize interventions.

Immunotherapy

Immunotherapy is an approach to cancer treatment that uses the body's own natural defenses. In immunotherapy, pharmaceuticals are used to stimulate the immune system to identify and kill cancer cells. *T cells,* a type of white blood cell that tailors the body's immune response to specific diseases, are key in immunotherapy treatments. Some T cells have proteins on their surface that act like a brake and prevent the cells from attacking cancer cells. When these proteins are blocked by immunotherapy drugs, the T cells can perform their duties and attack cancer cells (MD Anderson Cancer Center, 2019c).

Adoptive cell therapy (ACT) is "a highly personalized cancer therapy that involves administration to the cancer-bearing host of immune cells with direct anticancer activity" (Rosenberg & Restifo, 2015, p. 62). With ACT, T cells are collected from a patient and grown in the laboratory. This increases the number of T cells that can kill cancer cells or fight infections. These T cells are given back to the patient to help the immune system fight disease; this is also called *cellular adoptive immunotherapy* (NCI, 2018a).

There are two common methods of ACT. In the first method, the patient's own immune cells recognize and attack cancer, but their volume in the patient's bloodstream is not enough to be successful; the immune cells are multiplied many times in a laboratory and then injected back into the patient. In the second method, a patient's immune cells are genetically altered in the laboratory to recognize a specific cancer. The cells are then multiplied and injected back into the patient. Both methods are currently being explored and developed through clinical trials to more effectively target solid tumors and blood cancers.

Other immunotherapies fall into two general categories. *Targeted immunotherapies* stimulate the body's immune system by targeting specific proteins on the surface of cells that help identify cancer and stimulate an immune response. *General immunotherapies* do not affect cancer itself but work on proteins called *cytokines* that send signals to stimulate the body's immune system to fight cancer cells (MD Anderson Cancer Center, 2019c).

The side effects of immunotherapies include fatigue; diarrhea; flulike symptoms; skin reactions, including rashes, blistering, and itching; and immune-mediated adverse reactions, including hepatitis, dermatitis, enterocolitis, and nerve or endocrine gland damage (Society for Immunotherapy of Cancer, 2018). Occupational therapy can assist cancer survivors undergoing immunotherapy treatment to manage fatigue and to decrease the negative impact of side effects on occupational performance.

Stem Cell Transplants (Cellular Therapy)

Stem cell transplants (also called *cellular therapy*) use immature cells from bone marrow that develop into mature platelets, red blood cells, and white blood cells. Umbilical cord blood may also be used in allogenic stem cell procedures (i.e., cells from a donor). Stem cell transplants are used to treat cancers of the blood and cancers that affect the lymphatic system, including leukemia and lymphoma (MD Anderson Cancer Center, 2019g).

During a stem cell transplant, damaged or defective cells are replaced with healthy cells. Stem cell transplants might be considered more like a transfusion than a surgical procedure. The first step of the process is referred to as *conditioning* and includes the use of radiation and chemotherapy to damage or destroy the existing immune system, including the defective cells. The damaged bone marrow is then replaced with the healthy stem cells that were harvested before the process began (Dana-Farber Cancer Institute, 2019). Stem cell transplants use *hematopoietic stem cells,* immature cells that begin life in the bone marrow and eventually develop into the various types of mature blood cells, including

- *Red blood cells,* which carry oxygen;
- *Platelets,* which help the blood clot; and
- *White blood cells,* which help fight infection.

There are two main types of stem cell transplant: (1) autologous and (2) allogeneic.

Autologous stem cell transplant

In an *autologous stem cell transplant,* a patient's own stem cells are harvested before the initiation of chemotherapy or radiation to destroy the remaining bone marrow; the stem cells are replaced after this treatment. An advantage to an autologous stem cell transplant is that there is less risk of serious side effects, including *graft-versus-host disease* (GVHD), a condition that occurs when the body's immune cells attack cells from the donor, or when the donor cells attack the patient's cells. GVHD can occur right after the transplant or more than a year later (Cleveland Clinic, 2018). GVHD is categorized as acute or chronic; symptoms of acute and chronic GHVD are presented in Exhibit 2.1 (Cleveland Clinic, 2018; National Marrow Donor Program, 2016).

Allogeneic stem cell transplant

In an *allogeneic stem cell transplant,* stem cells are harvested from a donor whose tissue most closely matches the patient's. These cells can also come from umbilical cord blood extracted from the placenta after birth and stored in a cord blood bank for future use. After the patient's immune system is destroyed, the new stem cells are introduced. An advantage of an allogeneic stem cell transplant is that the process promotes a new immune system response to fight the cancer. The disadvantage of this type of stem cell transplant is an increased risk of rejection or GVHD (Memorial Sloan Kettering Cancer Center, 2018).

EXHIBIT 2.1.	Signs and Symptoms of Acute and Chronic GVHD

ACUTE GVHD	CHRONIC GVHD
Skin	**Skin and Nails**
▪ Rashes	▪ Rashes
▪ Blisters	▪ Skin thickening
▪ Yellow discoloration	▪ Nail thickening
Intestines and Digestive System	▪ Hair loss
▪ Nausea	▪ Itchy skin
▪ Vomiting	**Intestines and Digestive System**
▪ Decreased appetite	▪ Nausea
▪ Diarrhea	▪ Vomiting
▪ Stomachaches	▪ Decreased appetite
▪ Cramping	▪ Diarrhea
Liver	▪ Stomachaches
▪ Jaundice	▪ Cramping
▪ Discolored urine	**Joints and Muscles**
	▪ Pain
	▪ Stiffness
	▪ Cramps
	▪ Weakness
	Eyes
	▪ Dry eyes
	▪ Blurred vision or vision changes
	Mouth
	▪ Sores
	▪ Pain/irritation
	▪ Difficulty swallowing
	▪ Decreased movement
	Respiratory System
	▪ Shortness of breath
	▪ Cough
	Genitourinary System
	▪ Increased need to urinate
	▪ Burning or bleeding with urination
	▪ Vaginal dryness

Note. GVHD = graft-versus-host disease.

Stem cell transplant side effects and occupational therapy intervention

Because the patient's immune system is wiped out before a stem cell transplant, it takes about 6 months to a year for the immune system to recover and start producing healthy new blood cells. Transplant patients are at increased risk for infections during this time and must take precautions. Other side effects include
▪ GVHD,
▪ Increased risk of bleeding,
▪ Anemia,
▪ Fatigue, and
▪ Mouth sores.

Occupational therapy addresses the side effects of stem cell transplant using the same strategies that are used when side effects present following other treatments. GVHD can be life threatening and requires aggressive treatment and intervention from the entire cancer treatment and rehabilitation teams. One unique feature of stem cell transplant is the extended hospital stay that may require a cancer survivor to be an inpatient for as long as 4 weeks. Occupational therapy practitioners are ideally suited for preparing the survivor for admission and the impact that it will have on role performance, the ability to maintain communication and contact with friends and family members, and the boredom and sleep disruption that can occur during long hospitalization. See Chapters 10, "Prehabilitation" and 11, "Acute Inpatient Rehabilitation" for further discussion.

Complementary Medicine and Integrative Medicine

The terms *complementary medicine* and *integrative medicine* are sometimes used interchangeably. However, each of these approaches to medicine is different, and they may be provided as a complement to conventional medicine. At times, the phrase *alternative medicine* is used interchangeably with complementary medicine, but at other times, it refers to non-evidence-based approaches for cancer treatment that are used as a replacement for conventional medicine.
▪ *Conventional medicine:* "Traditional" medicine as practiced by a medical doctor, a doctor of osteopathy, and other allied health professionals.
▪ *Complementary medicine:* A group of mostly nonmedical approaches to help patients cope with cancer and treatment side effects, pain, depression, and anxiety. Research data have verified the benefits of many complementary therapies, including acupuncture, yoga, massage, stress-reduction techniques, and nutritional supplements.
▪ *Integrative medicine:* The practice of combining scientifically proven complementary therapies with conventional medicine as part of a comprehensive plan to treat both the disease and its physical and emotional side effects (adapted from MD Anderson Cancer Center, 2019b).

Cancer survivors may benefit from complementary medicine and integrative medicine approaches. However, the primary oncologist should evaluate all treatments carefully to assure that there is no risk.

Supportive Treatment

Palliative care (sometimes called *supportive care*) is a holistic approach to decreasing the negative effects of cancer and its treatments and improving the comfort and QoL of cancer survivors. Palliative care may be provided alongside active curative treatment. At times, the term *palliative care* has been used interchangeably with the term *hospice,* but this is not accurate. When a cancer survivor enters **hospice,** also referred to as **end-of-life care,** they are deciding to end efforts for a cure and to focus on minimizing symptoms and maximizing comfort and QoL. The goal of palliative care is to provide the best possible QoL at every stage of treatment, starting at diagnosis.

Palliative care can include
▪ Management of pain, fatigue, nausea, loss of appetite, and other treatment-related symptoms;

- Treatment of depression and anxiety; and
- End-of-life or hospice care.

According to the American Occupational Therapy Association (2015),

> Occupational therapy with an emphasis on palliative and hospice care can be provided in a hospital setting, a specialized hospice facility, an individual's home, or an outpatient setting. Occupational therapy practitioners use a client-centered approach to evaluate of the needs of the client in his or her occupational roles (e.g., parent, spouse, worker), identify current and potential abilities, and determine barriers to engaging in occupations, including activities of daily living, instrumental ADLs, rest and sleep, leisure, and social participation. They also help prevent contractures and maintain joint integrity with stretching routines or splints that don't interfere with daily activities. (para. 4)

Hospice may be appropriate if the cancer can no longer be treated; the focus shifts to providing end-of-life care. Palliative care specialists can help determine the patient's needs and create a plan to address them. End-of-life planning should include these components:

- *Patient comfort:* Treat symptoms, such as pain, fatigue, breathing difficulties, and other problems.
- *Advance care planning:* Discuss decisions about wills, funeral arrangements, and other details with family members. The palliative care team can help with advance care planning, including living wills and medical power of attorney.
- *Deciding where and how care will be provided:* Help a patient and their family decide whether to begin hospice care. Hospice care can be provided at home, in the hospital, in assisted-care communities, or in nursing homes. Some hospice organizations have inpatient facilities where patients can stay for a short time for treatment of uncontrolled symptoms.

Eligibility for hospice services requires a doctor's certification that the patient's life expectancy is 6 months or less.

CANCER TREATMENT AND CANCER REHABILITATION TEAMS

A *cancer rehabilitation team* comprises members from a range of medical and health disciplines that address all aspects of cancer treatment and the side effects of treatment. The members of a cancer rehabilitation team are described below.

Case Managers

Case managers are health professionals who work in

> hospital and health care systems in a collaborative practice model including patients, nurses, social workers, occupational therapy practitioners, physicians, other practitioners, caregivers, and the community. The case management process encompasses communication and facilitates care along a continuum through effective resource coordination. The goals of case management include the achievement of optimal health, access to care, and appropriate utilization of resources, balanced with the patient's right to self-determination. (American Case Management Association, 2018, para. 2)

The case manager's role on the cancer rehabilitation team is to facilitate the process of care for cancer survivors and their families, advocate for the survivor and their families, and triage and coordinate the provision of care. Case managers are often nurses or social workers but can hold other health degrees at the bachelor's or graduate levels. Certified case managers pass a certification process coordinated by the American Case Management Association.

Chaplains and Spiritual Care Counselors

Chaplains and other spiritual care counselors in oncology settings provide pastoral care to cancer survivors, their families, and staff. The chaplain or spiritual care counselor's role on the cancer rehabilitation team is to provide prayer or spiritual counseling and guidance; provide spiritual support; arrange communion, baptism, and the sacrament of the sick; and assist survivors who are wrestling with issues, such as unresolved grief, lack of faith, or loss of hope or meaning of life (Denham & Humbert, 2016; MD Anderson, 2019d). Chaplains in health care settings typically have a master's or doctoral degree.

Child Life Specialists

Child life specialists are health professionals who help children and their families manage the stress and symptoms of acute and chronic illnesses. Child life specialists "provide evidence-based, developmentally and psychologically appropriate interventions including therapeutic play, preparation for procedures, and education to reduce fear, anxiety, and pain" (Association of Child Life Professionals [ACLP], 2018, para. 3). The child life specialist's role on the cancer rehabilitation team is to help children with cancer and their families cope with the sometimes difficult process of undergoing cancer treatment. This may include fostering the student role, promoting normal development, and supporting family members. Child life specialists may be educated at the bachelor's or master's level and may pursue a voluntary certification by ACLP.

Clinical Dietitians or Nutritionists

Clinical dietitians, also called *nutritionists,* are health professionals who

> provide medical nutrition therapy for patients in institutions such as hospitals and nursing care facilities. They assess patients' nutritional needs, develop and implement nutrition programs, and evaluate and report the results. They confer with doctors and other health care professionals in order to coordinate medical and dietary needs. (Explorehealthcareers.org, 2018, para. 2)

The clinical dietitian or nutritionist's role is to promote a healthy diet and to assure adequate nutrition for the cancer patient. This includes providing a dietary prescription and recommending strategies when cancer survivors experience side effects that make eating difficult, such as mucositis. Clinical dietitians may be educated at the bachelor's or master's level. Certifications can be obtained as a certified nutritional specialist, a certified clinical nutritionist, and registered dietitian among others available through the American Nutrition Association (2018).

Clinical Psychologists

Clinical psychologists are health professionals who provide

> continuing and comprehensive mental and behavioral health care for individuals and families; consultation to agencies and communities; training, education, and supervision; and research-based practice. It is a specialty in breadth—one that is broadly inclusive of severe psychopathology—and marked by comprehensiveness and integration of knowledge and skill from a broad array of disciplines within and outside of psychology proper. (American Psychological Association, 2018, para. 1)

The clinical psychologist's role on the cancer rehabilitation team is to support the mental health of the cancer survivor, their family, and their significant other. They provide assessments, diagnostic interviews, behavioral assessments, and individual consultation to promote intellectual, emotional, and psychological well-being. Clinical psychologists are educated at the master's or doctoral level; most have doctoral degrees.

Nurses

Nurses are health professionals who provide services to maintain and restore the health of people of all ages. Nurses provide assessment, diagnosis, outcomes planning, care implementation, and evaluation of health conditions (American Nurses Association, 2018). The nurse's role on the cancer rehabilitation team is to coordinate the nursing care of the cancer survivor and collaborate with the oncologist and other team members. Nurses may be educated at the associate's, bachelor's, or graduate level and may practice as a registered nurse (RN), a licensed practical nurse who performs tasks under the supervision of an RN, a clinical nurse specialist (CNS), or a nurse practitioner (NP). *CNSs* and *NPs* are nursing specialists who work under the supervision of a physician and take on some roles of physicians, such as prescribing medications and ordering medical tests and assessments (Nurse Practitioner Schools, 2018; Santiago, 2018).

Occupational Therapy Practitioners

Occupational therapists and *occupational therapy assistants* are health care providers who specialize in helping individuals across the lifespan participate in society and perform their most valued occupations, regardless of whether they have an illness, disease, or disability (American Occupational Therapy Association, 2019). Occupations are the familiar everyday activities we perform as we go about our daily lives. Occupational therapists may have a bachelor's degree or postbachelor's degree, although postbachelor's-only programs have been accredited and required since 2007. Occupational therapy assistants require education at the associate's degree level, and beginning in 2020, educational programs for the occupational therapy assistant may also be offered at the bachelor's level.

Oncologists

Oncologists are physicians who specialize in the treatment and medical care of a person diagnosed with cancer. Oncologists typically specialize in one of three major areas:
- A medical oncologist uses chemotherapy, targeted therapy, or immunotherapy to treat a patient's cancer.
- A surgical oncologist performs surgery to remove the cancer tumor and nearby tissue and performs biopsies to diagnose cancer.
- A radiation oncologist uses radiation therapy to treat cancer. (American Society of Clinical Oncology, 2018b)

The oncologist's role on the cancer rehabilitation team is to coordinate treatment of the survivor's cancer. During the course of treatment, cancer survivors may have one oncologist or several involved in their care.

Pharmacists

Pharmacists are health professionals who

> provide patient care that optimizes medication therapy and promotes health, wellness, and disease prevention. The practice of clinical pharmacy embraces the philosophy of pharmaceutical care; it blends a caring orientation with specialized therapeutic knowledge, experience, and judgment for the purpose of ensuring optimal patient outcomes. (American College of Clinical Pharmacy, 2018, para. 3)

The pharmacist's role on the cancer rehabilitation team is to prepare and dispense medications, including chemotherapy, to cancer survivors. They assess whether prescribed medications are meeting the patient's needs, recognize untreated conditions that could improve with medication, provide patient and caregiver education, alert the patient and physician to potential drug interactions, and consult with the physician and other team members to select medication that best meets the patient's needs. Pharmacists are educated at the doctoral level (Pharm.D) and must pass the North American Pharmacist Licensure Examination (National Association of Boards of Pharmacy, 2018).

Physiatrists

Physiatrists are physicians who specialize in physical medicine and rehabilitation. The physiatrist's role is to collaborate with and coordinate the cancer rehabilitation team to "maximize what a patient can do and assist the patient in adapting to what he or she cannot. A physiatrist should be consulted when pain, weakness, or disability is preventing a patient from achieving their desired level of independence" (American Academy of Physical Medicine and Rehabilitation, 2018, para. 1).

Physiatrists hold a graduate degree from a medical school. Most physiatrists become board certified, which indicates advanced knowledge. Board certification is required by some hospitals and health care organizations. Board certification is also available in a variety of specialties within physiatry, such as pain, palliative care, and sports medicine.

Physical Therapists and Physical Therapist Assistants

Physical therapists and *physical therapist assistants* are health professionals

> who diagnose and treat individuals of all ages, from newborns to the very oldest, who have medical problems or other health-related conditions that limit their abilities to move and perform functional activities in their daily lives.
>
> [Physical therapists] examine each individual and develop a plan using treatment techniques to promote the ability to move, reduce pain, restore function, and prevent disability. In addition, they work with individuals to prevent the loss of mobility before it occurs by developing fitness- and wellness-oriented programs for healthier and more active lifestyles. (American Physical Therapy Association, 2018, para. 1–2)

The physical therapist and physical therapist assistant's role on the cancer rehabilitation team is to promote functional movement and mobility. Physical therapists are educated at the doctoral level (since 2017), and physical therapist assistants are educated at the associate's degree level.

Social Workers

Social workers are professionals who work to enhance the well-being and help to meet the basic needs of all people, especially the most vulnerable in society (National Association of Social Workers, 2017). The social worker's role on the cancer rehabilitation team is to help patients and caregivers cope with the impact of a cancer diagnosis. Social work counselors provide counseling, advance care planning, resource linkage, and support groups, among other services. Social workers may hold a bachelor's or master's degree, depending on the level of services offered.

SUMMARY

The impact of treating cancer and the side effects on occupational performance can range from minor to severe. At their worst, the side effects can cause major disruptions to occupational performance and the ability to maintain habits, routines, and familiar roles.

Although occupational therapy practitioners do not have a role in the direct administration of treatments for cancer, they work alongside the oncologist and the rest of the cancer rehabilitation team to help cancer survivors ameliorate the negative effects and to maintain and improve their QoL. Later chapters focus on the most significant side effects and complications of cancer treatment.

REFERENCES

American Academy of Physical Medicine and Rehabilitation. (2018). *What does a physiatrist do?* Retrieved from https://www.aapmr.org/career-center/medical-students/a-medical-student%27s-guide-to-pm-r/what-does-a-physiatrist-do

American Cancer Society. (2018). *Risks of cancer surgery.* Retrieved from https://www.cancer.org/treatment/treatments-and-side-effects/treatment-types/surgery/risks-of-cancer-surgery.html

American Cancer Society. (2019). *Targeted therapy side-effects.* Retrieved from https://www.cancer.org/treatment/treatments-and-side-effects/treatment-types/targeted-therapy/side-effects.html

American Case Management Association. (2018). *What is case management?* Retrieved from https://www.acmaweb.org/section.aspx?sID=136

American College of Clinical Pharmacy. (2018). *Clinical pharmacy defined.* Retrieved from https://www.accp.com/about/clinicalPharmacyDefined.aspx

American Nurses Association. (2018). *What is nursing?* Retrieved from http://www.nursingworld.org/EspeciallyForYou/What-is-Nursing

American Nutrition Association. (2018). *Description of degrees/credentials.* Retrieved from http://americannutritionassociation.org/toolsandresources/descriptiondegreescredentials

American Occupational Therapy Association. (2015). *The role of occupational therapy in palliative and hospice care.* Retrieved from https://www.aota.org/~/media/Corporate/Files/AboutOT/Professionals/WhatIsOT/PA/Facts/FactSheet_Palliative-Care.pdf

American Occupational Therapy Association. (2019). *Resources for beginning your OT career.* Retrieved from https://www.aota.org/Education-Careers/Considering-OT-Career/Resources.aspx

American Physical Therapy Association. (2018). *Role of a physical therapist.* Retrieved from http://www.apta.org/PTCareers/RoleofaPT/

American Psychological Association. (2018). *Clinical psychology.* Retrieved from https://www.apa.org/ed/graduate/specialize/clinical

American Society of Clinical Oncology. (2018a). *Proton therapy.* Retrieved from https://www.cancer.net/navigating-cancer-care/how-cancer-treated/radiation-therapy/proton-therapy

American Society of Clinical Oncology. (2018b). *Types of oncologists.* Retrieved from https://www.cancer.net/navigating-cancer-care/cancer-basics/cancer-care-team/types-oncologists

Association of Child Life Professionals. (2018). *What is a certified child life specialist?* Retrieved from https://www.childlife.org/the-child-life-profession

Barton, M. B., Jacob, S., Shafiq, J., Wong, K., Thompson, S. R., Hanna, T. P., & Delaney, G. P. (2014). Estimating the demand for radiotherapy from the evidence: A review of changes from 2003 to 2012. *Radiotherapy Oncology, 112,* 140–144. https://doi.org/10.1016/j.radonc.2014.03.024

Cleveland Clinic. (2018). *Graft vs host disease: An overview in bone marrow transplant.* Retrieved from https://my.clevelandclinic.org/health/diseases/10255-graft-vs-host-disease-an-overview-in-bone-marrow-transplant

Cleveland Clinic. (2019). *Radiofrequency ablation.* Retrieved from https://my.clevelandclinic.org/health/treatments/17411-radiofrequency-ablation

Dana-Farber Cancer Institute. (2019). *What happens during the stem cell transplant process?* Retrieved from http://www.dana-farber.org/health-library/articles/what-happens-during-the-stem-cell-transplant-process-/

Denham, P., & Humbert, T. K. (2016). Spirituality through the lens of health care chaplaincy. In T. K. Humbert (Ed.), *Spirituality and occupational therapy: A model for practice and research* (pp. 59–75). Bethesda, MD: AOTA Press.

Explorehealthcareers.org. (2018). *Dietitian nutritionists.* Retrieved from https://explorehealthcareers.org/career/nutrition-dietetics/dietitian-nutritionist/

Gelet, A., Crouzet, S., Rovuiere, O., & Chapelon, J. Y. (2017). High-intensity focused ultrasound (HIFU) for prostate cancer. In M. Bolla & H. van Poppel (Eds.), *Management of prostate cancer: A multidisciplinary approach* (pp. 251–271). Cham, Switzerland: Springer.

Kamen, C., Tejani, M. A., Chandwani, K., Janelsins, M., Peoples, A. R., Roscoe, J. A., & Morrow, G. R. (2014). Anticipatory nausea and vomiting due to chemotherapy. *European Journal of Pharmacology, 722,* 172–179. https://doi.org/10.1016/j.ejphar.2013.09.071

Mayo Clinic. (2019). *Ablation therapy.* Retrieved from https://www.mayoclinic.org/tests-procedures/ablation-therapy/about/pac-20385072

MD Anderson Cancer Center. (2019a). *Chemotherapy.* Retrieved from https://www.mdanderson.org/treatment-options/chemotherapy.html

MD Anderson Cancer Center. (2019b). *Complimentary, alternative & integrative medicine.* Retrieved from https://www.mdanderson.org/treatment-options/complementary-and-integrative-medicine.html

MD Anderson Cancer Center. (2019c). *Immunotherapy.* Retrieved from https://www.mdanderson.org/treatment-options/immunotherapy.html

MD Anderson Cancer Center. (2019d). *Radiation therapy.* Retrieved from https://www.mdanderson.org/treatment-options/radiation-therapy.html

MD Anderson Cancer Center. (2019g). *Stem cell transplants.* Retrieved from https://www.mdanderson.org/treatment-options/stem-cell-transplantation.html

MD Anderson Cancer Center. (2019h). *Surgery.* Retrieved from https://www.mdanderson.org/treatment-options/surgery.html

MD Anderson Cancer Center. (2019i). *Targeted therapies (precision medicine).* Retrieved from https://www.mdanderson.org/treatment-options/targeted-therapy.html

Medical News Today. (2018). *Proton therapy as an option for treating cancer.* Retrieved from https://www.medicalnewstoday.com/articles/268629.php

MedicineNet.com. (2019). *Medical definition of surgery.* Retrieved from https://www.medicinenet.com/script/main/art.asp?articlekey=5603

Memorial Sloan Kettering Cancer Center. (2018). *Blood & marrow stem cell transplantation.* Retrieved from https://www.mskcc.org/cancer-care/diagnosis-treatment/cancer-treatments/blood-stem-cell-transplantation

National Association of Boards of Pharmacy. (2018). *NAPLEX.* Retrieved from https://nabp.pharmacy/programs/naplex

National Association of Social Workers. (2017). *Social work month 2017.* Retrieved from https://www.socialworkers.org/events/campaigns/social-work-month/social-work-month-2017

National Cancer Institute. (2018a). *NCI dictionary of terms: Adoptive cellular therapy.* Retrieved from https://www.cancer.gov/publications/dictionaries/cancer-terms/def/adoptive-cellular-therapy

National Cancer Institute. (2018b). *NCI dictionary of terms: Targeted therapy.* Retrieved from https://www.cancer.gov/publications/dictionaries/cancer-terms/def/targeted-therapy

National Cancer Institute. (2018c). *Radiation therapy side effects.* Retrieved from https://www.cancer.gov/about-cancer/treatment/types/radiation-therapy/side-effects

National Cancer Institute. (2018d). *Targeted cancer therapies.* Retrieved from https://www.cancer.gov/about-cancer/treatment/types/targeted-therapies/targeted-therapies-fact-sheet

National Marrow Donor Program. (2016). *GVHD signs and symptoms.* Retrieved from https://bethematch.org/patients-and-families/life-after-transplant/physical-health-and-recovery/gvhd-signs-and-symptoms/

Nurse Practitioner Schools. (2018). *What is a nurse practitioner?* Retrieved from https://www.nursepractitionerschools.com/faq/what-is-np

Pearce, A., Haas, M., Viney, R., Pearson, S. A., Haywood, P., Brown, C., & Ward, R. (2017). Incidence and severity of self-reported chemotherapy side effects in routine care: A prospective cohort study. *PloS One, 12*(10), e0184360. https://doi.org/10.1371/journal.pone.0184360

RadiologyInfo.org. (2018). *Cryotherapy.* Retrieved from https://www.radiologyinfo.org/en/info.cfm?pg=cryo

Rosenberg, S. A., & Restifo, N. P. (2015). Adoptive cell transfer as personalized immunotherapy for human cancer. *Science, 348*(6230), 62–68. https://doi.org/10.1126/science.aaa4967

Santiago, A. C. (2018). Different types and roles of nurses. *Verywell Health.* Retrieved from https://www.verywellhealth.com/what-are-the-different-types-of-nurses-1736354

Scripps. (2014). *How does pencil-beam scanning treat cancer?* Retrieved from https://www.scripps.org/news_items/4740-scripps-opens-region-s-first-proton-therapy-center-for-cancer-care/scripps-opens-region-s-first-proton-therapy-center-for-cancer-care

Society for Immunotherapy of Cancer. (2018). *Side effects.* Retrieved from http://www.sitcancer.org/clinician/resources/melanoma/side-effects

Applying the *Occupational Therapy Practice Framework* With Cancer Survivors

3

Brent Braveman, OTR, PhD, FAOTA

LEARNING OBJECTIVES

After completing this chapter, readers should be able to
- Describe the purpose of the *Occupational Therapy Practice Framework: Domain and Process,*
- Explain the application of the occupational therapy process to occupational therapy clients with cancer, and
- Identify and describe examples of occupational therapy intervention with cancer survivors across the lifespan.

KEY TERMS AND CONCEPTS

- Activity analysis
- Analysis of occupational performance
- Body functions
- Body structures
- Cancer care continuum
- Cancer survivor
- Client
- Client-centered care

- Client factors
- Context
- Domain
- Environment
- Evaluation
- Occupation
- Occupational performance
- Occupational profile

- *Occupational Therapy Practice Framework: Domain and Process*
- Participation
- Patient
- Performance patterns
- Performance skills
- Professional reasoning
- Therapeutic use of self

INTRODUCTION

An official document of the American Occupational Therapy Association (AOTA), the **Occupational Therapy Practice Framework: Domain and Process** (3rd ed.; *OTPF*; AOTA, 2014) "presents a summary of interrelated constructs that describe occupational therapy practice" that "was developed to articulate occupational therapy's contribution to promoting the health and participation of people, organizations, and populations through engagement in occupation" (p. S1). The *OTPF* can be used to conceptualize and guide occupational therapy practice alongside the use of evolving occupational therapy evidence and related knowledge.

This chapter describes applying the *OTPF* and its key concepts to occupational therapy intervention with cancer survivors. Those interested in understanding the *OTPF* more deeply should refer to the full document and supplementary resources, such as online courses on the application of the *OTPF* available from AOTA through its website (www.aota.org) and online store (store.aota.org).

HISTORY OF THE *OTPF*, USE, AND LIMITATIONS

Prior to developing the *OTPF* (also referred to as the *Framework*), AOTA (1994) relied on the *Uniform Terminology for Occupational Therapy (UT–III)* to provide "a generic outline of the domain of concern of occupational therapy" and "to create common terminology for the profession and to capture the essences of occupational therapy succinctly for others" (p. 1047). In 1999, AOTA's Commission on Practice was charged with reviewing the *UT–III;* the Commission determined that a new document was needed that would meet the original goals of *UT–III* but centralize the importance of occupation (Pendleton & Schultz-Krohn, 2018).

The first edition of the *OTPF* was published in 2002. It was then revised and updated in 2008. The third edition was published in 2014 (AOTA, 2002, 2008, 2014). The *OTPF* is a tool developed by the occupational therapy profession to

more clearly articulate and enhance the understanding of what OT [occupational therapy] practitioners do (occupational therapy domain) and how they do it (occupational therapy process). The intended beneficiaries of all three editions of the *OTPF* were as envisioned as including not only OT practitioners (an internal audience), but also the recipients of OT services (referred to as clients), other health professionals, and those providing reimbursement for OT services (an external audience). (Pendleton & Schultz-Krohn, 2018, p. 2)

The *OTPF* has become widely used as a guide for terminology use and a reference that describes the occupational therapy domain and process in various arenas, including textbooks and other publications. AOTA (2014) describes the *OTPF* as an "ever evolving document," and it is reviewed and updated every 5 years (p. S2).

Although the *OTPF* is a useful tool to structure thinking and communication about the domain and process of occupational therapy, it also has limitations. These limitations include its theoretical nature, evidence, and U.S.-based perspective:

- The *OTPF* may be considered essentially atheoretical because it pulls from a wide range of occupational therapy conceptual practice models, theories, and frames of references as well as related knowledge. AOTA (2014) states that the *OTPF* "does not serve as a taxonomy, theory, or model" (p. S3).
- The OTPF reflects both current and evolving practices that are not necessarily evidence based.
- Because the *OTPF* is written by volunteer occupational therapy practitioners of AOTA, it may not fully or accurately represent occupational therapy practice outside of the United States.

DOMAIN

Exhibit 3.1 identifies the aspects of occupational therapy's **domain,** which is the scope of influence of the profession and the area in which its members have an established body of knowledge and expertise (AOTA, 2014). "All aspects of the domain, including occupations, client factors, performance skills, performance patterns, and context and environment, are of equal value, and together they interact to affect the client's occupational identity, health, well-being, and participation in life" (AOTA, 2014, p. S4).

Providing comprehensive occupational therapy intervention with cancer survivors at any point in the lifespan and in any practice setting requires that occupational therapy practitioners consider all aspects of the domain. Although each aspect of the domain is of equal value, some aspects may have more relevance for the occupational therapy practitioner at a particular time given the specific cancer diagnosis, the survivor's occupational profile, and the specific practice setting in which the survivor is receiving intervention.

For example, a newly diagnosed client may have significant concerns about the ability to continue to work and may be more focused on IADLs related to parenting or managing the home. Alternatively, a client undergoing active treatment in an inpatient medical facility may be more focused on rest and sleep and the impact of cancer and its treatments on client factors such as body functions and body structures. Other chapters in this book focus more specifically on occupations, client factors, and other aspects of the domain. Figure 3.1 reflects the major components of the domain and their dynamic interrelationship as well as the influence of context and environment.

The terms **client,** *patient,* and *cancer survivor* may all be used to refer to a person with cancer. In this text, we often use the term *client* to emphasize the importance of client-centered care. **Client-centered care** is defined in the *OTPF* as an "approach to service that incorporates respect for and partnership with clients as active participants in the therapy process. This approach emphasizes clients' knowledge and experience, strengths, capacity for choice, and overall autonomy" (Boyt Schell et al., 2014, p. 1230, referenced in AOTA, 2014, p. S41). At times, the term **patient** may be used if specifically referencing care provided in a medical model setting, such as a hospital or outpatient center.

The term **cancer survivor** can be used to refer more generally to any person with cancer at any point in their cancer journey. We use the term widely throughout this text when referring to the provision of occupational therapy services in general. In 1986, the founders of the National Coalition for Cancer Survivorship (NCCS) sought to "replace the words 'cancer victim' with 'cancer survivor' and bring about a different notion of the cancer experience" (NCCS, 2018, para. 2). The term *survivor* is defined as "from the time of diagnosis and for the balance of life" and is used in this text to represent that view of the person with cancer (NCCS, 2018, para. 1).

EXHIBIT 3.1.   Aspects of Occupational Therapy Domain

OCCUPATIONS	CLIENT FACTORS	PERFORMANCE SKILLS	PERFORMANCE PATTERNS	CONTEXTS AND ENVIRONMENTS
ADLs*	Values, beliefs, and spirituality	Motor skills	Habits	Cultural
IADLs	Body functions	Process skills	Routines	Personal
Rest and sleep	Body structures	Social interaction skills	Rituals	Physical
Education			Roles	Social
Work				Temporal
Play				Virtual
Leisure				
Social participation				

*Also referred to as *basic activities of daily living (BADLs)* or *personal activities of daily living (PADLs).*

Note. All aspects of the domain transact to support engagement, participation, and health. This exhibit does not imply a hierarchy.

Source. From "Occupational Therapy Practice Framework: Domain and Process (3rd ed.)," by American Occupational Therapy Association, 2014, *American Journal of Occupational Therapy,* Vol. 68, Suppl. 1, p. S5. Copyright © 2014 by the American Occupational Therapy Association. Used with permission.

FIGURE 3.1 Occupational therapy's domain.

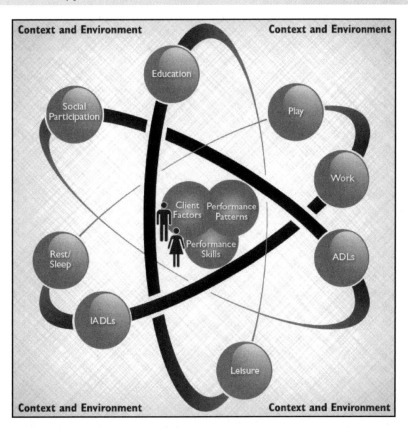

Note. ADLs = activities of daily living; IADLs = instrumental activities of daily living.
Source. From "Occupational Therapy Practice Framework: Domain and Process (3rd ed.)," by American Occupational Therapy Association, 2014, *American Journal of Occupational Therapy,* Vol. 68, Suppl. 1, p. S5. Copyright © 2014 by the American Occupational Therapy Association. Used with permission.

Occupations

Multiple definitions of the term *occupation* can be found in the occupational therapy literature, and the *OTPF* includes several. At times, the term *occupation* has been used interchangeably with the term *activity.* This text uses the term **occupation** generally to refer to the everyday important things that people want to or need to perform in the course of their daily lives. In the second edition of the *OTPF, areas of occupation* were identified and included ADLs, IADLs, rest and sleep, education, work, play, leisure, and social participation (AOTA, 2008). These areas of occupation are referred to simply as *occupations* in the third edition (AOTA, 2014).

Occupational therapy practitioners may address any or all of the occupations identified in the *OTPF* when providing occupational therapy intervention to cancer survivors. The age of the cancer survivor and their developmental stage (e.g., child, adolescent, young adult, adult, older adult) will guide the process of gathering information on how cancer and its treatments are affecting each cancer survivor as an individual.

Client Factors

Client factors are defined in the *OTPF* as "specific capacities, characteristics, or beliefs that reside within the person and that influence performance in occupations" (AOTA, 2014, p. S7).

Client factors include values, beliefs and spirituality, body functions, and body structures. **Body functions** include the physiologic functions of body systems (e.g., mental functions, sensory functions, neuromusculoskeletal and movement-related functions, cardiovascular and respiratory functions). **Body structures** are anatomical parts of the body, such as organs, limbs, and their components that support body function.

Cancer and its treatments may affect all types of client factors. Clients may perceive challenges to their values, beliefs, and spirituality as they face a life-threatening disease and their own mortality. Both cancer and its treatments may affect body functions and body structures, and the effects can vary widely from minor to major. Understanding the specific potential impact of the type and stage of cancer a particular client has and the treatments chosen to combat the cancer is critical to effectively applying the occupational therapy process. Gaining such clinical knowledge can only come with experience, and newer practitioners with limited exposure to cancer must be both diligent and patient as they learn about the various forms of cancer and the many complex treatments.

Performance Skills

Performance skills are defined in the *OTPF* as "goal-directed actions that are observable as small units of engagement in daily life occupations" (AOTA, 2014, p. S7). Performance skills include motor skills demonstrated when a person interacts with and moves objects about; process skills demonstrated when a person selects, interacts with, and uses task tools and materials and modifies performance when problems are encountered; and social interaction skills demonstrated when a person interacts with others (Boyt Schell et al., 2014). Cancer and its treatments can have negative effects on all types of performance skills, such as decreases in strength or endurance, limited range of motion, difficulty processing information, reduced cognitive capacity, and decreased social interaction as work and other social occupations are affected. Some cancer survivors may experience issues with body image and changes in appearance that can also affect social interactions.

Performance Patterns

Performance patterns are defined in the *OTPF* as "the habits, routines, roles, and rituals used in the process of engaging in occupations or activities that can support or hinder occupational performance" (AOTA, 2014, p. S8). *Habits* are automatic behaviors demonstrated in response to environmental stimuli and demands; routines are sequenced patterns of occupations that structure everyday life; *roles* are interconnected occupations that are performed to meet the expectation of society and others and can be socially identified and named (e.g., parent) or can be individually constructed and understood (e.g., appreciator of art); and *rituals* are symbolic actions with spiritual, cultural, or social meaning to an individual or group. Performance patterns support occupational performance and help individuals manage interactions with their environments.

Performance patterns are often disrupted by cancer and its treatments. Familiar routines may be replaced by new routines related to multiple medical interventions, and new habits may be required to support occupational performance. Well-established roles may be challenged as the symptoms of cancer and the side effects of treatment interfere with a survivor's capacity to perform familiar occupations. The focus of occupational therapy intervention may vary widely depending on the setting in which the practitioner is seeing the client. Unfortunately, roles such as worker or parent may receive little attention as intervention is consumed by a focus on more basic occupations such as self-care and movement and mobility.

Context and Environment

The *OTPF* states, "Engagement and participation in occupation take place within the social and physical environment situated within context" (AOTA, 2014, p. S8). Although the terms *environment* and *context* are often used interchangeably, in the *OTPF*, "both terms are used to reflect the importance of considering the wide array of interrelated variables that influence performance" (AOTA, 2014, p. S8).

The *environment* includes both the physical environment (e.g., plants, terrain, objects, buildings) and the social environment, including people, groups, and populations. *Context* refers to "elements within and surrounding a client that are often less tangible than physical and social environments but nonetheless exert a strong influence on performance. Contexts . . . are cultural, personal, temporal, and virtual" (AOTA, 2014, p. S9). Alterations in context and environment can foster improved occupational performance or have a negative effect on performance. The performance of familiar occupations may become more challenging when clients must perform in an unfamiliar environment, such as a hospital room.

Occupational Performance and Participation

Occupational performance is defined in the *OTPF* as the "act of doing and accomplishing a selected action (performance skill), activity, or occupation that results from the dynamic transaction among the client, the context, and the activity" that improves or enables skills and patterns for engagement or activities (AOTA, 2014, p. S34). Improving occupational performance is often the articulated goal of occupational therapy intervention. However, although not always explicitly identified, the ultimate goal of occupational therapy intervention is to increase or maintain participation. Participation may be thought of as a broader concept than that of occupational performance.

The *OTPF* frequently mentions **participation.** It is included as an element of the *OTPF's* definition of *occupational therapy:* "The therapeutic use of everyday life activities (occupations) with individuals or groups for the purpose of enhancing or enabling participation in roles, habits, and routines in home, school, workplace, community, and other settings" (AOTA, 2014, p. S1). However, participation is not richly defined within the *OTPF,* and the definition provided is from the World Health Organization's (2001) International Classification of Function, Disability and Health, which is, "*Participation*—involvement in a life situation" (p. 10).

Full participation is challenging for cancer survivors. There is a need for occupational therapy practitioners to help survivors of cancer maximize participation in activities that reflect their life roles and life situations because an exclusive focus on symptom management and impairment reduction may not automatically improve participation (Newman et al., 2019). Recent models of cancer rehabilitation acknowledge that participation in life situations and roles is also affected by personal factors, environmental factors, and activity demands (Campbell et al., 2012). As you read later chapters, especially those focused on impairments such as lymphedema or fatigue, you are encouraged to remember the complexity of promoting full participation beyond occupational performance.

PROCESS

Exhibit 3.2 includes the three major components of the occupational therapy process: (1) evaluation, (2) intervention, and (3) targeting of outcomes. In addition to these components, enduring elements of the occupational therapy process, such as therapeutic use of self, activity analysis, professional reasoning, and service delivery models, must be considered.

EXHIBIT 3.2.	Process of Occupational Therapy Service Delivery. The process of service delivery is applied within the profession's domain to support the client's health and participation.

Evaluation

Occupational profile—The initial step in the evaluation process, which provides an understanding of the client's occupational history and experiences, patterns of daily living, interests, values, and needs. The client's reasons for seeking services, strengths, and concerns in relation to performing occupations and daily life activities, areas of potential occupational disruption, supports and barriers, and priorities are also identified.

Analysis of occupational performance—The step in the evaluation process during which the client's assets and problems or potential problems are more specifically identified. Actual performance is often observed in context to identify supports for and barriers to the client's performance. Performance skills, performance patterns, context or environment, client factors, and activity demands are all considered, but only selected aspects may be specifically assessed. Targeted outcomes are identified.

Intervention

Intervention plan—The plan that will guide actions taken and that is developed in collaboration with the client. It is based on selected theories, frames of reference, and evidence. Outcomes to be targeted are confirmed.

Intervention implementation—Ongoing actions taken to influence and support improved client performance and participation. Interventions are directed at identified outcomes. The client's response is monitored and documented.

Intervention review—Review of the intervention plan and progress toward targeted outcomes.

Targeting of Outcomes

Outcomes—Determinants of success in reaching the desired end result of the occupational therapy process. Outcome assessment information is used to plan future actions with the client and to evaluate the service program (i.e., program evaluation).

The process of service delivery is applied within the profession's domain to support the client's health and participation.

Source. From "Occupational Therapy Practice Framework: Domain and Process (3rd ed.)," by American Occupational Therapy Association, 2014, *American Journal of Occupational Therapy*, Vol. 68, Suppl. 1, p. S10. Copyright © 2014 by the American Occupational Therapy Association. Used with permission.

Enduring Elements of the Occupational Therapy Process

Therapeutic use of self

The therapeutic use of self is a key tool in developing and managing therapeutic relationships between occupational therapy practitioners and clients with cancer; it also promotes a client-centered and collaborative approach to service delivery (AOTA, 2014). Punwar and Peloquin (2000) defined **therapeutic use of self** as a practitioner's "planned use of his or her personality, insights, perceptions, and judgments as part of the therapeutic process" (p. 285).

Providing occupational therapy intervention to cancer survivors can be emotionally taxing because clients are facing life-threatening illness and, in fact, many die from their cancer. Therapeutic use of self can help practitioners provide appropriate occupational therapy intervention while taking care of themselves and addressing their own emotional needs.

Activity analysis

Activity analysis is a process used by occupational therapy practitioners to determine the demands of an activity or occupation so it may be used therapeutically in occupational therapy intervention or so the occupation or its context can be adapted to improve the functional outcome (Wilson & Landry, 2014). Occupational therapy practitioners use activity analysis to obtain information to guide intervention planning and promote participation in occupations that are meaningful to the cancer survivor. Activity demands are specific to each occupation and can influence the meaning of the occupation for the client. Examples of activity demands include the amount and type of energy required to perform the occupation as well as the various skills required (e.g., cognitive or physical skills). Activity demands can be altered by changing the occupation itself or by using adaptive equipment to lessen or increase the demands. Examples include eliminating steps, incorporating opportunities for rest, and changing characteristics of objects such as weight, size, shape, color, and texture.

Professional reasoning

Professional reasoning (also referred to as *critical reasoning* or *clinical reasoning*) is "the process that practitioners use to plan, direct, perform, and reflect on client care" (Boyt Schell, 2014, p. 384). Professional reasoning develops over time with experience and is supplemented by the use of evidence. Occupational therapy practitioners rely on multiple forms of professional reasoning, including narrative, pragmatic, ethical, and interactive (Boyt Schell & Schell, 2018). Occupational therapy intervention with cancer survivors can be complex because of the various ways that cancer and its treatments affect individuals and their physical, cognitive, and psychosocial functioning.

Cancer care continuum and service delivery models

Rehabilitation professionals including occupational therapy practitioners commonly refer to the **cancer care continuum** to identify the stages of the cancer experience at which various interventions can be provided. The stages of the cancer care continuum include
- Primary prevention,
- Detection,
- Diagnosis,

- Treatment, and
- Survivorship.

Services are also provided as part of end-of-life care (National Cancer Institute, 2012). Examples of occupational therapy interventions at each stage of the cancer care continuum are included in Table 3.1. End-of-life care, or hospice, has been added as an additional stage of occupational therapy intervention with some cancer survivors.

People with cancer receive occupational therapy in a variety of intervention settings (e.g., intensive care, acute care, inpatient rehabilitation, skilled nursing, and long-term-care hospitals; outpatient clinics; home health care) for various lengths of time. Several of these settings are explored in more depth in Section III of this textbook, "Cancer Care Continuum and Cancer Rehabilitation." Common settings for intervention are also briefly described in Table 3.2.

Evaluation

The *OTPF* states that ***evaluation*** focuses on

finding out what a client wants and needs to do; determining what a client can do and has done; and identifying supports and barriers to health, well-being, and participation. Evaluation occurs during the initial and all subsequent interactions with a client. The type and focus of the evaluation differ depending on the practice setting. (AOTA, 2014, p. S13)

TABLE 3.1.   Examples of Occupational Therapy Interventions at Each Cancer Care Continuum Stage

STAGE OF CARE	EXAMPLE OF OCCUPATIONAL THERAPY INTERVENTION
Prevention	Lifestyle redesign, including adoption of healthy behaviors, such as incorporating a healthy diet and exercise, to prevent or decrease the chance of cancer
Early detection and screening	Patient education and strategies focused on primary and secondary prevention of functional deficits because of the cancer and its treatments
Diagnosis	Prehabilitation to prepare the cancer survivor for treatment and possible side effects. Education on cancer and work such as reasonable accommodations or strategies for managing fatigue to allow the survivor to continue to work.
Treatment	A wide variety of interventions targeting the impact of the cancer and its treatments on occupational performance such as fatigue, cognition, body image, ADLs, IADLs, mobility, symptom management, medication management, and fall reduction
Survivorship	Lifestyle redesign to incorporate occupations focused on preventing the recurrence of cancer and to minimize the impact of cancer and its treatments once curative treatment is stopped
End-of-life care	Assisting the dying person to achieve goals such as the creation of legacy documents or recordings for family and friends, planning burial ceremonies, and continuing to perform enjoyed occupations as the person is able

Note. ADLs = activities of daily living; IADLs = instrumental activities of daily living.

Table 3.2   Common Settings for Cancer Care

SETTING	DESCRIPTION
Physician offices/Physician-owned practices	Care provided by general practitioners, primary care providers, or oncologic specialists in private offices or group practices
Acute care	Small community-based hospitals to large research and treatment hospitals. Includes intensive care unit for critical care. Care is focused on immediate medical needs or interventions such as surgery. Lengths of stay are typically short (2–5 days). Cancer survivors may have multiple acute care admissions because their cancer care may extend over years.
Inpatient rehabilitation (IRFs)	Intensive rehabilitation of 3 hours or more, including occupational therapy, physical therapy, speech therapy, and other services. Lengths of stay typically vary from 7 to 14 days.
Post-acute care (LTAC, SNF)	Care for cancer survivors who are not yet ready to return home and do not qualify for or are unable to tolerate intensive acute rehabilitation
Home health care	Nursing and rehabilitative care provided in the cancer survivor's home. Home health care is often provided when the patient is too ill to frequently leave the home for outpatient treatment.
Hospice	Compassionate care for people facing a life-limiting illness or injury, hospice care involves a team-oriented approach to expert medical care, pain management, and emotional and spiritual support expressly tailored to the cancer survivor's needs and wishes when the survivor decides to end efforts at curative care

Note. IRF = inpatient rehabilitation facility; LTAC = long-term acute care hospital; SNF = skilled nursing facility.

The evaluation includes developing the occupational profile and analyzing occupational performance.

Occupational profile

The ***occupational profile*** is "a summary of a client's occupational history and experiences, patterns of daily living, interests, values, and needs" (AOTA, 2014, p. S13). It is central to a client-centered approach to occupational therapy intervention (AOTA, 2017). A comprehensive occupational profile provides a clear understanding of the client's perspective including the following:

- Why is the client seeking occupational therapy services?
- What concerns does the client have regarding occupational performance and performance of rituals, routines, and roles?
- What does the client value?
- What are the client's interests?
- What are the client's priorities and goals for occupational therapy intervention and targeted outcomes?
- How can you improve the client's quality of life, well-being, and health and wellness?

Analysis of occupational performance

Through ***analysis of occupational performance,*** occupational therapy practitioners can learn about a client's strengths and limitations. This is accomplished through the use of assessment tools chosen specifically for the client's situation and the factors that may be promoting or limiting occupational performance. At this point in the process, the practitioner begins to collaborate with the client to identify targeted outcomes. According to the *OTPF* (AOTA, 2014), the following strategies can be used to assess occupational performance:

- "Synthesizing information from the occupational profile to focus on specific occupations and contexts that need to be addressed
- "Observing a client's performance during activities relevant to desired occupations, noting effectiveness of performance skills and performance patterns
- "Selecting and using specific assessments to measure performance skills and performance patterns, as appropriate
- "Selecting and administering assessments, as needed, to identify and measure more specifically the contexts or environments, activity demands, and client factors that influence performance skills and performance patterns
- "Selecting outcome measures
- "Interpreting the assessment data to identify supports and hindrances to performance
- "Developing and refining hypotheses about the client's occupational performance strengths and limitations
- "Creating goals in collaboration with the client that address the desired outcomes
- "Determining procedures to measure the outcomes of intervention
- "Delineating a potential intervention approach or approaches based on best practices and available evidence" (p. S14).

A variety of approaches may be used to measure and gather data from the client and members of their support network. Examples include structured and nonstructured interviews and standardized criterion or norm-referenced assessment tools. Table 3.3 includes a nonexhaustive list

Table 3.3   Selected Assessments Commonly Used With Cancer Survivors

ASPECT OF THE DOMAIN OF OT	CATEGORIES WITHIN EACH ASPECT	EXAMPLES OF ASSESSMENTS USED IN OT PRACTICE	BRIEF DESCRIPTION OF ASSESSMENT
Areas of occupation	ADLs IADLs Rest and sleep Education Work Leisure Social participation	Activity Card Sort (Baum & Edwards, 2008)	Flexible and useful measure of occupation that helps clients describe their IADLs
		Activity Measure for Post-Acute Care Short Forms for Inpatient and Outpatient Settings (Jette et al., 2015)	Activity limitations instrument that examines functional activities most adults are likely to encounter during daily routines
		Child and Adolescent Scale of Participation (Bedell, 2008)	Measures the extent to which children participate in home, school, and community activities compared with children of the same age, as reported by family caregivers.
		FIM (Uniform Data System for Medical Rehabilitation, 2016)	Rating tool for functional performance in self-care, sphincter control, transfers, locomotion, communication, and social cognition
		Instrumental Activities of Daily Living Scale (Lawton & Brody, 1969)	Tool to assess IADLs necessary for functioning in community settings (e.g., shopping, cooking, finances)

(Continued)

Table 3.3 Selected Assessments Commonly Used With Cancer Survivors *(Cont.)*

ASPECT OF THE DOMAIN OF OT	CATEGORIES WITHIN EACH ASPECT	EXAMPLES OF ASSESSMENTS USED IN OT PRACTICE	BRIEF DESCRIPTION OF ASSESSMENT
		Katz Index of Independence in Activities of Daily Living (Katz et al., 1963)	Graded assessment of bathing, dressing, toileting, transfers, feeding, and continence
		Kohlman Evaluation of Living Skills (Kohlman-Thomson & Robnett, 2016)	Assessment of ability to function in basic living skills
		Physical Self-Maintenance Scale (Lawton & Brody, 1969)	Tool to gauge disability in older adults in a community or institution for use in assessment and treatment planning; items target observable behaviors
		Test of Grocery Shopping Skills (Brown et al., 2009)	Performance-based measure of how accurately and efficiently clients can locate items in a grocery store
		Worker Role Interview (Braveman et al., 2005)	Assessment of the psychosocial variables that predict return to work
Performance skills	Motor skills	Brief Fatigue Inventory (Mendoza et al., 1999)	Short assessment of the severity of fatigue experienced over the past 24 hours and its impact on function
	Motor skills	Peabody Developmental Motor Scales, Second Edition (Folio & Fewell, 2000)	Assesses reflexes, stationary, locomotion, object manipulation, grasping, and visual–motor integration
	Balance and functional mobility	Lower Extremity Functional Scale (Binkley et al., 1999)	Questionnaire assessing a person's ability to perform everyday tasks that can be used to measure clients' initial function, ongoing progress, and outcomes and to set functional goals
	Process skills (e.g., attends, initiates, uses, sequences, organizes, searches/locates, navigates, adjusts)	Assessment of Motor and Process Skills (Fisher & Jones, 2012)	Measure of the quality of a person's performance of functional tasks assessed by rating the effort, efficiency, safety, and independence of motor and process skills
	Social interaction skills (e.g., produces speech, speaks fluently, questions, replies, expresses emotion)	Assessment of Communication and Interactions Skills (Forsyth et al., 1998)	Observational assessment that gathers data on communication and interaction skills in 3 domains: physicality, information exchange, and relationships
	Visual motor skills	Beery Buktenica Developmental Test of Visual Motor Integration (Beery et al., 2010)	Screen for visual–motor deficits with norms for ages 2–18 and 19 and above

(Continued)

Table 3.3 Selected Assessments Commonly Used With Cancer Survivors *(Cont.)*

ASPECT OF THE DOMAIN OF OT	CATEGORIES WITHIN EACH ASPECT	EXAMPLES OF ASSESSMENTS USED IN OT PRACTICE	BRIEF DESCRIPTION OF ASSESSMENT
Performance patterns	Habits, routines, rituals, roles	Canadian Occupational Performance Measure (Law et al., 2019)	Client-centered tool to enable clients to identify and prioritize everyday issues that restrict or affect their performance in everyday living
		Occupational Circumstances Assessment Interview and Rating Scale (Forsyth et al., 2005)	Tool that provides a structure for gathering, analyzing, and reporting the extent and nature of a client's occupational participation
		Occupational Performance History Interview (Kielhofner et al., 2004)	Semistructured interview that explores a client's life history in the areas of work, play, and self-care
		Model of Human Occupation Screening Tool (Parkinson et al., 2006)	Screening assessment that addresses the majority of Model of Human Occupation concepts (volition, habituation, skills, and environment), yielding an overview of the client's occupational functioning
Context and environments	Cultural, personal, temporal, and virtual contexts and physical and social environments influencing performance	Work Environment Impact Scale (Moore-Corner et al., 1998)	Semistructured interview and rating scale that assesses how clients with physical or psychosocial disabilities experience and perceive their work environments
Client factors	Body functions Mental functions (e.g., attention, memory, higher-level cognition, perception)	A–ONE (Árnadóttir, 2011)	Cognitive assessment that directly links functional performance (ADLs and mobility) to neurobehavioral deficits, including cognitive–perceptual and motor impairments, in clients with damage to the central nervous system
		Children's Kitchen Task Assessment (Rocke et al., 2008)	Assesses EF in children ages 8–12 years through the novel task of making play dough
		Executive Function Performance Test (Baum et al., 2008)	Performance-based standardized assessment of cognitive function
		Kettle Test (Hartman-Maeir et al., 2009)	Performance-based assessment of cognitive functional performance
		Multiple Errands Test–Revised (Morrison et al., 2013)	Tool that evaluates the effect of EF deficits on everyday functioning through a number of real-world tasks
		Montreal Cognitive Assessment (Nasreddine et al., 2005)	Brief screening tool for mild cognitive impairment
		Test of Everyday Attention (Robertson et al., 1994)	Measure of selective attention, sustained attention, and attentional switching

(Continued)

Table 3.3   Selected Assessments Commonly Used With Cancer Survivors *(Cont.)*

ASPECT OF THE DOMAIN OF OT	CATEGORIES WITHIN EACH ASPECT	EXAMPLES OF ASSESSMENTS USED IN OT PRACTICE	BRIEF DESCRIPTION OF ASSESSMENT
		Rivermead Behavioral Memory Test (Clare et al., 2008)	Assessment of visual, verbal, recall, recognition, immediate, and delayed everyday memory
		Weekly Calendar Planning Activity (Toglia, 2015)	Screening tool for EF, higher-level cognitive ADLs, and the underlying nature of performance problems
	Sensory functions	Pain visual analog scales	Visual or spoken scales for rating pain (e.g., 0 = *no pain* to 10 = *worst pain imaginable,* Wong–Baker FACES Scale that uses pictures to express *no hurt* to *worst hurt*)
	Sensory functions	The Pediatric-Modified Total Neuropathy Score (Gilchrist & Tanner, 2013)	Pediatric modified scale to measure chemotherapy-induced peripheral neuropathy in school-age children
	Respiratory system function	UCSD Shortness of Breath Questionnaire (Eakin et al., 1998)	Assessment of shortness of breath during ADLs
	Control of voluntary movement (e.g., gross and fine motor control, eye–hand coordination, oral–motor control, oculomotor control)	Disabilities of the Arm, Shoulder and Hand (Gummesson et al., 2003)	Self-report questionnaire to measure physical function and symptoms in clients with musculoskeletal disorders of the upper limb
		Manual Ability Measure (Chen & Bode, 2010)	Occupation-based assessment of manual ability
Outcomes	Quality of life	Functional Assessment of Cancer Therapy (Cella et al., 1993)	General assessment of quality of life for clients with cancer
		Functional Assessment of Chronic Illness Therapy (Webster et al., 2003)	Collection of health-related quality of life questionnaires targeted to the management of chronic illness
		Patient-Reported Outcomes Measurement Information System (Cella et al., 2007)	System of measures of client-reported physical, mental, and social well-being
		Pediatric Quality of Life Inventory Multidimensional Fatigue Scale (PedsQL Multidimensional Fatigue Scale; Varni et al., 2002)	Designed as a generic symptom-specific instrument to measure fatigue in patients with acute and chronic health conditions as well as healthy school and community populations
		Pediatric Quality of Life Inventory (PedsQL) Generic Core Scales (Varni et al., 2002)	23-item scale designed to measure the core dimensions of health and role functioning

Note. ADLs = activities of daily living; EF = executive functioning; IADLs = instrumental activities of daily living; OT = occupational therapy; UCSD = University of California, San Diego.

Source. Adapted from *Occupational Therapy Practice Guidelines for Cancer Rehabilitation With Adults* by B. Braveman & E. G. Hunter, 2017, p. 13. Bethesda, MD: AOTA Press. Copyright © 2017 by the American Occupational Therapy Association. Used with permission.

of assessments commonly used with cancer survivors to evaluate occupational performance. Many later chapters in this text include references to multiple assessments that can be used with clients at various points across the lifespan to measure various elements of occupational performance.

Intervention

Occupational therapy intervention with cancer survivors is focused on counteracting the negative effects of cancer and its treatments on occupational performance. The *OTPF* describes various approaches to intervention that may be used. These approaches include: (1) create and promote, (2) prevent, (3) establish and restore, (4) modify, and (5) maintain. Table 3.4 includes examples of each of these types of occupational therapy intervention related to the common problem of cancer-related fatigue.

Intervention plan

The intervention plan includes goals focused on the client's current and potential capacity and desire to perform occupations and considers the potential discharge setting and context. The type of cancer, the stage of the cancer care continuum that the client is in, and the treatment the client is undergoing will heavily influence the occupational therapy intervention plan. Evidence-based strategies to reach these goals are chosen based on the occupational therapy practitioner's knowledge and in collaboration with the client. According to the *OTPF,* the plan includes

- "Objective and measurable occupation-focused goals and related time frames;
- "The occupational therapy intervention approach or approaches, such as create or promote, establish or restore, maintain, modify, and prevent; and
- "Methods for service delivery, including who will provide the intervention, types of interventions, and service delivery models to be used" (AOTA, 2014, p. S15).

Intervention implementation

Intervention implementation is the process of carrying out the implementation plan. Occupational therapy interventions can include:

- The therapeutic use of occupations related to the goals established in collaboration with the client and considering the context and demands of the occupation.
- Preparatory methods and preparatory tasks to prepare the client for participation in occupation. Examples include the use of modalities, splinting, use of assistive technology, and components of occupations that challenge the client in specific ways and simulate occupation but that may not hold inherent meaning.
- Education and training. Education is the "imparting of knowledge and information about occupation, health,

well-being, and participation that enables the client to acquire helpful behaviors, habits, and routines that may or may not require application at the time of the intervention session" (AOTA, 2014, p. S30). Training is "the facilitation of the acquisition of concrete skills for meeting specific goals in a real-life applied situation. In this case, skills refer to measurable components of function that enable mastery" (AOTA, 2014, p. S30).

- Advocacy by the practitioner and self-advocacy by the client supported by the practitioner.
- Group interventions with a variety of foci to promote successful occupational performance.

Intervention implementation also includes monitoring a client's response to specific interventions on the basis of ongoing evaluation and reevaluation of their progress toward goals.

Intervention review

Intervention review is the continuous process of reevaluating and reviewing the effectiveness of the intervention plan and determining if adequate progress is being made toward achieving the targeted outcomes. If adequate progress is not being made, the practitioner must make adjustments to the plan in collaboration with the client.

The intervention review includes the following steps (AOTA, 2014):

1. "Reevaluating the plan and how it is implemented relative to achieving outcomes
2. "Modifying the plan as needed
3. "Determining the need for continuation or discontinuation of occupational therapy services and for referral to other services" (p. S16).

Targeting of Outcomes

Outcomes are the direct result of occupational therapy intervention and can be driven by the intervention. According to AOTA (2014, p. S16), "outcomes may also be traced to the improved transactional relationship among the areas of the domain that result in clients' ability to engage in desired occupations secondary to improved abilities at the client factor and performance skill level." Outcomes may be objective, or

Table 3.4 Examples of Occupational Therapy Interventions for Cancer-Related Fatigue

OT INTERVENTION APPROACH	EXAMPLE
Create and promote	Create educational materials to guide patients in management of cancer-related fatigue or cognitive impairment.
Prevent	Screen for early signs of lymphedema and instruct patients and family members in prevention strategies and wrapping techniques.
Establish and restore	Examine daily routines and establish habits and patterns that incorporate rest and exercise to minimize cancer-related fatigue.
Modify	Simplify ADL and IADL tasks and add cueing strategies to compensate for cancer-related cognitive impairment such as impaired short-term memory and lowered attention span.
Maintain	Identify occupations and roles important to the patient and prioritize involvement in meaningful occupations that will allow the patient to continue role fulfillment. Use lifestyle redesign approaches to maintain strength, endurance, and mobility during and after treatment.

Note. ADL = activity of daily living; IADL = instrumental activity of daily living; OT = occupational therapy.

Table 3.5 Case Study: Occupational Therapy Process Applied to a 55-Year-Old Woman With Breast Cancer

COMPONENT	ACTIVITIES
Evaluation	
Occupational profile	■ **Ellen,** a woman age 55, was diagnosed with invasive cancer of the right breast after finding a lump on a routine mammogram. ■ Oncological treatment included chemotherapy, modified radical mastectomy, sentinel lymph node biopsy, breast tissue reconstruction, and radiation therapy targeting the right axilla and chest wall, 5 days a week for 4 weeks. The biopsy revealed Stage III breast cancer. ■ Two days after surgery, Ellen developed an infection requiring a prolonged hospital stay to manage the infection and prepare her for radiation simulation. A referral for occupational therapy services was received in the acute care setting 2 days post-operatively. ■ The occupational profile was developed using the COPM (Law et al., 2019). Ellen lived in a two-story townhouse in an urban area. She was married and had two children, ages 25 and 27. She was employed full-time as a lawyer. Ellen's prior level of function was independent with all ADLs and IADLs, including home management, meal preparation, and medication management. Ellen typically took public transportation (bus or subway) to work. Leisure occupations included reading, listening to music, walking, knitting, and playing golf.
Analysis of occupational performance	■ Evaluation consisted of clinical observation of Ellen in the hospital room, transition from supine to sitting, and quality of right and left upper-extremity movement in a functional context. ■ The Quick DASH (Gummesson et al., 2003) was used to identify the impact of Ellen's upper-extremity symptoms on her physical function and activity participation. ■ A structured interview using the OPHI–II (Kielhofner et al., 2004) was completed to identify and understand Ellen's occupational roles. ■ ADL and IADL performance was assessed using the Katz ADL Index (Katz et al., 1963) and the Lawton IADL Scale (Lawton & Brody, 1969), with a specific focus on Ellen's ability to complete self-care tasks and work-related responsibilities while undergoing cancer treatment. ■ Fatigue levels were affecting Ellen's daily activity participation and relationship with her husband and children. ■ Fatigue was measured using the FACIT–F (Webster et al., 2003) and the BFI (Mendoza et al., 1999). ■ ROM of bilateral shoulder joints in all planes was measured using goniometry. ■ Measurements of the operated side vs. the contralateral side were compared. ■ Circumferential measurements of the upper arm, elbow, wrist, and MCP joint of the right arm were taken to monitor edema over time. ■ Clinical observations were noted about Ellen's right upper-extremity tissue texture (i.e., pitting vs. nonpitting; normal, soft, or hard tissue), skin integrity, and skin temperature.
Intervention	
Intervention plan	■ Occupational therapy services were provided 4 days a week for 1.5 weeks while Ellen was in the hospital. ■ Radiation simulation was performed to configure the radiation machine for Ellen's individual treatment settings. She was required to remain supine with her right shoulder externally rotated and abducted for approximately 45 minutes. Ellen demonstrated limited right shoulder flexibility and limited tolerance for maintaining her arm in the required position. ■ Fatigue limited Ellen's ability to complete daily activities, and she was concerned about the possibility of developing subclinical lymphedema in the right arm.
Intervention implementation	■ Occupation-based intervention was focused on improving Ellen's occupational performance in everyday activities that support leisure activity, reengagement, return to work, and resumption of meaningful occupational roles. ■ Ellen prioritized specific activities to be incorporated into treatment sessions to increase her occupational engagement, including dressing, knitting, and vocational tasks (e.g., computer setup and use). ■ Fatigue management included activity modification and education, use of a journal to monitor activity patterns throughout the day or week, incorporation of stress management and mindfulness techniques into Ellen's daily routine, and an exercise program (e.g., daily walking or yoga) to improve occupational performance and engagement (Jacobsen et al., 2007; Kuchinski et al., 2009). ■ Symptom management included incorporation of therapeutic exercises to maintain and improve upper-extremity flexibility, strength, and coordination; education and instruction about energy conservation techniques and body mechanics principles so Ellen could be successful with ADLs, IADLs, and work-related activities (e.g., sitting at a computer for lengthy periods, typing emails and legal documents, attending meetings, carrying large and heavy files to and from the courthouse); and training in stress management and relaxation techniques to successfully manage pain, fatigue, distress, and other side effects associated with cancer treatment (Cramer et al., 2012). ■ Lymphedema education was provided to increase Ellen's understanding of the risks and precautions associated with lymphedema, and instruction was provided on how to incorporate good skin care and general self-care principles into her daily routine (Chan et al., 2010; Oremus et al., 2012).

(Continued)

Table 3.5   Case Study: Occupational Therapy Process Applied to a 55-Year-Old Woman With Breast Cancer *(Cont.)*

COMPONENT	ACTIVITIES
Intervention review	<ul><li>The intervention plan was reviewed 1.5 weeks before discharge to assess Ellen's progress and remaining limitations.</li><li>Ellen improved in the following ways:<ul><li>Dressed and showered with modified independence;</li><li>Independently used energy conservation techniques and coping skills to manage fatigue throughout the day;</li><li>Independently performed general shoulder AROM exercises and activities to improve flexibility and decrease muscle tightness with ADL performance; and</li><li>Independently maintained good skin care and gentle self-massage to improve lymphatic flow.</li></ul></li><li>Ellen's progress was limited by fatigue, complicated medical status, and development of a new infection. Additional healing time was required after surgery to regain full functional right shoulder AROM.</li><li>The intervention plan was revised to recommend continuation of occupational therapy services with an outpatient occupational therapist. Ellen's primary medical oncologist provided a referral.</li></ul>
	Targeting of Outcomes
Outcomes	<ul><li>The intervention plan was reviewed at hospital discharge.</li><li>The Katz ADL Index was readministered, showing that Ellen demonstrated full independence with ADLs.</li><li>The Lawton IADL Scale was readministered, showing that Ellen continued to require assistance with meal preparation and laundry tasks.</li><li>The BFI was readministered, and Ellen continued to report that fatigue affected daily activity participation.</li><li>The occupational therapist made the following recommendations:<ul><li>Client to continue to incorporate energy conservation techniques and stress management strategies in her home environment and daily routines.</li><li>Client to complete home exercise program daily to further improve right shoulder and upper-extremity function in daily occupations.</li><li>Client to follow up with outpatient occupational therapy evaluation and continuation of occupational therapy services as an outpatient.</li></ul></li></ul>

Note. ADLs = activities of daily living; AROM = active range of motion; BFI = Brief Fatigue Inventory; COPM = Canadian Occupational Performance Measure; DASH = Disabilities of the Shoulder, Arm and Hand; FACIT–F = Functional Assessment of Chronic Illness Therapy–Fatigue; IADLs = instrumental activities of daily living; MCP = metacarpophalangeal; OPHI–II = Occupational Performance History Interview–II; ROM = range of motion.
Source. Adapted from *Occupational Therapy Practice Guidelines for Cancer Rehabilitation With Adults* by B. Braveman & E. G. Hunter, 2017, p. 20. Bethesda, MD: AOTA Press. Copyright © 2017 by the American Occupational Therapy Association. Used with permission.

Table 3.6   Case Study: Occupational Therapy Process Applied to a 13-Year-Old Girl With Osteosarcoma

Evaluation	Occupational profile	<ul><li>**Alicia** is a 13-year-old adolescent girl diagnosed with osteosarcoma in the left hemipelvis.</li><li>A referral for occupational therapy services was received postsurgery (left external hemipelvectomy and partial sacrectomy).</li><li>Oncologic medical treatment had included chemotherapy and 6 weeks of radiation therapy treatments (5 days per week) prior to resection.</li><li>Alicia lived in a suburban one-story home with a walk-in shower and three steps to enter the home. Her family consisted of her mother, father, and two siblings, ages 8 and 3.</li><li>She attended a public school but as behind academically because of extended absences.</li><li>Prior level of function was independent with all age-appropriate BADLs and IADLs.</li><li>Leisure occupations included shopping, hanging out with her friends and siblings, and participating in gymnastics.</li><li>The occupational profile as developed using the Canadian Occupational Performance Measure (Law et al., 2019) and interview.</li></ul>
	Analysis of occupational performance	<ul><li>Evaluation consisted of clinical observation of Alicia in the pediatric intensive care unit for evaluation for early mobilization.</li><li>The initial interview as conducted with Alicia and her parents, who provided information about roles and routines.</li><li>Alicia was observed on a low-air loss hospital bed, which limited her mobility.</li><li>The Short Child Occupational Profile (SCOPE; Bowyer et al., 2005) provided information on the effects of volition, habituation, and the environment on occupational performance.</li><li>ROM, MMT, and sensation (via monofilament) were assessed.</li><li>Pain was assessed, and Alicia reported her pain level at 3 out of 10 located at the incision site at the lower back.</li></ul>

(Continued)

Table 3.6   Case Study: Occupational Therapy Process Applied to a 13-Year-Old Girl With Osteosarcoma *(Cont.)*

Intervention	Intervention plan	▪ Occupational therapy services were provided 5 times weekly for 4 weeks. ▪ Bed rest continued for 2–3 days when early mobilization and out-of-bed activity was approved, allowing for additional evaluation. ▪ Goals developed for the inpatient hospitalization included ADLs, functional mobility including transfers and wheelchair, ostomy care, and body image.
	Intervention implementation	▪ Occupation-based intervention focused on improving occupational performance in self-care, including bowel and bladder management, bathing, hygiene and proper skin care, ostomy care, care of skin flap, and functional mobility. ▪ Graded body image activities included observation of the incision, coping strategies for addressing emotions, exposure to social situations (e.g., going to the cafeteria for a snack), explaining what happened, and describing her new body to family and friends (developing a short story and a long story of her illness). ▪ Skin care education included education and instruction to increase understanding of the risks and precautions to promote flap viability.

	Intervention review	• Intervention plan was reviewed after 2 weeks at the 10th session via formal reevaluation.
		• Alicia had demonstrated improvements with
		  • Ostomy care with minimal assistance,
		  • Sponge bathing in the hospital bed with minimal assistance,
		  • LE dressing with moderate assistance using adaptive equipment (supervision with UE dressing),
		  • Grooming with supervision for safety at the sink,
		  • Transferring from bed to chair with minimal assistance, and
		  • Comfort with presenting herself in social situations (e.g., going to the hospital hair salon to have her hair washed).
		• Progress was limited by
		  • Increased pain with removal of the epidural (she reported 6 out of 10) at incision site,
		  • Lowered activity tolerance with fatigue upon exertion, and
		  • Significant hesitation to interact with friends in person or via social media.
		• The intervention plan was revised to increase the focus on family training and education, home assessment including adaptations (e.g., a ramp), durable medical equipment for bathing, and a reclining wheelchair and pressure-relieving air cushion.

Targeting of outcomes	Outcomes	• The intervention plan was reviewed at time of hospital discharge.
		• Self-care and functional mobility were reassessed in the hospital room and in public areas. Alicia achieved her goals for self-care and community mobility at the hospital level.
		• Progress with acceptance of body changes as assessed through observation and self-report. Alicia became gradually more comfortable in public and initiated contact with friends and her social network via social media.
		• The occupational therapist made the following recommendations:
		  • Client to continue with outpatient occupational therapy for more advanced self-care, continued client and family education and IADLs, and return to school.
		  • Client to be assessed for powered mobility.
		  • Client to follow precautions during community mobility, transfers, and ADLs/IADLs.
		  • Client to begin exploration of leisure activities.
		  • Client to continue to address body image.

Note. ADLs = activities of daily living; BADLs = basic activities of daily living; IADLs = instrumental activities of daily living; LE = lower extremity; MMT = manual muscle testing; ROM = range of motion; UE = upper extremity.

Acknowledgment given to Asfia Mohammed for contribution to this case example.

they can be subjective and related to the client or caregiver's perception of the impact of intervention. Effectively targeting outcomes requires that the desired outcomes be identified at initiation of intervention and that the mode of measurement of each outcome be clearly defined. The use of psychometrically valid tools consistent with the focus of intervention can facilitate the process of targeting and measuring outcomes.

CASE EXAMPLES

Table 3.5 is presented as a case study of the occupational therapy process with a 55-year-old woman with breast cancer. Table 3.6 is presented as a case study of the occupational therapy process with a 13-year-old girl with osteosarcoma.

SUMMARY

The third edition of the *Occupational Therapy Practice Framework: Domain and Process* can be applied to all clients, including cancer survivors. Key concepts of both the occupational therapy domain and process are important considerations when establishing occupational therapy interventions and goals. The impact of cancer and its treatments on occupational performance, client factors, performance skills, performance patterns, and contexts and environments can be addressed by occupational therapy as part of the cancer team. The wide variation in impact based on the type of cancer each client has, its stage, and the treatments the client is receiving dictate the type of occupational therapy interventions provide. Many components of the *OTPF* are explored in more depth in later chapters.

REFERENCES

American Occupational Therapy Association. (1994). Uniform terminology for occupational therapy—Third Edition. *American Journal of Occupational Therapy, 48,* 1047–1054. https://doi.org/10.5014/ajot.48.11.1047

American Occupational Therapy Association. (2002). Occupational therapy practice framework: Domain and process. *American Journal of Occupational Therapy, 56,* 609–639. https://doi.org/10.5014/ajot.56.6.609

American Occupational Therapy Association. (2008). Occupational therapy practice framework: Domain and process (2nd ed.). *American Journal of Occupational Therapy, 62,* 625–683. https://doi.org/10.5014/ajot.62.6.625

American Occupational Therapy Association. (2014). Occupational therapy practice framework: Domain and process (3rd ed.). *American Journal of Occupational Therapy, 68*(Suppl. 1), S1–S48. https://doi.org/10.5014/ajot.2014.682006

American Occupational Therapy Association. (2017). AOTA occupational profile template. *American Journal of Occupational Therapy, 71,* 7112420030. https://doi.org/10.5014/ajot.2017.716S12

Árnadóttir, G. (2011). Impact of neurobehavioral deficits on activities of daily living. In G. Gillen (Ed.), *Stroke rehabilitation: A function-based approach* (3rd ed., pp. 456–500). St. Louis: Mosby.

Baum, C. M., Connor, L. T., Morrison, T., Hahn, M., Dromerick, A. W., & Edwards, D. F. (2008). Reliability, validity, and clinical utility of the Executive Function Performance Test: A measure of executive function in a sample of people with stroke. *American Journal of Occupational Therapy, 62,* 446–455. https://doi.org/10.5014/ajot.62.4.446

Baum, C., & Edwards, D. (2008). *Activity Card Sort* (2nd ed., ACS). Bethesda, MD: AOTA Press.

Bedell, G. (2008). The Child and Adolescent Scale of Participation (CASP): Further psychometric testing. *Journal of Head Trauma Rehabilitation, 23,* 341. https://doi.org/10.1097/01.HTR.0000336850.29574.7a

Beery, K. E., Buktenica, N. A., Beery, N. A., & Keith, E. (2010). *Developmental Test of Visual-Motor Integration* (6th ed.). Minneapolis, MN: NSC Pearson.

Binkley, J. M., Stratford, P. W., Lott, S. A., Riddle, D. L., & North American Orthopaedic Rehabilitation Research Network. (1999). The Lower Extremity Functional Scale (LEFS): Scale development, measurement properties, and clinical application. *Physical Therapy, 79*(4), 371–383.

Bowyer, P. L., Kramer, J., Kielhofner, G., Ploszaj, A., Ross, M., Schwartz, O., & Kramer, K. (2005). *A user's manual for the Short Child Occupational Profile (SCOPE)*. Chicago: Model of Human Occupation Clearinghouse, Department of Occupational Therapy, College of Applied Health Sciences, University of Illinois at Chicago.

Boyt Schell, B. A. (2014). Professional reasoning in practice. In B. A. Boyt Schell, G. Gillen, & M. Scaffa (Eds.), *Willard and Spackman's occupational therapy* (12th ed., pp. 384–397). Philadelphia: Lippincott Williams & Wilkins.

Boyt Schell, B. A., Gillen, G., & Scaffa, M. (2014). Glossary. In B. A. Boyt Schell, G. Gillen, & M. Scaffa (Eds.), *Willard and Spackman's occupational therapy* (12th ed., pp. 1229–1243). Philadelphia: Lippincott Williams & Wilkins.

Boyt Schell, B. A., & Schell, J. W. (2018). *Clinical and professional reasoning in occupational therapy* (2nd ed.). Philadelphia: Wolters Kluwer Health/Lippincott Williams & Wilkins.

Braveman, B., & Hunter, E. G. (2017). *Occupational therapy practice guidelines for cancer rehabilitation with adults*. Bethesda, MD: AOTA Press.

Braveman, B., Robson, M., Velozo, C., Kielhofner, G., Fisher, G., Forsyth, K., & Kerschbaum, J. (2005). *Worker Role Interview (WRI) (Version 10.0)*. Chicago: Model of Human Occupation Clearinghouse, Department of Occupational Therapy, College of Applied Health Sciences, University of Illinois at Chicago.

Brown, C., Rempfer, M., & Hamera, E. (2009). *The Test of Grocery Shopping Skills*. Bethesda, MD: AOTA Press.

Campbell, K. L., Pusic, A. L., Zucker, D. S., McNeely, M. L., Binkley, J. M., Cheville, A. L., & Harwood, K. J. (2012). A prospective model of care for breast cancer rehabilitation: Function. *Cancer, 118*(S8), 2300–2311. https://doi.org/10.1002/cncr.27464

Cella, D. F., Tulsky, D. S., Gray, G., Sarafian, B., Linn, E., Bonomi, A., . . . Eckberg, K. (1993). The Functional Assessment of Cancer Therapy scale: Development and validation of the general measure. *Journal of Clinical Oncology, 11,* 570–579. https://doi.org/10.1200/JCO.1993.11.3.570

Cella, D., Yount, S., Rothrock, N., Gershon, R., Cook, K., Reeve, B., . . . Rose, M.; PROMIS Cooperative Group. (2007). The Patient-Reported Outcomes Measurement Information System (PROMIS): Progress of an NIH Roadmap cooperative group during its first two years. *Medical Care, 45*(Suppl. 1), S3–S11. https://doi.org/10.1097/01.mlr.0000258615.42478.55

Chan, D. N. S., Lui, L. Y. Y., & So, W. K. W. (2010). Effectiveness of exercise programmes on shoulder mobility and lymphoedema after axillary lymph node dissection for breast cancer: Systematic review. *Journal of Advanced Nursing, 66,* 1902–1914. https://doi.org/10.1111/j.1365-2648.2010.05374.x

Chen, C. C., & Bode, R. K. (2010). Psychometric validation of the Manual Ability Measure–36 (MAM–36) in patients with neurologic and musculoskeletal disorders. *Archives of Physical Medicine and Rehabilitation, 91,* 414–420. https://doi.org/10.1016/j.apmr.2009.11.012

Clare, L., Crawford, J., Wilson, B. A., Cockburn, J., Baddeley, A., Watson, P., . . . Greenfield, E. (2008). *Rivermead Behavioral Memory Test*. Bury St. Edmunds, UK: Thames Valley Test Co.

Cramer, H., Lauche, R., Paul, A., & Dobos, G. (2012). Mindfulness-based stress reduction for breast cancer—A systematic review and meta-analysis. *Current Oncology, 19,* e343–e352. https://doi.org/10.3747/co.19.1016

Eakin, E. G., Resnikoff, P. M., Prewitt, L. M., Ries, A. L., & Kaplan, R. M. (1998). Validation of a new dyspnea measure: The UCSD Shortness of Breath Questionnaire. *Chest, 113,* 619–624. https://doi.org/10.1378/chest.113.3.619

Fisher, A. G., & Jones, K. B. (2012). *Assessment of Motor and Process Skills: Development, standardizations, and administration manual* (7th ed., rev.). Fort Collins, CO: Three Star Press.

Folio, M. R., & Fewell, R. R. (2000). *Peabody Developmental Motor Scales* (2nd ed.). Austin, TX: PRO-ED, Inc.

Forsyth, K., Deshpande, S., Kielhofner, G., Henriksson, C., Haglund, L., Olson, L., . . . Kulkarni, S. (2005). *The Occupational Circumstances Assessment Interview and Rating Scale (OCAIRS). Version 4.0.* Chicago: Model of Human Occupation Clearinghouse, Department of Occupational Therapy, College of Applied Health Sciences, University of Illinois at Chicago.

Forsyth, K., Salamy, M., Simon, S., & Kielhofner, G. (1998). *The Assessment of Communication and Interaction Skills (ACIS). Version 4.* Chicago: Model of Human Occupation Clearinghouse, Department of Occupational Therapy, College of Applied Health Sciences, University of Illinois at Chicago.

Gilchrist, L. S., & Tanner, L. (2013). The Pediatric-Modified Total Neuropathy Score: A reliable and valid measure of chemotherapy-induced peripheral neuropathy in children with non-CNS cancers. *Supportive Care in Cancer, 21,* 847–856. https://doi.org/10.1007/s00520-012-1591-8

Gummesson, C., Atroshi, I., & Ekdahl, C. (2003). The Disabilities of the Arm, Shoulder, and Hand (DASH) outcome questionnaire: Longitudinal construct validity and measuring self-rated health change after surgery. *BMC Musculoskeletal Disorders, 4,* 11. https://doi.org/10.1186/1471-2474-4-11

Hartman-Maeir, A., Harel, H., & Katz, N. (2009). Kettle Test—A brief measure of cognitive functional performance: Reliability and validity in stroke rehabilitation. *American Journal of Occupational Therapy, 63,* 592–599. https://doi.org/10.5014/ajot.63.5.592

Jacobsen, P. B., Donovan, K. A., Vadaparampil, S. T., & Small, B. J. (2007). Systematic review and meta-analysis of psychological and activity-based interventions for cancer-related fatigue. *Health Psychology, 26,* 660–667. https://doi.org/10.1037/0278-6133.26.6.660

Jette, A., Haley, S. M., Coster, W., & Ni, P. S. (2015). *AM-PAC Short Forms for Inpatient and Outpatient Settings: Instruction manual.* Boston: Boston University.

Katz, S., Ford, A. B., Moskowitz, R. W., Jackson, B. A., & Jaffe, M. W. (1963). Studies of illness in the aged: The Index of ADL: A standardized measure of biological and psychosocial function. *JAMA, 185,* 914–919. https://doi.org/10.1001/jama.1963.03060120024016

Kielhofner, G., Mallinson, T., Crawford, C., Nowak, M., Rigby, M., Henry, A., & Walens, D. (2004). *Occupational Performance History Interview–II (OPHI–II)* (Version 2.1). Chicago: Model of Human Occupation Clearinghouse, Department of Occupational Therapy, College of Applied Health Sciences, University of Illinois at Chicago.

Kolhman-Thomson, L., & Robnett, R. (2016). *Kohlman Evaluation of Living Skills* (4th ed.). Bethesda, MD: AOTA Press.

Kuchinski, A. M., Reading, M., & Lash, A. A. (2009). Treatment-related fatigue and exercise in patients with cancer: A systematic review. *Medsurg Nursing, 18,* 174–180.

Law, M., Baptiste, S., Carswell, A., McColl, M., Polatajko, H. & Pollock, N. (2019). *Canadian Occupational Performance Measure* (5th ed., rev.). Altona, Canada: COPM, Inc.

Lawton, M. P., & Brody, E. M. (1969). Assessment of older people: Self-maintaining and instrumental activities of daily living. *Gerontologist, 9,* 179–186. https://doi.org/10.1093/geront/9.3_Part_1.179

Mendoza, T. R., Wang, X. S., Cleeland, C. S., Morrissey, M., Johnson, B. A., Wendt, J. K., & Huber, S. L. (1999). The rapid assessment of fatigue severity in cancer patients: Use of the Brief Fatigue Inventory. *Cancer, 85,* 1186–1196. https://doi.org/10.1002/(SICI)1097-0142(19990301)85:5<1186::AID-CNCR24>3.0.CO;2-N

Moore-Corner, R. A., Kielhofner, G., & Olson, L. (1998). *A user's guide to Work Environment Impact Scale (WEIS) (Version 2.0).* Chicago: University of Illinois.

Morrison, M. T., Giles, G. M., Ryan, J. D., Baum, C. M., Dromerick, A. W., Polatajko, H. J., & Edwards, D. F. (2013). Multiple Errands Test–Revised (MET–R): A performance-based measure of executive function in people with mild cerebrovascular accident. *American Journal of Occupational Therapy, 67,* 460–468. https://doi.org/10.5014/ajot.2013.007880

Nasreddine, Z. S., Phillips, N. A., Bédirian, V., Charbonneau, S., Whitehead, V., Collin, I., … Chertkow, H. (2005). The Montreal Cognitive Assessment, MoCA: A brief screening tool for mild cognitive impairment. *Journal of the American Geriatrics Society, 53,* 695–699. https://doi.org/10.1111/j.1532-5415.2005.53221.x

National Cancer Institute. (2012). End-of-life care for people who have cancer. Retrieved from https://www.cancer.gov/about-cancer/advanced-cancer/care-choices/care-fact-sheet

National Coalition for Cancer Survivorship. (2018). *The National Coalition for Cancer Survivorship.* Retrieved from https://www.canceradvocacy.org/about-us/our-history/.

Newman, R. M., Alfano, C. M., Radomski, M. V., Pergolotti, M., Wolf, T. J., Sleight, A. G., … Daniels, E. (2019). Catalyzing research to optimize cancer survivors' participation in work and life roles. *OTJR: Occupation, Participation and Health,* 1539449219844749. https://doi.org/10.1177/1539449219844749

Oremus, M., Dayes, I., Walker, K., & Raina, P. (2012). Systematic review: Conservative treatments for secondary lymphedema. *BMC Cancer, 12,* 6. https://doi.org/10.1186/1471-2407-12-6

Parkinson, S., Forsyth, K., & Kielhofner, G. (2006). *The Model of Human Occupation Screening Tool* (Version 2). Chicago: Model of Human Occupation Clearinghouse, Department of Occupational Therapy, College of Applied Health Sciences, University of Illinois at Chicago.

Pendleton, H. M., & Schultz-Krohn, W. (2018). The *Occupational Therapy Practice Framework* and the practice of occupational therapy for people with physical disabilities. In H. M. Pendleton & W. Schultz-Krohn (Eds.), *Pedretti's occupational therapy: Practice skills for physical dysfunction* (8th ed., pp. 1–15). St. Louis: Mosby.

Punwar, A. J., & Peloquin, S. M. (2000). *Occupational therapy: Principles and practice.* Lippincott Williams & Wilkins.

Robertson, I. H., Nimmo-Smith, I. N., Ward, T., & Ridgeway, V. (1994). *The Test of Everyday Attention: TEA.* Bury St. Edmunds, UK: Thames Valley Test Co.

Rocke, K., Hays, P., Edwards, D., & Berg, C. (2008). Development of a performance assessment of executive function: The Children's Kitchen Task Assessment. *American Journal of Occupational Therapy, 62,* 528–537. https://doi.org/10.5014/ajot.62.5.528

Toglia, J. (2015). *Weekly Calendar Planning Activity (WCPA): A performance test of executive function.* Bethesda, MD: AOTA Press.

Uniform Data System for Medical Rehabilitation. (2016). *About the FIM System*. Buffalo, NY: University of Buffalo.

Varni, J. W., Burwinkle, T. M., Katz, E. R., Meeske, K., & Dickinson, P. (2002). The PedsQL in pediatric cancer: Reliability and validity of the Pediatric Quality of Life Inventory Generic Core Scales, Multidimensional Fatigue Scale, and cancer module. *Cancer, 94,* 2090–2106. https://doi.org/10.1002/cncr.10428

Webster, K., Cella, D., & Yost, K. (2003). The Functional Assessment of Chronic Illness Therapy (FACIT) Measurement System: Properties, applications, and interpretation. *Health and Quality of Life Outcomes, 1,* 79. https://doi.org/10.1186/1477-7525-1-79

Wilson, S. A., & Landry, G. (2014). *Task analysis: An individual, group, and population approach* (3rd ed.). Bethesda, MD: AOTA Press.

World Health Organization. (2001). *International classification of functioning, disability and health*. Geneva: Author.

PART II.

Impact of Common Forms of Cancer Across the Lifespan

Special Considerations for Children With Cancer

Jessica Sparrow, OTD, OTR/L, BCP

LEARNING OBJECTIVES

After completing this chapter, readers should be able to

- Describe the unique factors that differentiate the role of occupational therapy provided to children with cancer from that provided to other onology populations;
- Describe evidence-based occupational therapy assessments that assist in identifying limitations in function, participation, and quality of life (QoL) for children with cancer; and
- Describe evidence-based occupational therapy interventions that improve function, participation, and QoL for children with cancer.

KEY TERMS AND CONCEPTS

- Cancer-related cognitive impairment
- Cancer-related fatigue
- Chemotherapy-induced peripheral neuropathy
- Graft-versus-host disease
- Immunocompromise
- Myelosuppression
- Occupational profile
- Pain
- Pediatric palliative care
- Posterior fossa syndrome
- Quality of life
- Stem cell transplant

INTRODUCTION

Childhood is a time of rapid development and acquisition of new occupational performance skills and occupational roles. The child's developing body and central nervous system (CNS) are highly vulnerable to the negative effects of cancer and related treatments. Children with cancer therefore are at substantial risk for experiencing limitations in performance skills and subsequent restrictions in participation and *quality of life* (QoL), the dynamic appraisal of life satisfaction, self-concept, health and functioning, and socioeconomic factors (American Occupational Therapy Association [AOTA], 2014). Many of these limitations are amenable to occupational therapy interventions.

Rehabilitation of children with cancer is unlike rehabilitation of adolescents and young adults with cancer because childhood cancer involves different diagnoses, which necessitate distinct treatments and result in distinct restrictions in performance skills and participation. This chapter helps occupational therapy practitioners identify children who may be at risk for occupational performance restrictions by describing lifespan considerations and cancer's impact on a child's physical, sensory, cognitive, and psychosocial functions. Additionally, the chapter lists recommendations for assessment and intervention strategies to promote age-appropriate development, participation, and QoL for this unique population.

WHO ARE CHILDREN? LIFESPAN AND DEVELOPMENTAL CHALLENGES

Developmental transitions and the related development of new occupational roles occur throughout life; however, development in early childhood is rapid, involving profound psychobiological changes (Case-Smith, 2010; National Research Council [NRC] & Institute of Medicine [IOM], 2000). The occupations of childhood include play, school participation, self-care, and social engagement. The development of these occupations is influenced by environmental, cultural, and physiological factors (Jaffe et al., 2010; NRC & IOM, 2000). Successful transitions from the occupations of infancy to those of toddlers, preschoolers, and school-age children require opportunities for play, social interaction, and exploration of and interaction with the environment (Jaffe et al., 2010; NRC & IOM, 2000). Health conditions and associated disability can affect a child's ability to fully participate in age-appropriate occupations and roles.

MOST COMMON FORMS OF CANCER AMONG CHILDREN

Pediatric cancer is rare, but it is the second leading cause of death among children in the United States (Siegel et al.,

CANCER TYPE	NO. CASES	%
Acute lymphocytic leukemia	2,670	26
Brain and CNS	2,240	21
Neuroblastoma (includes ganglioneuroblastoma)	710	7
Non-Hodgkin lymphoma	620	6
Wilms tumor	510	5
Acute myeloid leukemia	500	5
Bone tumors	450	4
Hodgkin lymphoma	380	3
Rhabdomyosarcoma	340	3
Retinoblastoma	280	3
All sites	**10,450**	**83**

Note. Estimates are for malignant cancers and are rounded to the nearest 10. In addition, 730 children will be diagnosed with benign and borderline brain tumors. CNS = central nervous system.
Source. Data from Ward et al. (2014).

2017). The most common type of pediatric cancer is acute lymphocytic leukemia (ALL), which accounts for 26% of all childhood cancers. Cancers of the brain and CNS are the second most common type of cancer (21%), followed by neuroblastoma (7%) and non-Hodgkin lymphoma (6%; Ward, et al., 2014; see Exhibit 4.1).

The number of childhood cancer survivors continues to rise with advances in treatment and supportive care, resulting in a more than 20% increase in overall pediatric survival rates since the mid-1970s (Howlader et al., 2019). The overall 5-year relative survival rates for children ages birth to 14 years for all International Classification of Childhood Cancer groups (a standardized method for categorizing childhood malignancies set forth by the World Health Organization; Steliarova-Foucher et al., 2005) is 83%. However, these rates vary substantially by cancer type. For example, the relative survival rates for lymphoid leukemia and Hodgkin lymphoma are 90.2% and 97.7%, but the relative survival rates for acute myeloid leukemia and osteosarcoma are 64.2% and 69.5%, respectively (Siegel et al., 2017).

FACTORS THAT MAY CONTRIBUTE TO OCCUPATIONAL DYSFUNCTION AMONG CHILDREN WITH CANCER

Exhibit 4.2 provides an overview of the various client factors and restrictions in performance skills that may contribute to occupational dysfunction in children with cancer.

Pediatric Cancer Treatment

Treatment of pediatric cancer may include surgery, chemotherapy, radiation therapy, immunotherapy, targeted

LEUKEMIA

- Cognitive impairment
- Gross and fine motor coordination impairment
- Chemotherapy-induced peripheral neuropathy
- Avascular necrosis
- Muscle weakness and fatigue
- Obesity
- Psychological distress
- Myelosuppression

STEM CELL TRANSPLANT

- GVHD, including skin breakdown, muscular fibrosis and contractures, weakness, cramping, fatigue, pain, edema (Armenian et al., 2011; Baird et al., 2010; Couriel et al., 2006; Gurney et al., 2006)
- Generalized weakness and fatigue
- Gross and fine motor coordination impairment
- Pain
- Cognitive impairment
- Psychological distress

CNS TUMORS

- Sensory impairments, including pain, vision loss, hearing loss, decreased sensation
- Chemotherapy-induced peripheral neuropathy
- Neuromuscular dysfunction, including impaired fine and gross motor coordination, ataxia, hemiplegia, and abnormalities in tone
- Muscle weakness and fatigue
- Obesity
- Cognitive impairment
- Behavioral changes
- Psychological distress
- Speech and language disorders
- Feeding and swallowing difficulties
- Myelosuppression

BONE AND SOFT TISSUE TUMORS

- Muscle weakness
- Limited ROM
- Pain
- Decreased sensation
- Chemotherapy-induced peripheral neuropathy
- Psychological distress
- Myelosuppression

RETINOBLASTOMA

- Vision impairment
- Sensory integration impairment
- Feeding difficulties
- Visual–motor integration impairment
- Psychological distress
- Pain

(Continued)

| EXHIBIT 4.2. | Factors Contributing to Occupational Dysfunction Among Children With Various Cancer Diagnoses *(Cont.)* |

NEUROBLASTOMA

- Feeding difficulties
- Psychological distress
- Sensory impairments, including hearing or vision loss
- Cognitive impairments
- Pain
- Fatigue

Any diagnosis among children 3 years old or younger

- Developmental delay

Note. CNS = central nervous system; GVHD = graft-versus-host disease; ROM = range of motion.

therapy, and stem cell transplantation (SCT). The treatment team considers the specific details of a child's cancer diagnosis, including stage (i.e., extent and severity of the disease), risk group (e.g., clinical features of the disease, child's age, results of laboratory tests), and grade (i.e., high vs. low grade), when determining the most effective treatment plan (National Cancer Institute, 2015). (See Chapter 2, "Cancer Treatment Approaches Across the Lifespan," for further discussion of treatment approaches.)

A child's age heavily influences the type of treatment they will receive, because young children are particularly vulnerable to the effects of toxic chemotherapy and radiation treatments. Occupational therapy practitioners must know the potential side effects of childhood cancer treatment and work with the child and family to determine optimal timing for interventions and to modify intervention activities when a child is ill or fatigued. Table 4.1 provides

TABLE 4.1. Pediatric Cancer Treatments and Potential Complications or Late Effects

TREATMENT OR INTERVENTION	POTENTIAL COMPLICATIONS OR LATE EFFECTS	OCCUPATIONAL THERAPY PRECAUTIONS
Radiation therapy	▪ Acute toxicities: insomnia, anorexia, nausea, vomiting, alopecia, fatigue, dermatitis (Ermoian et al., 2016; Suneja et al., 2013) ▪ Long-term effects: neurologic, musculoskeletal, endocrine, and cognitive deficits; secondary malignancies (Antonini et al., 2017; Ermoian et al., 2016) ▪ Other symptoms may emerge relative to the area of the body radiated	▪ If sedation is required for radiation therapy, it may inhibit the child from immediate participation in therapy after treatment. ▪ Activity precautions are based on the area of the body radiated.

Chemotherapy (overview in Table 4.2)	▪ Acute toxicities (usually reversible):
	  • Myelosuppression
	  • Nausea and vomiting
	  • Alopecia
	  • Oral and intestinal mucositis
	  • Liver function abnormalities
	  • Allergic reactions
	▪ Incompletely reversible toxicities (e.g., late-onset cardiovascular complications due to anthracycline administration)
	▪ Additional side effects from drugs required to control the side effects of chemotherapy
		Be aware of the possible side effects and related precautions of all of a child's current medications, including those used to treat chemotherapy toxicities.

Surgery	▪ Limitations in performance skills and participation (vary with the type and extent of tumor resection, amputation, or other surgery required)	Modify the therapy plan as needed to accommodate postoperative precautions and functional limitations.
Central line	▪ Line damage or dislodgement ▪ High risk of infection ▪ Pain or discomfort	▪ Ensure that the line is secure. ▪ Keep the area clean and dry. ▪ Follow infection control precautions. ▪ Use equipment (e.g., pillows, blankets) for positioning when working in prone to ensure the child's comfort. ▪ Do not push the child past the point of comfort during upper extremity ROM activities. ▪ Avoid contact sports and heavy lifting.
Stem cell transplant	▪ Low blood cell count (thrombocytopenia) ▪ High risk of infections ▪ Fatigue and weakness ▪ Reduced appetite ▪ Pain ▪ GVHD	Follow infection control precautions.

Note. GVHD = graft-versus-host disease; ROM = range of motion.

TABLE 4.2. Common Pediatric Cancer Chemotherapeutic Agents and Side Effects Pertinent to Occupational Therapy

CLASS	AGENT	SIDE EFFECTS
Antimetabolite	Methotrexate	*Occasional:* Learning disability *Rare:* Leukoencephalopathy, seizures, acute neurotoxicity, lung damage, osteoporosis, osteonecrosis and soft tissue necrosis, progressive CNS deterioration
	Cytarabine	*Occasional:* Flulike symptoms *Rare:* Encephalopathy, cerebellar dysfunction; learning disability, convulsions, ataxia when given intrathecally
Plant alkaloid	Vincristine	*Common:* Loss of deep tendon reflexes *Occasional:* Pain, numbness, weakness, tingling, clumsiness, peripheral neuropathy *Rare:* Ptosis, vocal cord suppression, CNS depression, seizures
	Etoposide	*Rare:* Hypotension, peripheral neuropathy
	Topotecan	*Common:* Fatigue *Occasional:* Weakness, dyspnea Rare: Myalgia, paresthesia
	Irinotecan	*Occasional:* Pain at infusion site *Rare:* Tremor, headache, dizziness, disorientation or confusion, pneumonitis, pulmonary infiltrates
	Vinblastine	*Occasional:* Loss of deep tendon reflexes, paresthesia *Rare:* Bone pain, peripheral neuropathy, ptosis, double vision
Alkylating agent	Cyclophosphamide	*Rare:* Transient blurred vision
	Cisplatin	*Common:* High-frequency hearing loss *Occasional:* Hearing loss in the normal hearing range *Rare:* Peripheral neuropathy, tinnitus, seizure
	Temozolomide	*Occasional:* Fatigue, CNS effects
	Ifosfamide	*Occasional:* Confusion, weakness, seizure, cardiac toxicities with arrhythmias at high doses, myocardial necrosis *Rare:* Encephalopathy, peripheral neuropathy, pulmonary fibrosis
	Carboplatin	*Rare:* Peripheral neuropathy, hearing loss
Antitumor or monoclonal antibiotics	Doxorubicin and Daunorubicin	*Occasional:* Cardiomyopathy (cumulative and dose dependent)
	Rituximab	*Occasional:* Dizziness, fatigue, insomnia, headache, neuropathy, pain, paresthesia, arthralgia, back pain, muscle spasm, myalgia, weakness *Rare:* Arthritis, encephalitis, optic neuritis, hypoxia
Biotherapeutic agent	Dasatinib	*Common:* Palpitations *Occasional:* Dizziness, fatigue, headache, insomnia, myasthenia, pain, peripheral neuropathy, muscle spasm, myalgia, stiffness, weakness, abnormal bone growth *Rare:* Anxiety, arthritis, ataxia, confusion, facial nerve palsy, dementia, malaise, hearing loss, dysphagia, equilibrium disturbance, osteonecrosis, osteopenia, optic neuritis, seizure, syncope, tendonitis, transient ischemic attack, vertigo, voice disorder
	Imatinib	*Common:* Fatigue, headache, dizziness *Rare:* Paresthesia, blurred vision, flulike syndrome
	Crizotinib	*Occasional:* Dizziness, fatigue, syncope, multiple neuropathies, limb pain, muscle spasms, visual disturbances
	Aldesleukin	*Occasional:* Confusion, dizziness, drowsiness, malaise, pain, psychosis, stupor, weakness *Rare:* Blindness (transient or permanent), myopathy, myositis, neuralgia, neuritis, neuropathy, CVA, delirium, syncope, seizure, transient ischemic attack, optic neuritis
Miscellaneous	Asparaginase Erwinia chrysanthemi	*Occasional:* Thrombosis *Rare:* Seizure, transient ischemic attacks
	Corticosteroids	*Common:* Increased appetite *Occasional:* Muscle weakness, osteonecrosis *Rare:* Aseptic necrosis of femoral head, growth retardation, cataracts, osteopenia

Note. CNS = central nervous system; CVA = cerebrovascular accident.
Sources. Children's Oncology Group (2013); Kline et al. (2014).

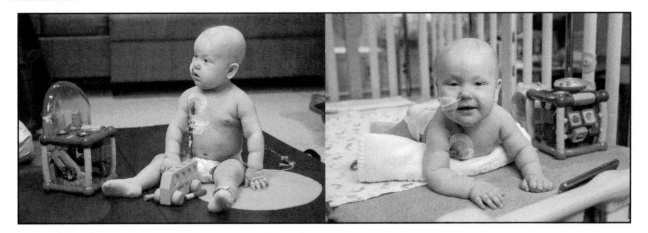

Source. Justin Veneman. Used with permission.

a summary of potential complications and late effects of pediatric cancer treatments.

Radiation therapy poses significant acute and long-term adverse effects for children because their developing tissues and cells are more sensitive to the late effects of irradiation than are mature adult tissues. Furthermore, children who receive CNS-directed radiation therapy are at risk for cognitive dysfunction and other late CNS effects, including radiation-induced necrosis. Additionally, increased intracranial pressure resulting from radiation-induced edema could cause headache, nausea, vomiting, seizures, or exacerbation of existing neurological symptoms. Similarly, children who require radiation therapy to the lungs are at risk for postradiation pulmonary toxicity (Ermoian et al., 2016). Such issues may make participating in school, ADLs, or play difficult.

The types of chemotherapy drugs commonly used to treat childhood cancers often differ from those used to treat adult cancers, so the type of side effects experienced may also differ. See Table 4.2 for a list of chemotherapies commonly used to treat childhood cancers and related toxicities.

Surgery for childhood cancer typically involves biopsy of the tumor, tumor resection, shunt placement, or limb-sparing or amputation procedures for children with an upper or lower extremity bone or soft-tissue tumor, all of which may affect performance and participation. Another common aspect of childhood cancer treatment is the placement of central lines to administer medications (e.g., chemotherapy), draw blood for laboratory tests, and transfuse blood products.

Placement of a central line requires a surgical procedure in which a catheter is inserted into a large vein in the neck or chest. Because central lines enable direct access to major blood vessels, they carry a high risk of potentially deadly infections; dislodgement of a central line is a medical emergency. Children with central lines should avoid contact sports and heavy lifting to protect the lines from damage or dislodgement. The occupational therapy practitioner can ensure patient comfort during therapy by using pillows, blankets, and other equipment or props for positioning

when working with children prone and by not pushing a child past the point of comfort during upper extremity range-of-motion activities (see Figure 4.1).

SCT is the replacement of stem cells when bone marrow is abnormal or has been destroyed by disease, chemotherapy, or radiation. Such transplantation is often used to treat pediatric cancers, particularly leukemias and lymphomas. (See Chapter 2, "Cancer Treatment Approaches Across the Lifespan," for an overview of the SCT process.) During the initial phases of the SCT process, the child is severely immunocompromised and remains as an inpatient for approximately 6 weeks. During this time, the child and all caregivers and medical staff must follow heightened infection-control precautions, including unit or room isolation, reverse isolation, dietary restrictions, meticulous cleaning of linens, and restrictions on the number of visitors and types of items that can enter the room (e.g., stuffed animals). At discharge, many of these infection-control precautions remain in place until the child's immune system is adequate to fight infection.

In addition to infection, development of *graft-versus-host disease* (GVHD) is a major concern after SCT. GVHD is a widespread immune response of donor tissue to the host, with features and symptoms similar to those of an autoimmune or immunodeficiency disorder (see Chapters 2 and 9, "Acute and Medically Complex Settings," for more information on GVHD). GVHD can cause significant morbidity and diminished QoL and is the most significant nonrelapse cause of morbidity and death after an allogeneic (hematopoietic) SCT. An estimated 20%–50% of children experience GVHD after an allogenic SCT; the risk is higher in cases of matched unrelated donors (Baird et al., 2010).

Myelosuppression

Immunological system functions are widely affected across many pediatric cancer diagnoses because of the myelosuppression caused by several chemotherapy agents and regimens. *Myelosuppression,* or bone marrow depression, results in decreased production of all blood components (i.e., red blood cells, white blood cells, platelets). The resulting immunosuppression, thrombocytopenia, and anemia place a child at risk for adverse events, and chronically low blood counts may significantly restrict a child's ability to participate in age-appropriate occupations. Children with thrombocytopenia are at risk for bleeds, including bleeds in muscles and joints. Children with anemia are at risk for periods of low oxygen saturation, cardiac arrhythmias, and tachycardia.

Occupational therapy practitioners working with a child with cancer should be acutely aware of the child's blood count values and related risk factors, because they may affect the therapist's evaluation and intervention. In the case of a child with critically low blood count values, the practitioner should regularly collaborate with the child's oncology team to determine the appropriateness of occupational therapy intervention.

Additionally, it is the practitioner's responsibility to continuously monitor a child with cancer for symptoms of low blood counts that would necessitate modification to evaluation or intervention activities or exercises. Modifications may need to be made, including

- When a child experiences pain, fatigue, headache, pallor indicating anemia, bruising, or petechia;
- When there is reported abnormal bleeding indicating thrombocytopenia;
- When there are abnormal resting vitals (e.g., heart rate, blood pressure, respiratory rate, oxygen saturation); or
- In the presence of other symptoms, including nausea (Gilchrist & Tanner, 2017).

Immunocompromise, a weakened immune system, resulting from neutropenia (i.e., abnormally low neutrophil count) is a common side effect of cancer treatment among children. Children with an absolute neutrophil count below 500/mm^3 are at increased risk for infection. Children with neutropenia must follow more stringent guidelines for infection control, including meticulous hand hygiene, enhanced personal hygiene, avoidance of people who are ill and large crowds of people (e.g., school, shopping, events), dietary restrictions, and restrictions on swimming. If neutropenia is accompanied by a fever, which indicates some type of infection, then medical attention will likely be required.

Certain populations, such as children receiving an SCT, may require additional or more explicit infection control precautions, because they are at substantial risk for life-threatening infections during the early phases of transplant. In general, occupational therapy practitioners should ensure thorough cleaning of equipment and the treatment environment, including toys, exercise equipment, ADL equipment, and mat surfaces, after every use. Only hard-surfaced, washable toys and equipment should be used. Occupational therapy practitioners are also responsible for their own meticulous hand hygiene and for being healthy when providing services to an immunocompromised child with cancer. Isolation and infection control procedures should be followed in accordance with the organization's policies and procedures.

Neuromusculoskeletal Issues

Children with cancer often have difficulties with fatigue, strength, range of motion (ROM), coordination, posture, and balance. For example, children with leukemia can experience muscle weakness, impaired gross motor coordination and balance, and impaired fine motor coordination (e.g., handwriting ability; Green et al., 2013; Hockenberry et al., 2007; Reinders-Messelink et al., 1999; Taverna et al., 2017; Wright et al., 2005). Children who receive SCT are also at risk for increased fatigue and limitations in strength, ROM, coordination, and visual–motor and visual–perceptual skills (Fahnehjelm et al., 2018; Graef et al., 2016; Taverna et al., 2017). These symptoms are likely exacerbated by prolonged hospitalization and the related deprivation of participation in meaningful childhood occupations.

Children with brain tumors can experience a wide range of neuromusculoskeletal deficits, including impaired coordination, hemiplegia, muscle weakness, fatigue, and speech and language disorder (Armstrong et al., 2009; Ness et al., 2010; Packer et al., 2003; Turner et al., 2009). The types of deficits experienced are related to the location of the tumor. For example, a tumor in the frontal lobe might result in behavioral or dysexecutive symptoms; a tumor in the parietal lobe may affect a child's handwriting ability and spatial awareness; and a tumor in the posterior fossa area might result in cerebellar symptoms, including ataxia.

As many as 60% of children with brain tumors experience coordination and motor control difficulties, including hemiplegia or ataxia, and 83% experience some level of balance impairment (Armstrong et al., 2009; Kuper et al., 2013). As many as 50% of child and adolescent survivors of posterior fossa tumors demonstrate significantly lower gross motor physical functioning, including impaired balance, coordination, strength, and agility. These issues limit performance skills and performance of occupations such as play, ADLs, IADLs, and school attendance (Demers et al., 2015; Hudson et al., 2003; Piscione et al., 2014). Because of these limitations, survivors of childhood brain tumors are less likely to be employed, attain education beyond high school, or live independently (Ness et al., 2010).

Posterior fossa syndrome (PFS) is a unique syndrome of neurobehavioral dysfunction resulting from surgical resection of an infratentorial tumor. Among children with medulloblastoma, researchers estimate that 25% of patients treated with surgery have PFS (Gelabert-González & Fernández-Villa, 2001; Pollack et al., 1995; Wells et al., 2008). Symptoms of PFS usually present 24–48 hours postsurgery and may include cerebellar mutism, apraxia (oromotor, oculomotor, limb), emotional lability, axial hypotonia, and cerebellar or brainstem dysfunction (e.g., ataxia). Tracheostomy placement may be required in severe cases. Mutism, severe ataxia, and emotional lability or irritability are considered to be three cardinal symptoms of PFS (Morris et al., 2009; Robertson et al., 2006). Mutism and emotional lability are generally transient, abating weeks to months after onset; however, cognitive speech and neuromuscular symptoms can persist more than 5 years postsurgery (Robertson et al., 2006).

Diagnosis and treatment-related factors, such as neurological dysfunction, may lead to feeding problems among young children with cancer. Children may experience neurotoxicity and resulting vocal cord paralysis, changes in tastes, vomiting, and mucositis, which can lead to prolonged periods of enteral nutrition (Fleming et al., 2015). These issues can lead to feeding dysfunction, including delays in oral motor development, oral hypersensitivity, and abnormalities in neuromuscular function.

Cancer-related fatigue is defined as "a distressing, persistent subjective sense of physical, emotional and/or cognitive tiredness or exhaustion related to cancer or cancer treatment that is not proportional to recent activity and interferes with usual functioning" (Berger et al., 2015, p. 1020). Such fatigue may limit a child's motivation or ability to participate in daily activities; play; and other meaningful, age-appropriate activities. (See Chapter 15, "Cancer-Related Fatigue," for more information.)

Mental Functions

Up to 40% of survivors of childhood cancer who receive CNS-directed therapy may experience cognitive deficits, with risk for associated academic problems, high unemployment rates, and decreased QoL (Gurney et al., 2009; Moleski, 2000; Mulhern et al., 1999). These neurocognitive late effects among children with cancer and long-term survivors of childhood cancer have been well documented. They manifest as global intellectual decline and impairments in attention, executive function (EF), processing speed, working memory, memory, visual–spatial skills, and visual–motor skills (Butler et al., 2008; Conklin et al., 2013; Palmer et al., 2013).

Chemotherapy alone is associated with cognitive dysfunction among children with cancer and childhood cancer survivors. *Cancer-related cognitive impairment* is defined as impairment in an individual's memory, learning, concentration, reasoning, EF, attention, and visuospatial skills during and after discontinuation of chemotherapy (Argyriou et al., 2011; see Chapter 17, "Cancer-Related Cognitive Impairment," for additional information on this topic). A meta-analysis in 2015 showed that children with ALL treated with chemotherapy but without radiation therapy had significantly impaired IQ and moderately impaired working memory and processing speed (Iyer et al., 2015).

Children treated with cranial irradiation, such as those with high-risk leukemia or brain tumors, are at significant risk for cognitive decline. Cognitive deficits manifest as an inability to acquire new information and skills at a rate comparable to that of healthy, same-age peers because of progressive deficits in underlying core abilities, such as memory, attention, and processing speed (Palmer et al., 2001). Significant risk factors for cognitive decline among children treated with radiation therapy include younger age at radiation treatment (younger than 5 years), higher dosage of radiation, and tumor location (because of potential damage to surrounding tissues; Duffner, 2004).

Sensory Functions

Sensory functions may also be disrupted among children with cancer. For example, certain types of cancers are associated with visual impairments. Retinoblastoma is a malignancy of the eye that originates in retinal cells of one or both eyes (Lohmann & Gallie, 1993). Possible treatments include enucleation (i.e., surgical removal of the eye), radiation therapy, chemotherapy (periocular injections or systemic), cryotherapy, and laser therapy, all of which can lead to vision loss. Because of their young age at diagnosis and the potential for diagnosis-related and treatment-related impairments, children with retinoblastoma are vulnerable to developmental delays and functional limitations (Willard et al., 2014).

Children with a brain tumor are also at risk for tumor-related visual deficits, depending on the location of the tumor. A brain tumor or related surgical intervention may cause cranial nerve damage, resulting in abnormal eye movements and subsequent difficulties with tracking, scanning, or double vision. Impairment in visual fields or acuity is common with certain brain tumor diagnoses. For example, as many as 40% of children with craniopharyngioma experience abnormal visual acuity, and 63% experience abnormal visual fields (Repka, 2006).

Optic pathway gliomas, which arise in or around the optic nerve or chiasm, are among the most frequent tumors affecting children who present with ophthalmologic signs (Binning et al., 2007). Specific clinical symptoms of brain tumor–related visual impairment vary depending on the particular tumor and its location; however, they may include

- Impaired visual acuity (mild loss to no functional vision),
- Impaired visual fields,
- Strabismus,
- Ptosis,
- Nystagmus, and
- Double vision.

Children with cancer diagnoses other than brain tumors are also at risk for visual impairment often related to cancer treatment. In particular, radiation and glucocorticoids are established risk factors for eye-related complications (commonly, cataracts; Whelan et al., 2010).

Certain cancers and treatments, including chemotherapy and radiation therapy, may lead to hearing loss or speech and speech-related disorders. The chemotherapy agents carboplatin and cisplatin are commonly used to treat childhood cancers and increase the risk of significant, permanent hearing loss (Brock et al., 2012; Qaddoumi et al., 2012). Younger age at exposure and higher cumulative dose of chemotherapy are associated with a higher risk for hearing loss (Li et al., 2004; Qaddoumi et al., 2012). Because of potential damage to auditory structures, children who undergo radiation therapy to the brain, head, or neck may also experience hearing loss (Bass et al., 2016; Hua et al., 2008). Ototoxicity monitoring before, during, and after treatment helps with early detection and management of hearing loss among children with cancer and mitigates the potential for related occupational performance restrictions (Bass & Bhagat, 2014). Survivors of childhood cancer with serious hearing loss have been found to be at increased risk for nonindependent living, unemployment, poor academic attainment (Brinkman et al., 2015; Schreiber et al., 2014), and deficits in EF (Orgel et al., 2016).

Some commonly used chemotherapeutic agents, including vincristine and cisplatin, damage children's peripheral nerves, resulting in *chemotherapy-induced peripheral neuropathy* (CIPN; see Chapter 19, "Chemotherapy-Induced

Peripheral Neuropathy," for more information on this topic). Symptoms of CIPN include numbness or tingling, loss of vibration sensation, impaired light-touch sensation, loss of position sense, pain, weakness, incoordination, and balance disturbance (Gilchrist, 2012; Gilchrist & Tanner, 2013). A child experiencing CIPN may have difficulty carrying out ADLs, IADLs, and school tasks (e.g., buttoning, handwriting). They may also have limited ability to complete age-appropriate play tasks. Performance skills that may become a challenge as a result of CIPN include grasping and manipulating objects, safely completing transfers, and ambulating (Hausheer et al., 2006).

Impact on Participation and QoL

Development

Very young children, particularly those age 3 years or younger, are at risk for delays in development because of their diagnosis and treatment. Prolonged periods of hospitalization, illness, and cancer-related precautions all restrict the child's access to age-appropriate environments, activities, and social experiences, which in turn limits opportunities for play and learning. Some young children with cancer may experience added developmental challenges, including cognitive, neuromuscular, or musculoskeletal impairments, which can further limit progression of age-appropriate developmental skills. Across nearly all pediatric cancer diagnoses and treatment types (e.g., chemotherapy, radiation therapy, SCT), young children with cancer are at risk for delays in cognitive development, fine motor and gross motor skills, social–emotional development, and behavioral functioning (Bornstein et al., 2012; Mulchay Levy et al., 2013; Quigg et al., 2013; Willard et al., 2014).

ADLs

Cancer complicates the development of new ADL skills among young children because illness, hospitalization, and limited exposure to natural environments, habits, roles, and routines limit opportunities for participation in typical occupations. These factors may restrict the child's development of new ADL skills.

For older children who demonstrated age-appropriate ADL skills before diagnosis and treatment, performance may be negatively affected by illness, depression, decreased motivation, fatigue, and weakness, and children may show a regression of skills. Consider, for example, an 8-year-old boy who is in the hospital for 30 days while receiving an SCT. His schedule varies substantially from day to day, or he may not have any schedule at all; he rarely leaves his hospital room and has multiple IV lines. These and other factors limit the boy's motivation and capacity to participate in dressing and self-care activities each day. (Chapter 21, "ADLs and IADLs," further discusses this topic.)

Education

Education is defined by the *Occupational Therapy Practice Framework: Domain and Process* (3rd ed.; AOTA, 2014) as activities involved in learning and participating in the educational environment. Because of advances in cancer treatments and an increasing number of childhood cancer

survivors, more children with cancer can return to school. However, children with recent cancer diagnoses and longer term survivors are at risk for performance restrictions that may affect their ability to participate in and maximally benefit from school.

Psychosocial factors, body image issues (e.g., worry about how other students will respond to hair loss, scars, significant weight change) and depression may reduce a child's readiness to return to school. Physical and cognitive factors, such as fatigue, illness, immunocompromise, limitations in executive processing, vision loss, or fine motor coordination deficits, may reduce a child's ability to participate in academic tasks, including carrying a book bag, walking to class, organizing the work space, completing written work, or eating lunch in a crowded cafeteria. Environmental safety and accessibility factors, such as crowded school settings and inaccessible physical environments, may limit a child's access to school environments. Additionally, frequent hospitalizations, illness, immunocompromise, limitations in mobility, and pain may limit some children with cancer from attending school.

Children may participate in a homebound schooling program or attend a hospital's in-house school program while they are unable to attend school. When children return to school, their successful transition may require educational and environmental supports, services, and accommodations and modifications through an individualized education program (IEP) or a 504 Plan (see the section "Educational and Developmental Achievement" for more details on school-related services). Indeed, it has been reported that as many as 23% of childhood cancer survivors use special education services. More than 50% of children with CNS disease and treatment require special education services to support them in school (Mitby et al., 2003). Case Example 4.1 provides an example of the role of occupational therapy in supporting successful educational participation for a child with cancer.

Health-related QoL

The symptoms and performance restrictions experienced by some children with cancer have been associated with adverse effects on QoL (Varni et al., 2004). Children in the acute phases of the cancer care continuum and long-term survivors have been reported to experience statistically significant differences in health-related QoL in the areas of physical health, psychosocial health, emotional functioning, school functioning, and social functioning (Graef et al., 2016; Macartney et al., 2014; Zheng et al., 2018). Parents of children with cancer also report worrying about the health, development, and social adjustment of their child (Long et al., 2014).

OCCUPATIONAL THERAPY EVALUATION OF CHILDREN WITH CANCER

Occupational Profile

The occupational therapist's evaluation of a child with cancer must include a detailed medical and social history and

CASE EXAMPLE 4.1 EMILY: OCCUPATIONAL THERAPY THROUGHOUT THE CANCER CARE CONTINUUM

Emily was 2 years old when her anaplastic ependymoma was diagnosed. She underwent a gross total resection of the tumor shortly after diagnosis, which was followed by a 1-year protocol of chemotherapy and radiation therapy. Because of her tumor and treatment, she experienced right hemiplegia, balance impairment, and visual deficits. During her treatment, she experienced periods of nausea and vomiting, immunosuppression, thrombocytopenia, anemia, fatigue, hearing loss, generalized muscle weakness, and intermittent hospitalizations.

Emily received occupational therapy, speech therapy, and physical therapy as well as neuropsychology services to address developmental delays, neurological impairments, and resulting restrictions in play and age-appropriate self-care tasks. Her occupational therapist identified Emily's performance strengths and weaknesses and monitored her function with the Pediatric Quality of Life Inventory Parent Report for Toddlers (ages 2–4 years; Varni et al., 2001), the Short Child Occupational Profile (Bowyer et al., 2005), and the Peabody Developmental Motor Scales (2nd ed.; Folio & Fewell, 2000).

At 3 years old, Emily completed treatment and returned home. Her hospital-based occupational therapy practitioner completed a referral for early intervention in Emily's home community and communicated with the early intervention occupational therapy provider before Emily's return home. She also provided Emily's parents with education and a home program focused on developmental and neurodevelopmental training.

At 4 years old, Emily began outpatient rehabilitation services, including occupational therapy. Occupational therapy goals focused on developing independence with age-appropriate daily activities and school readiness skills through neuromuscular training, strengthening, functional–cognitive skill development, and visual–motor integration training.

At 5 years old, Emily made the transition to kindergarten with collaboration among her oncology clinic rehabilitation team, neuropsychology team, outpatient rehabilitation providers, school team, and parents. A school-based occupational therapy evaluation was completed, consisting of the Bruininks–Oseretsky Test of Motor Proficiency (Bruininks, 2005) and the School Function Assessment (Coster et al., 1998). On assessment, Emily demonstrated gross and fine motor weaknesses and visual–motor integration weaknesses. Her writing and copying abilities were below a 3-year, 7-month level.

Recommendations from her hospital-based rehabilitation team, outpatient team, school occupational therapy team, and neuropsychology team were used to create an IEP, which Emily qualified for through the primary eligibility category of "Other Health Impaired." Occupational therapy–related components of the IEP included occupational therapy services to address fine motor and visual–motor impairments, including writing and copying skills and functional school-based daily activities. Accommodations through her IEP included preferential seating and reduced or modified paper–pencil tasks and scissor-skills tasks.

When she was 14 years old (11 years from completion of treatment), Emily's family moved to a new city, and she attended a new high school. A teacher quickly noticed that Emily had difficulty organizing her assignments and meeting assignment deadlines, had poor handwriting, and often seemed to be tired by the end of the day. An occupational therapy evaluation was recommended. The evaluation included the Child Occupational Self-Assessment (Kramer et al., 2014), the Beery–Buktenica Developmental Test of Visual–Motor Integration (Beery et al., 2010), the Behavior Rating Inventory of Executive Function (Strauss et al., 2006), and the Weekly Calendar Planning Activity assessment (Toglia, 2015).

The occupational therapist also recommended that Emily participate in neuropsychology testing because it had been more than 2 years since her most recent testing was completed. Results of occupational therapy assessments and observations indicated that Emily had difficulty with working memory (e.g., when asked to hold information in mind to complete a task), planning and organizing (e.g., when asked to manage current or future-oriented task demands), and self-monitoring (e.g., when required to monitor her own behavior). Her visual–motor integration skills were also noted to be below age level.

Occupational therapy recommendations included conducting a morning review of each day's schedule; minimizing classroom noise (visual and auditory); providing a quiet place for testing and work; having the teacher check in with Emily regarding her fatigue and provide breaks as needed; and giving her shortened assignments to preserve her stamina and frustration tolerance, especially when writing was involved. The occupational therapist also recommended that Emily's family seek direct occupational therapy services to help Emily develop and use cognitive strategies that would support independence with her daily schedule, use a simple planner or assistive technology with similar functionality, and explore using alternative means of written production (e.g., speech-to-text technologies).

information about the child's cancer treatment plan—the *occupational profile*. A medical history provides information about prior treatment (e.g., surgery, chemotherapy, radiation therapy), any recurrences, and secondary diagnoses (e.g., other cancers, other conditions). For example, children with Down syndrome or neurofibromatosis are more likely to develop certain types of cancers than children without these conditions (Scheurer et al., 2015). The occupational therapy practitioner needs information about the child's current medical status (e.g., blood count values, precautions) and cancer treatment (e.g., type of treatment, time frame, potential acute and long-term side effects) to develop a safe plan that meets the child's current and future rehabilitation needs.

A detailed psychosocial history is also a critical piece of the occupational profile. Intense treatment protocols; frequent hospital visits; financial burden; multiple home and family demands, including the care of other children (sometimes from afar); and worries about their child's health and prognosis affect the entire family system (Pai et al., 2007). These client factors may influence the parents' priorities with regard to occupational therapy services, their readiness to take in new information, and their ability to actively participate in the occupational therapy process. Background information may be obtained from a medical chart review. Other opportunities for obtaining this information include communicating with the child's oncology team (e.g., oncologist, nurse practitioner, social worker) or parents. The occupational profile should include information about the child's preferences, roles, routines, functional strengths and limitations, and participation in a variety of environments, as assessed by methods described in Table 4.3. (See Chapter 20, "Psychosocial Issues," and Chapter 26, "Social Participation," for discussions of the psychosocial and social participation issues experienced by cancer survivors and relevant assessment tools.)

Analysis of Occupational Performance and Participation

In addition to the occupational profile, the occupational therapist's evaluation plan should be guided by the child's specific diagnoses and known treatment-related side effects. Commonly used assessments recommended for children with cancer can be found in Table 4.3 and Appendix 4.A.

Certain diagnoses and treatment protocols may have predictable periods of risk for functional decline and performance restrictions that can guide the occupational therapy evaluation schedule. For example, in the case of a child being treated for leukemia who received chemotherapy agents that increase the child's risk for experiencing CIPN, the evaluating occupational therapist should identify potentially neurotoxic chemotherapy agents that are part of the child's treatment plan and the schedule of administration.

Chemotherapy

Children receiving chemotherapy treatment for leukemia typically follow a standard protocol of treatment. This protocol includes three periods of intense weekly vincristine treatments that correspond to increased incidence of neuropathic pain (Week 4 of the protocol [during remission induction], Week 16 [after Reinduction 1], and Week 26 [after Reinduction 2]) and may also correspond to increased incidence of other CIPN symptoms (Anghelescu et al., 2011). Assessment of functional performance is recommended at baseline before the start of treatment, at the three periods of intense weekly vincristine administration, and posttreatment.

Assessment tools valuable for identifying signs and symptoms of CIPN are listed in Table 4.3. The Pediatric-Modified Total Neuropathy Score is a valid, reliable, and clinically feasible assessment tool that has been developed to assess CIPN among school-age children with cancer (Gilchrist & Tanner, 2013). The scale consists of sensory, motor function, and autonomic symptom questions as well as a 5-part neurologic examination that includes light-touch testing, pin sensibility, vibration sensibility, distal strength assessment, and deep tendon reflexes.

Formal testing for symptoms of CIPN among very young children (younger than 3 years) may not be feasible because of their inability to report symptoms and comply with instructions and procedures. It is important in such a case to obtain a detailed parental report of any changes in the child's functional abilities. Observation of the child during self-care tasks (e.g., finger feeding), transitional movements, and play tasks (e.g., stacking blocks, stringing beads) is also necessary. The child may have difficulty grasping objects because of limited ROM or weakness, be limited in their ability to fully extend the digits and wrists while crawling, or frequently drop objects because of loss of sensation.

SCT

Children who receive SCT may also experience predictable periods of risk for occupational performance restrictions. It is important for children undergoing SCT to maintain high levels of functional performance before transplant, during the initial hospitalization, and through the posttransplant phase (Steinberg et al., 2015). The first 100 days after an SCT is the period with the greatest risk for critical side effects, because the stem cells have typically engrafted and begun making new blood cells after this period. As such, monitoring children for limitations in occupational performance and performance skills (e.g., developmental delays, weakness, fatigue, limitations in ADL performance) during this phase is important. A recommended assessment schedule for children undergoing an SCT includes a pretransplant evaluation of the child's performance skills, weekly monitoring during the acute inpatient phase (Day 0 through discharge), and an outpatient occupational therapy evaluation at discharge.

Long-term monitoring is also recommended for up to 1 year posttransplant because the child remains at risk for complications that may negatively affect performance during this phase (primarily chronic GVHD [C-GVHD]). Monitoring for C-GVHD may occur through the use of an evaluation tool such as the National Institutes of Health C-GVHD Clinical Scoring System (Filipovich et al., 2005), which is completed by the child's oncology team. Monitoring should be combined with close collaboration between the medical team and rehabilitation providers at the first signs of C-GVHD in the skin or joints.

Monitoring is also important during this long-term follow-up phase, because children are preparing for several

TABLE 4.3. **Recommended Occupational Therapy Evaluation Tests and Assessments**

ASSESSMENT DOMAIN	TESTS AND ASSESSMENTS
Neuromusculoskeletal	<ul><li>ROM (direct assessment or observation)</li><li>Manual muscle testing (or observation of functional strength)</li><li>Fine motor and gross motor coordination<ul><li>9-Hole Peg Test (Wang et al., 2015)</li><li>Bruininks–Oseretsky Test of Motor Proficiency (Bruininks, 2005)</li><li>Peabody Developmental Motor Scales (Folio & Fewell, 2000)</li></ul></li><li>Grooved Pegboard Test (Wang et al., 2011)</li><li>NIH C-GVHD Clinical Scoring System Skin and Joints sections (Filipovich et al., 2005)</li><li>Photographic Range of Motion (Carpenter, 2011)</li><li>Feeding<ul><li>Assessment of mealtime participation and feeding history</li><li>Assessment of feeding-related sensory or behavioral issues</li></ul></li></ul>
Mental functions	<ul><li>Children's Kitchen Task Assessment (Rocke et al., 2008)</li><li>Weekly Calendar Planning Activity (Toglia, 2015)</li><li>Beery–Buktenica Developmental Test of Visual–Motor Integration (Beery et al., 2010)</li><li>Behavior Rating Inventory of Executive Function (Strauss et al., 2006)</li><li>Screen of cognitive function<ul><li>Digit Span Test (Wechsler, 1991)</li><li>Verbal Fluency Test (Benton et al., 1983)</li><li>Trail Making Test (Trites, 1977)</li></ul></li></ul>
Sensory	<ul><li>Sensation<ul><li>Monofilament testing, sharp–dull discrimination, vibration sense</li><li>Pediatric-Modified Total Neuropathy Score (Gilchrist & Tanner, 2013)</li><li>Close observation during functional grasping, holding, reaching, and upper extremity weight-bearing tasks</li></ul></li><li>Sensory Profile (Dunn, 2014)</li><li>Vision<ul><li>Screen of visual acuity (e.g., LEA Symbols Test; Hyvärinen et al., 1980)</li><li>Screen of visual fields and ocular motility</li><li>Oregon Project for Visually Impaired and Blind Preschool Children (Anderson et al., 2007)</li></ul></li></ul>
Pain	<ul><li>Faces Pain Scale (Hicks et al., 2001)</li><li>FLACC Pain Scale (Manworren & Hynan, 2003)</li></ul>
Developmental	<ul><li>Battelle Developmental Inventory (Newborg, 2005)</li><li>Peabody Developmental Motor Scales (2nd ed., Folio & Fewell, 2000)</li><li>Bayley Scales of Infant and Toddler Development (3rd ed., Bayley, 2005)</li><li>Ages and Stages Questionnaires (Squires et al., 2009)</li><li>Sensory Profile (Dunn, 2014)</li></ul>
Occupational performance, participation, and QoL	<ul><li>Pediatric Evaluation of Disability Inventory (Haley, 1992)</li><li>Pediatric Quality of Life Inventory<ul><li>Generic Core scales (Varni et al., 2001)</li><li>Cancer Module (Varni et al., 2002)</li><li>Brain Tumor Module (Palmer et al., 2007)</li><li>Stem Cell Transplant Module (Lawitschka et al., 2014)</li><li>Multidimensional Fatigue Scale (Varni et al., 2002)</li></ul></li><li>Miller Function and Participation Scales (Miller, 2006)</li><li>PROMIS Pediatric Fatigue Measure (Lai et al., 2013)</li><li>Paediatric Activity Card Sort (Mandich et al., 2004)</li><li>Preschool Activity Card Sort (Berg & LaVesser, 2006)</li><li>Canadian Occupational Performance Measure (Law et al., 2019)</li><li>Short Child Occupational Profile (Bowyer et al., 2005)</li><li>Child Occupational Self-Assessment (Kramer et al., 2014)</li><li>School Function Assessment (Coster et al., 1998)</li></ul>

Note. C-GVHD = chronic graft-versus-host disease; FLACC = Face, Legs, Activity, Cry, Consolability; NIH = National Institutes of Health; PROMIS = Patient-Reported Outcomes Measurement Information System; QoL = quality of life; ROM = range of motion.

important transitions. Occupational therapy practitioners can play an important role in evaluating children's adaptive, fine motor, visual–motor, gross motor, and cognitive skills as they transition back to school. Occupational therapy practitioners may recommend accommodations, modifications, or direct services that support successful participation in educational activities.

Endurance

Because children with cancer are at risk for cardiopulmonary complications as a result of treatment, myelosuppression, prolonged hospitalizations, and fatigue, evaluation of endurance and related occupational performance is recommended. The Patient-Reported Outcomes Measurement Information System (PROMIS) Pediatric Fatigue Measure (Hinds et al., 2013) and the Pediatric Quality of Life Inventory Multidimensional Fatigue Scale (Varni et al., 2004) are clinically feasible and valid indicators of child or proxy parent report of fatigue for children with cancer. (Chapter 15, "Cancer-Related Fatigue," provides additional information on cancer-related fatigue and related assessments.)

Pain

Pain, defined as an unpleasant feeling indicating potential or actual damage to some body structure (AOTA, 2014), may also limit the ability of a child with cancer to participate in meaningful activities and negatively affect their QoL. Cancer-related pain is a common distressing symptom reported by children and parents of children with cancer (Jibb et al., 2015). As many as 52%–60% of children with various diagnoses have been reported to experience pain during the course of their treatment (Heden et al., 2013). Suggested assessments for evaluating and monitoring pain among children with cancer can be found in Table 4.3. (Chapter 16, "Cancer-Related Pain," provides a more detailed discussion of pain, occupational therapy assessment, and intervention for individuals with cancer.)

Cognitive deficits

The high prevalence of cognitive deficits among children with cancer and the fact that these deficits may emerge over the course of the cancer care continuum highlight the importance of repeated monitoring of a child's cognitive abilities and related occupational performance across multiple contexts, including school and home. Comprehensive neurocognitive evaluation and follow-up are recommended for children with cancer who are at risk for cognitive impairments. However, this may not always be available or feasible.

Feasible and reliable neurocognitive screening batteries that are effective in screening for neuropsychological deficits among children with cancer (Krull et al., 2008) include the Digit Span Test (Wechsler, 1991), the Verbal Fluency Test (Benton et al., 1983), the Grooved Pegboard Test (Wang et al., 2011), and the Trail Making Test (Trites, 1977). Additionally, occupational therapy practitioners have access to several performance-based cognitive assessments designed to assess functional–cognitive skills among children with cancer. These measures (listed in Table 4.3) assess the child's capacity to participate in relevant everyday life activities, such as school-related and ADL tasks, and can provide valuable insight into a child's cognitive functioning. For example, the Children's Kitchen Task Assessment (Rocke et al., 2008) can be used with children ages 7–12 years to measure EF through the child's completion of the real-world, functional task of following a recipe to make play dough. Results of these occupational performance assessments can be combined with neuropsychological assessments of attention, EF, and memory for intervention planning.

Educational and developmental achievement

Because children with cancer are at substantial risk for difficulties with educational activities, occupational therapy practitioners should begin addressing a child's school participation at diagnosis with continued monitoring through all phases of the cancer treatment continuum. This includes reintegration to school in the treatment or acute post-treatment phases and into the survivorship phase as the child advances into higher grades, which may present new challenges.

Assessments effective in identifying school-based performance restrictions and performance-based strengths and weaknesses are listed in Table 4.3. The assessment's emphasis for occupational therapy practitioners should include performance skills, such as

- Neuromusculoskeletal functions (e.g., activity tolerance, impairments in balance or coordination),
- Sensory performance (e.g., visual impairments, neuropathy), and
- Mental functions (e.g., functional–cognitive skills, social preparedness).

These assessments—as well as communication with the child and the child's family, medical team, and school team—assist the occupational therapy practitioner in developing a plan to facilitate the child's reintegration to school, including recommendations for accommodations, modifications, special education services, or therapy services.

Children with cancer may qualify for educational supports, including accommodations or modifications through Section 504 of the Rehabilitation Act of 1973 (P. L. 93-112). Other children may be eligible for educational services under the "Other Health Impairment" category of an IEP through the Individuals With Disabilities Education Improvement Act of 2004 (P. L. 108-446). As with other aspects of a child's functional abilities, the child's school performance and related support needs may change over time and should be monitored closely (Barkon et al., 2007; Flegle & Edelbrock, 2019).

Because of the known risk of developmental delays resulting from cancer diagnosis and treatment, all children with cancer who are younger than 3 years should be referred for evaluation for early intervention services as early as possible in the cancer care continuum (Harman, 2018). Developmental assessments outlined in Table 4.3 will assist the occupational therapy practitioner in identifying a child who might have or be at risk for developmental delays so that appropriate recommendations for therapy services, caregiver education, or other developmental programming can be provided. Case Example 4.2 provides an

CASE EXAMPLE 4.2. CALEB: EARLY OCCUPATIONAL THERAPY INTERVENTION FOR AN INFANT WITH CANCER

Caleb was 2 months old when he was diagnosed with infantile acute lymphoblastic leukemia. Leading up to diagnosis, he had a short history of irritability, fever, and poor breastfeeding. He was taken to a local hospital, and his complete blood count showed a white blood cell count of 125,000 and thrombocytopenia.

Shortly after diagnosis, Caleb was transferred to a specialty children's hospital 4 hours away from his family's home, underwent surgical replacement of a central line, and began a chemotherapy treatment protocol that required him to be hospitalized frequently for treatment and management of treatment-related side effects. Within a few days of treatment initiation, he experienced neutropenia and immunosuppression, which necessitated strict infection control precautions. He also required red blood cell and platelet transfusions intermittently as a result of low hemoglobin and thrombocytopenia; his platelet transfusion threshold was more than 20,000. He experienced pain and nausea and received medications, including morphine, gabapentin, ondansetron, and Benadryl, some of which made him sleepy.

Supportive care services were consulted, including child life, psychology, music therapy, speech therapy, physical therapy, and occupational therapy. At the occupational therapy evaluation, Caleb's mother reported that she felt that Caleb had been developing good head and neck control and kicked his legs frequently before starting chemotherapy, but he seemed weak and tired all the time and did not kick his legs as much since chemotherapy. She also reported that he did not seem to be attending to objects and noises as well as he had been.

The occupational therapist completed selected subtests of the Peabody Developmental Motor Scales (PDMS; Folio & Fewell, 2000). Although results indicated that Caleb's gross motor and fine motor skills were within the average range (composite Fine Motor Quotient of 91, within 1.5 standard deviations from the mean), many diagnosis- and treatment-related factors increased Caleb's risk for developmental delays, including his age, active chemotherapy treatment, illness (e.g., nausea, pain, fatigue), frequent hospitalizations, limited opportunities for participation in age-appropriate play, and separation from family (Caleb's father and older brother remained at home so that his father could work and his brother could attend school).

The occupational therapist developed a care plan that included direct therapy services once per week. Occupational therapy sessions focused on promoting Caleb's fine motor, visual–motor integration, and adaptive skills by educating caregivers and closely monitoring for developmental delay and restrictions in occupational performance. The therapist monitored Caleb's medical treatment course, laboratory values, and

activity and behavior during sessions to guide clinical decision making about the need for occupational therapy modifications.

Nine months postdiagnosis, Caleb was cleared to return home and complete his cancer treatment on an outpatient basis through a local children's hospital. Before his return home, the hospital-based rehabilitation team made a referral for early intervention services, including occupational therapy, physical therapy, and speech therapy, in Caleb's community. Once home, Caleb received early intervention services and continued to achieve age-appropriate developmental skills. His parents appreciated having the services to monitor Caleb's skills closely while he continued to receive chemotherapy and to guide the family in their interactions and play with him.

Unfortunately, Caleb developed pneumonia while he was at home, so he required a 2-week stay in the intensive care unit at a specialty children's hospital, which included intubation and placement of a nasogastric (NG) tube. After extubation, rehabilitation services were consulted. The occupational therapist evaluated Caleb's developmental skills using subtests of the PDMS. Results indicated that Caleb had below-average skills in the areas of grasping and visual–motor integration (composite Fine Motor Quotient score of 85, greater than 1.5 standard deviations below the mean). The therapist also noted poor endurance, which limited Caleb's participation in age-appropriate play and self-care activities.

Direct occupational therapy services were initiated 3–5 times per week while Caleb remained in the hospital to recuperate and receive chemotherapy treatment. The occupational therapist was mindful of Caleb's central line and NG tubing during sessions and adhered to infection control precautions. Because of Caleb's ongoing risk of thrombocytopenia and low hemoglobin as well as periods of illness, the therapist monitored Caleb, his laboratory values, and his activity level and behaviors closely, modifying sessions as needed.

For example, on days when Caleb was nauseous and had critically low platelet levels, the occupational therapist focused the session more on education and demonstrating for Caleb's mother activities that they could complete when he was feeling better. Goals developed by the therapist in collaboration with the family focused on Caleb's return to baseline visual–motor integration and fine motor skills, improved activity tolerance, and increased upper-body and proximal strength to promote participation in age-appropriate self-care and play activities.

During this episode of care, Caleb experienced chemotherapy-related neuropathic pain, which was managed with gabapentin and massage therapy. He received high doses of steroids, which resulted in irritability and

(Continued)

CASE EXAMPLE 4.2. CALEB: EARLY OCCUPATIONAL THERAPY INTERVENTION FOR AN INFANT WITH CANCER *(Cont.)*

reluctance to engage in therapy sessions. The occupational therapy team collaborated with Caleb's parents to identify a therapy schedule that worked best for Caleb (he was more active and playful in the mornings) and to identify activities that were highly motivating for him. For example, Caleb was highly motivated by music, so the occupational therapist and music therapist collaborated frequently during sessions.

At just over a year postdiagnosis, Caleb experienced a relapse of his disease. His medical team determined that he required an SCT. At 1.5 years old, Caleb received an allogeneic haploidentical hematopoietic SCT. His father was his donor.

Caleb's father and brother moved to live near the hospital and join Caleb's mother while he underwent the transplant. Caleb participated in a pretransplant occupational therapy evaluation focused on

- Family education in the role of occupational therapy services during transplant,
- Direct assessment of Caleb's adaptive and social skills development, and
- Ongoing assessment of his fine motor skills and visual–motor integration.

His scores on the PDMS Grasping and Visual–Motor Integration subtests were in the *poor* category, with a composite Fine Motor Quotient score of 70 (more than 1.5 standard deviations below the mean).

The occupational therapist's plan of care included direct sessions 3–5 times per week to address ongoing developmental delays, feeding-related sensory and behavioral challenges, muscle weakness, and decreased endurance. During the acute inpatient transplant phase, Caleb experienced pancytopenia and ongoing nutritional support through his NG tube because of poor intake by mouth. Occupational therapy practitioners monitored Caleb for symptoms that would necessitate modification of occupational therapy sessions, including nausea, new-onset weakness or fatigue, petechiae, palor, and tachycardia.

On Day 20, Caleb experienced tachycardia, tachypnea, and fever and was transferred to the pediatric intensive care unit for monitoring. The occupational therapist observed further regression of Caleb's developmental skills and his upper body and proximal strength. After discussion with the medical team and Caleb's parents, occupational therapy services were continued with careful monitoring of vital signs and laboratory values and regular collaboration with the medical team.

On Day 42, Caleb was discharged from the inpatient transplant unit and referred to outpatient occupational therapy because of continued developmental delays and ongoing restrictions in age-appropriate activities. He continued to received therapy 2–3 times per week and progressed toward developmental visual–motor integration, fine motor, and strength goals. He enjoyed playing with his big brother and was motivated by his brother during his occupational therapy sessions and home programing.

At Day 100, Caleb's medical team deemed him healthy enough to return home. He was reevaluated with the PDMS. Results of both the Grasping and the Visual–Motor Integration subtests indicated that he had improved in specific aspects of his visual–motor integration and grasping performance but remained in the below-average range (Fine Motor Quotient score of 83, more than 1.5 standard deviations below the mean). A referral was made to a pediatric outpatient clinic in Caleb's home community where he could receive occupational therapy, physical therapy, and speech therapy services twice per week. The hospital-based occupational therapy practitioner provided the new outpatient occupational therapy practitioner with information on Caleb's medical history, evaluation results, current goals, and goal progress as well as infection control guidelines and the potential for symptom-based activity modifications. By 1 year posttransplant, Caleb was making great progress in therapies and enjoying being at home with his family.

---

example of the occupational therapist's role in monitoring and supporting the development of an infant with cancer.

OCCUPATIONAL THERAPY INTERVENTIONS FOR CHILDREN WITH CANCER

Table 4.4 provides an overview of the role of occupational therapy across the pediatric cancer care continuum. The need for rehabilitation services for children with cancer has been well established; however, because of the relative novelty of the role of occupational therapy in pediatric oncology, published evidence describing effective occupational therapy intervention programs for this population is limited. In the absence of specific descriptions of

pediatric oncology occupational therapy interventions, the evidence-based principles that guide intervention for other conditions can be used. For example, children with brain tumors who experience hemiplegia may benefit from neuromuscular interventions that are similar to those designed for children with acquired brain injuries (Sparrow et al., 2017).

Additionally, occupational therapy practitioners can draw on relevant established interventions from other disciplines to guide practice. For instance, exercise and physical activity reduce fatigue and increase strength and QoL for children with cancer (Baumann et al., 2013; see Table 4.4), and nonpharmacological pain management strategies, including distraction, cognitive–behavioral therapy, and deep breathing exercises, are effective in managing pain among children with cancer (Jibb et al., 2015).

TABLE 4.4.   Overview of the Role of Occupational Therapy Across the Cancer Care Continuum Among Children With Cancer

STAGE OF CANCER CARE CONTINUUM	ROLE OF OCCUPATIONAL THERAPY
Prevention	▪ Be aware of the signs and symptoms of pediatric cancer and advocate for medical evaluation if concerns arise. ▪ Advocate for health care programs and systems that promote early detection and for screening and wellness programs for children who are at risk for cancer.
Diagnosis	▪ Provide direct occupational therapy services, if needed. ▪ Provide anticipatory guidance and education about the function and role of occupational therapy. ▪ Discuss diagnosis-related or treatment-related risk factors for functional limitations. ▪ Prescribe a prehabilitative therapy program.

Treatment	▪ Identify and mitigate the negative effects of the diagnosis and related treatments on occupational performance.
	▪ Prevent performance restrictions and support age-appropriate development and participation by
	  • Closely monitoring children with known risk factors,
	  • Providing preventive education and direct interventions to promote typical development, and
	  • Supporting participation in age-appropriate occupations.
	▪ For children who experience functional limitations, provide rehabilitative, habilitative, and compensatory intervention.

Survivorship	▪ Provide rehabilitative management of occupational performance restrictions that result from the long-term sequelae of childhood cancer. ▪ Help the child and family navigate occupational transitions from childhood through adolescence across environments, including home, community, and school.

End-of-life care	▪ Use a holistic and family-centered approach.
	▪ Identify needs of children and their families at end of life to
	  • Improve symptom management,
	  • Facilitate participation in meaningful activities, and
	  • Improve QoL of the child and family.

Note. QoL = quality of life.

Generally, occupational therapy interventions for children with cancer may include rehabilitative, habilitative, or preventative services focused on mitigating negative effects of treatment. In particular, a focus of intervention may include

▪ ADL training and use of adaptive equipment;
▪ Early intervention services;
▪ Nonpharmacologic pain management;
▪ Sensory interventions;
▪ Visual–motor integration training;
▪ Fine motor training;
▪ Functional–cognitive intervention;
▪ School liaising;
▪ Therapeutic exercise (see Figure 4.2)
▪ Compensatory visual training;
▪ Neuromuscular reeducation and motor learning training; and
▪ Upper-extremity orthotic, wheelchair, or prosthesis fitting and training.

Table 4.5 provides additional occupational therapy intervention resources for children with cancer.

Exhibit 4.3 summarizes precautions that occupational therapy practitioners should take when providing services to children with cancer. Unlike a child with a brain injury or orthopedic injury whose function is generally expected to continue to improve with rehabilitation, a child with cancer may have multiple changes in functional abilities during the treatment continuum. Periods of illness, side effects of treatment, and recurrences of disease can limit a child's

function and disrupt their rehabilitation progress. In these instances, it is important for occupational therapy practitioners to be flexible and modify interventions and goals to reflect the child's current occupational performance levels.

Additionally, the occupational therapy practitioner should closely monitor the child's medical status for symptoms that would necessitate modifying occupational therapy interventions or placing them on hold, such as critically low laboratory values, illness, or pain. Acute incidences of severe pain, neurological changes, or extreme illness are indicative of a medical emergency or recurrence of disease and require immediate medical attention.

The duration of occupational therapy involvement differs depending on the length of a child's treatment protocol, side effects of treatment, and severity of functional impairment. Children with PFS and significant neurological compromise, for example, may require years of intensive occupational therapy services followed by long-term follow-up as they transition through childhood (Robertson et al., 2006).

Family-Centered Services and Education

Important components of occupational therapy intervention for the child with cancer are family-centered services and education. Provision of family-centered services (services that are consumer driven and competency enhancing; Case-Smith, 2010) and provision of education to the child and family serve to motivate and empower the family to take an active role in their child's rehabilitation and wellness.

FIGURE 4.2. A 5-year-old survivor of pineoblastoma with severe ataxia participates in yoga during occupational therapy.

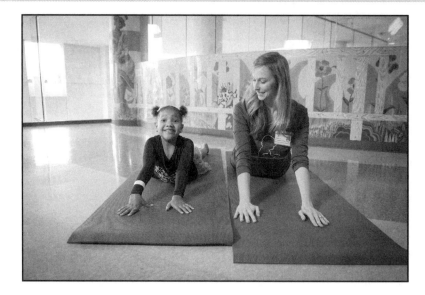

Source. Jere Parobeck. Used with permission.

TABLE 4.5. Suggested Occupational Therapy Interventions for Children With Cancer

PROBLEM	INTERVENTION (RESOURCE)
Pain	■ Mirror therapy (Anghelescu et al., 2016) ■ Physical positioning ■ Distraction ■ Cognitive–behavioral therapy ■ Deep breathing (Jibb et al., 2015) ■ Child and parent education
Developmental delay	■ Developmentally structured and sequenced play tasks ■ Environmental supports for hospital rooms or housing facilities (e.g., floor mats, developmentally appropriate toys and books) ■ Parent education
Chemotherapy-induced peripheral neuropathy	■ Gentle stretching and active ROM, including weight bearing, if tolerated ■ Desensitization ■ Fine motor coordination and strengthening through play-based tasks ■ Handwriting training ■ Massage ■ Compensatory training, including task or environmental modification ■ Education on home exercise programs, self-management strategies, and symptoms to watch for
Weakness, fatigue, and poor endurance	■ Exercise (Baumann et al., 2013) ■ Yoga (Wurz et al., 2014) ■ Play ■ ADL participation (Bauman et al., 2010) ■ Child and parent education in energy conservation and self-management strategies
Sensory impairment, including vision and hearing loss	■ Compensatory training ■ Equipment training (low-vision equipment, FM systems) ■ School recommendations ■ Referrals to ophthalmology and certified low-vision specialists ■ Referrals to audiology specialists

(Continued)

TABLE 4.5.   Suggested Occupational Therapy Interventions for Children With Cancer *(Cont.)*

PROBLEM	INTERVENTION (RESOURCE)
C-GVHD	■ Stretching ■ Exercise and strengthening, including education in home exercise programs ■ Orthotics ■ Massage ■ Use of topical ointments ■ Functional motor training and dexterity training, splinting (Carenzio et al., 2007; Couriel et al., 2006; Smith et al., 2015) ■ Education in use of adaptive equipment or compensatory strategies ■ Education in positioning techniques
Neuromuscular impairment	■ Seating and positioning ■ Feeding interventions, including positioning, adaptive equipment, oral sensory exploration through play, and neuromuscular interventions ■ Stretching ■ Weight bearing ■ ADL training ■ Motor learning (Sparrow et al., 2017)
Cognitive impairments	■ Mass practice, metacognitive strategy training, and cognitive–behavioral training (Butler et al., 2008) ■ Cognitive training (Castellino et al., 2014) ■ Computerized, home-based cognitive training programs (Conklin et al., 2017; Kesler et al., 2011)
Psychosocial issues	■ Cognitive–behavioral therapy (Kazak et al., 2004) ■ Exercise (National Comprehensive Cancer Network, 2017) ■ Yoga (Thygeson et al., 2010)

Note. ADL = activities of daily living; C-GVHD = chronic graft-versus-host disease; FM = fine motor; ROM = range of motion.

EXHIBIT 4.3.   Pediatric Oncology Occupational Therapy Considerations

■ Diagnoses, treatments, and contextual influences can result in restrictions in occupational performance and quality of life (QoL) for a child with cancer.
■ Multidisciplinary collaboration with the child's medical providers, rehabilitation providers, and other members of the child's care team is best practice.
■ Adhere strictly to infection control procedures.
■ During assessment and intervention, continuously monitor for illness (e.g., nausea, pain, headache, pallor, bruising, petechia, abnormal resting vitals, fatigue), and modify interventions as needed.
■ A child's occupational performance may fluctuate, so the occupational therapy plan of care should include ongoing monitoring of the child's participation and QoL, coordination with other care providers as needed, and adjustments made to reflect the child's current performance and needs.
■ Because of the known risk of developmental delays after a cancer diagnosis and treatment, all children with cancer under the age of 3 years should be referred for early intervention screenings as early as possible in the cancer care continuum (Harman, 2018).
■ Cancer treatment may result in prolonged hospitalization or time away from home and school. Promote normalization of the unnatural environment by recommending supplies and equipment and providing child and parent education to support optimal development and to maximize age-appropriate participation.
■ Develop a rapport with the parent and child to promote their active participation in the rehabilitation process.

Occupational therapy practitioners should have compassionate, supportive, and honest conversations with children and families about risk factors and functional implications of the child's disease, the child's rehabilitation prognosis, the role of occupational therapy in the child's cancer care continuum, goal setting, and progress toward goals.

Education for the child should be in keeping with the child's level of understanding of the illness and should be respectful of the level of information that parents would like the child to have. Awareness of and sensitivity to optimal timing for education are also central to ensure that the family and child are ready to receive the information. For example, addressing ADLs or transfer training may not be a priority for a family right after an oncologist reviews unfavorable test results with them.

End-of-Life Care

At the end of life, children with cancer may experience symptoms such as pain, fatigue, reduced mobility, anxiety, depression, and fear (Jalmsell et al., 2006). During this time, high symptom burden and substantial suffering are possible (Wolfe et al., 2000). All occupational therapy services for children with cancer should include a blend of holistic, occupation-based models, including family-centered care, occupation as an intervention means, and neurodevelopmental treatment. However, this is particularly important during end-of-life care.

The World Health Organization (2019) defines *pediatric palliative care* as the active total care of the child's body, mind, and spirit and also involves giving support to the family. Occupational therapy practitioners' role in palliative care is to support the child's participation in activities that are meaningful, including those related to school activities, community activities, play, and mobility. To enable participation, practitioners may build on existing skills or facilitate maintenance of current skills, provide pain management services, support physical and psychosocial needs, provide education in energy conservation strategies, adapt the environment to compensate for loss of physical or cognitive skills, and support meaningful family interactions (Tester, 2006). Chapter 13, "Palliative Care and Hospice," provides an overview of end-of-life services and the role of occupational therapy.

SUMMARY

Children with cancer and long-term survivors of childhood cancer are at risk for performance restrictions throughout the cancer care continuum and across multiple settings and environments. Occupational therapy practitioners have a valuable role in monitoring for such restrictions and in providing timely and evidence-based services that support-age appropriate development and participation in meaningful ADLs, play, and educational activities, which should result in improved QoL for the child with cancer. To be maximally effective, occupational therapy practitioners should work to increase clients' and oncology providers' awareness of available occupational therapy services and help develop evidence-based programming and interventions specifically designed for children with cancer.

ACKNOWLEDGMENTS

Thank you to Cherise Guess for her assistance with editing the content.

REFERENCES

American Occupational Therapy Association. (2014). Occupational therapy practice framework: Domain and process (3rd ed.). *American Journal of Occupational Therapy, 68*(Suppl. 1), S1–S48. https://doi.org/10.5014/ajot.2014.682006

Anderson, S., Boigon, S., Davis, K., & DeWaard, C. (2007). *The Oregon Project for Visually Impaired and Blind Preschool Children* (6th ed.). Medford: Southern Oregon Education Service District.

Anghelescu, D. L., Faughnan, L. G., Jeha, S., Relling, M. V., Hinds, P. S., Sandlund, J. T., . . . Pui, C.-H. (2011). Neuropathic pain during treatment for childhood acute lymphoblastic leukemia. *Pediatric Blood and Cancer, 57,* 1147–1153. https://doi.org/10.1002/pbc.23039

Anghelescu, D. L., Kelly, C. N., Steen, B. D., Wu, J., Wu, H., DeFeo, B. M., . . . Burgoyne, L. (2016). Mirror therapy for phantom limb pain at a pediatric oncology institution. *Rehabilitation Oncology, 34,* 104–110. https://doi.org/10.1097/01.reo.0000000000000022

Antonini, T. N., Ris, M. D., Grosshans, D. R., Mahajan, A., Okcu, M. F., Chintagumpala, M., . . . Kahalley, L. S. (2017). Attention, processing speed, and executive functioning in pediatric brain tumor survivors treated with proton beam radiation therapy. *Radiotherapy and Oncology, 124,* 89–97. https://doi.org/10.1016/j.radonc.2017.06.010

Argyriou, A. A., Assimakopoulos, K., Iconomou, G., Giannakopoulou, F., & Kalofonos, H. P. (2011). Either called "chemobrain" or "chemofog," the long-term chemotherapy-induced cognitive decline in cancer survivors is real. *Journal of Pain and Symptom Management, 41,* 126–139. https://doi.org/10.1016/j.jpainsymman.2010.04.021

Armenian, S. H., Sun, C.-L., Kawashima, T., Arora, M., Leisenring, W., Sklar, C. A., . . . Mills, G. (2011). Long-term health-related outcomes in survivors of childhood cancer treated with HSCT versus conventional therapy: A report from the Bone Marrow Transplant Survivor Study (BMTSS) and Childhood Cancer Survivor Study (CCSS). *Blood, 118,* 1413–1420. https://doi.org/10.1182/blood-2011-01-331835

Armstrong, G. T., Liu, Q., Yasui, Y., Huang, S., Ness, K. K., Leisenring, W., . . . Stovall, M. (2009). Long-term outcomes among adult survivors of childhood central nervous system malignancies in the Childhood Cancer Survivor Study. *Journal of the National Cancer Institute, 101,* 946–958. https://doi.org/10.1093/jnci/djp148

Baird, K., Cooke, K., & Schultz, K. R. (2010). Chronic craft-versus-host disease (GVHD) in children. *Pediatric Clinics of North America, 57,* 297–322. https://doi.org/10.1016/j.pcl.2009.11.003

Barkon, B., Scheboth, S., & Jackacki, R. (2007). Characterizing neurobehavioral and social causes of school problems in survivors of pediatric brain tumors: The Survivor Education and Reintegration Support Program [Abstract]. *Neuro-Oncology, 9,* 569.

Bass, J. K., & Bhagat, S. P. (2014). Challenges in ototoxicity monitoring in the pediatric oncology population. *Journal of the American Academy of Audiology, 25,* 760–774. https://doi.org/10.3766/jaaa.25.8.6

Bass, J. K., Hua, C.-H., Huang, J., Onar-Thomas, A., Ness, K. K., Jones, S., . . . Merchant, T. E. (2016). Hearing loss in patients who received cranial radiation therapy for childhood cancer. *Journal of Clinical Oncology, 34,* 1248–1255. https://doi.org/10.1200/JCO.2015.63.6738

Baumann, F. T., Bloch, W., & Beulertz, J. (2013). Clinical exercise interventions in pediatric oncology: A systematic review. *Pediatric Research, 74,* 366–374. https://doi.org/10.1038/pr.2013.123

Baumann, F. T., Kraut, L., Schule, K., Bloch, W., & Fauser, A. A. (2010). A controlled randomized study examining the effects of exercise therapy on patients undergoing haematopoietic stem cell transplantation. *Bone Marrow Transplant, 45,* 355–362. https://doi.org/10.1038/bmt.2009.163

Bayley, N. (2005). *Bayley Scales of Infant and Toddler Development* (3rd ed.). San Antonio: Pearson.

Beery, K. E., Buktenica, N. A., & Beery, N. A. (2010). *Beery–Buktenica Developmental Test of Visual–Motor Integration* (6th ed.). New York: Pearson Assessments.

Benton, A. L., Hamsher, K. D., & Sivan, A. (1983). *Multilingual Aphasia Examination* (3rd ed.). Iowa City, IA: AJA Associates.

Berg, C., & LaVesser, P. (2006). The Preschool Activity Card Sort. *OTJR: Occupation, Participation and Health, 26,* 143–151. https://doi.org/10.1177/153944920602600404

Berger, A. M., Mooney, K., Alvarez-Perez, A., Breitbart, W. S., Carpenter, K. M., Cella, D., . . . Smith, C. (2015). Cancer-related fatigue, Version 2.2015. *Journal of the National Comprehensive Cancer Network, 13,* 1012–1039. https://doi.org/10.6004/jnccn.2015.0122

Binning, M. J., Liu, J. K., Kestle, J. R. W., Brockmeyer, D. L., & Walker, M. L. (2007). Optic pathway gliomas: A review. *Neurosurgical Focus, 23,* E2. https://doi.org/10.3171/FOC-07/11/E2

Bornstein, M. H., Scrimin S., Putnik, D., Capello, F., Haynes, O. M., de Falco, S., . . . Pillon, M. (2012). Neurodevelopmental functions in very young children undergoing treatment for non-CMS cancers. *Journal of Pediatric Psychology, 37,* 660–673. https://doi.org/10.1093/jpepsy/jss003

Bowyer, P., Ross, M., Schwartz, O., Kielhofner, G., & Kramer, J. (2005). *The Short Child Occupational Profile (Version 2.1).* Chicago: Model of Human Occupation Clearinghouse.

Brinkman, T. M., Bass, J. K., Li, Z., Ness, K. K., Gajjar, A., Pappo, A. S., . . . Gurney, J. G. (2015). Treatment-induced hearing loss and adult social outcomes in survivors of childhood CNS and non-CNS solid tumors: Results from the St. Jude Lifetime Cohort Study. *Cancer, 121,* 4053–4061. https://doi.org/10.1002/cncr.29604

Brock, P. R., Knight, K. R., Freyer, D. R., Campbell, K. C. M., Steyger, P. S., Blakley, B. W., . . . Neuwelt, E. A. (2012). Platinum-induced ototoxicity in children: A consensus review on mechanisms, predisposition, and protection, including a new International Society of Pediatric Oncology Boston Ototoxicity Scale. *Journal of Clinical Oncology, 30,* 2408–2417. https://doi.org/10.1200/JCO.2011.39.1110

Bruininks, R. H. (2005). *Bruininks–Oseretsky Test of Motor Proficiency.* Circle Pines, MN: AGS Publishing.

Butler, R. W., Copeland, D. R., Fairclough, D. L., Mulhern, R. K., Katz, E. R, Kazak, A. E., . . . Sahler, O. J. Z. (2008). A multicenter, randomized clinical trial of a cognitive remediation program for childhood survivors of a pediatric malignancy. *Journal of Consulting and Clinical Psychology, 76,* 367–378. https://doi.org/10.1037/0022-006X.76.3.367

Carenzio, G., Gherardi, P., Bardoni, M. T., Zecca, M., Bonetti, F., Locatelli, F., & Dalla, E. T. (2007). Rehabilitation of chronic graft versus host disease in children: A clinical series. *Europa Medicophysica, 43*(4), 445–450.

Carpenter, P. A. (2011). How I conduct a comprehensive chronic graft-versus-host disease assessment. *Blood, 118,* 2679–2687. https://doi.org/10.1182/blood-2011-04-314815

Case-Smith, J. (2010). Development of childhood occupations. In J. Case-Smith & J. O'Brien (Eds.), *Occupational therapy for children* (6th ed., pp. 56–83). St. Louis: Mosby.

Castellino, S. M., Ullrich, N. J., Whelen, M. J., & Lange, B. J. (2014). Developing interventions for cancer-related cognitive dysfunction in childhood cancer survivors. *Journal of the National Cancer Institute, 106,* dju186. https://doi.org/10.1093/jnci/dju186

Children's Oncology Group. (2013). *Long-term follow-up guidelines for survivors of childhood, adolescent and young adult cancers, Version 4.0.* Monrovia, CA: Author. Retrieved from www.survivorshipguidelines.org.

Conklin, H. M., Ashford, J. M., Clark, K. N., Martin-Elbahesh, K., Hardy, K. K., Merchant, T. E., . . . & Zhang, H. (2017). Long-term efficacy of computerized cognitive training among survivors of childhood cancer: A single-blind randomized controlled trial. *Journal of Pediatric Psychology, 42,* 220–231. https://doi.org/10.1093/jpepsy/jsw057

Conklin, H. M., Ashford, J. M., Di Pinto, M., Vaughan, C. G., Gioia, G. A., Merchant, T. E., . . . Wu, S. (2013). Computerized assessment of cognitive late effects among adolescent brain tumor survivors. *Journal of Neuro-Oncology, 113,* 333–340. https://doi.org/10.1007/s11060-013-1123-5

Coster, W., Coster, W., Deeney, T. A., Haley, S., & Haltiwanger, J. (1998). *School Function Assessment.* San Antonio: Psychological Corporation.

Couriel, D., Carpenter, P. A., Cutler, C., Bolaños-Meade, J., Treister, N. S., Gea-Banacloche, J., . . . Flowers, M. E. D. (2006). Ancillary therapy and supportive care of chronic graft-versus-host disease: National Institutes of Health Consensus Development Project on Criteria for Clinical Trials in Chronic Graft-Versus-Host Disease: V. Ancillary Therapy and Supportive Care Working Group report. *Biology of Blood and Marrow Transplantation, 12,* 375–396. https://doi.org/10.1016/j.bbmt.2006.02.003

Demers, C., Gélinas, I., & Carret, A.-S. (2015). Activities of daily living in survivors of childhood brain tumor. *American Journal of Occupational Therapy, 70,* 7001220040. https://doi.org/10.5014/ajot.2016.014993

Duffner, P. K. (2004). Long-term effects of radiation therapy on cognitive and endocrine function in children with leukemia and brain tumors. *Neurologist, 10,* 293–310. https://doi.org/10.1097/01.nrl.0000144287.35993.96

Dunn, W. (2014). *Sensory Profile 2 user's manual.* Bloomington, MN: Pearson.

Ermoian, R., Fogh, S. E., Braunstein, S., Mishra, K. M., Kun, L. E., & Haas-Kogan, D. A. (2016). General principles of radiation oncology. In R. Pizzo & D. Poplack (Eds.), *Principles and practice of pediatric oncology* (6th ed., pp. 362–377). Philidapha: Wolters Kluwer.

Fahnehjelm, K. T., Törnquist, A. L., Olsson, M., Winiarski, J., & Ek, U. (2018). Visual perceptual skills and visual motor integration in children and adolescents after allogeneic hematopoietic stem cell transplantation. *Pediatric Transplantation, 22,* e13117. https://doi.org/10.1111/petr.13117

Filipovich, A. H., Weisdorf, D., Pavletic, S., Socie, G., Wingard, J. R., Lee, S. J., . . . Cowen, E. W. (2005). National Institutes of Health Consensus Development Project on Criteria for Clinical Trials in Chronic Graft-Versus-Host Disease: I. Diagnosis and Staging Working Group report. *Biology of Blood and Marrow Transplantation, 11,* 945–956. https://doi.org/10.1016/j.bbmt.2005.09.004

Flegle, J. H., & Edelbrock, C. M. (2019). Best practices for supporting students with other health impairments. In G. Frolek Clark, J. Rioux, & B. E. Chandler (Eds.), *Best practices for occupational therapy in schools* (2nd ed., pp. 289–295). Bethesda, MD: AOTA Press.

Fleming, C. A. K., Cohen, J., Murphy, A., Wakefield, C. E., Cohn, R. J., & Naumann, F. L. (2015). Parent feeding interactions and practices during childhood cancer treatment: A qualitative investigation. *Appetite, 89,* 219–225. https://doi.org/10.1016/j.appet.2014.12.225

Folio, M. R., & Fewell, R. R. (2000). *Peabody Developmental Motor Scales: Examiner's manual.* Austin, TX: Pro-Ed.

Gelabert-González, M., & Fernández-Villa, J. (2001). Mutism after posterior fossa surgery: Review of the literature. *Clinical Neurology and Neurosurgery, 103*(2), 111–114. https://doi.org/10.1016/s0303-8467(01)00125-1

Gilchrist, L. (2012). Chemotherapy-induced peripheral neuropathy in pediatric cancer patients. *Seminars in Pediatric Neurology, 19,* 9–17. https://doi.org/10.1016/j.spen.2012.02.011

Gilchrist, L. S., & Tanner, L. (2013). The Pediatric-Modified Total Neuropathy Score: A reliable and valid measure of chemotherapy-induced peripheral neuropathy in children with non-CNS cancers. *Support Care Cancer, 21,* 847–856. https://doi.org/10.1007/s00520-012-1591-8

Gilchrist, L., & Tanner, L. R. (2017). Safety of symptom-based modification of physical therapy interventions in pediatric oncology patients with and without low blood counts. *Rehabilitation Oncology, 35,* 3–8. https://doi.org/10.1097/01.REO.0000000000000042

Graef, D. M., Phipps, S., Parris, K. R., Martin-Elbahesh, K., Huang, L., Zhang, H., & Crabtree, V. M. (2016). Sleepiness, fatigue, behavioral functioning, and quality of life in survivors of childhood hematopoietic stem cell transplant. *Journal of Pediatric Psychology, 4,* 600–609. https://doi.org/10.1093/jpepsy/jsw011

Green, J. L., Knight, S. J., McCarthy, M., & De Luca, C. R. (2013). Motor functioning during and following treatment with chemotherapy for pediatric acute lymphoblastic leukemia. *Pediatric Blood and Cancer, 60,* 1261–1266. https://doi.org/10.1002/pbc.24537

Gurney, J. G., Krull, K. R., Kadan-Lottick, N., Nicholson, H. S., Nathan, P. C., Zebrack, B., . . . Ness, K. K. (2009). Social outcomes in the Childhood Cancer Survivor Study cohort. *Journal of Clinical Oncology, 27,* 2390–2395. https://doi.org/10.1200/JCO.2008.21.1458

Gurney, J. G., Ness, K. K., Rosenthal, J., Forman, S. J., Bhatia, S., & Baker, K. S. (2006). Visual, auditory, sensory, and motor impairments in long-term survivors of hematopoietic stem cell transplantation performed in childhood. *Cancer, 106,* 1402–1408. https://doi.org/10.1002/cncr.21752

Haley, S. M. (1992). *Pediatric Evaluation of Disability Inventory (PEDI): Development, standardization and administration manual.* Boston: PEDI Resarch Group.

Harman, J. L., Wise, J., & Willard, V. W. (2018). Early intervention for infants and toddlers: Applications for pediatric oncology. *Pediatric Blood and Cancer, 65,* e26921. https://doi.org/10.1002/pbc.26921

Hausheer, F. H., Schilsky, R. L., Bain, S., Berghorn, E. J., & Lieberman, F. (2006). Diagnosis, management, and evaluation of chemotherapy-induced peripheral neuropathy. *Seminars in Oncology, 33,* 15–49. https://doi.org/10.1053/j.seminoncol.2005.12.010

Heden, L., Poder, U., von Essen, L., & Ljungman, G. (2013). Parents' perceptions of their child's symptom burden during and after cancer treatment. *Journal of Pain and Symptom Management, 46,* 366–375. https://doi.org/10.1016/j.jpainsymman.2012.09.012

Hicks, C. L., von Baeyer, C. L., Spafford, P. A., van Korlaar, I., & Goodenough, B. (2001). The Faces Pain Scale–Revised: Toward a common metric in pediatric pain measurement. *Pain, 93,* 173–183. https://doi.org/10.1016/s0304-3959(01)00314-1

Hinds, P. S., Nuss, S. L., Ruccione, K. S., Withycombe, J. S., Jacobs, S., DeLuca, H., . . . DeWalt, D. A. (2013). PROMIS pediatric measures in pediatric oncology: Valid and clinically feasible indicators of patient-reported outcomes. *Pediatric Blood and Cancer, 60,* 402–408. https://doi.org/10.1002/pbc.24233

Hockenberry, M., Krull, K., Moore, K., Gregurich, M. A., Casey, M. E., & Kaemingk, K. (2007). Longitudinal evaluation of fine motor skills in children with leukemia. *Journal of Pediatric Hematology/Oncology, 29,* 535–539. https://doi.org/10.1097/MPH.0b013e3180f61b92

Howlader, N., Noone, A., Krapcho, M., Miller, D., Brest, A., Yu, M., . . . Croning, K. A. (Eds). (2019). *SEER cancer statistics review, 1975–2016.* Bethesda, MD: National Cancer Institute. Retrieved from https://seer.cancer.gov/csr/1975_2016

Hua, C., Bass, J. K., Khan, R., Kun, L. E., & Merchant, T. E. (2008). Hearing loss after radiotherapy for pediatric brain tumors: Effect of cochlear dose. *International Journal of Radiation Oncology, Biology, Physics, 72,* 892–899. https://doi.org/10.1016/j.ijrobp.2008.01.050

Hudson, M. M., Mertens, A. C., Yasui, Y., Hobbie, W., Chen, H., Gurney, J. G., . . . Robison, L. R. (2003). Health status of adult long-term survivors of childhood cancer: A report from the Childhood Cancer Survivor Study. *JAMA, 290,* 1583–1592. https://doi.org/10.1001/jama.290.12.1583

Hyvärinen, L., Näsänen, R., & Laurinen, P. (1980). New visual acuity test for preschool children. *Acta Ophthalmologica, 58,* 507–511. https://doi.org/10.1111/j.1755-3768.1980.tb08291.x

Individuals With Disabilities Education Act of 1990, Pub. L. 101–476, renamed the Individuals With Disabilities Education Improvement Act, codified at 20 U.S.C. §§ 1400–1482.

Iyer, N. S., Balsamo, L. M., Bracken, M. B., & Kadan-Lottick, N. S. (2015). Chemotherapy-only treatment effects on long-term neurocognitive functioning in childhood ALL survivors: A review and meta-analysis. *Blood, 126,* 346–353. https://doi.org/10.1182/blood-2015-02-627414

Jaffe, L., Humphry, R., & Case-Smith, J. (2010). Working with families. In J. Case-Smith & J. O'Brien (Eds.), *Occupational therapy for children* (6th ed., pp. 108–145). St. Louis: Mosby.

Jalmsell, L., Kreicbergs, U., Onelov, E., Steineck, G., & Henter, J. I. (2006). Symptoms affecting children with malignancies during the last month of life: A nationwide follow-up. *Pediatrics, 117,* 1314–1320. https://doi.org/10.1542/peds.2005-1479

Jibb, L. A., Nathan, P. C., Stevens, B. J., Seto, E., Cafazzo, J. A., Stephens, N., . . . Stinson, J. N. (2015). Psychological and physical interventions for the management of cancer-related pain in pediatric and young adult patients: An integrative review. *Oncology Nursing Forum, 42,* E339–E357. https://doi.org/10.1188/15.ONF.E339-E357

Kasch, M., & Walsh, J. (2013). Hand and upper extremity injuries. In H. M. Pendleton & W. Schultz-Krohn (Eds.), *Pedretti's occupational therapy practice skills for physical dysfunction* (7th ed., pp. 1045–1046). St. Louis: Elsevier Mosby.

Kazak, A. E., Alderfer, M. A., Streisand, R., Simms, S., Rourke, M. T., Barakat, L. P., . . . Cnaan, A. (2004). Treatment of posttraumatic stress symptoms in adolescent survivors of childhood cancer and their families: A randomized clinical trial. *Journal of Family Psychology, 18,* 493–504. https://doi.org/10.1037/0893-3200.18.3.493

Kesler, S. R., Lacayo, N. J., & Jo, B. (2011). A pilot study of an online cognitive rehabilitation program for executive function skills in children with cancer-related brain injury. *Brain Injury, 25*(1), 101–112. https://doi.org/10.3109/02699052.2010.536194

Kline, N., Bryant, R., Carlson, C., Hooke, M., & Nixon, C. (Eds.). (2014). *Essentials of pediatric hematology/oncology nursing: A core curriculum* (4th ed.). Chicago: Association of Pediatric Hematology/Oncology Nurses.

Kramer, J., Ten Velden, M., Kafkes, A., Basu, S., Federico, J., & Kielhofner, G. (2014). *Child Occupational Self-Assessment* (Version 2.2). Chicago: Model of Human Occupation Clearinghouse.

Krull, K. R., Okcu, M. F., Potter, B., Jain, N., Dreyer, Z., Kamdar, K., & Brouwers, P. (2008). Screening for neurocognitive impairment in pediatric cancer long-term survivors. *Journal of Clinical Oncology, 26,* 4138–4143. https://doi.org/10.1200/jco.2008.16.8864

Kuper, M., Doring, K., Spangenberg, C., Konczak, J., Gizewski, E. R., Schoch, B., & Timmann, D. (2013). Location and restoration of function after cerebellar tumor removal: A longitudinal study of children and adolescents. *Cerebellum, 12*(1), 48–58. https://doi.org/10.1007/s12311-012-0389-z

Lai, J. S., Stucky, B. D., Thissen, D., Varni, J. W., DeWitt, E. M., Irwin, D. E., . . . & DeWalt, D. A. (2013). Development and psychometric properties of the PROMIS® pediatric fatigue item banks. *Quality of Life Research, 22,* 2417–2427. https://doi.org/10.1007/s11136-013-0357-1

Law, M., Baptiste, S., Carswell, A., McColl, M., Polatajko, H. & Pollock, N. (2019). *Canadian Occupational Performance Measure* (5th ed., rev.). Altona, Canada: COPM, Inc.

Lawitschka, A., Güclü, E. D., Varni, J. W., Putz, M., Wolff, D., Pavletic, S., . . . Felder-Puig, R. (2014). Health-related quality of life in pediatric patients after allogeneic SCT: Development of the PedsQL Stem Cell Transplant Module and results of a pilot study. *Bone Marrow Transplantation, 49*(8), 1093–1097. https://doi.org/10.1038/bmt.2014.96

Li, Y., Womer, R. B., & Silber, J. H. (2004). Predicting cisplatin ototoxicity in children: The influence of age and the cumulative dose. *European Journal of Cancer, 40,* 2445–2451. https://doi.org/10.1016/j.ejca.2003.08.009

Lohmann, D. R., & Gallie, B. L. (1993). Retinoblastoma. In M. P. Adam, H. H. Ardinger, R. A. Pagon, et al. (Eds.), *GeneReviews.* Seattle: University of Washington. Retrieved from http://www.ncbi.nlm.nih.gov/books/NBK1452/

Long, K. A., Keeley, L., Reiter-Purtill, J., Vannatta, K., Gerhardt, C. A., & Noll, R. B. (2014). Child-rearing in the context of childhood cancer: Perspectives of parents and professionals. *Pediatric Blood and Cancer, 61,* 326–332. https://doi.org/10.1002/pbc.24556

Macartney, G., Harrison, M. B., VanDenKerkhof, E., Stacey, D., & McCarthy, P. (2014). Quality of life and symptoms in pediatric brain tumor survivors: A systematic review. *Journal of Pediatric Oncology Nursing, 31,* 65–77. https://doi.org/10.1177/1043454213520191

Mandich, A., Polatajko, H. J., Miller, L., & Baum, C. (2004). *Paediatric Activity Card Sort.* Ottawa, Canada: CAOT Publications.

Manworren, R. C., & Hynan, L. S. (2003). Clinical validation of FLACC: Preverbal patient pain scale. *Pediatric Nursing, 29,* 140–146.

Miller, L. J. (2006). *Miller Function and Participation Scales: Examiner's manual.* San Antonio: Pearson.

Mitby, P. A., Robison, L. L., Whitton, J. A., Zevon, M. A., Gibbs, I. C., Tersak, J. M., . . . Mertens, A. C. (2003). Utilization of special education services and educational attainment among long-term survivors of childhood cancer: A report from the Childhood Cancer Survivor Study. *Cancer, 97,* 1115–1126. https://doi.org/10.1002/cncr.11117

Moleski, M. (2000). Neuropsychological, neuroanatomical, and neurophysiological consequences of CNS chemotherapy for acute lymphoblastic leukemia. *Archives of Clinical Neuropsychology, 15,* 603–630. https://doi.org/10.1016/S0887-6177(99)00050-5

Morris, E. B., Phillips, N. S., Laningham, F. H., Patay, Z., Gajjar, A., Wallace, D., . . . Ogg, R. J. (2009). Proximal dentatothalamocortical tract involvement in posterior fossa syndrome. *Brain, 132,* 3087–3095. https://doi.org/10.1093/brain/awp241

Mulchay Levy, J. M., Tello, T., Giller, R., Wilkening, G., Quinones, R., Keating, A. K., Liu, A. K. (2013). Late effects of total body irradiation and hematopoietic stem cell transplant in children under 3 years of age. *Pediatric Blood and Cancer, 60,* 700–704. https://doi.org/10.1002/pbc.24252

Mulhern, R. K., Reddick, W. E., Palmer, S. L., Glass, J. O., Elkin, T. D., Kun, L. E., . . . Gajjar, A. (1999). Neurocognitive deficits in medulloblastoma survivors and white matter loss. *Annals of Neurology, 46*(6), 834–841. https://doi.org/10.1002/1531-8249(199912)46:6<834::aid-ana5>3.0.co:2-m

National Cancer Institute. (2015). *Children with cancer: A guide for parents.* Bethesda, MD: Author.

National Comprehensive Cancer Network. (2017). *Distress management guidelines.* Retrieved from https://www.nccn.org/store/login/login.aspx?ReturnURL=https://www.nccn.org/professionals/physician_gls/pdf/distress.pdf

National Research Council & Institute of Medicine. (2000). *From neurons to neighborhoods: The science of early childhood development.* Washington, DC: National Academy Press.

Ness, K. K., Morris, E. B., Nolan, V. G., Howell, C. R., Gilchrist, L. S., Stovall, M., . . . Neglia, J. P. (2010). Physical performance limitations among adult survivors of childhood brain tumors. *Cancer, 116,* 3034–3044. https://doi.org/10.1002/cncr.25051

Newborg, J. (2005). *Battelle Developmental Inventory* (2nd ed.). Itasca, IL: Riverside Publishing.

Orgel, E., O'Neil, S. H., Kayser, K., Smith, B., Softley, T. L., Sherman-Bien, S., . . . Freyer, D. R. (2016). Effect of sensorineural hearing loss on neurocognitive functioning in pediatric brain tumor survivors. *Pediatric Blood and Cancer, 63,* 527–534. https://doi.org/10.1002/pbc.25804

Packer, R. J., Gurney, J. G., Punyko, J. A., Donaldson, S. S., Inskip, P. D., Stovall, M., . . . Zeltzer, L. K. (2003). Long-term neurologic and neurosensory sequelae in adult survivors of a childhood brain tumor: Childhood cancer survivor study. *Journal of Clinical Oncology, 21,* 3255–3261. https://doi.org/10.1200/JCO.2003.01.202

Pai, A. L., Greenley, R. N., Lewandowski, A., Drotar, D., Youngstrom, E., & Peterson, C. C. (2007). A meta-analytic review of the influence of pediatric cancer on parent and family functioning. *Journal of Family Psychology, 21,* 407–415. https://doi.org/10.1037/0893-3200.21.3.407

Palmer, S. L., Armstrong, C., Onar-Thomas, A., Wu, S., Wallace, D., Bonner, M. J., . . . Mabbott, D. (2013). Processing speed, attention, and working memory after treatment for medulloblastoma: An international, prospective, and longitudinal study. *Journal of Clinical Oncology, 31,* 3494–3500. https://doi.org/10.1200/JCO.2012.47.4775

Palmer, S. L., Goloubeva, O., Reddick, W. E., Glass, J. O., Gajjar, A., Kun, L., . . . Mulhern, R. K. (2001). Patterns of intellectual development among survivors of pediatric medulloblastoma: A longitudinal analysis. *Journal of Clinical Oncology, 19,* 2302–2308. https://doi.org/10.1200/JCO.2001.19.8.2302

Palmer, S. N., Meeske, K. A., Katz, E. R., Burwinkle, T. M., & Varni, J. W. (2007). The PedsQL™ Brain Tumor Module: Initial reliability and validity. *Pediatric Blood and Cancer, 49,* 287–293. https://doi.org/10.1002/pbc.21026

Piscione, P. J., Bouffet, E., Mabbott, D. J., Shams, I., & Kulkarni, A. V. (2014). Physical functioning in pediatric survivors of childhood posterior fossa brain tumors. *Neuro-Oncology, 16,* 147–155. https://doi.org/10.1093/neuonc/not138

Pollack, I. F., Polinko, P., Albright, L. A., Towbin, R., & Fitz, C. (1995). Mutism and pseudobulbar symptoms after resection of posterior fossa tumors in children: Incidence and pathophysiology. *Neurosurgery, 37,* 885–892. https://doi.org/10.1097/00006123-199605000-00051

Qaddoumi, I., Bass, J. K., Wu, J., Billups, C. A., Wozniak, A. W., Merchant, T. E., . . . Rodriguez-Galindo, C. (2012). Carboplatin-associated ototoxicity in children with retinoblastoma. *Journal of Clinical Oncology, 30,* 1034–1041. https://doi.org/10.1200/jco.2011.36.9744

Quigg, T. C., Mahajerin, A., Sullivan, P. D., Pradhan, K., & Bauer, N. S. (2013). Ages and Stages Questionnaire—3 developmental screening of infants and young children with cancer. *Journal of Pediatric Oncology Nursing, 30,* 235–241. https://doi.org/10.1177/1043454213493510

Rehabilitation Act of 1973, Pub. L. 93–112, 29 U.S.C. §§ 701–7961.

Reinders-Messelink, H., Schoemaker, M., Snijders, T., Goeken, L., van Den Briel, M., Bokkerink, J., & Kamps, W. (1999). Motor performance of children during treatment for acute lymphoblastic leukemia. *Medical and Pediatric Oncology, 33,* 545–550. https://doi.org/10.1002/(sici)1096-911x(199912)33:6<545::aid-mpo4>3.0.co;2-y

Repka, M. X. (2006). Brain lesions with ophthalmological manifestations. In K. W. Wright, P. H. Spiegel, & L. S. Thompson (Eds.), *Handbook of pediatric neuro-opthalmology* (pp. 255–288). New York: Springer.

Robertson, P. L., Muraszko, K. M., Holmes, E. J., Sposto, R., Packer, R. J., Gajjar, A., . . . Allen, J. C. (2006). Incidence and severity of postoperative cerebellar mutism syndrome in children with medulloblastoma: A prospective study by the Children's Oncology Group. *Journal of Neurosurgery: Pediatrics, 105,* 444–451. https://doi.org/10.3171/ped.2006.105.6.444

Rocke, K., Hays, P., Edwards, D., & Berg, C. (2008). Development of a performance assessment of executive function: The Children's Kitchen Task Assessment. *American Journal of Occupational Therapy, 62,* 528–537. https://doi.org/10.5014/ajot.62.5.528

Scheurer, M., Lupo, P., & Bondy, M. (2015). Epidemiology of childhood cancer. In R. Pizzo & D. Poplack (Eds.), *Principles and practice of pediatric oncology* (6th ed., pp. 1–10). Philadelphia: Wolters Kluwer.

Schreiber, J. E., Gurney, J. G., Palmer, S. L., Bass, J. K., Wang, M., Chen, S., . . . Mabbott, D. J. (2014). Examination of risk factors for intellectual and academic outcomes following treatment for pediatric medulloblastoma. *Neuro-Oncology, 16,* 1129–1136. https://doi.org/10.1093/neuonc/nou006

Siegel, R. L., Miller, K. D., & Jemal, A. (2017). Cancer statistics, 2017. *CA: A Cancer Journal for Clinicians, 67,* 7–30. https://doi.org/10.3322/caac.21387

Smith, S. R., Haig, A. J., & Couriel, D. R. (2015). Musculoskeletal, neurologic, and cardiopulmonary aspects of physical rehabilitation in patients with chronic graft-versus-host disease. *Biology of Blood and Marrow Transplantation, 21,* 799–808. https://doi.org/10.1016/j.bbmt.2014.10.019

Sparrow, J., Zhu, L., Gajjar, A., Mandrell, B. N., & Ness, K. K. (2017). Constraint-induced movement therapy for children with brain tumors. *Pediatric Physical Therapy, 29,* 55–61. https://doi.org/10.1097/pep.0000000000000331

Squires, J., Bricker, D., Twombly, E., Nickel, R., Clifford, J., Murphy, K., . . . Farrell, J. (2009). *Ages and Stages Questionnaires* (3rd ed.). Baltimore: Brookes.

Steinberg, A., Asher, A., Bailey, C., & Fu, J. B. (2015). The role of physical rehabilitation in stem cell transplantation patients. *Support Care Cancer, 23,* 2447–2460. https://doi.org/10.1007/s00520-015-2744-3

Steliarova-Foucher, E., Stiller, C. A., Lacour, B., & Kaatsch, P. (2005). International Classification of Childhood Cancer, third edition. *Cancer, 103,* 1457–1467. https://doi.org/10.1002/cncr.20910

Strauss, E., Sherman, E. M. S., & Spreen, O. (2006). *Behavior Rating Inventory of Executive Function (BRIEF): A compendium of neuropsychological tests, administration, norms, and commentary* (3rd ed.). New York: Oxford University Press.

Suneja, G., Poorvu, P. D., Hill-Kayser, C., & Lustig, R. A. (2013). Acute toxicity of proton beam radiation for pediatric central nervous system malignancies. *Pediatric Blood and Cancer, 60,* 1431–1436. https://doi.org/10.1002/pbc.24554

Taverna, L., Tremolada, M., Bonichini, S., Tosetto, B., Basso, G., Messina, C., & Pillon, M. (2017). Motor skill delays in preschool children with leukemia one year after treatment: Hematopoietic stem cell transplantation therapy as an important risk factor. *PloS One, 12*(10), e0186787. https://doi.org/10.1371/journal.pone.0186787

Tester, C. (2006). Occupational therapy in paedatric oncology and palliative care. In J. Cooper (Ed.), *Occupational therapy in oncology and palliative care* (pp. 107–124). West Sussex, England: Whurr Publishers.

Thygeson, M. V., Hooke, M. C., Clapsaddle, J., Robbins, A., & Moquist, K. (2010). Peaceful play yoga: Serenity and balance for children with cancer and their parents. *Journal of Pediatric Oncology Nursing, 27,* 276–284. https://doi.org/10.1177/1043454210363478

Toglia, J. (2015). *Weekly Calendar Planning Activity: A performance test of executive function.* Bethesda, MD: AOTA Press.

Trites, R. L. (1977). *Neuropsychological test manual.* Ottawa, Canada: Royal Ottawa Hospital.

Turner, C. D., Rey-Casserly, C., Liptak, C. C., & Chordas, C. (2009). Late effects of therapy for pediatric brain tumor survivors. *Journal of Child Neurology, 24*(11), 1455–1463. https://doi.org/10.1177/0883073809341709

Varni, J. W., Burwinkle, T. M., & Katz, E. R. (2004). The PedsQL™ in Pediatric Cancer Pain: A prospective longitudinal analysis of pain and emotional distress. *Journal of Developmental and Behavioral Pediatrics, 25,* 239–246.

Varni, J. W., Burwinkle, T. M., Katz, E. R., Meeske, K., & Dickinson, P. (2002). The PedsQL™ in pediatric cancer: Reliability and validity of the Pediatric Quality of Life Inventory™ Generic Core Scales, Multidimensional Fatigue Scale, and Cancer Module. *Cancer, 94*(7), 2090–2106. https://doi.org/10.1002/cncr.10428

Varni, J. W., Seid, M., & Kurtin, P. S. (2001). PedsQL™ 4.0: Reliability and validity of the Pediatric Quality of Life Inventory™ Version 4.0 Generic Core scales in healthy and patient populations. *Medical Care, 39,* 800–812. https://doi.org/10.1097/00005650-200108000-00006

Wang, Y., Magasi, S. R., Bohannon, R. W., Reuben, D. B., & McCreath, H. E. (2011). Assessing dexterity function: A comparison of two alternatives for the NIH toolbox. *Journal of Hand Therapy, 24,* 313–320. https://doi.org/10.1016/j.jht.2011.05.001

Wang, Y. C., Bohannon, R. W., Kapellusch, J., Garg, A., & Gershon, R. C. (2015). Dexterity as measured with the 9-Hole Peg Test (9-HPT) across the age span. *Journal of Hand Therapy, 28,* 53–60. https://doi.org/10.1016/j.jht.2014.09.002

Ward, E., DeSantis, C., Robbins, A., Kohler, B., & Jemal, A. (2014). Childhood and adolescent cancer statistics, 2014. *CA: A Cancer Journal for Clinicians, 64,* 83–103. https://doi.org/10.3322/caac.21219

Wechsler, D. (1991). *WISC–III: Wechsler Intelligence Scale for Children: Manual* (3rd ed.). San Antonio: Psychological Corporation.

Wells, E. M., Walsh, K. S., Khademian, Z. P., Keating, R. F., & Packer, R. J. (2008). The cerebellar mutism syndrome and its relation to cerebellar cognitive function and the cerebellar cognitive affective disorder. *Developmental Disabilities Research Reviews, 14,* 221–228. https://doi.org/10.1002/ddrr.25

Whelan, K. F., Stratton, K., Kawashima, T., Waterbor, J. W., Castleberry, R. P., Stovall, M., . . . Mertens, A. C. (2010). Ocular late effects in childhood and adolescent cancer survivors: A report from the Childhood Cancer Survivor Study. *Pediatric Blood and Cancer, 54,* 103–109. https://doi.org/10.1002/pbc.22277

Willard, V. W., Qaddoumi, I., Chen, S., Zhang, H., Brennan, R., Rodriguez-Galindo, C., . . . Phipps, S. (2014). Developmental and adaptive functioning in children with retinoblastoma: A longitudinal investigation. *Journal of Clinical Oncology, 32,* 2788–2793. https://doi.org/10.1200/JCO.2013.53.1996

World Health Organization. (2019). *WHO definition of palliative care.* Retrieved from http://www.who.int/cancer/palliative/definition/en

Wolfe, J., Grier, H. E., Klar, N., Levin, S. B., Ellenbogen, J. M., Salem-Schatz, S., . . . Weeks, J. C. (2000). Symptoms and suffering at the end of life in children with cancer. *New England Journal of Medicine, 342,* 326–333. https://doi.org/10.1056/nejm200002033420506

Wright, M. J., Galea, V., & Barr, R. D. (2005). Proficiency of balance in children and youth who have had acute lymphoblastic leukemia. *Physical Therapy, 85,* 782–790. https://doi.org/10.1093/ptj/85.8.782

Wurz, A., Chamorro-Vina, C., Guilcher, G. M. T., Schulte, F., & Culos-Reed, S. N. (2014). The feasibility and benefits of a 12-week yoga intervention for pediatric cancer out-patients. *Pediatric Blood and Cancer, 61,* 1828–1834. https://doi.org/10.1002/pbc.25096

Zheng, D. J., Lu, X., Schore, R. J., Balsamo, L., Devidas, M., Winick, N. J., . . . Kadan-Lottick, N. S. (2018). Longitudinal analysis of quality-of-life outcomes in children during treatment for acute lymphoblastic leukemia: A report from the Children's Oncology Group AALL0932 trial. *Cancer, 124,* 571–579. https://doi.org/10.1002/cncr.31085

APPENDIX 4.A. Assessments for Children With Cancer

9-Hole Peg Test: Wang, Y. C., Bohannon, R. W., Kapellusch, J., Garg, A., & Gershon, R. C. (2015). Dexterity as measured with the 9-Hole Peg Test (9-HPT) across the age span. *Journal of Hand Therapy, 28,* 53–60. https://doi.org/10.1016/j.jht.2014.09.002

Ages and Stages Questionnaires: Squires, J., Bricker, D., Twombly, E., Nickel, R., Clifford, J., Murphy, K., . . . Farrell, J. (2009). *Ages and Stages Questionnaires* (3rd ed.). Baltimore: Brookes.

Battelle Developmental Inventory: Newborg, J. (2005). *Battelle Developmental Inventory* (2nd ed.). Itasca, IL: Riverside Publishing.

Bayley Scales of Infant and Toddler Development: Bayley, N. (2005). *Bayley Scales of Infant and Toddler Development* (3rd ed.). San Antonio: Pearson.

Beery–Buktenica Developmental Test of Visual–Motor Integration: Beery, K. E., Buktenica, N. A., & Beery, N. A. (2010). *Beery–Buktenica Developmental Test of Visual–Motor Integration* (6th ed.). New York: Pearson Assessments.

Behavior Rating Inventory of Executive Function: Strauss, E., Sherman, E. M. S., & Spreen, O. (2006). *Behavior Rating Inventory of Executive Function (BRIEF): A compendium of neuropsychological tests, administration, norms, and commentary* (3rd ed.). New York: Oxford University Press.

Bruininks–Oseretsky Test of Motor Proficiency: Bruininks, R. H. (2005). *Bruininks–Oseretsky Test of Motor Proficiency.* Circle Pines, MN: AGS Publishing.

Canadian Occupational Performance Measure: Law, M., Baptiste, S., Carswell, A., McColl, M., Polatajko, H. & Pollock, N. (2019). *Canadian Occupational Performance Measure* (5th ed., rev.). Altona, Canada: COPM, Inc.

Child Occupational Self-Assessment: Kramer, J., Ten Velden, M., Kafkes, A., Basu, S., Federico, J., & Kielhofner, G. (2014). *Child Occupational Self-Assessment* (Version 2.2). Chicago: Model of Human Occupation Clearinghouse.

Children's Kitchen Task Assessment: Rocke, K., Hays, P., Edwards, D., & Berg, C. (2008). Development of a performance assessment of executive function: The Children's Kitchen Task Assessment. *American Journal of Occupational Therapy, 62,* 528–537. https://doi.org/10.5014/ajot.62.5.528

Digit Span Test: Wechsler, D. (1991). *WISC–III: Wechsler Intelligence Scale for Children: Manual* (3rd ed.). San Antonio: Psychological Corporation.

Faces Pain Scale: Hicks, C. L., von Baeyer, C. L., Spafford, P. A., van Korlaar, I., & Goodenough, B. (2001). The Faces Pain Scale–Revised: Toward a common metric in pediatric pain measurement. *Pain, 93,* 173–183. https://doi.org/10.1016/s0304-3959(01)00314-1

FLACC Pain Scale: Manworren, R. C., & Hynan, L. S. (2003). Clinical validation of FLACC: Preverbal patient pain scale. *Pediatric Nursing, 29,* 140–146.

LEA Symbols: Hyvärinen, L., Näsänen, R., & Laurinen, P. (1980). New visual acuity test for preschool children. *Acta Ophthalmologica, 58,* 507–511. https://doi.org/10.1111/j.1755-3768.1980.tb08291.x

Miller Function and Participation Scales: Miller, L. J. (2006). *Miller Function and Participation Scales: Examiner's manual.* San Antonio: Pearson.

(Continued)

APPENDIX 4.A.   Assessments for Children With Cancer *(Cont.)*

Monofilament testing, sharp–dull discrimination, vibration sense: Kasch, M., & Walsh, J. (2013). Hand and upper extremity injuries. In H. M. Pendleton & W. Schultz-Krohn (Eds.), *Pedretti's occupational therapy practice skills for physical dysfunction* (7th ed., pp. 1045–1046). St. Louis: Elsevier Mosby.

National Institutes of Health Chronic Graft-Versus-Host Disease Clinical Scoring System: Filipovich, A. H., Weisdorf, D., Pavletic, S., Socie, G., Wingard, J. R., Lee, S. J., . . . Cowen, E. W. (2005). National Institutes of Health Consensus Development Project on Criteria for Clinical Trials in Chronic Graft-Versus-Host Disease: I. Diagnosis and Staging Working Group report. *Biology of Blood and Marrow Transplantation, 11,* 945–956. https://doi.org/10.1016/j.bbmt.2005.09.004

Oregon Project for Visually Impaired and Blind Preschool Children: Anderson, S., Boigon, S., Davis, K., & DeWaard, C. (2007). *The Oregon Project for Visually Impaired and Blind Preschool Children* (6th ed.). Medford: Southern Oregon Education Service District.

Patient-Reported Outcomes Measurement Information System (PROMIS) Pediatric Fatigue Measure: Lai, J. S., Stucky, B. D., Thissen, D., Varni, J. W., DeWitt, E. M., Irwin, D. E., . . . & DeWalt, D. A. (2013). Development and psychometric properties of the PROMIS® pediatric fatigue item banks. *Quality of Life Research, 22,* 2417–2427. https://doi.org/10.1007/s11136-013-0357-1

Peabody Developmental Motor Scales: Folio, M. R., & Fewell, R. R. (2000). *Peabody Developmental Motor Scales: Examiner's manual.* Austin, TX: Pro-Ed.

Pediatric Activity Card Sort: Mandich, A., Polatajko, H. J., Miller, L., & Baum, C. (2004). *Paediatric Activity Card Sort.* Ottawa, Canada: CAOT Publications.

Pediatric Evaluation of Disability Inventory: Haley, S. M. (1992). *Pediatric Evaluation of Disability Inventory (PEDI): Development, standardization and administration manual.* Boston: PEDI Research Group.

Pediatric-Modified Total Neuropathy Scale: Gilchrist, L. S., & Tanner, L. (2013). The Pediatric-Modified Total Neuropathy score: A reliable and valid measure of chemotherapy-induced peripheral neuropathy in children with non-CNS cancers. *Supportive Care in Cancer, 21,* 847–856. https://doi.org/10.1007/s00520-012-1591-8

Pediatric Quality of Life Inventory Brain Tumor Module: Palmer, S. N., Meeske, K. A., Katz, E. R., Burwinkle, T. M., & Varni, J. W. (2007). The PedsQL™ Brain Tumor Module: Initial reliability and validity. *Pediatric Blood and Cancer, 49,* 287–293. https://doi.org/10.1002/pbc.21026

Pediatric Quality of Life Inventory Generic Core scales: Varni, J. W., Seid, M., & Kurtin, P. S. (2001). PedsQL™ 4.0: Reliability and validity of the Pediatric Quality of Life Inventory™ Version 4.0 Generic Core scales in healthy and patient populations. *Medical Care, 39,* 800–812. https://doi.org/10.1097/00005650-200108000-00006

Pediatric Quality of Life Inventory Multidimensional Fatigue Scale: Varni, J. W., Burwinkle, T. M., Katz, E. R., Meeske, K., & Dickinson, P. (2002). The PedsQL™ in pediatric cancer: Reliability and validity of the Pediatric Quality of Life Inventory™ Generic Core scales, Multidimensional Fatigue Scale, and Cancer Module. *Cancer, 94,* 2090–2106. https://doi.org/10.1002/cncr.10428

Preschool Activity Card Sort: Berg, C., & LaVesser, P. (2006). The Preschool Activity Card Sort. *OTJR: Occupation, Participation and Health, 26,* 143–151. https://doi.org/10.1177/153944920602600404

School Function Assessment: Coster, W., Coster, W., Deeney, T. A., Haley, S., & Haltiwanger, J. (1998). *School Function Assessment.* San Antonio: Psychological Corporation.

Sensory Profile: Dunn, W. (2014). *Sensory Profile 2 user's manual.* Bloomington, MN: Pearson.

Short Child Occupational Profile: Bowyer, P., Ross, M., Schwartz, O., Kielhofner, G., & Kramer, J. (2005). *The Short Child Occupational Profile (Version 2.1).* Chicago: Model of Human Occupation Clearinghouse.

Trail Making Test: Trites, R. L. (1977). *Neuropsychological test manual.* Ottawa, Canada: Royal Ottawa Hospital.

Verbal Fluency Test: Benton, A. L., Hamsher, K. D., & Sivan, A. (1983). *Multilingual Aphasia Examination* (3rd ed.). Iowa City, IA: AJA Associates.

Weekly Calendar Planning Activity: Toglia, J. (2015). *Weekly Calendar Planning Activity: A performance test of executive function.* Bethesda, MD: AOTA Press.

Special Considerations for Adolescents and Young Adults With Cancer

5

Donna Kelly, OTR/L, MED, CLT

LEARNING OBJECTIVES

After completing this chapter, readers should be able to

- Understand specific lifespan and developmental challenges experienced by adolescent and young adult (AYA) cancer survivors and their impact on age-appropriate roles, habits, and routines;
- Identify cancer-related impairments and their effect on occupational performance across the cancer care continuum in the AYA population;
- Comprehend the specific role education plays in the AYA population, including caregiver education and how to advance therapeutic interventions to support assimilation of cancer survivors into normative educational environments;
- Differentiate the specific needs of the AYA population in comparison with pediatric, adult, and older adult populations; and
- Formulate specialized interventions to support occupational engagement, prevent latency effects of treatment, and deter social isolation.

KEY TERMS AND CONCEPTS

- Adolescent and young adult cancer survivors
- Avascular necrosis
- Body image
- Cancer-related fatigue
- Chemotherapy-induced peripheral neuropathy
- Cognitive impairments
- Early young adulthood
- Environmental impact
- Healthy lifestyle
- Late effects
- Late young adulthood
- Learned dependency
- Occupational competence
- Performance capacity
- Prehabilitation
- Transformational change
- Young adulthood

INTRODUCTION

About 5,000 adolescents and 60,000 young adults are diagnosed with cancer each year in the United States (American Cancer Society [ACS], 2017, 2018). Although nearly 70% of all adolescents and young adults (AYAs) survive at least 5 years beyond initial diagnosis, cancer remains a leading cause of death in the AYA population, following only suicide and homicide (National Cancer Institute [NCI], 2018). Despite increasing rates of diagnosis and survival, AYA-related cancers continue to display significant disparities when compared to the pediatric population. These disparities include lack of health insurance, differences in disease biology, delay of diagnosis and treatment, increased toxicities, lower socioeconomic status, and overall lack of awareness in the medical field as to the special needs of this population (Isenalumhe et al., 2016). Given that 1 in 570 young adults will be long-term survivors of childhood cancer, occupational therapy practitioners may interact with survivors of cancer throughout

the cancer care continuum and well into survivorship (Berg & Hayashi, 2013).

The immediate and late effects of a cancer diagnosis greatly affect self-image and body awareness, role identification, and quality of life (QoL), because adolescence and young adulthood are times of self-discovery through normative rites of passage, such as moving away to attend college, getting a first job, dating and getting married, and starting a family. **Body image,** or *body awareness,* can be defined as thoughts or perceptions related to the person's physical appearance and the resultant feelings associated with those perceptions. Feelings related to body image can be positive or negative and can be influenced by individual or environmental factors. **Late effects** of cancer treatment are side effects of treatment that become apparent after treatment has ended. Late effects of cancer can include impaired cognition (e.g., attention, concentration), fatigue, hearing loss, skin changes, and generalized weakness. Recent studies have found that many AYA survivors underestimate their risk for late effects of cancer treatment and

5

underreport these late effects, assuming they are unrelated to prior treatment (Berg et al., 2008).

It is also important to note that in the adult population, caregivers often overestimate and physicians often underestimate the degree of symptom burden. Agreement on symptom burden, which includes these late effects of cancer, is more common with visible symptoms, such as immobility, and less frequent with symptoms in the psychosocial domains, such as pain and impaired coping (Zhukovsky et al., 2015). Reliance on symptom reports by medical professionals is higher among children than it is among adults; however, this area requires further research specific to the AYA population.

Additional late effects of treatments can include shortness of breath, impaired balance, chemotherapy-induced peripheral neuropathy (CIPN), and lack of interest in activity engagement (Berg et al., 2008). Survivors often cite multiple late effects or symptoms affecting QoL and occupational engagement. Poor symptom management in these areas can be distressing not only for the survivor but also for caregivers, which is discussed further in the "Survivorship" section. Lack of research in symptom management, in conjunction with the underreporting of symptoms, adds an additional barrier to treatment, including misinterpretation of clinical presentation, delay in appropriate treatment interventions, and impaired rate of goal attainment, all of which can lead to further distress for the cancer survivor and compound symptoms of social isolation, anxiety, and depression.

The AYA population faces critical lifespan and developmental challenges regarding role development that can be negatively affected by cancer and its treatment:

- Transition to adult roles for independent living
- Achievement of societal autonomy
- Selection of occupation and achievement of higher education
- Engagement in social activities and social milestones.

Cancer-related fatigue (CRF), chronic pain, lower engagement and social isolation, cognitive impairments (e.g., memory, attention), peripheral neuropathy, and body image impairments are just some of the effects of cancer and its treatments that can negatively affect typical development. Impairments left unaddressed in these areas have the potential to lead to impaired developmental milestones, such as higher education achievements, employment, independent living, and marital status (Berg et al., 2008). This chapter discusses both current and late effects of AYA treatment on both participation and QoL. It also addresses how occupational therapy practitioners can positively affect occupational performance, QoL, and participation.

WHO ARE AYAs?

The National Cancer Society and the *Journal of Adolescent and Young Adult Oncology* have defined *AYA cancer survivors* as those ages 15–39 years. Within this range, survivors are categorized into the following subgroups: *early young adulthood* (ages 15–18 years), *young adulthood* (ages 19–24 years), and *late young adulthood* (ages 25–39 years; Liebert, 2011; NCI, 2018). These smaller age groups make it easier to identify and understand the specific potential toxic effects that cancer treatments have that increase a survivor's risk for chronic disease and lower life expectancy.

Cancer treatments can lead to a disruption in day-to-day functioning, and approximately two-thirds of survivors experience one or more late effects (Berg & Hayashi, 2013).

Adolescence and young adulthood are continuously evolving periods when people transition between highly structured environments (e.g., school and pediatric health care systems) to a world where they are expected to navigate environments independently, with consistent self-directed and goal-oriented behavior. Work and health care environments require a higher level of self-management as people age and transition into new roles and relationships. The *environmental impact*—that is, the opportunity, support, demand, and constraint that the environment has (i.e., Model of Human Occupation)—on a person in this age range can vary, but more often than not, the environment requires a higher cognitive and physical competency for successful navigation (Taylor, 2017).

In early young adulthood (15–18 years of age), cancer survivors face many social situations that may affect their self-esteem and body image. These include dating, learning to drive or navigate in a community with independence, and transitioning to higher education. School events often highlight these situations with age-related rites of passage, such as prom and homecoming, which place a higher level of importance on personal appearance.

Students need higher levels of cognitive functioning to move seamlessly to higher education environments or roles within the workforce. For many survivors, early young adulthood may be the first time they notice impaired attention or memory: Their peers are moving forward with college and employment opportunities, whereas they struggle to follow the same path.

In young adulthood (19–24 years old), individuals may face recurrent issues with the aforementioned impairments, in addition to new ones. During this time of life, most people transition into changing life stages and familial roles. This can include transitioning to living on their own, managing their own finances for the first time, maintaining full-time employment, and getting married or starting their own family, all while also being responsible for managing their own health care. These roles challenge clients to self-address personal care skills, IADLs (many AYA individuals have not previously been required to complete any type of home management skill), vocational needs, and changing social skills.

Because many late effects present themselves years after cancer treatment, it is important that long-term follow-up continues to be a priority. Research suggests, however, that as survivors age and transition to handling their medical care on their own, there is often limited follow-up with specialized cancer centers because survivors are unaware of the relationship between problems they are currently experiencing and their prior cancer history (Berg & Hayashi, 2013). This knowledge gap can be significantly narrowed through an improved multidisciplinary approach among health care providers, occupational therapy practitioners, and young survivors.

In late young adulthood (25–39 years old), occupational therapy practitioners not only see recurrence of previously identified impairments but also see onset of new difficulties as adolescents move into parenthood, join the workforce, display continued community involvement, and venture into new leisure pursuits. Compared with normative groups within the same age ranges, survivors have indicated specific occupation-based tasks limiting their full engagement in ADLs. Some of these task-specific impairments include carrying groceries, lifting heavy objects (in particular with visual field blocked, e.g., with a large box or piece of furniture), bending, and walking one block (Berg & Hayashi, 2013).

Despite some variability in life experiences, certain late effects seem to resonate consistently throughout this population. These themes are in the areas of pain, fatigue, body image distortion, depression, sensation impairments, impaired physical performance, impaired cognition, and social isolation. Research in these areas continues to be limited despite the growing number of survivors. Occupational therapy practitioners are in the unique role of being able to assist young adult survivors through the process of transitioning to adult roles through occupational therapy interventions.

MOST COMMON FORMS OF CANCER IN THE AYA POPULATION

The most common forms of cancer diagnosed in the AYA population are brain and central nervous system tumors; breast, cervical, colorectal, and germ cell tumors; leukemia; lymphoma; melanoma; sarcomas (both bony and soft tissue); and testicular and thyroid cancers. Despite the rather long list of common forms of cancer in this population, the incidence of cancer varies according to age. The most common forms of cancer diagnosed in young adulthood include leukemia, lymphoma, testicular cancers, and thyroid cancers (NCI, 2018). In late young adulthood, the most common types of cancer are breast cancer and melanoma. This wide and varied list leaves multiple areas of treatment opportunities and focus areas for occupational therapy practitioners.

OVERVIEW OF OCCUPATIONAL THERAPY'S ROLE ACROSS THE CANCER CARE CONTINUUM WITH AYA CLIENTS WITH CANCER

AYA cancer survivors present a particularly interesting role for occupational therapy practitioners because adolescents as a whole struggle with identity and daily judgment as they transition into productive societal roles. AYAs with cancer tend to present at more advanced stages of disease compared with older populations, possibly related to feelings of invincibility, lifestyle, lack of or inconsistent medical care and screenings, and lack of awareness of their cancer risk (Keegan et al., 2012). An additional barrier to preventative screening and consistent health care follow-ups for many types of cancer, including human papillomavirus and melanoma, is the lack of medical coverage because many young adults are no longer covered by their parents' insurance plans. The same can be said for follow-up with outpatient therapy services.

The role of occupational therapy practitioners in health management is largely in education. This education should focus on modifiable factors of cancer risk while promoting a healthy lifestyle. A *healthy lifestyle* can include various facets, such as fitness, leisure pursuits and participation, healthy eating (to include healthy meal preparation), and engagement in self-advocacy as it pertains to symptom management as the cancer survivor transitions to independent handling of their health care needs.

This type of education is beneficial for cancer survivors at any point on the care continuum because engagement in health management helps establish consistent routines and aids in transition to adult roles. In the context of prevention, occupational therapy practitioners can look to community models for improving the education of the AYA population on preventative testing, self-management strategies, nutrition and weight loss, and the importance of consistent medical care (Berg & Hayashi, 2013).

Research has consistently shown that early intervention and involvement of occupational therapy practitioners has increased engagement in and self-initiation of personal care, leisure interests, and school-based tasks; return to work; and prevention of cognitive decline (i.e., deficits in attention and concentration associated with the cognitive effects of chemotherapy; Keegan et al., 2012). Despite this research, however, more than half of cancer survivors have unmet informational or service needs.

The informational needs of this population relate to education about their cancer treatment, the effects of their cancer treatment, and the likelihood of recurrence. A total of 56%–75% of AYA cancer survivors who would benefit from occupational therapy do not receive these services (Keegan et al., 2012). More research is needed to further meet the needs of this population.

Prehabilitation

Over the past several years, there has been growing interest in the incorporation of prehabilitation (i.e., "prehab") programs in the cancer population, including the AYA population. *Prehabilitation* is defined as

> a process on the cancer continuum of care that occurs between the time of cancer diagnosis and the beginning of acute treatment and includes physical and psychological assessments that establish a baseline functional level, identify impairments, and provide interventions that promote physical and psychological health to reduce the incidence and/or severity of future impairments. (Silver, 2015, p. 14; Silver et al., 2013)

Prehabilitation helps practitioners to intervene with survivors at a point at which they are not yet overwhelmed with the burdens of symptom management. (See Chapter 10, "Prehabilitation," for more information.)

Despite increasing survival rates in the AYA population, mortality rates among AYA survivors related to recurrence, secondary cancer, and cardiovascular and lung disease surpass rates among both the general population and those individuals diagnosed with cancer later in life. Given the known risks of mortality, fostering healthy lifestyles through incorporation of exercise is crucial in both combating late effects of cancer treatment and promoting healthy aging across the continuum of care (Barnes et al., 2016).

The inclusion of a prehab program helps articulate the distinct value and the specific role of occupational therapy in the context of cancer rehabilitation. Prehab is a key component in facilitation of *transformational change.* This type of change refers to fundamentally altering an established pattern of thinking, feeling, and doing. It helps clearly define expectations for the course of treatment, benefits of engagement in out-of-bed activities (e.g., participation in self-care, leisure, health management, school- and work-based tasks), and prevention of latency effects of treatment before treatment initiation. Prehab supports the fundamental change away from prior theories of rest as a way to promote healing to the contemporary understanding of the value of physical engagement and participation to prevent functional decline.

Prehab is steadily gaining ground, and many institutions are incorporating prehab programs into their acute-based settings. One unique area for prehab intervention is the hematology population. On the basis of knowledge already discussed in this chapter, the general AYA population exhibits difficulties in the areas of health maintenance, fitness engagement, and healthy lifestyle. Carrying these poor habits through a long treatment course (e.g., stem cell transplant [SCT], chimeric antigen receptor T-cell therapy) could further exacerbate treatment-induced impairments. Furthermore, cancer survivors display higher levels of depression, disengagement from personal care, impaired coping related to length of treatment, and social isolation (which limits occupational demands and participation in leisure activities), and prehab is a key component in combating these problems (Barnes et al., 2016).

Inclusion of prehab services with AYA clients has improved self-advocacy, increased awareness of and incorporation of coping strategies throughout the course of prolonged hospitalizations, and improved awareness of potential latency symptoms, assisting with continuity of care in the survivorship stage (Shun, 2016). Prehab services have further improved participation in mobilization to include ambulation, self-care engagement, and participation in fitness routines.

Prehab also helps clients understand how consistent participation in activity affects both cognition and physical performance. This understanding can be vital to promoting consistent engagement in activity (e.g., occupations, roles, routines, habits) as it helps clients to connect their engagement to the continued ability to do the things important to them. It also fosters follow up with home exercise program reassessments and consistency in tracking changes over time (Barnes et al., 2016). Education on potential treatment side effects while engaging in activities also plays a large role in any prehab program.

Often in a prehab program, patients are treated prior to initiation of various treatment interventions (e.g., chemotherapy, radiation, surgery), so they arrive feeling well and functioning near or at their baseline, wondering why they were referred to occupational therapy. Providing education on the course of treatment, its potential side effects, and its potential latent symptoms helps to make clients aware of the potential for decline in function and what signs and symptoms to be aware of, for both clients and caregivers. Such information helps patients feel more control and aids in more consistent participation in home exercise programs and attendance of therapy appointments and aids the caregivers in understanding the role of therapy services, further supporting the patient in therapeutic engagement.

Consistent engagement in prehab has been shown to decrease length of hospital admissions, improve mental and physical preparation for treatment initiation (which leads to improved outcomes), and increase engagement in therapeutic interventions throughout the course of treatment (Shun, 2016).

Occupational Therapy Intervention

There are many opportunities across the cancer care continuum for occupational therapy services. Depending on the type of cancer and the specific course of treatment, occupational therapy practitioners can see any number of limitations, including impaired ADL and IADL performance, decreased cognitive function, significant pain and fatigue levels that impede occupational engagement, impaired health management (e.g., fitness routines, medication management, fall prevention, energy conservation), and impaired mobility (in both home and community settings). Many survivors also experience impaired sleep–wake cycles, social isolation, and muscle weakness, which lead to impaired balance and endurance.

As AYA clients approach the later course of their treatment, occupational therapy practitioners may see an increase in pain, weight gain or loss, and generalized edema. These can all lead to a decline in occupational engagement associated with prolonged or extensive exposure to steroids.

Steroids

Many clients in the AYA population have had exposure to steroids over the course of many months or even many years. Prolonged exposure to steroids can cause additional symptoms such as pain, fluid retention, and impaired memory. Prolonged steroid exposure can also be associated with diagnoses such as avascular necrosis (AVN). *AVN* refers to the death of bone tissue due to an interruption in blood supply, and it commonly affects the ends of the long bones. Treatment for symptoms evolved from AVN can often lead to joint replacements, requiring further occupational therapy intervention for task modification, adaptive equipment use, education and carryover of surgical precautions, and improved mobilization.

Chemotherapy-induced peripheral neuropathy

In the AYA population, occupational therapy practitioners also see a large number of cancer survivors with symptoms of CIPN associated with exposure to chemotherapy agents. *CIPN* is defined by a set of symptoms caused by damage to the nerves outside the brain and spinal cord. These symptoms can often include numbness, tingling, burning, and pain. CIPN is often chronic and irreversible (ACS, 2017, 2018). These symptoms can range from mild numbness and tingling to immobilizing sensations of burning or extreme sensitivity that impair the client's ability to don or tolerate footwear and ambulate even short household distances. CIPN also can further enhance social isolation secondary to inability to tolerate vertical positioning or out-of-bed engagement. (See Chapter 19, "Chemotherapy Induced Peripheral Neuropathy," for more in-depth information on CIPN.)

Some common chemotherapy agents used specifically with the AYA population known to cause CIPN are carboplatin, cisplatin, doxorubicin, methotrexate, vincristine, and etoposide. The Pediatric Modified Total Neuropathy Scale is a helpful assessment to use with the early young adult population to accurately measure CIPN (Gilchrist et al., 2013). Treatment for CIPN continues to evolve, with varying success rates, and is an area that requires further research in the context of occupational therapy.

Many clients find improvements with therapeutic use of Kinesio tape, acupuncture, yoga, and other relaxation techniques, and strengthening exercises have been shown to reduce neuropathic pain when completed regularly. Desensitization techniques, such as gentle soft tissue massage, contrast baths, and stretching, have also been shown to be helpful.

Cancer-related fatigue

CRF plays a large role in the treatment of cancer survivors as a whole, and the AYA population is no exception. **CRF** is defined as a distressing, persistent, subjective sense of physical, emotional, or cognitive tiredness or exhaustion related to cancer or cancer treatment that is not proportional to recent activity and interferes with a person's usual functioning. CRF is the number one side effect of cancer treatment and can often plague an individual for months to years following treatment (NCI, 2018).

Fatigue is part of typical development for many people in the early young adult or young adult stage. Four or more times a week, even in the absence of a pathology or illness, one-third of both young men and young women have symptoms of substantial fatigue. Fatigue becomes even more burdensome after the introduction of CRF and compounding treatment. Higher levels of fatigue are also associated with poorer QoL, disengagement from coping strategies, and higher rates of depression. All of these issues can lengthen an acute inpatient stay, resulting in further muscle atrophy and weakness; coping impairments; and hospital-acquired illnesses, such as pneumonia and infection.

Levels of CRF can be further affected by impaired sleep–wake cycles in hospital settings. Sleep–wake cycles can be inhibited by frequent interruptions to sleep, such as health care professionals taking vital signs and administering medications in late evening or early morning hours when an individual would normally be sleeping. Premedication for chemotherapy agents or blood products (e.g., diphenhydramine for platelet administration) can cause increased drowsiness and sleep during day hours. Altered scheduling for procedures and tests during acute stays can further exacerbate this issue (e.g., magnetic resonance imaging).

In conjunction with higher levels of depression, CRF can further be exacerbated with prolonged supine positioning; disengagement from roles, routines, and habits; and impaired self-management of symptom burden. Treatment interventions for fatigue and fatigue management often include initiation of and engagement in sleep preparation; work with interdisciplinary team members to cluster care to allow prolonged periods of uninterrupted sleep; and incorporation of rest periods focused on quiet periods, relaxation, and calming engagement in interests. Occupational therapy can also intervene with strategies for energy conservation, task prioritization, routine establishment and carryover, and self-awareness.

The AYA population and those providing care to these clients often benefit from further education on the role of physical activity in the management of CRF. Clients often feel that engagement in activity or physical fitness is counterintuitive to the management of fatigue. For many, this could not be further from the truth. Promotion of physical fitness can be vital in this population. See Exhibit 5.1 for further information on education about CRF.

Engagement in physical activity has been shown to reduce symptoms of CRF both during and after cancer treatment (Brown et al., 2012). Occupational therapy practitioners can often provide home exercise programs in the areas of aerobic exercise, stretching, flexibility, strengthening, and range of motion (ROM) based on the needs of each cancer survivor. Activity engagement can also be graded to promote routine establishment, engagement in routine completion, and advancement to participation in home exercise programs or ambulation once the client feels consistently able to complete the tasks that are most meaningful to them within a manageable fatigue level.

Interventions and education in the area of fatigue can also include energy conservation and fatigue management techniques developed around school and work-based tasks within self-management. These can include techniques for self-reflection or use of fatigue scales, such as the Brief Fatigue Inventory, to identify burdensome tasks for appropriate incorporation of self-initiated breaks or pacing (MD Anderson Cancer Center, 2020). Scales can also be helpful for task prioritization before fatigue levels peak and for understanding metabolic equivalences in relation to functional activities. This type of education can improve both engagement in function and self-awareness, which can further improve clients' independence level. (See Chapter 15, "Cancer Related Fatigue," for more in-depth information.)

Cancer-related cognitive impairment

Cognitive impairments play a unique role in occupational participation in the AYA population. Cancer is a chronic illness, and the AYA population must self-manage symptoms across various phases of treatment and into survivorship. To address self-management needs, Lorig and Holman (2003) identified five core skills for success:
1. Problem solving,
2. Decision making,

EXHIBIT 5.1. Educating Caregivers on CRF

Clinicians treating the AYA population are often sandwiched between clients and their caregivers. In this stage of life, clients often battle with varying levels of self-advocacy versus regression toward being cared for. Educating caregivers and survivors alike on CRF and its implications for roles and routines posttreatment can significantly improve carryover. This carryover can be linked to improved consistency in follow-up appointments, increased reporting of symptoms, and full engagement in therapeutic interventions.

Note. AYA = adolescent and young adult; CRF = cancer-related fatigue.

3. Formation of client–provider relationships,
4. Action planning, and
5. Self-tailored programs.

These skills are often impaired related to exposure to chemotherapy agents, impaired self-responsibility or management of care, social limitations, and impaired goal-oriented behavior. As core skills become impaired, so, in turn, does clients' **occupational competence,** or their ability to perform occupations and skills with ease. Self-management programs involving individual or group treatments focused on improving these cognitive deficits are another area of education applicable to young adults.

Cognitive function or limitation also affects a client's ability to return to work roles as well as actively engage in an educational environment. This relates to impairments in **performance capacity,** or one's ability to complete tasks in relation to underlying physical and mental components and their subjective experience. When we discuss a person's capacity to do things in relation to an impairment in cognitive function, we can also discuss and understand how chronic disease is experienced and how it affects performance. Impairments in development and cognitive performance have been shown to affect clients into later stages of adulthood and survivorship.

Developmental and cognitive effects are evident when the cancer AYA population is compared with healthy control participants. Survivors of childhood cancers achieve fewer social milestones, such as higher education, employment, independent living, and marriage (Berg et al., 2008). In a study assessing AYA participants' ability to engage in self-management, out of 42 participants (with a mean age of 20 years), only 2 reported a personal income over $20,000. Many of these survivors cited memory impairments as a contributing factor related to their inability to be successful in a work environment and in educational activities (Berg & Hayashi, 2013).

SURVIVORSHIP

Survivorship and cancer care in the AYA population are quite different than survivorship in other age ranges. With improvements in cancer care, approximately 70% of young adult survivors are living at least 5 years into survivorship, and this number continues to grow (Armenian et al., 2019). As adolescent survivors transition into a self-mastery stage of life, late effects can limit their ability to engage in occupation. Survivors may struggle with a decline in capacity that affects both performance and identity and thus requires adaptation (Taylor, 2017). In many cases, AYA clients have spent months to years in treatment, which has caused social isolation and continued delay in achievement of adult roles. This delay places the AYA survivorship population at further risk for impaired health-related QoL and impaired participation in occupation, work roles, educational achievements, and social engagements.

Survival rates for the AYA population have improved vastly over the past 30 years; however, rates of survival vary widely by the type of cancer being treated and the age of the individual at diagnosis. AYA cancer survivors may also be diagnosed with secondary cancers during their survivorship. These secondary cancers are often directly correlated to the client's prior lifesaving treatment. Typical treatment in this age range includes a combination of chemotherapies, radiation, and surgical interventions to improve survivorship. These combinations in treatment also contribute to the varying survival rate among this age group. However, the types of treatment used and combined to cure cancer can also be linked to potential areas of impairment.

Many survivors who report latency symptoms have never received occupational therapy intervention for these symptoms, which further inhibits the survivors' achievement of societal expectations compared with healthy, normative populations. In addition to late effects of cancer treatment, AYA survivors are also working against lack of familial expectations (e.g., decreased or lack of participation in age-appropriate chores, social engagements, and community mobility activities), lack of environmental adaptations, and decreased participation in vigorous leisure activities. These limitations inhibit a transition to adulthood roles, including participating in exercise for health maintenance, navigating independently in a community setting, and performing home maintenance responsibilities. These latency effects translate to fewer survivors having paid employment, a greater percentage of survivors living with their parents, and fewer survivors having romantic relationships (Stam et al., 2005).

Education about and incorporation of self-management strategies into roles and routines are critical for the AYA population to reduce the impact of late effects on their transition to adult roles. The first step is to identify personal goals in relation to home management, educational or job pursuits, and independent living. Intervention may include working with school districts or employment agencies for appropriate modifications to environments as needed.

End-of-life care can be difficult with this population because occupational therapy practitioners must address both the survivor's needs and the caregivers' needs as appropriately as possible. In some cases, the survivor's goals may not match the caregivers' goals. Many interventions are based on comfort, and adaptive equipment needs to easily transition the client and their family members to their home environment in a safe and functional manner. See Exhibit 5.2 for further understanding of caregiver burden. End-of-life care can incorporate aspects of family training, environmental modification, social and leisure participation, and legacy completion. Examples of rehabilitative interventions across the cancer care continuum are included in Table 5.1.

EXHIBIT 5.2.   Caregiver Burden in the AYA Population

Caring for a young adult can create considerable strain on a caregiver in the areas of finance; time; and mental, physical, and social health. These strains can often result in sleep disturbance, depression, anxiety, and social isolation. It is important to incorporate the caregiver as part of treatment interventions in the psychosocial realm of treatment to aid in the care of cancer survivors and their families. (See Chapter 27, "Caregiving," for more information on caregiving.)

Note. AYA = adolescent and young adult.

TABLE 5.1. Examples of Rehabilitation Care for Adolescents and Young Adults Across the Cancer Care Continuum

STAGE OF CARE	REHABILITATIVE INTERVENTIONS EXAMPLES
Prevention and early detection	<ul><li>Education to include fitness routine, weight management, medical screening, sun exposure</li><li>Empowerment and engagement in health management</li></ul>
Diagnosis	<ul><li>Early therapeutic intervention (e.g., coping strategies, relaxation techniques, self-advocacy)</li><li>Prehabilitation</li></ul>
Treatment	<ul><li>Self-management</li><li>Fatigue, pain, peripheral neuropathy</li><li>Return to work or school</li><li>ADLs and IADLs</li><li>Cognition</li><li>Health management (e.g., medication management, fitness routine, fall prevention, energy conservation)</li><li>Social engagement</li><li>Adaptive equipment</li></ul>
Survivorship	<ul><li>Environmental modifications in school and work settings</li><li>Self-management techniques, often extending out from treatment</li><li>Health management</li><li>Social and leisure engagement</li></ul>
End-of-life care	<ul><li>Legacy completion</li><li>Family training</li><li>Adaptive equipment as needed</li></ul>

Note. ADLs = activities of daily living; IADLs = instrumental activities of daily living.

FACTORS CONTRIBUTING TO OCCUPATIONAL DYSFUNCTION AMONG AYAs WITH CANCER

Client Factors

Many factors may contribute to occupational dysfunction in the AYA population. One such factor is personal growth and aging. Behaviors often occur in the context of *learned dependency*. Many AYA survivors have been sick for a large portion of their childhood or young adulthood and have relied on the care, nurturing, and advice of others. This can be very detrimental, because the survivor continues to engage in thought behaviors such as, "Someone else will help me with this task because I am sick." Self-management has consistently been perceived as being of lesser value, and adolescents often struggle to take responsibility for actions that will lead to financial independence (Stam et al., 2005).

Research has shown that AYA survivors display a pattern of limited or restricted engagement and participation in both client factors and skills as they move into more independent life roles without the constant supervision or advice of parents or guardians (Barrera et al., 2005; Mulrooney et al., 2008; Ness et al., 2008; Pang et al., 2008). These activities of limited engagement include, but are not limited to, personal grooming and hygiene tasks, social activities, employment, chores, and school pursuits. The AYA population struggles as a whole with transitions from structured and coordinated environments, and this struggle is amplified in the AYA cancer population.

The influence of body functions and body structures on occupational dysfunction is varied. Depending on the type of cancer, the stage of cancer at diagnosis, and the course of treatment experienced by a client, multiple body functions and structures can be impaired at the same time, which can greatly affect occupational performance.

One issue highlighted earlier in this chapter is body image. Varying body functions and structures are affected throughout the course of cancer treatment and can include change in skin color or texture; change in mobility related to resection or loss of limb; changes to hair or loss of hair; and visual, auditory, and vocal changes. All of these functions and structures can have a lasting effect on communication, interaction, engagement, participation, and role establishment. This can be further compounded by cognitive impairments related to treatment-associated "chemo brain." In an acute-based setting, occupational therapy practitioners often treat not one impairment or one diagnosis but multiple body limitations that may actually be changing or evolving at a rapid rate because of disease progression. This requires practitioners to be adaptable in their treatment planning and interventions. Body image is explored in Case Example 5.1.

Performance Skills

The primary limiting factor in performance skills stems from social isolation and impaired social interaction skills, including social–emotional skills such as coping skills, communication skills, and appropriate behaviors. Many survivors have been on treatment-required isolation for an impaired immune system, which affects the skills acquired through day-to-day interaction with peers and older adults. This limits the normative progression and growth of social skills.

CASE EXAMPLE 5.1. ISABELLA: BODY IMAGE IMPAIRMENT ASSOCIATED WITH HEAD AND NECK SURGERY

Isabella is a 16-year-old girl with history of pharyngeal carcinoma. She presented for radical neck dissection after recurrence of her first neck dissection, completed at age 9 years. Isabella was referred to occupational therapy on Postoperative Day 1. During her evaluation, it was revealed that she took a long break from school during her initial treatment and was coping with body image impairments before her second resection, which created a much larger surgical area on her face and neck.

Isabella reported that her leisure engagement included being the school mascot. She revealed that once she placed the bulldog mask over her head, she "enjoyed being able to pretend to be someone else for a while." The mask allowed her to shield her scars and communicate more openly with her peers in socially acceptable situations. Being the mascot allowed Isabella to engage more frequently with her athletic peers but also kept her protected from feelings of shame, self-doubt, and the perceptions of others based on her visual appearance.

Isabella worked through her first two sessions by discussing ways she could plan to maintain control over the visual images presented to her peers during an upcoming FaceTime session with the athletes at her school. She worked to place scarves strategically over her new incisions to protect areas she felt unsure of, and she was able to appropriately problem solve how to manipulate her coverings to reveal her surgical incisions to her peers during their conversation as she felt more comfortable. Unique to this situation was that Isabella was very self-motivated and self-aware of how her visual appearance affected her engagement in daily interactions.

Social impairments can affect multiple areas of occupational engagement in the AYA population, including communication, work, education, and dating and relationships. Further impairments to appropriate social interaction can be lack of self-monitoring, learned dependency behaviors, and treatment-associated anxiety and depression. Occupational therapy practitioners can use various treatment interventions to meet these needs, including behavior journals, task modification, task initiation, and activities focused on initiation and self-responsibility. Tasks focused on improved responsibility and decreased dependency can vary. On the basis of the level of impairment, intervention can focus on initiation and setup of hygiene tasks once weekly, with limited cueing to self-management of fatigue for initiation of appropriate rest periods during work or school-related tasks to manage deadlines appropriately.

Cognitive functioning after treatment, including memory, attention, processing, safety, and perception, must be assessed. Cancer survivors' perception of impairments and how they relate to decline in function in one or many areas of routine completion often greatly affect engagement and carryover of therapeutic tasks. Occupational therapy practitioners see this frequently with clients who are higher functioning or those who have not returned to age-appropriate roles (e.g., living on their own, driving, returning to school or work), which limits their awareness of how subtle impairments can affect daily functioning.

Similar to client factors, it is difficult to isolate one or two performance skills because chronic illness can change clinical presentation or latency effects of treatment across the continuum of care. Any change in one performance skill can affect several other performance skills. This furthers the needs for consistent education on latency effects of cancer treatment. It also further highlights the need for consistent or strategic reassessments after completion of cancer treatment to monitor survivors as they return to precancer roles, routines, and habits.

Performance Patterns

Performance patterns are often the first area of impairment noted because treatment immediately begins to affect one's normative roles, routines, and habits. Survivors undergoing SCTs are typically independent in ADLs and function with appropriate strength, ROM, social skills, and cognitive abilities at initial evaluation. This is typical at the start of treatment. As the transplant process unfolds, it is common to disengage from roles and routines, and occupational therapy practitioners see a drop in therapeutic engagement as well as physical ability to engage. Cancer survivors who have the skills to complete specific ADL tasks, such as dressing, bathing, and toileting, but do not consistently engage in a specific routine can suffer from poor nutrition, social isolation, and decline in functional performance. Case Example 5.2 explores the effects of decline in performance patterns and therapeutic engagement during an inpatient hospital admission for a patient undergoing SCT.

Context and Environment

Environments play a very important role in the treatment and outcomes of the AYA cancer population. A typical day for an AYA individual in the normative population might include waking up in a home or apartment, completing their morning ADL routine, and perhaps making a meal. They may take public transportation or drive to a school or work environment. After work- or school-based tasks, they return home, perhaps do laundry, make dinner, take care of young children, and complete a bedtime routine.

At the start of cancer treatment, this entire routine may change, and the client's environments change from home, school, work, and community settings to hospitals, day clinics, diagnostic imaging rooms, and perhaps hotels or extended-stay environments if they are traveling for treatment. Changes in physical environments may also change their social environments. Cancer survivors undergoing treatment may

CASE EXAMPLE 5.2. PATRICK: COMPLICATIONS RESULTING FROM IMPAIRED PERFORMANCE PATTERNS

Patrick is a 23-year-old man with newly diagnosed acute lymphoblastic leukemia. On initial admission to the hospital, he was evaluated for baseline performance before autologous SCT. Patrick was initially very resistant to engaging in services, despite education provided to him and his parents by the therapy practitioners and the medical team. However, with encouragement, he completed his assessments.

Despite education from multiple team members on the importance of routine completion and engagement, leisure participation, and completion of his home exercise program, Patrick consistently deferred all out-of-bed activities, although he had the physical ability to complete these tasks. This resulted in many complications, including bilateral pleural effusions muscle atrophy, and sepsis resulting in an admission to the intensive care unit.

Patrick continued to defer engaging in self-care tasks, moving out of bed to a chair, and participating in therapy sessions, which led to further complications. His length of stay significantly increased, from an estimated 3 weeks to an actual stay of 5 months.

---

no longer have access to close family or friends, supportive colleagues, or their religious or spiritual supports. These significant changes can lead to social isolation, impaired engagement in functional activities, and decreased self-management of care related to depression and anxiety.

Another important environment to consider when working with the AYA population is the virtual environment. We are in an age when phones, tablets, and communication applications are prominent, which can be magnified in a controlled environment, such as a hospital room. Combining occupational therapy interventions into a variety of environments or worlds can improve functional outcomes and overall engagement in occupational interventions, especially with regard to routine establishment in new environments.

OCCUPATIONAL THERAPY EVALUATION OF AYA CLIENTS

When developing an occupational profile during an AYA evaluation, occupational therapy practitioners should include many factors, such as:

- What does a typical day in the life of this client look like?
- What types of roles and responsibilities does this client need to participate in?
- How is current or prior treatment affecting this client? (Does the survivor suffer from fatigue, neuropathy, cognitive impairments, weakness, or isolation?)
- Who is the primary caregiver for the individual? Does the client self-manage needs?
- What is the survivor's prior level of function?
- What are the survivor's and family's goals for improved engagement, participation, and QoL?
  See Table 5.2 for assessment tool examples.

Occupational Therapy Interventions Focused on AYA Clients

There are many areas in which occupational therapy practitioners can make an impact in the care and treatment of the AYA population. Treatment interventions vary widely on the basis of type of cancer, stage of cancer treatment, and location of interventions (i.e., hospital-based vs.

TABLE 5.2. Examples of Appropriate Assessment Tools in the AYA Population

ASSESSMENT	SPECIFIC USE, BENEFIT TO TREATMENT
Adolescent/Adult Sensory Profile (Brown & Dunn, 2002)	Identifies sensory-processing patterns and effects on functional patterns
Adolescent Role Assessment (Black, 1976)	Gathers information on the adolescent's role involvement over time and across domains
Arnadottir Occupational Therapy–ADL Neurobehavioral Evaluation (Arnadottir, 2019)	Identifies neurobehavioral deficits, the impact they have on functional performance of ADLs, and how they relate to the location of cortical lesions
Canadian Occupational Performance Measure (Law et al., 2019)	Detects change in a client's self-perception of occupational performance over time
Child and Adolescent Social Perception Measure (Magill-Evans et al., 1995)	Measures a child's sensitivity to nonverbal aspects of communication
Pediatric Quality of Life Inventory (Varni, 2019)	Measures health-related QoL (pediatric, AYA, and adults) with acute and chronic health conditions; also has specific modules to assess fatigue, SCT, and brain cancer
Functional Independence Measure (Uniform Data System for Medical Rehabilitation, 2012)	Measures independent performance in self-care, toileting, transfers, locomotion, communication, and social cognition

Note. ADLs = activities of daily living; AYA = adolescents and young adults; QoL = quality of life; SCT = stem cell transplant.

outpatient clinic). Education is a vast component of occupational therapy treatment and includes benefits of out-of-bed activity, functional engagement in self-management, cognitive functions (and awareness of challenges), home exercise programs for strengthening, and potential latency symptoms.

Adolescence presents with a wide array of challenges and opportunities surrounding growth and development. These challenges require occupational therapy practitioners to be creative and diligent in meeting the unique needs of this population. The psychosocial needs of this population are defined by development of identity, sexual maturity, and formation of relationships. To fully support survivors in this age range, occupational therapy practitioners must also address coping skills (surrounding anxiety and depression), communication, social isolation, chronic pain, body image, and CRF. Interventions in these areas can be focused individually or in group settings to include skills training sessions, activity analysis, community reintegration, and cognitive functioning.

Another area critical to the AYA population is return to work and school environments. Social isolation, impaired endurance, decline in cognitive functions, CRF, muscle weakness, and other impairments can prove challenging. Interventions vary on the basis of the type of cancer and resulting impairments; however, they focus largely on improved attention and concentration, energy conservation, task modification, and self-regulation for incorporation of rest periods as needed.

Reinforcement of education to family and friends of clients in this age range is critical to improve outcomes and prevent latent effects because survivors are more likely to suffer from learned dependency. As survivors are continually encouraged and presented with improved results, carryover of interventions outside of therapy sessions becomes more consistent.

SUMMARY

In work with the AYA population, many facets affect occupational engagement and functional outcomes. These facets can vary from a prehab course of treatment to inpatient acute treatment and outpatient and follow-up assessments. Clients' success after cancer treatment can be greatly affected by completion of age-appropriate tasks to include normative roles within established routines and by being adaptable to new roles, routines, and habits as the course of treatment changes performance.

It is vital that occupational therapy practitioners consistently monitor their clients across the cancer continuum of care from prehab to survivorship. Practitioners must continually adapt to the changes that survivors face as they move through early young adulthood to late young adulthood. Practitioners must identify changes and challenges as roles, routines, and environments change and help to guide their clients through these areas. Given that clients experience changes in intervention plans and interventions on the medical end as well, it is important to anticipate changes in functional performance and expected impairments to aid survivors in return to their prior level of functioning before the cancer diagnosis.

REFERENCES

American Cancer Society. (2017). *Key statistics for cancers in adolescents.* Retrieved from https://www.cancer.org/cancer/cancer-in-adolescents/key-statistics.html

American Cancer Society. (2018). *Key statistics for cancers in young adults.* Retrieved from https://www.cancer.org/cancer/cancer-in-young-adults/key-statistics.html

Armenian, S. H., Gibson, C. J., Rockne, R. C., & Ness, K. K. (2019). Premature aging in young cancer survivors. *JNCI: Journal of the National Cancer Institute, 111,* 226–232. https://doi.org/10.1093/jnci/djy229

Arnadottir, G. (2019). *A-ONE: The ADL-Focused Occupation-Based Neurobehavioral Evaluation.* Retrieved from http://www.a-one.is/index.html

Barnes, M., Plaisance, E., Hanks, L., & Casazza, K. (2016). Pre-habilitation: Promoting exercise in adolescent and young adult cancer survivors for improving lifelong health: A narrative review. *Cancer Research Frontiers, 2,* 22–32. https://doi.org/10.17980/2016.22

Barrera, M., Shaw, A., Speechley, K., Maunsell, E., & Pogany, L. (2005). Educational and social late effects of childhood cancer and related clinical, personal, and familial characteristics. *Cancer, 104,* 1751–1760. https://doi.org/10.1002/cncr.21390

Berg, C., & Hayashi, R. (2013). Participation and self-management strategies of young adult childhood cancer survivors. *OTJR: Occupation, Participation, and Health, 33,* 21–30. https://doi.org/10.3928/15394492-20120607-01

Berg, C., Neufeld, P., Harvey, J., Downes, A., & Hayashi, R. (2008). Late effects of childhood cancer, participation, and quality of life of adolescents. *OTJR: Occupation, Participation, and Health, 29,* 116–124. https://doi.org/10.3928/15394492-20090611-04

Black, M. M. (1976). Adolescent Role Assessment. *American Journal of Occupational Therapy, 30,* 73–79.

Brown, C., & Dunn, W. (2002). *Adolescent/Adult Sensory Profile.* Toronto: Pearson.

Brown, J. C., Winters-Stone, K., Lee, A., & Schmitz, K. H. (2012). Cancer physical activity, and exercise. *Comprehensive Physiology, 2,* 2775–2809. https://doi.org/10.1002/cphy.c12d005

Gilchrist, L., & Tanner, L. (2013). The Pediatric-Modified Total Neuropathy Score: A reliable and valid measure of chemotherapy-induced peripheral neuropathy in children with non-CNS cancers. *Supportive Care in Cancer, 21,* 847–856. https://doi.org/10.1007/s00520-012-1591-8

Isenalumhe, L., Fridgen, O., Beaupin, L. K., Quinn, G. P., & Reed, D. R. (2016). Disparities in adolescents and young adults with cancer. *Cancer Control, 23,* 424–433. https://doi.org/10.1177/107327481602300414

Keegan, T., Lichtensztajn, D., Kato, I., Kent, E., Wu, X. C., West, M. W., . . . AYA Hope Study Collaborative Group. (2012). Unmet adolescent and young adult cancer survivors' information and service needs: A population-based cancer registry study. *Journal of Cancer Survivorship, 6,* 239–250. https://doi.org/10.1007/s11764-012-0219-9

Law, M., Baptiste, S., Carswell, A., McColl, M. A., Polatajko, H., & Pollock, N. (2019). *Canadian Occupational Performance Measure* (5th ed., rev.). Altona, MB, Canada: COPM, Inc.

Liebert, M. A. (2011). What should the age range be in adolescent oncology? *Journal of Adolescent and Young Adult Oncology, 1.* https://doi.org/10.1089/jayao.2011.1505

Lorig, K., & Holman, H. (2003). Self-management education: History, definitions, outcomes, and mechanisms. *Annals of Behavioral Medicine, 26,* 1–7. https://doi.org/10.1207/S15324796ABM2601_01

Magill-Evans, J., Koning, C., Cameron-Sadava, A., & Manyk, K. (1995). The Child and Adolescent Social Perception Measure. *Journal of Nonverbal Behavior, 19,* 151–169. https://doi.org/10.1007/BF02175502

MD Anderson Cancer Center. (2020). *Brief Fatigue Inventory.* Retrieved from https://www.mdanderson.org/research/departments-labs-institutes/departments-divisions/symptom-research/symptom-assessment-tools/brief-fatigue-inventory.html

Mulrooney, D., Neglia, J., & Hudson, M. (2008). Caring for adult survivors of childhood cancer. *Current Treatment Options in Oncology, 9,* 51–66. https://doi.org/10.1007/s11864-008-0054-4

National Cancer Institute. (2018). *Adolescents and young adults with cancer.* Retrieved from https://www.cancer.gov/types/aya

Ness, K. K., Gurney, J. G., Zeltzer, L., Leisenring, W., Mulrooney, D., & Nathan, P. (2008). The impact of limitations in physical, executive, and emotional function on health-related quality of life among adult survivors of childhood cancer: A report from the Childhood Cancer Survivors Study. *Archives of Physical Medicine and Rehabilitation, 89,* 128–136. https://doi.org/10.1016/j.apmr.2007.08.123

Pang, J. W., Friedman, D. L., Whitton, J. A., Stovall, M., Mertens, A. C., Robinson, L. L., & Weiss, N. S. (2008). Employment status among adult survivors in the Childhood Cancer Survivor Study. *Pediatric Blood & Cancer, 50,* 104–110. https://doi.org/10.1002/pbc.21226

Shun, S. (2016). Cancer prehabilitation for patients starting from active treatment to surveillance. *Asia Pacific Journal of Oncology Nursing, 3,* 37–40. https://doi.org/10.4103/2347-5625.178169

Silver, J. K. (2015). Cancer prehabilitation and its role in improving health outcomes and reducing health care costs. *Seminars in Oncology Nursing, 31*(1), 13–30. https://doi.org/10.1016/j.soncn.2014.11.003

Silver, J. K., Baima, J., & Mayer, R. S. (2013). Impairment-driven cancer rehabilitation: An essential component of quality care and survivorship. *CA: A Cancer Journal for Clinicians, 63,* 295–317. https://doi.org/10.3322/caac.21186

Stam, H., Grootenhuis, M., & Last, B. (2005). The course of life of survivors of childhood cancer. *Psycho-Oncology, 14,* 227–238. https://doi.org/10.1002/pon.839

Taylor, R. (2017). *Kielhofner's Model of Human Occupation* (5th ed.). Alphen aan den Rijn, the Netherlands: Wolters Kluwer.

Uniform Data System for Medical Rehabilitation. (2012). *The FIM® instrument: Its background, structure, and usefulness.* Buffalo, NY: Author.

Varni, J. W. (2019) *The PedsQL™: Measurement model for the Pediatric Quality of Life Inventory™.* Retrieved from https://www.pedsql.org/index.html

Zhukovsky, D., Rozmus, C., Robert, R., Bruera, E., Wells, R., Chisholm, G., . . . Cohen, M. (2015). Symptom profiles in children with advanced cancer: Patient, family caregiver, and oncologist ratings. *Cancer, 121,* 4080–4087. https://doi.org/10.1002/cncr.29597

Special Considerations for Adults With Cancer

6

Claudine Campbell, OTD, OTR/L, CLT

LEARNING OBJECTIVES

After completing this chapter, readers should be able to

- Summarize how adults with cancer are susceptible to an overall decrease in activity participation secondary to cancer-associated side effects across the continuum of care;
- Understand salient developmental issues for adults who may be affected by a cancer diagnosis;
- Analyze the impact of cancer treatment–associated side effects and related factors on occupational performance and on the development of the occupational profile, analysis of occupational performance, and occupational therapy plan of care; and
- Describe the occupational therapy evaluation process and interventions relevant to adults with cancer, including considerations involving special precautions and contraindications that may affect occupational performance.

KEY TERMS AND CONCEPTS

- Adult life course
- Analysis of occupational performance
- Cancer care continuum
- Client factors
- Complications
- Contexts
- Education
- Environments
- Financial burden
- Group interventions
- Isolation precautions
- Modifiable risk factors
- Pain and fatigue
- Performance patterns
- Psychosocial sequelae
- Return-to-work programs

INTRODUCTION

Adults who are diagnosed with cancer and receive treatment are at risk for developing alterations in emotional, cognitive, physical, social, and financial capacities that can limit activity and participation (Baxter et al., 2017). Decreased participation in meaningful occupations can result from the cancer itself, from the disease progression, and from the side effects of the treatment modalities used to minimize or eradicate the cancer (Pergolotti et al., 2016). This chapter focuses on special considerations, developmental issues, and occupational therapy's role with adults with cancer.

Depending on the primary cancer diagnosis (i.e., type), the stage and extent of the disease (i.e., metastatic vs. local), and the specific treatment modalities or medications they receive, adults with cancer may experience complications and obstacles that interfere with personally meaningful occupations. *Complications* resulting from cancer diagnosis and treatment include organ dysfunction; cardiac, hematological, renal, and orthopedic complications; communication and swallowing difficulties; metastatic disease (including osseous disease); neurological dysfunction, including changes in cognition or perception; cancer-related fatigue; peripheral neuropathy; psychosocial

sequelae, including depression and anxiety; lymphedema; and cancer-related pain (Cristian et al., 2012). Complications can potentially arise throughout the life course, and their severity and intensity may increase as adult clients age.

Treatment-related cognitive and physical impairments in adults with cancer have been associated with higher health care costs and hospital readmissions. Availability and use of rehabilitation services, including occupational therapy, across the cancer care continuum can lower costs and readmissions by minimizing occupational performance limitations, promoting activity engagement, and increasing role resumption (Pergolotti et al., 2016). For example, occupational therapy practitioners can address consistent, ongoing management of lymphedema, a chronic condition that may occur any time after cancer treatment. Lymphedema has been associated with elevated health care costs and decreased quality of life (QoL) because of delayed return to work and inability to fulfill necessary life roles (Pergolotti et al., 2016).

Psychosocial sequelae commonly associated with a cancer diagnosis include anxiety, distress, and depression; role disruption caused by this life-altering illness; the *financial burden* of cancer treatment and its effect on occupational engagement; and the impact of compromised or lost employment. The cost of cancer treatment and associated

---

follow-up medical care and surveillance can create special challenges for young adults, who may not have the financial security older adults typically acquire over the course of their lifespan (Landwehr et al., 2016). Cancer treatment side effects can affect clients' ability to perform their routine job responsibilities, engage in certain types of work, or even continue to work full-time, further compromising financial security (Mullen & Mistry, 2017).

Returning to work and other meaningful life roles in some capacity can assist adult clients in regaining a sense of normalcy and reclaiming confidence in their abilities to perform desired and necessary occupations after a cancer diagnosis (Désiron et al., 2013). Adults with cancer can benefit from comprehensive **return-to-work programs** with targeted strategies addressing cancer-specific issues such as clinical factors, client-related factors such as ability to work and overall work performance during and after treatment, and environmental modifications; such programs present an opportunity for occupational therapy practitioners to fill a gap by providing valuable services to this client population. (For more information, see Chapter 25, "Work.")

Understanding the cancer disease process and potential treatment side effects can enable clinicians to anticipate and identify occupational engagement limitations adult clients with cancer may face throughout the cancer continuum. Proper identification of cancer treatment consequences and occupational performance limitations as early as the time of initial diagnosis is essential for the development of client-centered occupational therapy treatment plans focused on safe and appropriate occupation-based interventions to maximize QoL and resumption of meaningful life roles.

LIFESPAN AND DEVELOPMENTAL CHALLENGES FOR ADULTS WITH CANCER

A cancer diagnosis often entails attention to comorbidities or lifestyle choices that are associated with **modifiable risk factors** (as opposed to nonmodifiable risk factors, such as genetics or family history of cancer). As explained in Chapter 1, "Cancer Demographics and Trends Across the Lifespan," the risk for developing cancer can be minimized by reducing unhealthy behaviors such as tobacco use, poor diet, lack of routine exercise, and excessive sun exposure (American Cancer Society [ACS], 2018). According to a recent study, approximately 42% of newly diagnosed cancers in the United States could be avoided or prevented with lifestyle changes, and routine screenings have been shown to assist in preventing colorectal and cervical cancers (ACS, 2018).

When they are diagnosed with cancer, adult clients may receive occupational therapy services to help them resume or maintain participation in daily activities and occupations or improve their level of occupational engagement (Braveman & Hunter, 2017). The focus of services depends on the client's specific stage of the **adult life course** when initially diagnosed; the individual may be focused on managing relationships (e.g., spouse or partner, family of origin), identifying a career

---

TABLE 6.1.   Developmental Challenges for Adults With Cancer

CHALLENGE	EXPLANATION
Managing relationships	Relationships with family members can become strained by the many decisions that need to be made regarding medical treatment schedules; selection of the best treatment options; payment for treatment; and the need to balance life responsibilities while coping with the psychosocial, cognitive, and physical side effects of treatment (Mullen & Mistry, 2017).
Identifying a career plan or obtaining a degree	For adults who are in the process of identifying a career plan or obtaining a degree, a cancer diagnosis can place additional strain on the individual and cause mental health issues such as depression and anxiety. A disruption in a client's educational coursework or a delay in obtaining a desired degree may contribute to a client's anxiety and distress about returning to normal roles and routines.
Managing a professional career	A lapse in education or work while undergoing treatment and the risk of unemployment present significant challenges for adults with cancer, including role disruption and occupational imbalance secondary to impaired ability to fulfill principal life roles. For clients who are the primary provider or decision maker in their family unit, the need to take a less active role can change or alter family dynamics, adding another source of stress (Mullen & Mistry, 2017). These stressors are explored in more depth in Chapter 20, "Psychosocial Issues."
Managing a family or household	Managing a household during cancer treatment can be extremely challenging for many adults. Caring for children or older family members, maintaining a home, and managing their own cancer treatment and regular medical appointments may become overwhelming in addition to their other responsibilities.
Achieving financial stability	One of the major challenges for adult clients is concern about the financial and economic burden of cancer treatment on the individual as well as the family unit. This burden includes the medical costs of cancer treatment; lost income as a result of absences from work; missed professional development opportunities; costs of follow-up care and insurance copayments; limited financial assistance resources; and the additional burden or strain placed on children, family members, and caregivers (Baxter et al., 2017; Landwehr et al., 2016). Approximately one-third of U.S. cancer survivors face unmet needs for financial assistance during their cancer treatment, and young adults are more likely to report financial barriers to their medical care than older adults (Landwehr et al., 2016). The stress associated with the financial burden of cancer treatment can manifest in anxiety and distress and is associated with decreased quality of life (Landwehr et al., 2016).

plan or obtaining a degree, managing a professional career, managing a family or household (e.g., planning to become a parent, expanding the family, caring for young children or older family members), or achieving financial stability (e.g., considering a career change or retirement after an established career). Table 6.1 describes the effects of a cancer diagnosis on each of these stages in the adult life course.

MOST COMMON FORMS OF CANCER AND RELATED HEALTH RISKS IN ADULTS

The most common types of cancer in men are prostate, lung, colon, bladder, and skin cancers, and the most common types of cancer in women are breast, lung, colon, uterine, and thyroid cancers (ACS, 2018). Adults with multiple comorbidities, lower socioeconomic status, and membership in ethnic minority groups are at greater risk for cancer mortality attributable to various social, economic, cultural, and environmental influences, including unemployment, early negative life experiences, high work-related stress, poor diets, and limited social support networks (Braveman & Hunter, 2017). Early onset of diabetes, hypertension, or heart disease can complicate a cancer diagnosis, and there is a significant relationship between cancer and psychosocial stressors, specifically the extent, number, and persistence of the stressors and the effectiveness of coping strategies.

ROLE OF OCCUPATIONAL THERAPY ACROSS THE CANCER CARE CONTINUUM

Occupational therapy practitioners provide rehabilitation interventions for adults with cancer across the cancer care continuum and over the life course. Clients may encounter an occupational therapy practitioner at any stage of the *cancer care continuum,* beginning with pretreatment, during early phases of treatment, during an acute hospital or post-acute rehabilitation admission, throughout post-treatment as an outpatient, and at the end stage of illness (Braveman & Hunter, 2017; Cristian et al., 2012). The role of occupational therapy practitioners with adults with cancer includes encouraging, supporting, and facilitating participation in meaningful and preferred occupations, including basic ADLs and IADLs, work and leisure, social participation, and rest and sleep as well as functional activities to maintain strength, coordination, endurance, cognitive function, and psychosocial well-being.

During active cancer treatment, the primary goal and focus of occupational therapy intervention may be to optimize clients' functional mobility, ability to complete basic self-care activities with or without family assistance, and participation in meaningful occupations through activity modifications or use of assistive devices (Stubblefield & O'Dell, 2009). When clients are receiving daily or weekly chemotherapy or daily radiation treatments, they may need to learn how to conserve their energy, prioritize meaningful daily activities, incorporate activity or environmental modifications, use adaptive equipment, develop more effective rest and sleep patterns or routines, complete familiar tasks

in new ways, and implement strategies for work simplification or modification (Braveman & Hunter, 2017).

Although many adult cancer survivors live normal lifespans with minimal cancer-related complications, some live the remainder of their lives with short-term and long-term consequences from the cancer diagnosis itself or their primary or secondary cancer treatment (Pergolotti et al., 2016). The severity of side effects may depend on the client's prognosis and cancer stage at the time of diagnosis. In a functional context, cancer survivors who develop emotional, cognitive, or physical sequelae from cancer treatment commonly report difficulty returning to normal roles and routines, including work, community involvement, and social functioning, resulting in decreased QoL (Baxter et al., 2017). Additionally, their ability to drive, care for others, and fulfill everyday responsibilities, such as paying bills and managing a household, may decrease, along with their independence with ADLs and IADLs (Braveman & Hunter, 2017). The combination of physical, cognitive, and spiritual challenges associated with cancer can result in a decreased sense of purpose and altered life roles.

During active treatment, adult clients may spend time thinking about their preferred roles and responsibilities and question whether they will be able to reintegrate into their meaningful roles and occupations. Occupational therapy practitioners can assist clients in identifying important present or future roles, facilitate realistic goal setting, and determine steps to work toward goal achievement. Practitioners can address occupational adaptation during cancer treatment by using the Model of Human Occupation (Kielhofner, 2008) and the Revised Role Checklist (Scott et al., 2019) to assess clients' volition, habituation, occupational skill, occupational performance and participation, and environment and then helping clients identify goals for all areas of their life (Bonsaksen et al., 2015; Désiron et al., 2013).

Occupational therapy practitioners can implement a range of adaptations, including adaptive equipment and devices and environmental modifications, to optimize clients' occupational performance and safety in the home and community during the diagnosis (i.e., pretreatment) and active treatment phases (Cheville & Basford, 2014). In addition, practitioners can incorporate compensatory strategies such as special positioning to minimize pain and discomfort and modification of ADLs to help clients with cognitive dysfunction or altered endurance levels maximize occupational engagement across the cancer care continuum (American Occupational Therapy Association [AOTA], 2011). Examples of rehabilitation interventions across the cancer care continuum are provided in Table 6.2.

FACTORS THAT MAY CONTRIBUTE TO OCCUPATIONAL DYSFUNCTION

Client Factors: Special Considerations With Adults

Client factors include values and beliefs, body functions, and body structures that influence motivation and participation in occupations (AOTA, 2014). The client factors most commonly affected by a cancer diagnosis and most critical to assess with adult clients include the client's values

TABLE 6.2.   Occupational Therapy Interventions for Adults Across the Cancer Care Continuum

STAGE OF CARE	INTERVENTIONS
Prevention	Adults with cancer can benefit from preventive education and training regarding modifiable risk factors, healthy behaviors to maximize energy levels and functional abilities, and appropriate exercise regimens that maintain safe blood pressure and resting and target heart rate during activity.
Early detection and screening	Early detection and screening may involve primary and secondary prevention of deficits in physical, cognitive, and emotional levels of function. Education can be provided about signs and symptoms of cancer and ways to minimize risk through routine screening and surveillance.
Diagnosis	At the time of diagnosis, adult clients may benefit from education and training to maintain function and promote psychological health throughout the course of treatment. Clients should receive education about potential side effects, precautions, and limitations to anticipate as they undergo various types of cancer treatment to effectively prepare them for the challenges they may face during and after treatment. Providing education on the benefits of regular exercise and continued participation in meaningful roles and routines can enable clients to sustain their emotional, cognitive, and physical abilities for a sense of overall well-being; this education is an important and valued role of occupational therapy practitioners and can be combined with prehabilitation programming.
Treatment	Adults with cancer require education about optimal symptom management during active cancer treatment. Suggestions for modifications to self-care routines when lab values are lower than normal can improve clients' health and safety; for example, when a client's platelet count is below 150,000–400,000 platelets per microliter, instruction can be provided to avoid using sharp objects (e.g., scissors, nail clippers) to prevent the risk of excessive bleeding. In addition, education about fall risk precautions in the home and community environments should address wearing proper footwear for maximal support, requesting assistance with daily activities from family members when necessary, and using energy conservation principles to avoid extreme fatigue.
Survivorship	Making adjustments in lifestyle, resuming healthy behaviors, and participating in community wellness activities to maintain health and wellness are important components of survivorship. At this stage, adult clients may benefit from education about safe and appropriate exercises and activities to participate in when energy levels fluctuate or are lower than baseline.
End-of-life care	Interventions in end-of-life care promote function and goal attainment. The focus is on modifying basic ADLs, positioning the client to maximize safety and comfort, and addressing the client's specific goals for engagement in day-to-day activities and meaningful occupations.

Note. ADLs = activities of daily living.

and commitments, cognitive beliefs, and spirituality; mental, sensory, motor, and muscle functions; cardiovascular, hematological, immunological, and respiratory functions; and body structures affected by the cancer diagnosis and treatment, which may include multiple systems and organs.

Using both subjective and objective measures to comprehensively assess client factors in adults is the optimal approach for analyzing the negative impact of cancer and its treatment on occupational performance. Subjective factors can be ascertained through the client interview, which should include questions about the client's current pain level, energy and activity tolerance levels, prior and current ability to complete ADLs and IADLs, and sensory changes such as visual, hearing, or vestibular affecting occupational performance (Stubblefield et al., 2013).

Pain and fatigue are common client factors that may contribute to occupational dysfunction in adults across the cancer care continuum. For example, pain and fatigue may affect a client's ability to attend school, work, or parent as well as to tolerate additional cancer treatment. Variability in blood pressure (e.g., hypotension, hypertension), respiratory system status (e.g., low blood oxygenation, shortness of breath), and aerobic capacity and stamina can compromise clients' full participation in home management tasks, meal preparation, and work and leisure activities (AOTA, 2014). Common side effects of daily radiation therapy, such as nausea, poor appetite, mental fatigue, and generalized muscle fatigue resulting in poor stamina, may reduce

clients' independence with daily self-care and work routines, ability to complete safe functional transfers in and out of a car, and ability to safely travel to and from the radiation therapy clinic every day via public transportation or car (Hwang et al., 2015).

Performance Patterns: Special Considerations With Adults

Performance patterns, which include habits, routines, roles, and rituals, can potentially change in clients with prolonged hospital stays. For example, adults who undergo a bone marrow transplant are typically admitted to the hospital for pretransplant conditioning in which they receive high doses of chemotherapy or radiation to rid the body of cancer cells, often killing healthy cells in the process. During this time, clients may be placed on *isolation precautions,* requiring the use of a mask, gown, and gloves, because they are susceptible to infection and treatment complications, limiting their normal activity and open access to visitors.

Such clients benefit from education and therapeutic interventions focused on maintaining activity engagement and preserving psychosocial well-being within the isolation parameters. Clients can be encouraged to uphold normal self-care routines and schedules for bathing, grooming, and dressing and to sustain social contact with family members, friends, and coworkers outside the hospital through regular phone calls, email, or social media. The Canadian

Occupational Performance Measure (Law et al., 2019) can be used with adults to assess performance of and satisfaction with routines and roles that are personally meaningful and to identify problems as they arise (Braveman & Hunter, 2017).

Context and Environment: Special Considerations With Adults

Contexts are the cultural, personal, temporal, and virtual conditions within and around the client, whereas *environments* are the external physical and social conditions surrounding the client; context and environment influence participation in meaningful occupations (AOTA, 2014). The contexts and environments of adults with cancer are important to consider when completing evaluations and providing treatment. Clients' preferred methods for completing meaningful occupations may be based on customs, beliefs, or socioeconomic status, and they may wish to continue performing these occupations in the same manner despite impairments caused by the cancer diagnosis and treatment.

For example, a client may be accustomed to kneeling or sitting on the floor to perform a daily prayer ritual, eat meals, or complete grooming tasks to embrace religious customs and rituals. However, if this client develops weakness, pain, and bone metastases secondary to the spread of cancer to the spine, the client's ability to safely kneel or sit on the floor without experiencing discomfort may be compromised. The occupational therapy practitioner can provide culturally sensitive care by using an adaptive approach to modify these activities by incorporating an alternative seating position or by adapting equipment or the environment (e.g., use of cushions or a small stool).

Clients who develop cognitive dysfunction from cancer treatment may benefit from grading the difficulty of daily activities or incorporating the use of familiar objects. For example, a client may demonstrate increased ability to shower or bathe when using soap or shampoo they typically use at home. Another may be able to complete a simple meal preparation task such as making a cup of coffee when using their preferred brand of coffee and favorite mug from home. This client may respond more positively to a group meal preparation activity than to a solo activity if cooking meals with family during holidays and get-togethers holds value and meaning.

OCCUPATIONAL THERAPY EVALUATION OF ADULTS WITH CANCER

Occupational Profile

To gain an understanding of an adult client's need for occupational therapy services, the reason for occupational therapy referral, and the client's occupational history and experiences, the following guiding questions can be used in the initial interview (AOTA, 2017):

- What is your primary occupation, and are you currently working?
- Explain what a typical day looks like for you from the time you wake up to the time you go to bed. What are your primary roles at home and at work or school?

- Do you have support from family and friends? Who is your primary support person?
- What are your greatest interests? What do you enjoy doing for fun or leisure?
- Why do you feel you need occupational therapy services?
- What physical, cognitive, and emotional symptoms have you experienced since your diagnosis and cancer treatment?
- Have you been informed about any special precautions or restrictions related to your cancer treatment and everyday activity performance? If you have, how do you think these precautions will affect how you perform your everyday activities at home, at work or school, and in the community?

Analysis of Occupational Performance

To complete the analysis of occupational performance, occupational therapy practitioners can use observation and objective measures to identify the client's strengths and problem areas (i.e., impairments) and potential problems. Table 6.3 includes a list of assessments appropriate for use with adults with cancer.

The *analysis of occupational performance* is a synthesis of both subjective information gathered from the client interview and occupational profile and observations of the client's performance during tasks or activities that are tied to meaningful or necessary occupations. Practitioners incorporate consideration of client factors, performance patterns, contexts and environments, and activity demands to provide an overall picture of the client's strengths and areas for improvement and establish goals that are meaningful to the client. Case Example 6.1 describes the evaluation and intervention process for a client with a brain tumor.

OCCUPATIONAL THERAPY INTERVENTIONS WITH ADULTS WITH CANCER

The occupational therapist develops an intervention plan and goals in collaboration with the client. Together, they take into consideration the occupations the client needs and wants to participate in and the client's individualized precautions, special considerations and treatment parameters, and limitations necessary to maximize safety and enhance occupational performance.

When feasible, occupational therapy practitioners should assess clients shortly after initial diagnosis or before the initiation of cancer treatment to provide surveillance and education about lifestyle modifications to enhance their tolerance of subsequent cancer treatment (Maltser et al., 2017). Identification of comorbidities and additional life stressors that may affect a client's ability to tolerate cancer treatment early on can have a direct impact on the client's QoL and overall survival. Education about minimizing stress, improving health and well-being in all realms of life, and making healthy diet and exercise choices can positively affect adult clients' ability to tolerate the recommended course of cancer treatment.

TABLE 6.3.   Assessments Commonly Used With Adults With Cancer

DOMAIN OF OCCUPATIONAL THERAPY	ASSESSMENTS

Occupations	▪ Activity Card Sort (Baum & Edwards, 2008)
	▪ Activity Measure for Post-Acute Care (AM–PAC) Short Forms for Inpatient and Outpatient Settings (Jette et al., 2015):
	  • Applied Cognitive
	  • Basic Mobility
	  • Daily Activity (Self-Care)
	▪ FIM® (Uniform Data System for Medical Rehabilitation, 1997)
	▪ Instrumental Activities of Daily Living Scale (Lawton & Brody, 1969)
	▪ Katz Index of Independence in Activities of Daily Living (Katz et al., 1963)
	▪ Physical Self-Maintenance Scale (Lawton & Brody, 1969)
	▪ Role Checklist (Kielhofner, 2008)
	▪ Worker Role Interview (Braveman et al., 2005)

Performance skills	▪ Activities-specific Balance Confidence (ABC) Scale (Powell & Myers, 1995) ▪ Assessment of Motor and Process Skills (AMPS; Fisher & Jones, 2012) ▪ Brief Fatigue Inventory (Mendoza et al., 1999) ▪ Treatment-Induced Neuropathy Assessment Scale (Galer & Jensen, 1997)
Performance patterns	▪ Canadian Occupational Performance Measure (COPM; Law et al., 2019) ▪ Model of Human Occupation Screening Tool (MOHOST; Parkinson et al., 2006) ▪ Occupational Performance History Interview–II (Kiehlhofner et al., 2004)

Targeted Occupations and Activities

Occupations and activities to be addressed in occupational therapy intervention sessions are selected on the basis of the client's primary roles and routines. For a client with a primary role of parent, one focus of intervention may be restoring body functions—for example, strength, coordination, endurance, or sensation, within treatment parameters—to promote engagement in caregiver roles and responsibilities. If resistive strengthening exercises are not feasible because of low laboratory values or bone disease, isometric exercises or functional tasks to enhance standing balance, strength, and general activity tolerance may be considered to promote increased independence with caring for children—for example, assisting them in and out of a car or helping them get ready for school in the morning.

Another focus of intervention may be environmental modifications or adaptive equipment provision and training to maximize clients' independence in occupational performance. For example, practitioners may modify clothing (e.g., T-shirt, pants) with hook-and-loop or other fasteners to increase clients' ability to don and doff clothing with greater ease or may modify clients' technique and method of getting in and out of a car to improve community access. Adaptive equipment may help compensate for impaired body functions; for example, for a client with decreased hand strength or coordination because of tremors, utensils with built-up handles, a universal cuff, or a supportive wrist brace may be recommended to improve engagement in meal preparation activities.

Clients with cancer of the central nervous system may require occupation-focused interventions similar to those for clients with stroke or traumatic brain injury. Therapeutic interventions such as functional transfer training, self-care adaptation, and IADL training might be the primary focus during active cancer treatment to ensure that clients

can perform their daily activities with the current level of support and caregiver assistance at home.

For a client who is focused on participating in household management responsibilities, reviewing safe body mechanics for shower transfers and bathroom negotiation and eliminating dangerous household obstacles may be necessary to maximize the client's safety. Clients may also benefit from the challenge of participating in a task that is novel to improve their ability to problem solve and sequence through a more familiar task; for example, to prepare a meal for a weekly family dinner, the client can first verbalize and write down the ingredients and steps of a recipe and then complete the steps.

For clients who want and need to return to work for psychosocial and financial benefits but who are experiencing significant cancer-related fatigue and peripheral neuropathy, an occupational therapy intervention plan may involve a range of occupation-focused modalities. Creating a self-management program that includes using a daily fatigue journal and daily mindfulness practice, practicing meaningful tasks with modifications to match energy demands (e.g., taking notes during a meeting, answering emails and phone calls, giving a presentation), identifying new habits and routines to achieve the goal of returning to work, and exploring the option to initially return with a flexible or modified schedule are a few examples of occupational therapy work-related interventions. The focus of the intervention plan would be on maximizing occupational performance and participation, role competence, and QoL to address management of a professional career.

Preparatory Methods and Tasks

Preparatory methods and tasks are used to prepare clients for participation in occupations and frequently involve a combination of low-tech and high-tech assistive technology

CASE EXAMPLE 6.1. SUSAN: AGE 45, WITH A BRAIN TUMOR

Background

- **Susan,** a woman, age 45 years, has been diagnosed with astrocytoma, a primary brain tumor. She has a history of hypertension and anxiety.
- Susan underwent several cycles of chemotherapy on an outpatient basis and then a craniotomy of the left temporoparietal region of the brain.
- Susan is hospitalized for 4 days postsurgery.

Occupational Profile

- Susan lives alone and is a high school French teacher. She is currently on short-term disability from her full-time teaching position. She enjoys gardening, reading, and socializing with friends. She has two sisters who live within a 30-minute drive of her house.
- Susan's house has two levels with a full bathroom on the second floor and a half bath on the first floor. Before her surgery, Susan was independent with basic ADLs but required assistance with IADL management because of generalized weakness, fatigue, and impaired balance resulting from her diagnosis and outpatient chemotherapy treatment.
- Susan's sisters have noticed that Susan is finding it increasingly difficult to go up and down the flight of stairs in her home and is becoming more forgetful. She does not consistently remember to take her medications and sometimes confuses the dates and times of her medical appointments. Susan has also experienced elevated blood pressure since receiving chemotherapy.

Analysis of Occupational Performance

- The occupational therapist assesses Susan's ADL and IADL performance using the Activity Measure for Post-Acute Care short form for inpatient self-care (Jette et al., 2015), Instrumental Activities of Daily Living Scale (Lawton & Brody, 1969), Canadian Occupational Performance Measure (Law et al., 2019), Revised Role Checklist (Scott et al., 2019), and Montreal Cognitive Assessment (Nasreddine et al., 2005).

- Assessment findings indicate that Susan has impaired balance and coordination, decreased endurance and activity tolerance, decreased strength in the upper and lower extremities, and impaired memory and attention that compromise her ability to safely complete self-care tasks (dressing, toileting, showering) and IADLs (community mobility and access, medication management, meal preparation, home management). Susan is having the most difficulty completing dressing and showering tasks, reading and writing, retaining new information, and safely moving about in the community.
- Susan reports a moderate level of distress related to her decline in function and new dependence on others to complete basic and instrumental ADLs. Susan's anxiety has increased in intensity and frequency as she questions when and whether she will return to work, either full-time or part-time, in the future.

Occupational Therapy Interventions

- The occupational therapist creates the intervention plan and treatment goals collaboratively with Susan, taking into consideration the occupations she needs and wants to be able to participate in.
- Occupational therapy treatment sessions are focused on restoring body functions such as strength, coordination, and endurance to promote occupational engagement in dressing, showering, completing home management tasks, and reading books of interest.
- Another focus of intervention includes providing Susan with education and instruction on coping skills she can implement to manage her distress related to her decline in function, stress management and mindfulness techniques to manage her anxiety and stress, and compensatory strategies to address her difficulty with retaining new information such as her new daily medication schedule.
- Susan is instructed on how to incorporate deep breathing exercises into her daily routine and to use her smartphone to set reminders for her medical appointments and daily medication schedule. She also learns how to use a goal-setting app on her phone to track daily goals such as drinking at least eight glasses of water each day and practicing 5 minutes of mindfulness.

and environmental modifications. For example, for a client with a wrist drop or a skin graft taken from the forearm and transferred to the head or neck region during cancer treatment, a splint can be fabricated to support and position the hand and wrist for optimal healing. Other examples include providing a built-up pen or modifying a computer workstation to facilitate writing or typing with greater ease and less discomfort for a client with peripheral neuropathy (Speck et al., 2012), improving visual input by providing large-print educational materials or a magnifying glass to increase a client's ability to read, or using a variety of simple or complex communication boards with as few as

4 or as many as 16 pictures to improve a client's ability to communicate needs and thoughts by pointing to an image or word. In addition, the use of a dry-erase board can be implemented to improve a nonverbal client's ability to communicate more effectively through writing.

Education

Education is a necessary component of the treatment plan for adults with cancer. Education may be needed on a variety of topics, including (but not limited to) energy conservation principles; task simplification; safe body mechanics for self-care tasks, functional transfers, and mobility; modified body mechanics after surgery (e.g., spine precautions, weight-bearing precautions, range of motion restrictions, lifting and carrying restrictions, specific activity restrictions); lymphedema prevention and management; proper use of adaptive equipment and assistive devices; compensatory strategies for impaired cognition; communication management and modified communication strategies; strategies to improve sleep preparation and participation; stress reduction and mindfulness practice to address anxiety and stress; and return-to-work modifications or adaptations.

Key components of education for adult clients with cancer include the importance of maintaining routine daily activity participation, the benefits of scheduling preferred activities throughout the day when energy levels are higher, and the use of compensatory or adaptive strategies, including technology or smartphone apps, to maximize occupational engagement. Cancer treatment and its side effects place overwhelming and competing demands on adult clients, and occupational therapy practitioners play an important role in educating clients about strategies and modifications that can help them maintain or resume their preferred and desired roles.

Group Interventions

Occupational therapy practitioners in a variety of settings provide *group interventions* that bring adults with cancer together to promote exploration and development of new skills to improve occupational performance. Therapeutic groups can cover a variety of topics, including cognitive strategies to improve memory and executive functions, energy conservation principles to improve stamina and activity tolerance, education about methods to prevent and manage lymphedema, and techniques to manage daily stress and improve organization and prioritization of daily activities and tasks to reduce stress (Lyons, 2006).

SUMMARY

Adults with cancer may experience myriad side effects and complications specific to their primary cancer diagnosis, the stage and extent of the disease, and the cancer treatment modalities and medications they receive. Adult clients are referred for occupational therapy services throughout the cancer care continuum to address complications that compromise occupational performance, including organ dysfunction; cardiac, hematological, renal, and orthopedic complications; communication and swallowing difficulties; metastatic disease; changes in cognition or perception; psychosocial sequelae, including depression and anxiety; lymphedema; peripheral neuropathy; and cancer-related pain and fatigue (Cristian et al., 2012). Occupational therapy practitioners play a key role with adult clients with cancer by promoting participation in daily activities and maintenance of or improvement in overall strength, coordination, endurance, cognitive function, and psychosocial well-being to maximize occupational engagement.

To provide optimal evaluation and intervention, occupational therapy practitioners must have general knowledge about cancer treatment principles, precautions, special considerations, and treatment parameters that may affect clients' ability to perform daily occupations and meaningful activities. Comorbidities and emotional and financial distress may negatively affect clients' ability to tolerate cancer treatment, QoL, and overall survival (Mullen & Mistry, 2017). By using a combination of subjective and objective measures to comprehensively assess client factors and performance patterns in adults with cancer, occupational therapy practitioners can implement individualized, safe, and effective client-focused occupational therapy treatment plans aimed at improving occupational performance and QoL across the cancer care continuum.

REFERENCES

American Cancer Society. (2018). *Cancer facts and figures 2018.* Retrieved from https://www.cancer.org/content/dam/cancer-org/research/cancer-facts-and-statistics/annual-cancer-facts-and-figures/2018/cancer-facts-and-figures-2018.pdf

American Occupational Therapy Association. (2011). The role of occupational therapy in end-of-life care. *American Journal of Occupational Therapy, 65*(Suppl.), S66–S75. https://doi.org/10.5014/ajot.2011.65S66

American Occupational Therapy Association. (2014). Occupational therapy practice framework: Domain and process (3rd ed.). *American Journal of Occupational Therapy, 68*(Suppl. 1), S1–S48. https://doi.org/10.5014/ajot.2014.682006

American Occupational Therapy Association. (2017). AOTA occupational profile template. *American Journal of Occupational Therapy, 71,* 7112420030. https://doi.org/10.5014/ajot.2017.716S12

Baum, C., & Edwards, D. (2008). *Activity Card Sort* (2nd ed.). Bethesda, MD: AOTA Press.

Baxter, M. F., Newman, R., Longpre, S. M., & Polo, K. M. (2017). Health Policy Perspectives—Occupational therapy's role in cancer survivorship as a chronic condition. *American Journal of Occupational Therapy, 71,* 7103090010. https://doi.org/10.5014/ajot.2017.713001

Bonsaksen, T., Meidert, U., Schuman, D., Kvarsnes, H., Haglund, L., Prior, S., . . . Scot, P. J. (2015). Does the Role Checklist measure occupational participation? *Open Journal of Occupational Therapy, 3*(3). https://doi.org/10.15453/2168-6408.1175

Braveman, B., & Hunter, E. G. (2017). *Occupational therapy practice guidelines for cancer rehabilitation with adults.* Bethesda, MD: AOTA Press.

Braveman, B., Robson, M., Velozo, C., Kielhofner, G., Fisher, G., Forsyth, K., & Kerschbaum, J. (2005). *Worker Role Interview (Version 10.0).* Chicago: Model of Human Occupation Clearinghouse.

Cheville, A. L., & Basford, J. R. (2014). Role of rehabilitation medicine and physical agents in the treatment of cancer-associated pain. *Journal of Clinical Oncology, 32,* 1691–1702. https://doi.org/10.1200/JCO.2013.53.6680

Cristian, A., Tran, A., & Patel, K. (2012). Patient safety in cancer rehabilitation. *Physical Medicine and Rehabilitation Clinics of North America, 23,* 441–456. https://doi.org/10.1016/j.pmr.2012.02.015

Désiron, H. A. M., Donceel, P., de Rijk, A., & Van Hoof, E. (2013). A conceptual-practice model for occupational therapy to facilitate return to work in breast cancer patients. *Journal of Occupational Rehabilitation, 23,* 516–526. https://doi.org/10.1007/s10926-013-9427-z

Fisher, A. G., & Jones, K. B. (2012). *Assessment of Motor and Process Skills: Development, standardizations, and administration manual* (7th ed., rev.). Fort Collins, CO: Three Star Press.

Galer, B. S., & Jensen, M. P. (1997). Development and preliminary validation of a pain measure specific to neuropathic pain. *Neurology, 48,* 332–338. https://doi.org/10.1212/wnl.48.2.332

Hwang, E. J., Lokietz, N. C., Lozano, R. L., & Parke, M. A. (2015). Functional deficits and quality of life among cancer survivors: Implications for occupational therapy in cancer survivorship care. *American Journal of Occupational Therapy, 69,* 6906290010. https://doi.org/10.5014/ajot.2015.015974

Jette, A., Haley, S. M., Coster, W., & Ni, P. S. (2015). *AM-PAC Short Forms for Inpatient and Outpatient Settings: Instruction manual.* Boston: Boston University.

Katz, S., Ford, A. B., Moskowitz, R. W., Jackson, B. A., & Jaffe, M. W. (1963). Studies of illness in the aged: The Index of ADL: A standardized measure of biological and psychosocial function. *JAMA, 185,* 914–919. https://doi.org/10.1001/jama.1963.03060120024016

Kielhofner, G. (2008). *Model of Human Occupation* (4th ed.). Baltimore: Lippincott Williams & Wilkins.

Kielhofner, G., Mallinson, T., Crawford, C., Nowak, M., Rigby, M., Henry, A., & Walens, D. (2004). *Occupational Performance History Interview–II (Version 2.1).* Chicago: Model of Human Occupation Clearinghouse.

Landwehr, M. S., Watson, S. E., Macpherson, C. F., Novak, K. A., & Johnson, R. H. (2016). The cost of cancer: A retrospective analysis of the financial impact of cancer on young adults. *Cancer Medicine, 5,* 863–870. https://doi.org/10.1002/cam4.657

Law, M., Baptiste, S., Carswell, A., McColl, M. A., Polatajko, H., & Pollock, N. (2019). *Canadian Occupational Performance Measure* (5th ed., rev.). Altona, Canada: COPM.

Lawton, M. P., & Brody, E. M. (1969). Assessment of older people: Self-maintaining and instrumental activities of daily living. *Gerontologist, 9,* 179–186. https://doi.org/10.1093/geront/9.3_Part_1.179

Lyons, K. D. (2006). Occupation as a vehicle to surmount the psychosocial challenges of cancer. *Occupational Therapy in Health Care, 20,* 799–809. https://doi.org/10.1080/J003v20n02_01

Maltser, S., Cristian, A., Silver, J. K., Morris, G. S., & Stout, N. L. (2017). A focused review of safety considerations in cancer rehabilitation. *Physical Medicine and Rehabilitation, 9*(Suppl. 2), S415–S428. https://doi.org/10.1016/j.pmrj.2017.08.403

Mendoza, T. R., Wang, X. S., Cleeland, C. S., Morrissey, M., Johnson, B. A., Wendt, J. K., & Huber, S. L. (1999). The rapid assessment of fatigue severity in cancer patients: Use of the Brief Fatigue Inventory. *Cancer, 85,* 1186–1196. https://doi.org/10.1002/(sici)1097-0142(19990301)85:5<1186::aid-cncr24>3.0.co;2-n

Mullen, E., & Mistry, H. (2017). Managing cancer survivorship issues. *Journal for Nurse Practitioners, 14,* 337–343. https://doi.org/10.1016/j.nurpra.2017.12.022

Nasreddine, Z. S., Phillips, N. A., Bédirian, V., Charbonneau, S., Whitehead, V., Collin I., . . . Chertkow, H. (2005). The Montreal Cognitive Assessment, MoCA: A brief screening tool for mild cognitive impairment. *Journal of the American Geriatrics Society, 53,* 695–699. https://doi.org/10.1111/j.1532-5415.2005.53221.x

Parkinson, S., Forsyth, K., & Kielhofner, G. (2006). *The Model of Human Occupation Screening Tool, Version 2.* Chicago: Model of Human Occupation Clearinghouse.

Pergolotti, M., Williams, G. R., Campbell, C., Munoz, L. A., & Muss, H. B. (2016). Occupational therapy for adults with cancer: Why it matters. *Oncologist, 21,* 314–316. https://doi.org/10.1634/theoncologist.2015-0335

Powell, L. E., & Myers, A. M. (1995). The Activities-specific Balance Confidence (ABC) Scale. *Journals of Gerontology: Series A: Biological Sciences and Medical Sciences, 50*(1), M28–M34. https://doi.org/10.1093/gerona/50a.1.m28

Scott, P. J., McKinney, K. G., Perron, J. M., Ruff, E. G., & Smiley, J. L. (2019). The Revised Role Checklist: Improved utility, feasibility, and reliability. *OTJR: Occupation, Participation and Health, 39,* 56–63. https://doi.org/10.1177/1539449218780618

Speck, R. M., DeMichele, A., Farrar, J. T., Hennessy, S., Mao, J. J., Stineman, M. G., & Barg, F. K. (2012). Scope of symptoms and self-management strategies for chemotherapy-induced peripheral neuropathy in breast cancer patients. *Support Care Cancer, 20,* 2433–2439.

Stubblefield, M. D., & O'Dell, M. W. (2009). *Cancer rehabilitation: Principles and practice.* New York: Demos Medical Publishing.

Stubblefield, M. D., Schmitz, K. H., & Ness, K. K. (2013). Physical functioning and rehabilitation for the cancer survivor. *Seminars in Oncology, 40,* 784–795. https://doi.org/10.1053/j.seminoncol.2013.09.008

Uniform Data System for Medical Rehabilitation. (1997). *Guide for the Uniform Data Set for Medical Rehabilitation (including the FIM instrument), Version 5.1.* Buffalo, NY: Author.

7

Special Considerations for Older Adults With Cancer

Alix G. Sleight, PhD, OTD, MPH, OTR/L, and Robin Newman, OTD, OT, OTR, CLT, FAOTA

LEARNING OBJECTIVES

After completing this chapter, readers should be able to
- Understand common conditions and developmental challenges affecting older adults with cancer and their effect on occupational performance,
- Explain client factors that may contribute to occupational dysfunction in older adult cancer survivors,
- Distinguish specific goals of occupational therapy for older adults with cancer, and
- Summarize the sequence of evaluation and treatment in a typical occupational therapy session for older adult cancer survivors.

KEY TERMS AND CONCEPTS

- Cancer-specific geriatric assessment
- Client factors
- Cultural contexts
- Frailty
- Lifestyle Redesign®
- Loss
- Older adults
- Performance patterns
- Performance skills
- Personal contexts

INTRODUCTION

More than half of all cancer survivors in the United States are older adults. In fact, approximately 62% of the 15.5 million cancer survivors living in the United States today are age 65 years or older. By 2040, the proportion of older adult survivors will rise to 73% (Bluethmann et al., 2016). Older adults face unique challenges during cancer survivorship that often can be ameliorated through occupational therapy. For example, more than half of older adults with cancer enter treatment with multimorbidity (Williams et al., 2016), which increases the risk of treatment-related side effects (Vissers et al., 2013). In addition, common lifespan and developmental changes experienced during this stage may include retirement, the addition of grandchildren or great-grandchildren, loss and bereavement, and altered physical and psychosocial function. These changes can affect—and be affected by—cancer and its treatment for older adults.

Given that older adults will continue to dominate the survivor population, occupational therapy practitioners need to understand the unique needs of this group as well as the important role of occupational therapy. This chapter provides an overview of the most common cancers in older adults and the key factors that can contribute to occupational dysfunction in older adult oncology patients. This chapter also outlines the role of occupational therapy across the cancer care continuum—from prevention and diagnosis through treatment, survivorship, and end-of-life care.

Finally, using a case study for context, this chapter guides readers through the essential aspects of occupational therapy evaluation and intervention for older adults with cancer.

WHO ARE OLDER ADULTS? LIFESPAN AND DEVELOPMENTAL CHALLENGES

For the purposes of this chapter, *older adults* are considered those age 65 and older. However, age is only a number, and there is no typical older adult per se. Some 65-year-olds are frail and live with multiple comorbid conditions, while some 99-year-olds live independently and report feeling healthy and strong. For many older adults, later life can present an opportunity to relax, spend time with loved ones, volunteer, travel, and participate in activities old and new. However, unique challenges during this life phase are also common and can complicate the experience of cancer and its treatment for some people. *Loss* is a common theme during older adulthood. Friends and family members can be lost through death or divorce, and loved ones can relocate or fall out of contact. Spiritual and existential distress can sometimes occur as older adults navigate the terrain of loss and face their own mortality. At the same time, older adulthood can come with new caregiving responsibilities. Caring for a partner who has an illness or disability can be overwhelming, and the accompanying loss of personal freedom is often challenging.

Changes in physical and mental health are also common during older adulthood. In addition to cancer, other chronic illnesses and conditions such as diabetes, hypertension, stroke, arthritis, and heart disease are most prevalent in individuals age 65 years and older. Changes in sexual function, cognitive function, and energy level can also occur as a normal part of aging, and mental health issues such as depression and anxiety sometimes accompany declines in physical health.

Other common conditions that may complicate occupational therapy treatment for older adult cancer survivors include

- Incontinence,
- Falls,
- Delirium,
- Decubitus ulcers, and
- Frailty (Hurria & Balducci, 2009).

Frailty is defined as an increased vulnerability as a result of overall aging-associated decline, leading to a decreased ability to manage everyday stressors. It is often characterized by diminished energy, decreased waking speed, low levels of physical activity, unintentional weight loss, and low grip strength (Xue, 2011). Frailty is particularly important for occupational therapy practitioners to be aware of because it can substantially affect the ability to tolerate therapy and adhere to home recommendations. Occupational therapy protocols for frail older adults should be modified to accommodate possible complications.

The plethora of physical, cognitive, and spiritual changes faced during older adulthood can also result in a loss of independence as older adults experience a diminished ability to safely drive and navigate the home and community. A decreased sense of purpose can occur as these valued roles and activities or occupations become magnified by retirement from jobs and decreased involvement in treasured activities. Nonetheless, new purpose can also emerge during this life phase as older adults become grandparents or great-grandparents, experience life beyond the confines of work or child rearing, and watch their legacies and contributions to society unfold.

MOST COMMON FORMS OF CANCER IN OLDER ADULTS

Increased age is associated with a higher risk of cancer; 87% of all cancers in the United States are diagnosed in adults over the age of 50 (American Cancer Society [ACS], 2017). The most commonly diagnosed cancers in women over the age of 60, in order of prevalence, are (1) breast, (2) lung, (3) colon/rectal, and (4) uterine. Men over the age of 60 are most likely to be diagnosed with cancers of the (1) prostate, (2) lung, (3) colon or rectum, and (4) skin (ACS, 2017). Despite the higher incidence of cancer in older adults, improvements in treatment and early diagnosis have contributed to a steady increase in survival rates. The 5-year relative survival rate for all cancers combined has increased across all sociodemographic groups over the past 3 decades (ACS, 2017).

Notably, however, racial and ethnic disparities in survival rates persist among cancer patients of all ages, including older adults (Aizer et al., 2014). Cancer mortality rates are lower among Asian/Pacific Islanders and Hispanics than among Whites, while cancer mortality remains highest among Blacks (Singh & Jemal, 2017). Cancer mortality rates in lower socioeconomic groups have also declined at a slower rate (Singh & Jemal, 2017). Ultimately, although racial/ethnic and socioeconomic disparities in cancer survivorship must be addressed, the overall decrease in cancer mortality creates a growing population of older adult cancer survivors requiring occupational therapy.

FACTORS THAT MAY CONTRIBUTE TO OCCUPATIONAL DYSFUNCTION IN OLDER ADULTS WITH CANCER

Client Factors

Older adult cancer survivors may present with unique *client factors* (i.e., specific capacities, characteristics, beliefs) that can influence occupational performance and affect the experience of cancer treatment and survivorship. (See Chapter 3, "Applying the *Occupational Therapy Practice Framework* With Cancer Survivors," for a more detailed description of the components of the *Occupational Therapy Practice Framework* (American Occupational Therapy Association, 2014.)

Values, beliefs, and spirituality

Client values and beliefs may evolve during later life, and these changes may affect health outcomes during cancer treatment and survivorship. For example, older adults with cancer are more likely than their younger counterparts to value life storytelling, legacy building, and making financial and logistical arrangements in anticipation of the end of life. Older adults with cancer may also value different cancer treatment options than they might have when they were younger, sometimes opting to forgo lengthy treatment regimens or to focus sooner on palliative care.

Spirituality also evolves throughout the lifespan and can provide a strong coping mechanism during older adulthood, particularly because a cancer diagnosis sometimes forces a confrontation with mortality. Occupational therapy practitioners should ask clients about any preexisting spiritual beliefs and determine whether older adults with cancer are interested in pursuing occupations related to spirituality or religiosity during or after cancer treatment.

Body functions and structures

Many of the human body's structures and functions may be affected by cancer and its treatment in older adults. Cognitive function may decrease as a result of cancer-related cognitive impairment (CRCI), a phenomenon sometimes known as "chemo brain" associated with memory deficits and other cognitive impairments in 15%–25% of cancer survivors (Ahles et al., 2012). Older adults, particularly postmenopausal women, are particularly at risk for CRCI during survivorship (Sleight, 2015). The diminished mental function associated with CRCI may be compounded by preexisting mild cognitive deficits in older adults that can occur as a normal part of the aging process. Sensory function can also be affected by cancer treatment in older adults; chemotherapy-induced peripheral neuropathy can cause weakness, tingling, numbness, and pain during and after treatment. Chemotherapy can also cause changes to sensory function; some cancer patients report loss in taste, smell, and other senses.

Depending on the cancer site, various changes in other body structures and functions may also occur in older adults. Neuromusculoskeletal structures and movement functions may be affected not only by older age but also cancer-related surgeries, radiation, lymphedema, and extended sedentary periods that may accompany cancer treatment. Certain cancers and their respective treatments may also prompt changes to cardiovascular, hematological, and respiratory structures or functions; voice and speech structures or functions; digestive, metabolic, and endocrine structures or functions; skin structures; and genitourinary and reproductive structures or functions. At the same time, changes to many body structures and functions may accompany the aging process (e.g., hypertension, arthritis, dysphagia) and can interact with cancer-related changes, creating a complex interplay of factors affecting occupational function.

Performance Skills

Performance skills, defined as observable elements of action with implicit functional purpose, may be affected by cancer and its treatment in older adult cancer survivors. Motor skills such as walking, lifting, and maintaining endurance may already be limited in some older adults and can be further compromised by cancer treatments such as chemotherapy that cause fatigue, nausea, and weakness. Process skills allow individuals to select, interact with, and use relevant tools and materials for everyday actions. These can also be affected by cancer treatments, both via physical limitations (e.g., lymphedema obstructing the ability to use scissors) and cognitive limitations (e.g., cancer-related cognitive impairment limiting the ability to recall where the can opener is). Social interaction skills can also be affected by cancer and its treatment during older adulthood, particularly with certain types of cancer—such as head or neck cancer—that can affect speech mechanisms.

Performance Patterns

Habits, routines, roles, and rituals (also known as *performance patterns*) are instrumental in the process of engaging in occupations and can both support and hinder occupational performance. A diagnosis of cancer and its subsequent treatment may disrupt performance patterns in older adults. Cognitive decline and physical disability—whether caused by the aging process or by cancer and its treatment—can render habits and routines more difficult to execute. For example, an older adult who always follows the same sequence for morning toileting, bathing, and hygiene may suddenly find herself needing to establish new ADL routines to accommodate pain and limited range of motion secondary to a mastectomy for breast cancer. Another older adult with cancer might experience extreme fatigue after chemotherapy treatments and find it difficult to complete his usual Saturday morning routine of picking up his grandchildren and going to a local park. Rituals such as attending a place of worship may be of particular importance to some older adults, particularly those who are retired and rely on these rituals for social interaction and engagement in meaningful occupation. These rituals may be disrupted after a cancer diagnosis by new routines surrounding health care appointments, medication management, and self-care. Returning to valued habits, rituals, roles, and routines—with or without accommodations—is an important goal for many older adults with cancer.

Role changes may also be an important consideration for older adults when they are diagnosed and treated for cancer. Roles that commonly emerge during older adulthood include grandparent, volunteer, caregiver, or widow, among many others. These roles may evolve after a cancer diagnosis because an individual might find it difficult to keep up with the demands of certain roles during treatment.

In addition, the role of cancer survivor may resonate with some individuals, and meaningful routines associated with this new role may emerge. For example, an older adult may begin mentoring younger people with cancer through a hospital-based buddy program or establish a patient advocate role with a cancer-related nonprofit.

Occupational therapy practitioners working with older adults with cancer should be aware of the potential for both positive and negative changes to occupational performance patterns in this population after a cancer diagnosis.

Context and Environment

Contexts that can be relevant to older adults with cancer may include *cultural contexts* (e.g., customs and beliefs that affect health care decisions) and *personal contexts* (e.g., age, gender, socioeconomic status, educational attainment). For example, women may experience cancer and its treatment differently than men, particularly surrounding fertility, body image, and life roles (Paterson et al., 2016).

Older individuals may be more at risk for complications during surgery, chemotherapy, and radiation than their younger counterparts. In addition, the environment in which each older adult lives, works, and seeks health care can affect occupational performance. The physical surroundings in a home, for example, will affect how well an individual can move around the house despite fatigue or movement restrictions occurring secondary to cancer treatment.

The social environment occupied by older adults is also an important consideration for occupational therapy practitioners working with this population. The presence or absence of people in the immediate environment, the quality of each individual's interpersonal relationships, and the expectations of other people will affect the experience of cancer and its treatment. For example, a person who is diagnosed with cancer may feel strain and discord in a caregiving relationship if they are no longer able to fulfill previous expectations as a caregiver. On the other hand, older adults who are surrounded by caring, attentive family members regularly may find that coping with cancer and its treatment is easier. Compensating for a lack of social contact during treatment or navigating new social situations that arise with illness may be tasks that an occupational therapy practitioner can address during treatment.

OCCUPATIONAL THERAPY EVALUATION OF OLDER ADULTS WITH CANCER

Geriatric Assessment

Although chronological age classifies cancer survivors by stage of the life course, it does not account for the functional abilities of older adults. Older adults of differing chronological ages vary in their functional abilities (Economou et al., 2012). In response to the need for a better understanding of the "functional age" of older adults living with cancer, oncology professionals developed a *cancer-specific geriatric assessment* (Hurria et al., 2005). The assessment includes a comprehensive overview of functional status, comorbidities, cognition, psychological state, social support, and nutritional status (Hurria et al., 2005). An understanding of each of these areas can help to target interventions to support the older adult survivor.

Table 7.1 identifies the major domains of a cancer-specific geriatric assessment, recommends screening tools that may be used to address these domains, and suggests possible roles for occupational therapy practitioners in treating older adults with cancer. Although any number of assessments may be relevant to older adult cancer survivors, Table 7.2 describes the most common assessments used with this population.

OCCUPATIONAL THERAPY INTERVENTIONS WITH OLDER ADULTS WITH CANCER

From diagnosis through survivorship or end-of-life care, occupational therapy interventions focus on maximizing the older adult's functional abilities to participate in meaningful occupations. This should begin with prehabilitation to minimize the risk or severity of functional deficits before the initiation of cancer treatment. (See Chapter 10, "Prehabilitation," for more information; Carli et al., 2017; Silver & Baima, 2013).

Next, the primary goal during treatment and survivorship should be to maximize functional abilities and prevent disability through the remainder of the lifespan. When end-of-life care is relevant, occupational therapy practitioners may apply a variety of rehabilitation approaches that focus on dignity, role preservation, maintenance of daily routines, and legacy making (Chochinov et al., 1995).

TABLE 7.1.   Cancer-Specific Geriatric Assessments

GERIATRIC SCREEN DOMAIN	RECOMMENDED SCREENING TOOLS	ROLE OF THE OCCUPATIONAL THERAPY PRACTITIONER
Functional status	▪ Activities of daily living (MOS physical health subscale; Stewart & Ware, 1992) ▪ Instrumental activities of daily living (subscale of OARS; Fillenbaum & Smyer, 1981) ▪ Timed Up & Go (Podsiadlo & Richardson, 1991) ▪ Number of falls in the prior 6 months ▪ Karnofsky Self-Reported Performance Rating Scale (Karnofsky & Burchenal, 1948) ▪ Karnofsky Physician-Rated Performance Rating Scale (Karnofsky & Burchenal, 1948)	▪ Assess the client's ability to perform ADLs and IADLs. ▪ Assess the functional impact of client factors on the client's occupational performance and participation in daily activities.
Comorbidities	▪ Chart review ▪ Self-report of comorbidities ▪ Medication review	▪ Perform an occupational profile and thorough chart review to appreciate comorbidities and their potential impact on the client's occupational performance and participation in daily activities.
Cognition	▪ Short Blessed Test of Memory and Concentration (Katzman et al., 1983)	▪ Assess the functional impact of cognitive dysfunction on occupational performance and participation in daily activities.
Psychological state	▪ Hospital Anxiety and Depression Scale (Zigmond & Snaith, 1983)	▪ Assess the functional impact of depression or anxiety on occupational performance and participation in daily activities.
Social support	▪ MOS Social Activity Limitation Measure (Stewart & Ware, 1992) ▪ MOS Social Support Survey (Stewart & Ware, 1992) ▪ Seeman and Berkman Social Ties (Seeman et al., 1993)	▪ Assess the functional impact of limited social support on occupational performance and participation in daily activities.
Nutritional status	▪ Percentage of unintentional weight loss in prior 6 months ▪ Body mass index	▪ Assess the functional impact of poor nutritional status on occupational performance and participation in daily activities.

Note. ADLs = activities of daily living; IADLs = instrumental activities of daily living; MOS = Medical Outcomes Study; OARS = Older Americans' Resources and Services.
Sources. Economou et al., 2012; Hurria et al., 2005.

TABLE 7.2.   Common Assessments Used for Older Adults With Cancer

AREA	ASSESSMENT TOOLS
Occupational performance	▪ Canadian Occupational Performance Measure (Law et al., 2019) ▪ Activity Card Sort (Baum & Edwards, 2008) ▪ Occupational Self-Assessment (Kielhofner et al., 1998)
ADL assessment	▪ Functional Independence Measure (Keith et al., 1987) ▪ Activity Measure for Post Acute Care (Haley et al., 2004) ▪ Assessment of Motor and Process Skills (Fisher & Jones, 2012) ▪ Performance Assessment of Self-Care Skills (PASS; Holm & Rogers, 2008) ▪ Home evaluation
IADL assessment	▪ PASS (Holm & Rogers, 2008) ▪ Assessment of Motor and Process Skills (Fisher & Jones, 2012) ▪ Home evaluation
Sleep	▪ Sleep diary ▪ Epworth Sleepiness Scale (Johns, 1991)
Falls	▪ Timed Up & Go (Podsiadlo & Richardson, 1991) ▪ Falls Efficacy Scale (Tinetti et al., 1990) ▪ Falls Risk Questionnaire (Braun, 1998) ▪ Sensory function ▪ Vision screen ▪ Cognitive screen
Cognition	▪ Short Blessed Test of Memory and Concentration (Katzman et al., 1983) ▪ Montreal Cognitive Assessment (Nasreddine et al., 2005) ▪ Mini Mental State Exam (Folstein et al., 1975) ▪ Functional Assessment of Cancer Therapy–Cognitive (FACT-Cog; Wagner et al., 2009)
Fatigue	▪ Brief Fatigue Inventory (Mendoza et al., 1999) ▪ Functional Assessment of Chronic Illness Therapy (FACIT–F; Yellen et al., 1997)
Psychological assessment	▪ NCCN Distress Thermometer (National Comprehensive Cancer Network, 2017) ▪ Geriatric Depression Screen (Yesavage et al., 1983)
Social support and social functioning	▪ Social Activity Limitations Measure (Sherbourne, 1992) ▪ Social Activity Log (Syrjala et al., 2010)
Lifestyle, health behaviors, roles, routines, individual patient goals	▪ Canadian Occupational Performance Measure (Law et al., 2019) ▪ Narrative evaluation (occupational storytelling and storymaking)

Note. ADL = activity of daily living; IADL = instrumental activity of daily living; NCCN = National Comprehensive Cancer Network.

TABLE 7.3.   Overview of Occupational Therapy Interventions by Stage of Care

STAGE OF CARE	EXAMPLE OF OCCUPATIONAL THERAPY INTERVENTIONS
Prevention	Lifestyle Redesign as a preventive measure, promoting healthy behaviors, exercise, stress management, weight loss, and so on.
Early detection and screening	Prehabilitation. Primary and secondary prevention of functional deficits.
Diagnosis	Prehabilitation. Early intervention to maintain function and promote psychosocial well-being. Prepare clients for intervention.
Treatment	Symptom management and promotion of participation in valued occupations. Intervention for fatigue, cognition, ADLs, IADLs, mobility, symptom management, medication management, falls reduction. Lifestyle Redesign to promote engagement in valued occupations and make adaptations to allow for everyday participation.
Survivorship	Lifestyle Redesign to promote healthy behaviors, return to work, resumption of valued occupations, and reassessment of life roles.
End-of-life care	Full range of interventions promoting function and self-determination, goal attainment.

Note. ADLs = activities of daily living; IADLs = instrumental activities of daily living.

Table 7.4.   Targeted Occupational Therapy Interventions for Specific Health Outcomes in Older Adults With Cancer

HEALTH OUTCOME	OCCUPATIONAL THERAPY INTERVENTION
Cognition	▪ Cognitive rehabilitation ▪ Meta cognitive strategy training ▪ Neuropsychological or cognitive training ▪ Cognitive–behavioral therapy (CBT) ▪ Use of compensatory strategies (e.g., memory aids) ▪ Environmental modification ▪ Occupation/activity

Falls	▪ Multifactorial interventions focused on:
	  • Environmental modification
	  • Vision
	  • Cognition
	  • Sensory function
	  • Functional mobility/balance
	  • Strengthening
	  • Occupation/activity

Psychosocial/mental health	▪ Self-management ▪ Legacy making ▪ Identification, discover, or engagement in new occupations ▪ Adaptation of previously valued occupations to accommodate health status ▪ Relaxation and stress management ▪ Building social support
Decubitus ulcers	▪ Education ▪ Positioning ▪ Cushions, mattresses, or floating heels (i.e., skin protective cushion) ▪ Timers ▪ Hand mirrors

Incontinence	▪ Behavioral strategies, including:
	  • Rethinking daily schedules
	  • Scheduling voiding
	  • Asking for assistance when necessary

Sources. Evers et al., 2015; Hunjan & Twiss, 2013.

An overview of occupational therapy interventions commonly provided in each stage of cancer care can be found in Table 7.3. Sometimes older adults with cancer will present with specific needs or impairments that require more tailored interventions. A list of interventions designed to target some of the most commonly encountered health outcomes in this population can be found in Table 7.4. Most important, throughout the spectrum of cancer care, occupational therapy interventions should revolve around the long- and short-term goals identified by each patient and take into consideration the unique environments, life roles, and values of the individual cancer survivor. Case Example 7.1 provides the story of a frail older adult who worked with an occupational therapy practitioner to resume her previous routines and activities.

LIFESTYLE REDESIGN FOR THE OLDER ADULT CANCER SURVIVOR

Lifestyle Redesign®, an approach within occupational therapy, enhances health and quality of life through emphasis on maintaining a life balance of work, rest, leisure, and self-care

(Clark et al., 1997, 2015; Jackson et al., 1998). Lifestyle Redesign focuses on positive coping strategies and may help patients adapt to cancer and its consequences. This treatment approach can address such diverse topics as weight management, smoking cessation, pain management, mental health, sexuality and intimacy, time management, lifestyle balance, and energy conservation. It can be provided in a group or one-on-one setting and revolves around the achievement of measurable, individualized health-related goals over time. Lifestyle Redesign is appropriate at any point along the cancer care continuum from diagnosis through survivorship.

Evaluation typically combines a narrative, occupational storytelling approach (Clark, 1993) with tailored assessments such as the COPM. Treatment often focuses more on psychosocial elements of survivorship than physical impairments. Sessions are conversation based and frequently comprise patient education, motivational interviewing, and problem solving to address internal and external barriers to goal achievement. For more information about Lifestyle Redesign, please see Clark et al. (2015). Case Example 7.2 illustrates a real-life example of Lifestyle Redesign for cancer survivorship.

CASE EXAMPLE 7.1. LINDA: OCCUPATIONAL THERAPY FOR THE FRAIL OLDER ADULT WITH CANCER

Linda is a 75-year-old cancer survivor who completed her treatment for Stage II breast cancer 3 months ago. She is a widow and lives alone in an apartment building with elevator access. She has a daughter who lives nearby, but Linda does not want to burden her because she has a young family of her own. Linda is a retired schoolteacher, and before her cancer diagnosis, she volunteered at the local library, participated in a monthly book club with her friends, and cared for her grandchildren occasionally after school. Linda misses the social connection she had with her grandchildren, the fellow volunteers at the library, and the children from the community who visited the library. Linda has lived with diabetes for 15 years prior to her cancer diagnosis and has since developed diabetic retinopathy with mild visual impairment and peripheral neuropathy. She was recently hospitalized for a fall in her home and for poor management of her diabetes medication regimen and was referred to home occupational therapy after discharge from the acute care hospital.

Linda reports that since her cancer diagnosis, she has noticed a significant change in her daily routine. She generally wakes up between 5 a.m. and 7 a.m., watches the news, and has a cup of coffee. She showers and gets dressed in time for lunch, and when she has enough energy, she does household chores, such as the laundry or light housekeeping. She usually takes a daily afternoon nap. In the late afternoon, she makes a light dinner, if she is not too tired, and watches television until she falls asleep. Occasionally she will meet a friend for lunch or visit her daughter at her home. She reports that the fall she experienced occurred while carrying the laundry basket to the washing machine. She is distressed by these changes in her functional abilities and quality of life because her ability to participate in meaningful activities has significantly slowed.

Upon initial occupational therapy evaluation, the occupational therapist asked Linda about her daily routine, occupational performance challenges, and goals for occupational therapy. Through administration of the Canadian Occupational Performance Measure (COPM; Law et al., 2019), the occupational therapist identified several occupational performance challenges that would be the focus of intervention. During the administration of the COPM, Linda was asked to identify the occupational performance challenges that were most salient to her currently on a scale of 1–10, with 10 being the most important. She was able to identify the specific barriers to occupational performance, such as difficulty reading the print on the medication labels and remembering to take her medication at scheduled times, as well as a fear of falling during mobility and physical and cognitive fatigue. She was then asked to rate her current performance in each occupation on a scale from 1–10, with 10 being the best performance. Finally, she was asked to rate her satisfaction with her current performance in each category on a scale from 1–10, with 10 being the most satisfied (Table 7.5).

The COPM was supplemented with a screening of visual acuity, subjective cognitive function (Fact–Cog; Wagner et al., 2009), falls history, balance and mobility

TABLE 7.5. Linda's Occupational Performance Challenges

OCCUPATIONAL PERFORMANCE CHALLENGES	PERFORMANCE	SATISFACTION
Medication management ▪ Difficulty reading print on medication labels ▪ Difficulty remembering to take pills	3	2
Cooking ▪ Too fatigued to prepare meals ▪ Difficulty safely using sharp utensils	3	2
Laundry ▪ Fear of falling ▪ Difficulty carrying laundry basket because of neuropathy ▪ Too fatigued to fold laundry	4	2
Volunteer work ▪ Fear of falling ▪ Too fatigued to complete a 4-hour shift ▪ Difficulty with concentration and memory	1	1
Caring for grandchildren ▪ Fear of falling ▪ Too fatigued to engage in play activities for greater than 1 hour	1	1

(Continued)

CASE EXAMPLE 7.1. LINDA: OCCUPATIONAL THERAPY FOR THE FRAIL OLDER ADULT WITH CANCER *(Cont.)*

(Timed Up and Go; Podsiadlo & Richardson, 1991), fatigue (Facit-F; Yellen et al., 1997) and distress (National Comprehensive Cancer Network Distress Thermometer [NCCN], 2017; see Table 7.6). Results suggest that Linda was experiencing challenges across all domains tested, with reduced visual acuity, severe fatigue, high risk of falls, and a significant impact of perceived cognitive impairments on her quality of life.

The occupational therapist began intervention by educating Linda on the multidimensional etiology of CRCI and how the challenge she is reporting with memory and concentration can affect her daily activities. This reassured Linda because she thought she was "losing her mind." The occupational therapist and Linda discussed the benefits of establishing some new habits and routines to support her ability to perform the occupations of medication management, laundry, cooking, volunteer work, and child care, with a focus on energy management, fall prevention, adaptive strategies (e.g., use of a rolling laundry cart), and cognitive support aids such as a pill box. Linda expressed an eagerness to learn strategies to increase her satisfaction and performance of these activities. The occupational therapist recommended interventions to support Linda's success in her selected goal areas (Table 7.6).

TABLE 7.6. Linda's Occupational Therapy Interventions

OCCUPATIONS	INTERVENTIONS
Medication management	▪ Request large-print medication labels from pharmacy. ▪ Use a magnifier to read medication bottles. ▪ Purchase a pillbox to organize medication or use an electronic reminder system.
Cooking	▪ Buy prepared meals or precut fruits and vegetables. ▪ Freeze prepared meals to have extra portions for the week. ▪ Engage in meal preparation while seated versus standing at the kitchen counter. ▪ Wear shoes (for secure footing) while cooking (and walking in the kitchen) to minimize fall risk. ▪ Order home delivery of groceries.
Laundry	▪ Use a rolling laundry cart instead of carrying a laundry basket. ▪ Sit while folding laundry. ▪ Wear shoes (for secure footing) while doing laundry to minimize fall risk.
Volunteer work	▪ Arrange a volunteer schedule for gradual return to volunteer work. ▪ Modify volunteer responsibilities to maximize energy and concentration (e.g., read to children while seated, arrange for shorter volunteer hours).
Caring for grandchildren	▪ Arrange for visits when daughter is home. ▪ Arrange for children to come over to her house.

CASE EXAMPLE 7.2. JUDY: LIFESTYLE REDESIGN

Judy is a 65-year-old molecular biologist who recently survived stomach, colorectal, and uterine cancer. She is on disability leave from work, having recently completed cancer treatment. She sought Lifestyle Redesign because she was concerned about many of the changes she had experienced postchemotherapy and radiation. The occupational therapist performed a narrative interview to determine Judy's key concerns and goals. Judy's primary concerns are

▪ Weight gain,
▪ Low energy levels,
▪ Lack of sleep,
▪ Anxiety and stress, and
▪ Lifestyle imbalance (lack of leisure time and self-care).

Judy typically spent time each day running errands for her daughter, who lived down the street; driving to doctor's appointments; and babysitting her grandchildren. She enjoyed these routines, but she also found herself neglecting her own self-care. She mentioned that she often ate lunch in her car in between doctor's appointments and running errands, and she hadn't engaged in a leisure activity since she began cancer

(Continued)

CASE EXAMPLE 7.2. JUDY: LIFESTYLE REDESIGN *(Cont.)*

treatment. Judy also mentioned that she had lingering lower back pain.

On the basis of Judy's stated concerns, she and her occupational therapist agreed that her Lifestyle Redesign sessions would focus on three long-term goals:

1. Establish a regimen of moderate physical activity three times per week to control weight, decrease anxiety, and improve sleep.
2. Engage in one leisure activity per week to improve lifestyle balance and decrease anxiety.
3. Schedule 30 minutes per day for a sit-down lunch to increase lifestyle balance, increase energy, and decrease anxiety.

Weekly sessions focused on breaking down these long-term goals into smaller, manageable short-term goals. For example, sessions were spent

- Identifying Judy's favorite leisure activities (watching movies, playing pickleball, and reading science fiction);
- Identifying strategies to incorporate favorite leisure activities back into her daily schedule;
- Discussing options for including physical activity regimens in Judy's current lifestyle, including adapting forms of exercise she used to enjoy (e.g., pickleball) to accommodate some of her cancer-related impairments (e.g., pain, fatigue);
- Identifying and strategizing about incorporating healthy lunches that are appealing to Judy and feasible to make and eat in 30 minutes;
- Teaching deep-breathing exercises and simple stretches for stress and anxiety management;
- Establishing a bedtime routine and a nightly relaxation regimen to improve quality of sleep; and
- Learning about the pain cycle and pain management techniques, including ergonomics for cooking, cleaning, and driving, to help with her lower back pain.

At the end of 10 weeks, Judy's pain had decreased, her weight had decreased, and she was sleeping 6–8 hours per night (up from 2–3 hours). She had spoken to her family about decreasing the amount of time that she spent running errands for them each week. Subsequently, she resumed a weekly pickleball game at her local community center. She was making and eating a healthy lunch most days (she preferred poached salmon, brown rice, and vegetables). She also started engaging in new physical activities and stress management techniques such as engaging in mindfulness meditation and taking daily walks. She reported feeling ready to begin thinking about going back to work. She and her occupational therapist agreed to continue to meet monthly to check in on her progress and solve any new concerns.

SUMMARY

Older adults with cancer face unique lifespan and developmental challenges, and they are more likely to develop certain conditions than other populations of cancer survivors. Occupational therapy for older adults with cancer should be tailored to the unique needs of each individual survivor while taking into account common impairments and needs experienced by this group. It is important to remember that chronological age is just a number and cannot be relied on to determine the functional abilities of a cancer survivor. Rather, older age should signify a need for diligence in screening for age-related impairments, as well as a respect for the unique possibilities for living life to its fullest during this stage.

REFERENCES

Ahles, T., Root, J., & Ryan, E. (2012). Cancer- and cancer treatment-associated cognitive change: An update on the state of the science. *Journal of Clinical Oncology, 30,* 3675–3686. https://doi.org/10.1200/JCO.2012.43.0116

Aizer, A. A., Wilhite, T. J., Chen, M. H., Graham, P. L., Choueiri, T. K., Hoffman, K. E., . . . Nguyen, P. L. (2014). Lack of reduction in racial disparities in cancer-specific mortality over a 20-year period. *Cancer, 120,* 1532–1539. https://doi.org/10.1002/cncr.28617

American Cancer Society. (2017). *Cancer facts & figures 2017.* Atlanta: American Cancer Society. https://www.cancer.org/content/dam/cancer-org/research/cancer-facts-and-statistics/annual-cancer-facts-and-figures/2017/cancer-facts-and-figures-2017.pdf

American Occupational Therapy Association. (2014). Occupational therapy practice framework: Domain and process (3rd ed.). *American Journal of Occupational Therapy, 68*(Suppl. 1), S1–S48. https://doi.org/10.5014/ajot.2014.682006

Baum, C. M., & Edwards, D. (2008). *Activity Card Sort* (2nd ed.). Bethesda, MD: AOTA Press.

Bluethmann, S. M., Mariotto, A. B., & Rowland, J. H. (2016). Anticipating the "Silver Tsunami": Prevalence trajectories and comorbidity burden among older cancer survivors in the United States. *Cancer Epidemiology, Biomarkers, & Prevention, 25,* 1029–1036. https://doi.org/10.1158/1055-9965.EPI-16-0133

Braun, B. L. (1998). Knowledge and perception of fall-related risk factors and fall-reduction techniques among community-dwelling elderly individuals. *Physical Therapy, 78,* 1262–1276. https://doi.org/10.1093/ptj/78.12.1262

Carli, F., Gillis, C., & Scheede-Bergdahl, C. (2017). Promoting a culture of prehabilitation for the surgical cancer patient. *Acta Oncologica, 56,* 128–133. https://doi.org/10.1080/0284186X.2016.1266081

Chochinov, H. M., Wilson, K. G., Enns, M., Mowchun, N., Lander, S., Levitt, M., & Clinch, J. J. (1995). Desire for death in the terminally ill. *American Journal of Psychiatry, 152,* 1185–1191. https://doi.org/10.1176/ajp.152.8.1185

Clark, F. (1993). Occupation embedded in a real life: Interweaving occupational science and occupational therapy. *American Journal of Occupational Therapy, 47,* 1067–1078. https://doi.org/10.5014/ajot.47.12.1067

Clark, F., Azen, S. P., Zemke, R., Jackson, J., Carlson, M., Mandel, D., & Palmer, J. (1997). Occupational therapy for independent-living older adults: A randomized controlled trial. *JAMA, 278*, 1321–1326.

Clark, F., Blanchard, J., Sleight, A., Cogan, A., Eallonardo, L., Florindez, L., . . . Vigen, C. (2015). *Lifestyle Redesign: Implementing the Well Elderly program* (2nd ed.). Bethesda, MD: AOTA Press.

Economou, D., Hurria, A., & Grant, M. (2012). Integrating a cancer-specific geriatric assessment into survivorship care. *Clinical Journal of Oncology Nursing, 16*(3), E78–E85. https://doi.org/10.1188/12.CJON.E78-E83

Evers, S., Anderson, K., & Pagel, L. (2015). Occupational therapy's role in pressure care. *OT Practice, 20*(2), 13–15.

Fillenbaum, G. G., & Smyer, M. A. (1981). The development, validity, and reliability of the OARS multidimensional Functional Assessment Questionnaire. *Journal of Gerontology, 36*, 428–434. https://doi.org/10.1093/geronj/36.4.428

Fisher, A. G. & Jones, K. B. (2012). *Assessment of Motor and Process Skills: Vol. 1. Development, standardization, and administration manual* (7th ed.). Fort Collins, CO: Three Star Press, Inc.

Folstein, M. F., Folstein, S. E., & McHugh, P. R. (1975). "Mini-mental state": A practical method for grading the cognitive state of patients for the clinician. *Journal of Psychiatric Research, 12*(3), 189–198. https://doi.org/10.1016/0022-3956(75)90026-6

Haley, S. M., Coster, W. J., Andres, P. L., Ludlow, L. H., Ni, P., Bond, T. L. Y., . . . Jette, A. M. (2004). Activity outcome measurement for post acute care. *Medical Care, 42*(1), 149–161. https://doi.org/10.1097/01.mlr.0000103520.43902.6c

Holm, M. B., & Rogers, J. C. (2008). The Performance Assessment of Self-Care Skills (PASS). In B. J. Hemphill-Pearson (Ed.), *Assessments in occupational therapy mental health* (2nd ed., pp. 101–112). Thorofare, NJ: Slack.

Hunjan, R., & Twiss, K. L. (2013). Urgent interventions: Promoting occupational engagement for clients with urinary incontinence. *OT Practice, 8*(21), 8–12.

Hurria, A., & Balducci, L. (Eds.). (2009). *Geriatric oncology: Treatment, assessment and management.* Boston: Springer-Verlag. https://doi.org/10.1007/978-0-387-89070-8

Hurria, A., Gupta, S., Zauderer, M., Zuckerman, E. L., Cohen, H. J., Muss, H., . . . Kornblith, A. B. (2005). Developing a cancer-specific geriatric assessment: A feasibility study. *Cancer, 104*, 1998–2005. https://doi.org/10.1002/cncr.21422

Jackson, J., Carlson, M., Mandel, D., Zemke, R., & Clark, F. (1998). Occupation in lifestyle redesign: The Well Elderly study occupational therapy program. *American Journal of Occupational Therapy, 52*(5), 326–336. https://doi.org/10.514/ajot.52.5.326

Johns, M. W. (1991). A new method for measuring daytime sleepiness: The Epworth Sleepiness Scale. *Sleep, 14*, 540–545. http://doi.org/10.1093/sleep/14.6.540

Karnofsky, D. A., & Burchenal, J. H. (1948). The clinical evaluation of chemotherapeutic agents in cancer. In C. M. Macleod (Ed.), *Evaluation of chemotherapeutic agents* (pp. 191–295). New York: Columbia University Press.

Katzman, R., Brown, T., & Fuld, P. (1983). Validation of a short Orientation-Memory-Concentration Test of cognitive impairment. *American Journal of Psychiatry, 140*, 734–739. https://doi.org/10.1176/ajp.140.6.734

Keith, R. A., Granger, C. V., Hamilton, B. B., & Sherwin, F. S. (1987). The Functional Independence Measure: A new tool for rehabilitation. *Advances in Clinical Rehabilitation, 1*, 6–18.

Kielhofner, G., Baron, K., Iyenger, A., Goldhammer, V., & Wolenski, J. (1998). *A user's manual for the Occupational Self Assessment (OSA) (Version 2.2).* Chicago: University of Illinois.

Law, M., Baptiste, S., Carswell, A., McColl, M., Polatajko, H. & Pollock, N. (2019). *Canadian Occupational Performance Measure* (5th ed., rev.). Altona, Canada: COPM.

Mendoza, T. R., Wang, X. S., Cleeland, C. S., Morrissey, M., Johnson, B. A., Wendt, J. K., & Huber, S. L. (1999). The rapid assessment of fatigue severity in cancer patients: Use of the Brief Fatigue Inventory. *Cancer, 85*, 1186–1196. https://doi.org/10.1002/(SICI)1097-0142(19990301)85:5<1186::AID-CNCR24>3.0.CO;2-N

Nasreddine, Z. S., Phillips, N. A., Bédirian, V., Charbonneau, S., Whitehead, V., Collin, I., . . . Chertkow, H. (2005). The Montreal Cognitive Assessment, MoCA: A brief screening tool for mild cognitive impairment. *Journal of the American Geriatrics Society, 53*, 695–699. https://doi.org/10.1111/j.1532-5415.2005.53221.x

National Comprehensive Cancer Network. (2017). *NCCN clinical practice guidelines in oncology: Distress management.* Retrieved from https://www.nccn.org/professionals/physician_gls/default.aspx

Paterson, C., Lengacher, C. A., Donovan, K. A., Kip, K. E., & Tofthagen, C. S. (2016). Body image in younger breast cancer survivors: a systematic review. *Cancer Nursing, 39*(1), E39. https://doi.org/10.1097/NCC.0000000000000251

Podsiadlo, D., & Richardson, S. (1991). The Timed "Up & Go": A test of basic functional mobility for frail elderly persons. *Journal of the American Geriatrics Society, 39*, 142–148. https://doi.org/10.1111/j.1532-5415.1991.tb01616.x

Seeman T. E., Berkman, L. F., Kohout, F., Lacroix, A., Glynn, R., & Blazer, D. (1993). Intercommunity variations in the association between social ties and mortality in the elderly: A comparative analysis of three communities. *Annals of Epidemiology, 3*, 325–335. https://doi.org/10.1016/1047-2797(93)90058-C

Sherbourne, C. D. (1992). Social functioning: Social Activity Limitations Measure. In A. L. Stewart & J. E. Ware (Eds.), *Measuring functioning and well-being: The Medical Outcomes Study approach* (pp. 173–193). Durham, NC: Duke University Press.

Silver, J. K., & Baima, J. (2013). Cancer prehabilitation: An opportunity to decrease treatment-related morbidity, increase cancer treatment options, and improve physical and psychological health outcomes. *American Journal of Physical Medicine & Rehabilitation, 92*, 715–727. https://doi.org/10.1097/PHM.0b013e31829b4afe

Singh, G. K., & Jemal, A. (2017). Socioeconomic and racial/ethnic disparities in cancer mortality, incidence, and survival in the United States, 1950–2014: Over six decades of changing patterns and widening inequalities. *Journal of Environmental and Public Health, 2017,* Article ID 2819372. https://doi.org/10.1155/2017/2819372

Sleight, A. (2015). Coping with cancer-related cognitive dysfunction: A scoping review of the literature. *Disability and Rehabilitation, 38*, 400–408. https://doi.org/10.3109/09638288.2015.1038364

Stewart, A. L., & Ware, J. E., Jr. (1992). *Measuring functioning and well-being: The Medical Outcomes Study approach.* Durham, NC: Duke University Press.

Syrjala, K. L., Stover, A. C., Yi, J. C., Artherholt, S. B., & Abrams, J. R. (2010). Measuring social activities and social function in long-term cancer survivors who received hematopoietic stem cell transplantation. *Psycho-Oncology, 19*, 462–471. https://doi.org/10.1002/pon.1572

Tinetti, M., Richman, D., & Powell, L. (1990). Falls efficacy as a measure of fear of falling. *Journal of Gerontology, 45*(6), P239–P243. https://doi.org/10.1093/geronj/45.6.P239

Vissers, P. A., Thong, M. S., Pouwer, F., Zanders, M. M. J., Coebergh, J. W. W., & Van De Poll-Franse, L. V. (2013). The impact of comorbidity on Health-Related Quality of Life among cancer survivors: Analyses of data from the PROFILES registry. *Journal of Cancer Survivorship, 7,* 602–613. https://doi.org/10.1007/s11764-013-0299-1

Wagner, L., Sweet, J., Butt, Z., Lai, J.-S., & Cella, D. (2009). Measuring patient self-reported cognitive function: Development of the Functional Assessment of Cancer Therapy Cognitive Function Instrument. *Journal of Supportive Oncology, 7,* W32–W39.

Williams, G. R., Mackenzie, A., Magnuson, A., Olin, R., Chapman, A., Mohile, S., . . . Holmes, H. (2016). Comorbidity in older adults with cancer. *Journal of Geriatric Oncology, 7,* 249–257. https://doi.org/10.1016/j.jgo.2015.12.002

Xue, Q. L. (2011). The frailty syndrome: Definition and natural history. *Clinics in Geriatric Medicine, 27*(1), 1–15. https://doi.org/10.1016/j.cger.2010.08.009

Yellen, S. B., Cella, D. F., Webster, K., Blendowski, C., & Kaplan, E. (1997). Measuring fatigue and other anemia-related symptoms with the Functional Assessment of Cancer Therapy (FACT) measurement system. *Journal of Pain Symptom Management, 13,* 63–74. https://doi.org/10.1016/S0885-3924(96)00274-6

Yesavage, J. A., Brink, T. L., Rose, T. L., Lum, O., Huang, V., Adey, M., & Leirer, V. O. (1983). Development and validation of a geriatric depression screening scale: A preliminary report. *Journal of Psychiatric Research, 17,* 37–49. https://doi.org/10.1016/0022-3956(82)90033-4

Zigmond, A., & Snaith, R. (1983). The Hospital Anxiety and Depression Scale. *Acta Psychiatrica Scandinavica, 67,* 361–370. https://doi.org/10.1111/j.1600-0447.1983.tb09716.x

PART III.

Cancer Care Continuum and Cancer Rehabilitation

Primary and Secondary Prevention

8

Amanda Wheeler, MOT, OTR/L

LEARNING OBJECTIVES

After completing this chapter, readers should be able to

- Comprehend primary prevention and health promotion as they apply to occupational therapy across the lifespan in oncology,
- Understand secondary prevention in occupational therapy across the lifespan in oncology,
- Recognize common health care settings where primary and secondary preventative occupational therapy services are provided,
- Distinguish between primary and secondary prevention strategies,
- Apply principles of primary and secondary prevention to oncology rehabilitation, and
- Analyze case scenarios to synthesize and implement learned primary and secondary prevention concepts.

KEY TERMS AND CONCEPTS

- Community-based practice
- Contexts
- Cultural context
- Disease prevention
- Ecology of Human Performance
- Environment
- Health promotion
- Interprofessional health care team
- Model of Human Occupation
- Personal context
- Person–Environment–Occupation Model
- Physical environment
- Primary care
- Primary prevention
- Secondary prevention
- Social environment
- Temporal context
- Virtual context
- Wellness

INTRODUCTION

The cancer care continuum begins with primary and secondary prevention. ***Primary prevention*** begins before an individual is diagnosed with cancer and encompasses actions to minimize potential modifiable risk factors such as maintaining a healthy diet, exercising, or reducing exposure to environmental toxins known to cause cancer. ***Secondary prevention*** is provided at the point of cancer screening and initial diagnosis to provide support and reduce the potential burden of symptoms and treatment side effects through activities such as strength training and cognitively stimulating worksheets and puzzles (Söderback, 2014). The preventative phases of the cancer care continuum are important because although there are known lifestyle choices that increase one's risk for the development of cancer, a growing body of evidence indicates that living a healthy, active lifestyle can actually reduce the risk of developing cancer (Lee & Loh, 2013).

Functional deficits must be properly assessed and treated early in the cancer care continuum to reduce significant long-term functional decline (Braveman, 2017; Dahl-Popolizio et al., 2016; Leland et al., 2017). Occupational therapy practitioners' unique focus on engagement in healthy occupation and its interconnection with the promotion of overall health and well-being puts the profession in an optimal position to target individuals who are at risk for developing cancer or are in the initial phases of diagnosis and treatment (American Occupational Therapy Association [AOTA], 2014b; Christiansen, 1999).

Over the past decade, health care legislation has shifted health care practices to focus on ***health promotion*** (i.e., encouraging positive habits such as routine exercise and healthy eating), ***wellness*** (i.e., ability to find balance and perceive satisfaction in one's overall health and quality of life; AOTA, 2014a; Boyt Schell et al., 2014; Brownson & Scaffa, 2001), and ***disease prevention*** (i.e., participation in programs designed to reduce unhealthy habits such as smoking). Actions and initiatives are occurring at individual, local, and national levels that promote health and reduce the risk for development of disease (Brownson & Scaffa, 2001; Centers for Disease Control and Prevention, 2019). Occupational therapy practitioners have an opportunity to make an initial impact in ***primary care*** settings, where individuals typically have first contact with a medical provider such as general medical practitioner offices or community clinics (AOTA, 2014b; Donnelly et al., 2014; Muir, 2012).

Although many potential opportunities for the integration of occupational therapy exist in primary and secondary prevention in oncology rehabilitation, integrating preventive practices continues to be an emerging practice area for the profession (Muir, 2012). If health care continues to be driven by preventive practices, future opportunity exists for occupational therapy practitioners to expand primary and secondary prevention for clients in the oncology rehabilitation continuum (Braveman, 2017; Scaffa & Reitz, 2014).

This chapter begins by defining key features of primary and secondary prevention within oncology. The majority of this chapter focuses on describing occupational therapy's specific role within the primary and secondary prevention phases of the cancer care continuum, highlighting unique strategies used for varying age groups. Concluding the chapter are primary and secondary prevention case examples for the reader to apply knowledge gained.

DEFINING FEATURES OF PRIMARY AND SECONDARY PREVENTION AND THE CANCER CARE CONTINUUM

Practice Settings

Primary and secondary prevention often occur in primary care and **community-based practice** settings (AOTA, 2014b), environments in which prevention and health promotion practices are supported within the community and can be found in health centers or clinics, individual homes, or within the workplace (Scaffa & Reitz, 2014). Occupational therapy services are provided to individuals, groups, and populations through both direct and indirect methods of service delivery (AOTA, 2014a). Occupational therapy services may be integrated into primary and secondary preventative cancer care plans initiated by primary care practitioners or primary oncologists.

Care Team Members

Key stakeholders in the preventative phases of the cancer care continuum are those who generate referrals to occupational therapy in primary health care settings; they include physicians, nurse practitioners, and physician assistants (American Academy of Family Physicians, 2018). Other potential team members who may communicate with the occupational therapy practitioner to develop a comprehensive care plan include family members, physical therapists, speech-language pathologists, psychologists, social workers, and educators (Scaffa & Reitz, 2014).

Guidelines, Policies, and Legislation

The concepts of *health promotion* and *disease prevention* through engagement in meaningful occupation have been embedded in the profession of occupational therapy since its inception (Schwartz, 2009). The belief in "*meaningful engagement* in occupation . . . creating a healthy body and mind" (Schwartz, 2010, p. 8; italics added) was shared by the founders of the profession and still holds true to the profession's ethos today. The concepts of health promotion, disease prevention, and wellness through occupational engagement are integrated throughout the *Occupational Therapy Practice Framework: Domain and Process* (3rd ed.; *OTPF*; AOTA, 2014a) and form the overarching theme in the profession's domain and process.

Besides falling within the occupational therapy scope of practice, primary and secondary prevention are supported by several government initiatives. The Patient Protection and Affordable Care Act (ACA) of 2010 (P. L. 111-148) was designed to expand current health care coverage through affordable insurance options to all Americans. The intention of this act was to increase health care access across the continuum of care and improve access to prevention and early screening of health issues to improve individual health outcomes and reduce overall costs of care (Braveman & Metzler, 2012). The ACA has recognized occupational therapy as part of the ***interprofessional health care team***, therefore strengthening opportunities for occupational therapy practitioners to gain recognition and provide intervention at the primary care level and allowing for reimbursable involvement in primary and secondary prevention (Braveman & Metzler, 2012). The creation of accountable care organizations and patient-centered medical home models through the ACA has broadened the potential for occupational therapy involvement (Dahl-Popolizio et al., 2016; Muir, 2012).

The U.S. Department of Health and Human Services' (DHHS) *Healthy People 2020* initiative has outlined specific objectives for reducing the incidence and death rate associated with cancer through implementation of health promotion and early-detection strategies (DHHS, 2018). Key modifiable risk factors, including the use of tobacco products, physical inactivity, obesity, ultraviolet light exposure, environmental toxins, and sexually transmitted diseases, are being targeted to reduce the incidence of certain types of cancer through health care literacy initiatives, primary care screening, and work and home environment safety assessments (DHHS, 2018).

The ACA provides Americans several benefits with respect to primary and secondary prevention, including access to affordable health insurance and primary care providers (Braveman & Metzler, 2012). Mandates on insurance coverage have improved what is covered by health care insurance; one important aspect is primary care and preventative services. An increased number of individuals are receiving annual wellness assessments, which include assessment of physical, cognitive, and mental health.

Because annual primary care visits allow for more thorough screening, they enable occupational therapy practitioners to access more referrals at the primary care level (Braveman & Metzler, 2012). Besides fostering greater access to clients in need of occupational therapy services, the ACA includes habilitative and rehabilitative services as mandatory in a basic insurance package, which further ensures therapy service coverage at the primary and secondary prevention levels of care (Braveman & Metzler, 2012).

OCCUPATIONAL THERAPY'S ROLE

Practice Models to Guide Primary and Secondary Prevention

Several occupational therapy conceptual practice models apply to the primary and secondary prevention phases of the cancer care continuum. Occupational therapy practitioners can partner with an individual or group in the community to identify potential occupational barriers and solutions to maximize functional performance, to either prevent the diagnosis of cancer or prevent functional deficits from limiting occupational engagement once an initial diagnosis has been made (Scaffa & Reitz, 2014).

Scaffa and Reitz (2014) described three occupational therapy conceptual practice models applicable to community-based practice: (1) the Ecology of Human Performance Model (EHP; Dunn et al., 1994), (2) Model of Human Occupation (MOHO; Kielhofner & Burke, 1980), and (3) Person–Environment–Occupation Model (PEO; Law et al., 1996). Although this is not an exhaustive list, EHP, MOHO, and PEO are applicable in primary care settings and allow focus on health promotion and disease prevention.

EHP

The **EHP**, developed by Dunn et al. (1994), is a model that considers the environment to be a critical factor in human performance. It allows occupational therapy practitioners to consider the cancer survivor's skills in conjunction with their perception of context, which influences choice of occupation and ability to perform a particular task (Scaffa et al., 2010). EHP applies to health promotion and disease prevention because specific interventions described in EHP target preventative practices by facilitating clients' recognition of health needs and helping them gain competent performance (Scaffa et al., 2010).

For example, a community center in a low-income area hosts a free multidisciplinary educational series on healthy eating and meal preparation for all members of the community. This offers residents the opportunity, within their own context, to achieve competency in meal preparation and feeding to prevent obesity, which, among other health issues, is a major risk factor for the development of cancer (De Pergola & Silvestris, 2013; Dunn et al., 1994).

MOHO

The **MOHO**, developed by Kielhofner and Burke (1980), is based on the principle that human beings have an innate need for participation in occupation and that occupation produces health and well-being. Occupational therapy practitioners can apply various strategies to maintain, restore, reorganize, or develop a client's capacity, motivation for a particular occupation, and lifestyle (Scaffa et al., 2010).

An example of integrating the MOHO within secondary prevention is an older adult recently diagnosed with Stage I lung cancer who has been told he must quit smoking after a 40-year smoking history; although he recognizes the need, he feels helpless to stop smoking. The client begins working with an occupational therapist in an outpatient clinic, and the occupational therapist provides him with a motivational inventory to determine his occupational interests to supplement the negative occupation of cigarette smoking. Once several occupations of interest are identified, the therapist facilitates development and mastery of these occupations as well as resources to enhance the environment.

PEO

Created by Mary Law and colleagues in 1996, the **PEO** is based on the concept that human behavior and occupational performance cannot be separated from contextual influence and that occupational performance is the outcome of the transaction among the person, environment, and occupation (Law et al., 1996; Letts et al., 2003; Strong et al., 1999). The PEO is applicable to primary and secondary prevention because it allows the occupational therapy practitioner to work with the cancer survivor in their natural environments and provide strategies for modification or adaptation to create the best fit within the person–environment–occupation relationship.

An example of integrating the PEO within secondary prevention is an occupational therapy practitioner's providing home modification and energy conservation strategies to a survivor of advanced age who has recently initiated chemotherapy treatment for newly diagnosed cancer. The occupational therapy practitioner provides strategies to prevent or limit the negative effects of fatigue and neuropathy that may develop from chemotherapy treatment. Strategies focus on health behaviors as well as ways to adapt the environment.

Other models

Other relevant models created outside the occupational therapy profession are applicable to primary and secondary prevention. Scaffa and Reitz (2014) highlighted the importance of understanding models used outside the profession, particularly when the occupational therapy practitioner is working in primary care settings that integrate a multiprofessional approach to health care, because it allows for a shared language and understanding among team members. Three examples of models applicable to primary and secondary prevention developed outside the occupational therapy profession are (1) the Health Belief Model (HBM; Rosenstock, 1974), (2) the Transtheoretical Model of Health Behavior Change (TMHBC; Prochaska & Velicer, 1997), and (3) the Ecological Approach to Health Promotion (EAHP; Scaffa & Reitz, 2014; Söderback, 2014).

HBM focuses on an individual's beliefs and attitudes to predict health behaviors (Rosenstock, 1974, 1990). This model is useful because an occupational therapy practitioner can apply it to a specific client to determine their level of understanding and buy-in to engage in wellness and preventative activities. For example, an occupational therapy practitioner can ask a cancer survivor what they perceive to be their likelihood of developing cancer or how serious it might be if they were to eat an unhealthy diet or routinely drink in excess. Responses to the HBM can help guide selected interventions and predict survivors' implementation of preventative behaviors (Rosenstock, 1974).

TABLE 8.1.   Primary and Secondary Prevention Guiding-Practice Models

PRACTICE MODEL	DEFINITION
Ecology of Human Performance (EHP)	EHP is a model that considers the environment to be a critical factor in human performance. It is applicable to health promotion and disease prevention because specific interventions described in EHP target preventative practices through facilitating client recognition of health needs and gaining competent performance (Dunn et al., 1994).
Model of Human Occupation (MOHO)	MOHO is based on the principle that human beings have an innate need for participation in occupation, which produces health and well-being. The occupational therapy practitioner can influence a client's lifestyle choices in both primary and secondary prevention using MOHO (Kielhofner & Burke, 1980).
Person–Environment–Occupation (PEO)	PEO is based on the concept that occupational performance is the outcome of the transaction among the person, environment, and occupation (Law et al., 1996; Letts et al., 2003; Strong et al., 1999). The PEO is applicable within primary and secondary prevention because it allows the practitioner to work with the client in their natural environments and provide strategies for modification or adaptation to create the best PEO fit.
Health Belief Model (HBM)	HBM predicts one's likelihood to participate in health behaviors on the basis of one's beliefs and attitudes (Rosenstock, 1974, 1990). An occupational therapy practitioner can apply HBM to a specific client to determine their level of understanding and buy-in to engage in wellness and preventative activities.
Transtheoretical Model of Health Behavior Change (TMHBC)	TMHBC is used to conceptualize the process of behavior change applicable to multiple environments, contexts, and behaviors (Prochaska & Velicer, 1997). The model is useful in preventative phases of care because it can assist the clinician in determining the client's readiness for change from unhealthy habits or occupations.
Ecological Approach to Health Promotion (EAHP)	EAHP focuses on the interrelationship between the individual and their surrounding environment (physical, social, organizational, cultural, and political). Understanding and implementing EAHP can serve as a common language among various health care professionals and allows the clinician to view the larger picture influencing client occupational engagement and health choices (Söderback, 2014).

TMHBC is a model used to conceptualize the process of behavior change applicable to multiple environments, contexts, and behaviors. The model encompasses 6 stages of change and associated processes that occur while individuals are working through each stage of change (Prochaska & Velicer, 1997). Integrating this model can assist the occupational therapy practitioner working in primary care settings to determine a client's readiness to change certain unhealthy habits, such as lack of physical activity, poor diet, or use of tobacco products, which are all linked to potential development of cancer (Prochaska, 2008; Scaffa & Reitz, 2014; Wright et al., 2009).

EAHP, which has been integrated into health promotion practices for more than 2 decades, places significant emphasis on the interrelationship between the individual and their surrounding environment. *Environment* in this model can be physical, social, organizational, cultural, or political (Söderback, 2014). Understanding and implementing EAHP can help the occupational therapy practitioner understand environmental factors that affect an individual or community at both the micro and the macro levels (Söderback, 2014). Table 8.1 provides a brief overview of each practice model and its application to the primary and secondary prevention phases of the cancer care continuum.

Occupational Therapy Across the Lifespan

Occupational therapy practitioners can interact with cancer survivors at the primary and secondary prevention phases of the cancer care continuum across the lifespan. The basic concepts of screening and early intervention remain the same at each stage of life despite the use of different age-specific assessments and treatment strategies. See Table 8.2 for specific examples of occupational therapy's role across the life course in primary and secondary prevention.

Future Opportunities for Occupational Therapy

Current health care practices and reimbursement models support targeting individuals at the primary care level, which includes habilitative and rehabilitative services (Braveman & Metzler, 2012). Evidence shows that occupational therapy services are cost-effective in treating and preventing injury and improving health outcomes in programs designed to address falls, early intervention in pediatrics, pulmonary rehabilitation, home care, and stroke rehabilitation (Rexe et al., 2013; Rogers et al., 2016).

Many successful programs are targeted toward the geriatric population to integrate Lifestyle Redesign® (Clark et al., 2015) concepts, driver rehabilitation programs, and occupational therapy practitioners working with individuals at risk for mental health issues (Bazyk et al., 2015; Cassidy et al., 2017; Golisz, 2014; Lee & Loh, 2013; Stav et al., 2012). Although individuals with a cancer diagnosis may attend and benefit from some of these programs, there is limited information available regarding their effectiveness for primary and secondary prevention in cancer rehabilitation. Additional investigations are underway, such as

TABLE 8.2.   Role of the Occupational Therapy Practitioner in Primary and Secondary Prevention Across the Lifespan

AGE	ROLE OF OCCUPATIONAL THERAPY PRACTITIONER
Pediatric	■ Early screening, assessment, and treatment of pediatric clients; education of caregivers on developmental milestones and possible changes that may occur because of a cancer diagnosis or associated treatment (Connelly, 2015; Ness et al., 2005) ■ Education and involvement of caregivers to implement strategies at home to reduce potentially limiting client performance factors
Adolescent and young adult	■ Early screening for risk factors (e.g., unhealthy eating habits, sedentary behaviors), education on healthy lifestyle choices for client and caregiver ■ Once a client has been diagnosed with cancer, early involvement to assess for potential limiting performance factors, education of the client on preventative strategies to reduce potential physical and cognitive limitations during and after treatment (Hallquist Viale, 2016)
Adult	■ Preventative screening and healthy lifestyle education in primary care and community settings ■ Education on potential physical, cognitive, and psychosocial implications of cancer treatment as well as long-term side effects and ways to manage participation in meaningful life roles while undergoing cancer treatment (e.g., care for others, work, home maintenance, self-care, social participation; Braveman & Hunter, 2017)
Older adult	■ Preventative screening and healthy lifestyle education in primary care and community settings ■ Education on common cancer symptoms that can cause functional decline and ways to combat negative effects of cancer and associated treatment (e.g., falls prevention, activity modification, community resources; Pergolotti et al., 2016; Williams et al., 2015)

a randomized controlled trial to determine the impact of occupational and physical therapy services provided in an outpatient rehabilitation clinic for older adults who have a diagnosis of cancer and present with at least one functional deficit identified through screening during outpatient oncology visits (Pergolotti, Deal, Williams, et al., 2015).

Because primary and secondary prevention continues to be an area for growth for occupational therapy, it is important to understand current successful models of service delivery and use strategies such as educating primary care providers about the services occupational therapy provides, establishing partnerships to increase referrals, and potentially performing screenings in primary care clinics or medical homes. Nyrop et al. (2016) highlighted the lack of consistent attention primary oncologists pay to the level of physical activity of individuals with early-stage cancer despite understanding the benefits it provides in combating cancer-related fatigue, improving physical function, and increasing overall survival. Nyrop et al.'s (2016) findings demonstrate an opportunity for occupational therapy involvement to perform screenings in oncology outpatient clinics or to provide routine education as reminders for oncology physicians.

COMMON CHALLENGES IN PRIMARY AND SECONDARY PREVENTION

Individuals with a cancer diagnosis face many challenges across the lifespan resulting from the disease itself and its associated treatments. Cancer and its treatments create several side effects that have a direct effect on patients' ability to perform at their baseline level of functioning before diagnosis. (Refer to Section IV, "Sequelae of Cancer and Interventions Across the Lifespan," for more information

on many of these side effects.) Individuals with cancer can experience a range of symptoms from time of diagnosis to the survivorship phase of the continuum; therefore, it is important to initiate occupational therapy services early on to reduce the potential challenges clients with cancer face across the continuum. Functional decline among the oncology population, particularly in individuals of an advanced age, is linked to higher health care costs and hospital readmissions; however, there continues to be a lack of rehabilitative services provided at the early phases of the cancer care continuum (Pergolotti, Deal, Lavery, et al., 2015).

Figure 8.1 illustrates the potential physical, emotional, cognitive, and social challenges an individual at any age may face once diagnosed with cancer. These challenges may arise at different phases of the continuum, so it is important that occupational therapy practitioners recognize these challenges and teach cancer survivors to use a proactive approach to manage and possibly prevent functional decline.

CONTEXT AND ENVIRONMENT IN PRIMARY AND SECONDARY PREVENTION

AOTA (2010) endorses the importance of one's environment and contexts and the influence they have on healthy participation in occupation. *Contexts,* as defined in the *OTPF,* are "elements within and surrounding a client . . . that have a strong influence on performance" (AOTA, 2014a, p. S9). Contexts can be cultural, personal, temporal, and virtual.

Environments refer to tangible physical and social surroundings that exist while a person is engaging in occupation (AOTA, 2014a). Occupational therapy practitioners can analyze, adapt, structure, or modify the environment, the context, or both to facilitate optimal occupational performance

FIGURE 8.1.   Potential challenges experienced by clients diagnosed with cancer across the care continuum.

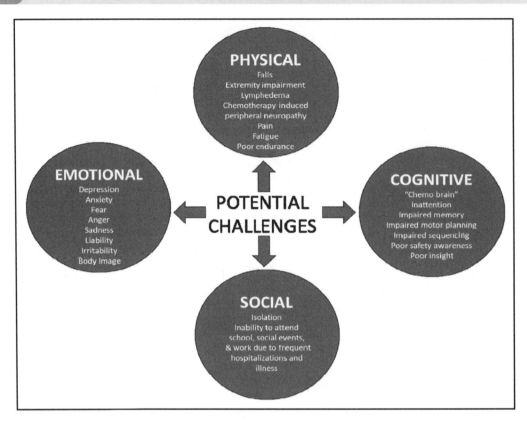

(AOTA, 2010). Assessing clients' contexts and environments is important during the primary and secondary prevention phases of the cancer care continuum across the lifespan. The guiding questions and examples in this section highlight potential interventions occupational therapy practitioners might use while working with clients during primary and secondary prevention phases of the cancer care continuum.

Physical Environment

The *physical environment* encompasses the physical space where an individual performs their daily occupations (AOTA, 2014a). To account for the physical environment, occupational therapy practitioners might ask, "Does the client's school, work, or home environment reduce potential barriers to participation in occupation? What are potential environmental modifications to maximize functional performance?" With this information, practitioners can offer appropriate interventions, such as

- Providing a chair or stool at a play table either at school or at home to allow for modified play as needed by the child to reduce fatigue,
- Suggesting classroom modifications to minimize distractions and increase students' attention in anticipation that they may experience cognitive difficulties from chemotherapy,
- Conducting a worksite analysis and providing suggestions for maximizing comfort and incorporating adequate rest breaks, and

- Providing home modification strategies to reduce the risk of falls for someone who is at risk for developing peripheral neuropathy or who has had impaired functional mobility since the onset of cancer diagnosis.

Social Environment

The *social environment* includes people or groups an individual has contact with while engaging in occupations. (AOTA, 2014a). Types of social environment and supports that foster preventative practices include

- Facilitating group play activities that are developmentally appropriate in a community center;
- For an adolescent client, encouraging communication (in person or web-based) with other adolescents through support groups for individuals recently diagnosed with cancer;
- Offering evening support groups for adults from a primary oncologist's office or in a primary care office or clinic; and
- Implementing social and networking groups for older adults in a senior center.

Cultural Context

Cultural context is any norms, customs, or beliefs associated with the individual's society (AOTA, 2014a). Occupational therapy practitioners can take cultural context into account by asking, "What are the cultural influences of the individual? What programs or activities would support wellness?" They can then use this information to determine appropriate interventions, such as

- Providing families with a low socioeconomic status with resources and education about healthy meal choices;
- Planning free sports and recreation activities at a local community center or park in a demographically low-income area with limited access to after-school recreational activities;
- Offering leisure activity workshops or classes at a local community center for individuals interested in smoking cessation; and
- For individuals recently diagnosed with cancer, providing a presentation on home safety modification to prevent falls in a local library or senior center, with an interpreter if the community's primary language is not the presenter's own.

Personal Context

The **personal context** is the demographic characteristics of an individual (AOTA, 2014a). When considering personal context, occupational therapy practitioners should ask, "How does the client's identity influence occupational engagement? What activities would fit the client's personal identity and unique roles?" Practitioners can then offer appropriate interventions, such as

- Offering educational sessions or support groups geared toward personal attributes of a particular client;
- Providing an educational series for mothers with breast cancer, providing strategies to conserve energy while completing child care tasks, or integrating compensatory strategies to keep track of schedules for those experiencing decreased memory and attention; and
- Running a support group for parents of children with cancer, with an emphasis on supporting the caregiver in performing the occupation of caregiving while maintaining self-care.

Temporal Context

The **temporal context** consists of the characteristics related to time associated with an individual (AOTA, 2014a). To account for the temporal context, occupational therapy practitioners should consider factors such as the client's life stage and the time of year. This information will help practitioners, for example, choose indoor bowling for teens during the winter or outdoor soccer in the summer, or select card games that are familiar to a geriatric client versus ones more familiar to a child.

Virtual Context

The **virtual context** is interaction that occurs without physical contact (AOTA, 2014a). In considering the virtual context, the occupational therapy practitioner should ask, "Does the individual have access to technology? What forms of technology is the client familiar with? How can technology be used to complement wellness and preventative strategies?" When selecting interventions that fit the client's virtual context, the practitioner might, for example,

- Schedule weekly virtual check-ins with parents of a child recently diagnosed with cancer to see how carryover of the occupational therapy home program is going and whether new issues have arisen with the child,
- Teach an adolescent with cancer how to mark daily progress on goals created in occupational therapy using a tablet or smart device,
- Show an adult recently diagnosed with cancer various internet-based chat groups and ways to access their personal medical information through hospital patient websites, or
- Educate an older adult on how to set reminders on a recently purchased cell phone to keep track of medical appointments and daily medications.

INTERVENTION APPROACHES IN PRIMARY AND SECONDARY PREVENTION

Occupational therapy services provided within primary prevention often focus on maintenance, health promotion, and prevention. Secondary prevention occupational therapy services include similar intervention approaches to primary prevention and may also include restorative and modification interventions, as defined in the *OTPF* (AOTA, 2014a).

Table 8.3 provides examples of types of interventions provided by occupational therapy practitioners within primary and secondary prevention working with clients who are at risk for or who were recently diagnosed with cancer. Case Examples 8.1 and 8.2 demonstrate occupational therapy evaluation, treatment plan development, treatment implementation, and targeted outcomes in the primary and secondary prevention phases of the cancer care continuum.

TABLE 8.3. **Intervention Strategies in Primary and Secondary Prevention**

STRATEGY	EXAMPLE
Health promotion	Provision of group classes along with other health professionals at a local community center for new parents to educate them on typical developmental patterns and when to seek further support if development seems delayed or has recently changed
Maintenance	Assessment of clients' functioning before and immediately after initiation of cancer treatment; provision of therapeutic exercises to maintain current level of functioning
Prevention	Individual consultation or group education session for individuals newly diagnosed with cancer requiring chemotherapy treatment; designed to educate individuals on chemotherapy treatment's potential impact on functional performance
Restorative	Therapeutic exercises for strengthening and increased activity tolerance before, during, and after initiation of cancer treatment
Modification	Individual training or group class offered to provide home modification strategies to reduce the risk of falls or training on energy conservation strategies to support successful functional participation

CASE EXAMPLE 8.1. RICHARD: PRIMARY PREVENTION

Occupational Profile

Richard is a 66-year-old recently retired steel pipe fitter who has a 40-year smoking history with several preexisting health conditions, including chronic obstructive pulmonary disease, hypertension, coronary artery disease, and Type 2 diabetes. Richard recently had an annual visit with his primary care provider, who recommended a chest X ray because of a persistent, worsening cough. The X ray revealed a lung nodule that needed further workup and biopsy. Richard underwent a minimally invasive procedure requiring an overnight stay in the hospital.

On discharge from the hospital, Richard returned to his primary care provider, who informed him that the biopsy was negative for cancer but that he would require annual assessments of the nodule and expressed concern for Richard's overall health and well-being. Richard's wife recently passed away, and he was finding it difficult to manage his day-to-day responsibilities since returning home from the hospital. The primary care provider referred Richard to outpatient occupational therapy for evaluation and treatment as part of a primary prevention care plan.

Guiding questions for Richard included:

- Tell me about a typical day for you. What activities do you find yourself engaging in every day? Has there been a change in what you do every day? What has changed?
- Are there activities that you find easy to do? How about activities that have been difficult in the past month or so?
- Have you been able to keep the house clean and run errands yourself?
- Are there things you enjoy doing or leisure activities that you have been having difficulty participating in?
- What do you find difficult about the tasks you've described? Do you feel tired or short of breath when you do them?
- What do you do to socialize with others? Do you belong to any clubs or speak to your neighbors or friends?

Analysis of Occupational Performance

After completing the occupational profile and obtaining information pertaining to Richard's concerns about his functional performance with basic ADLs, home maintenance, health management, and leisure participation, the occupational therapist performed an assessment of Richard's upper-extremity (UE) range of motion (ROM), strength, grip strength, sensation, and coordination through use of goniometer, manual muscle testing, monofilaments, and dynamometer. The occupational therapist also assessed Richard's ability to perform ADLs, such as donning and doffing socks and shoes, getting up and down from a low-surface chair, retrieving items from refrigerator shelves below waist level and above head level, and preparing a cup of tea.

On completion of the assessment, the occupational therapist noted that Richard had decreased UE strength, diminished hand sensation and fine motor coordination, shortness of breath on exertion while completing all functional tasks, and fair activity tolerance for both seated and standing activities, which limited his overall functional performance.

Intervention

Intervention plan

The occupational therapist implemented restorative, preventative, and education approaches to the treatment plan (AOTA, 2014a). The therapy plan consisted of weekly visits to the outpatient clinic, and recommendations for modification of Richard's home were also provided. The occupational therapist gave Richard community resources for assistance with home maintenance tasks as well as local senior classes offered for various leisure interests.

Intervention implementation

The intervention implementation consisted of weekly therapy sessions, during which Richard participated in a variety of activities to address his identified impairments. The occupational therapist used preparatory methods to provide environmental and activity modifications to allow Richard to successfully complete his daily activities that involved fine motor coordination; UE strength; and energy, including incorporation of energy conservation strategies and use of tools (e.g., electronic can opener, reacher). Besides using preparatory methods, the occupational therapist educated Richard on energy conservation strategies and gave him resources to increase his independence in the community and to successfully complete ADLs, home maintenance chores, and health management tasks.

The occupational therapist also referred Richard to a falls prevention series offered at the local senior center in town. This series of classes, offered for free to seniors in the community, recommends environmental modification strategies and physical activities for overall muscle strengthening and balance training. Last, while attending his weekly therapy sessions, Richard engaged in therapeutic activities and exercises selected to work specifically on his activity tolerance, upper-body strength, and fine motor coordination.

Intervention review

Richard and his occupational therapist continually reviewed his goals and modified the selected interventions each session on the basis of his progression in therapy. The occupational therapist saw Richard for 8 weekly visits before he achieved all of his established goals, at which time he was discharged from the current occupational therapy program and instructed to report to his doctor if he noticed any changes in his current abilities.

(Continued)

CASE EXAMPLE 8.1. RICHARD: PRIMARY PREVENTION *(Cont.)*

Targeting Outcomes

The primary goals Richard expressed were to sustain independence in completion of his meaningful daily activities and the tasks that were required to maintain his health and home. Richard found an overall improvement in his ability to care for himself and engage in meaningful occupation, which improved his quality of life and well-being.

CASE EXAMPLE 8.2. JASMINE: SECONDARY PREVENTION

Occupational Profile

Jasmine is a 5-year-old girl who lives with her mother and three older siblings in a walk-up apartment building in an urban community. She was meeting all developmental milestones and recently began kindergarten. About halfway through the school year, Jasmine's mother noticed over a few weeks' time that Jasmine frequently fell asleep as soon as she came home from school, lacked appetite, and reported that her body hurt all over. Jasmine's teacher also recognized similar symptoms at school and reported to the mother that Jasmine was having difficulty manipulating small items and sustaining a firm grasp while holding her pencil.

Jasmine was seen by a primary care physician, who had further concerns from returned lab reports. Jasmine was referred to a pediatric oncologist, who confirmed a diagnosis with pre-B-cell standard-risk acute lymphocytic leukemia, which required initiation of chemotherapy treatment. Among other supportive services, Jasmine was immediately referred to outpatient occupational therapy for evaluation and treatment because of her mother's expressed concern about Jasmine's ability to engage at school and during play activities as well as about anticipated further deficits that might occur during chemotherapy treatment. Jasmine was seen for initial occupational therapy evaluation in an outpatient pediatric clinic as part of her secondary prevention care plan.

Guiding questions for Jasmine's mother included:

- Tell me about a typical day for Jasmine. What types of activities does she do?
- What activities do you find to be most difficult for Jasmine to do right now when you think about the things she needs and typically wants to do throughout the day?
- What does Jasmine enjoy doing most? Have any of those things been difficult for her recently?
- What are some of your concerns related to Jasmine's recent participation at school and when playing with her siblings at home?
- Do you find she has an easier time when playing in certain environments versus others or at particular times of day?

Analysis of Occupational Performance

After completing the occupational profile and obtaining information pertaining to the mother's concerns about Jasmine's functional performance with basic ADLs, her ability to play with her siblings, and her difficulty participating in fine motor tasks at school, the occupational therapist performed an assessment of Jasmine's UE ROM, strength, grip strength, and coordination through use of goniometer, manual muscle testing, and dynamometer. The occupational therapist also assessed Jasmine's ability to perform age-appropriate basic ADLs (e.g., putting on a pullover shirt, brushing teeth), play in a standing position to put a puzzle together, and write her name, which her mother had indicated she was able to do. On completion of the assessment, Jasmine was noted to have limited UE and grip strength and fair activity tolerance for both seated and standing activities, which limited her ability to participate in basic ADLs, school, and play tasks.

Intervention

Intervention plan

The occupational therapist implemented restorative, modification, and preventative approaches to the treatment plan (AOTA, 2014a). The therapy plan consisted of weekly visits to the outpatient clinic and recommendations for modification of the home and school environment to maximize Jasmine's performance. The occupational therapist recommended that Jasmine's mother work with the school to determine whether school-based therapy services were needed and to discuss accommodations for Jasmine to be successful in class.

Intervention implementation

The intervention implementation consisted of weekly therapy sessions, during which Jasmine participated in a variety of activities to address her identified impairments. The occupational therapist used preparatory methods to provide environmental and activity modification to allow Jasmine to be successful while writing in class with use of an adapted writing implement and slant

(Continued)

CASE EXAMPLE 8.2. JASMINE: SECONDARY PREVENTION *(Cont.)*

board. The therapist also provided Jasmine's mother with energy conservation strategies to allow Jasmine to be successful in completing basic ADLs at home.

Besides using preparatory methods, the occupational therapist educated Jasmine and her mother on the importance of Jasmine's continued participation in meaningful play activities and self-care despite feelings of fatigue. Last, while attending her weekly therapy sessions, Jasmine engaged in play-based activities that were selected to work on her activity tolerance, upper body strength, and fine motor coordination.

Intervention review

The occupational therapist continuously reviewed Jasmine's goals and modified the selected interventions on the basis of her progression in therapy and response to her cancer treatment. Jasmine and her mother quickly achieved their goals to implement energy conservation

strategies, but Jasmine continued to require therapy services throughout her course of chemotherapy because it created ongoing fatigue and overall weakness as well as presented a new challenge of peripheral neuropathy, which caused discomfort and further fine motor difficulties. The occupational therapist updated the plan of care to incorporate goals to address Jasmine's peripheral neuropathy.

Targeting Outcomes

The primary goals Jasmine and her mother expressed were to allow Jasmine to continue engaging in school, playing with friends and siblings, and completing age-appropriate basic ADL tasks as independently as possible. Because ongoing factors might influence Jasmine's occupational performance throughout her course of treatment, the occupational therapist focused on targeting continued participation, quality of life, and occupational performance.

SUMMARY

Occupational therapy involvement in the cancer care continuum begins with primary and secondary prevention. Occupational therapy practitioners are well suited to address the needs of cancer survivors within primary and secondary prevention because the profession's focus on meaningful occupational engagement to promote overall health and well-being goes hand in hand with preventative care needs (AOTA, 2014b; Christiansen, 1999). The preventative phases of the cancer care continuum are of growing significance because timely recognition of potential risk factors or functional impairments allows clinicians to make an early impact and potentially prevent functional decline and maximize quality of life (Braveman, 2017; Dahl-Popolizio et al., 2016; Lee & Loh, 2013; Leland et al., 2017).

Current health care practices and insurance coverage support occupational therapy services provided in the community and at the primary care level (AOTA, 2014b; Donnelly et al., 2014; Muir, 2012). Understanding the potential impact occupational therapy practitioners can have within primary and secondary prevention in oncology as well as identifying applicable practice models and treatment approaches are the first steps toward developing and implementing primary and secondary prevention programs. It is important for occupational therapy practitioners to recognize opportunities for growth in the cancer care continuum, particularly within primary and secondary prevention and using existing models that have been successful with other client populations (Braveman, 2017; Scaffa & Reitz, 2014). Further development of occupational therapy's role is needed within primary and secondary prevention in oncology rehabilitation.

REFERENCES

American Academy of Family Physicians. (2018). *Primary care.* Retrieved from https://www.aafp.org/about/policies/all/primary-care.html

American Occupational Therapy Association. (2010). Occupational therapy's perspective on the use of environments and contexts to support health and participation in occupations. *American Journal of Occupational Therapy, 64,* S57–69. https://doi.org/10.5014/ajot.2010.64s57-64s69

American Occupational Therapy Association. (2014a). Occupational therapy practice framework: Domain and process (3rd ed.). *American Journal of Occupational Therapy, 68*(Suppl. 1), S1–S48. https://doi.org/10.5014/ajot.2014.682006

American Occupational Therapy Association. (2014b). The role of occupational therapy in primary care. *American Journal of Occupational Therapy, 68*(Suppl. 3), S25–S33. https://doi.org/10.5014/ajot.2014.686S06

Bazyk, S., Demirjian, L., LaGuardia, T., Thompson-Repas, K., Conway, C., & Michaud, P. (2015). Building capacity of occupational therapy practitioners to address the mental health needs of children and youth: A mixed-methods study of knowledge translation. *American Journal of Occupational Therapy, 69,* 6906180060. https://doi.org/10.5014/ajot.2015.019182

Boyt Schell, B. A., Gillen, G., & Scaffa, M. (Eds.). (2014). *Willard and Spackman's occupational therapy* (12th ed.). Philadelphia: Lippincott Williams & Wilkins.

Braveman, B. (2017a). Cancer and employment: Opportunities for occupational therapy in the coming decade. *SIS Quarterly Practice Connections, 2*(2), 27–29.

Braveman, B. (2017b). *Occupational therapy practice guidelines for cancer rehabilitation with adults.* Bethesda, MD: AOTA Press.

Braveman, B., & Metzler, C. A. (2012). Health care reform implementation and occupational therapy. *American Journal of Occupational Therapy, 66,* 11–14. https://doi.org/10.5014/ajot.2012.661001

Brownson, C. A., & Scaffa, M. E. (2001). Occupational therapy in the promotion of health and the prevention of disease and disability statement. *American Journal of Occupational Therapy, 55,* 656–660. https://doi.org/10.5014/ajot.55.6.656

Cassidy, T. B., Richards, L. G., & Eakman, A. M. (2017). Feasibility of a Lifestyle Redesign®–inspired intervention for well older adults. *American Journal of Occupational Therapy, 71,* 7104190050. https://doi.org/10.5014/ajot.2017.024430

Centers for Disease Control and Prevention. (2019). *How we prevent chronic diseases and promote health.* Retrieved from https://www.cdc.gov/chronicdisease/center/nccdphp/how.htm

Christiansen, C. H. (1999). Defining lives: Occupation as identity: An essay on competence, coherence, and the creation of meaning (Eleanor Clarke Slagle Lecture). *American Journal of Occupational Therapy, 53,* 547–558. https://doi.org/10.5014/ajot.53.6.547

Clark, F., Blanchard, J., Sleight, A., Cogan, A., Florindez, L., Gleanson, S., Heymann, R., . . . Vigen, C. (2015). *Lifestyle Redesign®: The intervention tested in the USC Well Elderly Studies* (2nd ed.). Bethesda, MD: AOTA Press.

Connelly, C. (2015). Pediatric oncology clients undergoing stem cell transplant: The impact on occupational performance. *OT Practice, 20*(9), 7–12.

Dahl-Popolizio, S., Manson, L., Muir, S., & Rogers, O. (2016). Enhancing the value of integrated primary care: The role of occupational therapy. *Families, Systems, & Health, 34,* 270–280. https://doi.org/10.1037/fsh0000208

De Pergola, G., & Silvestris, F. (2013). Obesity as a major risk factor for cancer. *Journal of Obesity, 2013,* 291546. https://doi.org/10.1155/2013/291546

Donnelly, C. A., Brenchley, C. L., Crawford, C. N., & Letts, L. J. (2014). The emerging role of occupational therapy in primary care. *Canadian Journal of Occupational Therapy, 81,* 51–61. https://doi.org/10.1177/0008417414520683

Dunn, W., Brown, C., & McGuigan, A. (1994). The Ecology of Human Performance: A framework for considering the effect of context. *American Journal of Occupational Therapy, 48,* 595–607. https://doi.org/10.5014/ajot.48.7.595

Golisz, K. (2014). Occupational therapy interventions to improve driving performance in older adults: A systematic review. *American Journal of Occupational Therapy, 68,* 662–669. https://doi.org/10.5014/ajot.2014.011247

Hallquist Viale, P. (2016). Late effects: Focus on adolescent and young adult cancer survivors. *Journal of the Advanced Practitioner in Oncology, 7,* 15–16. https://doi.org/10.6004/jadpro.2016.7.1.1

Kielhofner, G., & Burke, J. P. (1980). A Model of Human Occupation, Part 1. Conceptual framework and content. *American Journal of Occupational Therapy, 34,* 572–581. https://doi.org/10.5014/ajot.34.9.572

Law, M., Cooper, B., Strong, S., Stewart, D., Rigby, P., & Letts, L. (1996). The Person–Environment–Occupation Model: A transactive approach to occupational performance. *Canadian Journal of Occupational Therapy, 63,* 9–23. https://doi.org/10.1177/000841749606300103

Lee, J. E., & Loh, S. Y. (2013). Physical activity and quality of life of cancer survivors: A lack of focus for lifestyle redesign. *Asian Pacific Journal of Cancer Prevention, 14,* 2551–2555. https://doi.org/10.7314/apjcp.2013.14.4.2551

Leland, N. E., Fogelberg, D. J., Halle, A. D., & Mroz, T. M. (2017). Occupational therapy and management of multiple chronic conditions in the context of health care reform. *American Journal of Occupational Therapy, 71,* 7101090010. https://doi.org/10.5014/ajot.2017.711001

Letts, L., Rigby, P., & Stewart, D. (2003). *Using environments to enable occupational performance.* Thorofare, NJ: Slack.

Muir, S. (2012). Occupational therapy in primary health care: We should be there. *American Journal of Occupational Therapy, 66,* 506–510. https://doi.org/10.5014/ajot.2012.665001

Ness, K. K., Bhatia, S., Baker, K. S., Francisco, L., Carter, A., Forman, S. J., . . . Gurney, J. G. (2005). Performance limitations and participation restrictions among childhood cancer survivors treated with hematopoietic stem cell transplantation: The Bone Marrow Transplant Survivor Study. *Archives of Pediatrics and Adolescent Medicine, 159,* 706–713. https://doi.org/10.1001/archpedi.159.8.706

Nyrop, K. A., Deal, A. M., Williams, G. R., Guerard, E. J., Pergolotti, M., & Muss, H. B. (2016). Physical activity communication between oncology providers and patients with early-stage breast, colon, or prostate cancer. *Cancer, 122,* 470–476. https://doi.org/10.1002/cncr.29786

Patient Protection and Affordable Care Act, Pub. L. 111–148, 42 U.S.C. §§ 18001–18121 (2010).

Pergolotti, M., Deal, A. M., Lavery, J., Reeve, B. B., & Muss, H. B. (2015). The prevalence of potentially modifiable functional deficits and the subsequent use of occupational and physical therapy by older adults with cancer. *Journal of Geriatric Oncology, 6,* 194–201. https://doi.org/10.1016/j.jgo.2015.01.004

Pergolotti, M., Deal, A. M., Williams, G. R., Bryant, A. L., Reeve, B. B., & Muss, H. B. (2015). A randomized controlled trial of outpatient CAncer REhabilitation for older adults: The CARE Program. *Contemporary Clinical Trials, 44,* 89–94. https://doi.org/10.1016/j.cct.2015.07.021

Pergolotti, M., Williams, G. R., Campbell, C., Munoz, L. A., & Muss, H. B. (2016). Occupational therapy for adults with cancer: Why it matters. *Oncologist, 21,* 314–319. https://doi.org/10.1634/theoncologist.2015-0335

Prochaska, J. O. (2008). Decision making in the Transtheoretical Model of Behavior Change. *Medical Decision Making, 28,* 845–849. https://doi.org/10.1177/0272989X08327068

Prochaska, J. O., & Velicer, W. F. (1997). The Transtheoretical Model of Health Behavior Change. *American Journal of Health Promotion, 12,* 38–48. https://doi.org/10.4278/0890-1171-12.1.38

Rexe, K., Lammi, B. M., & Zweck, C. (2013). Occupational therapy: Cost-effective solutions for changing health system needs. *Healthcare Quarterly, 16*(1), 69–75. https://doi.org/10.12927/hcq.2013.23329

Rogers, A. T., Bai, G., Lavin, R. A., & Anderson, G. F. (2016). Higher hospital spending on occupational therapy is associated with lower readmission rates. *Medical Care Research and Review, 74,* 668–686. https://doi.org/10.1177/1077558716666981

Rosenstock, I. M. (1974). The Health Belief Model and preventive health behavior. *Health Education Monographs, 2,* 354–386. https://doi.org/10.1177/109019817400200405

Rosenstock, I. M. (1990). The Health Belief Model: Explaining health behavior through expectancies. In K. Glanz, F. M. Lewis, & B. K. Rimer (Eds.), *The Jossey-Bass health series. Health behavior and health education: Theory, research, and practice* (pp. 39–62). San Francisco: Jossey-Bass.

Scaffa, M. E., & Reitz, S. M. (2014). *Occupational therapy in community-based practice settings* (2nd ed.). Philadelphia: Davis.

Scaffa, M. E., Reitz, S. M., & Pizzi, M. (2010). *Occupational therapy in the promotion of health and wellness.* Philadelphia: Davis.

Schwartz, K. B. (2009). Eleanor Clarke Slagle Lecture—Reclaiming our heritage: Connecting the *Founding Vision* to the *Centennial Vision*. *American Journal of Occupational Therapy, 63,* 681–690. https://doi.org/10.5014/ajot.63.6.681

Schwartz, K. B. (2010). The history of occupational therapy. In E. Crepeau, E. Cohn, & B. Schell (Eds.), *Willard & Spackman's occupational therapy* (pp. 5–13). New York: Lippincott Williams & Wilkins.

Söderback, I. (2014). *International handbook of occupational therapy interventions.* New York: Springer.

Stav, W. B., Hallenen, T., Lane, J., & Arbesman, M. (2012). Systematic review of occupational engagement and health outcomes among community-dwelling older adults. *American Journal of Occupational Therapy, 66,* 301–310. https://doi.org/10.5014/ajot.2012.003707

Strong, S., Rigby, P., Stewart, D., Law, M., Letts, L., & Cooper, B. (1999). Application of the Person–Environment–Occupation Model: A practical tool. *Canadian Journal of Occupational Therapy, 66,* 122–133. https://doi.org/10.1177/000841749906600304

U.S. Department of Health and Human Services. (2018). *Healthy People 2020 topics and objectives: Cancer.* Retrieved from https://www.healthypeople.gov/2020/topics-objectives/topic/cancer

Williams, G. R., Deal, A. M., Nyrop, K. A., Pergolotti, M., Guerard, E. J., Jolly, T. A., & Muss, H. B. (2015). Geriatric assessment as an aide to understanding falls in older adults with cancer. *Supportive Care in Cancer, 23,* 2273–2280. https://doi.org/10.1007/s00520-014-2598-0

Wright, J. A., Velicer, W. F., & Prochaska, J. O. (2009). Testing the predictive power of the Transtheoretical Model of Behavior Change applied to dietary fat intake. *Health Education Research, 24,* 224–236. https://doi.org/10.1093/her/cyn014

9

Acute and Medically Complex Settings

Vi Nguyen, OTR/L, BSRC, MOT

LEARNING OBJECTIVES

After completing this chapter, readers should be able to
- Explain the relevance of acute and medically complex settings along the cancer rehabilitation continuum,
- Explain the distinct value of occupational therapy in acute and medically complex settings,
- Understand factors that contribute to occupational performance in acute and medically complex settings, and
- Apply strategies to enhance occupational performance and participation in acute and medically complex settings.

KEY TERMS AND CONCEPTS

- ABCDEF bundle
- Acute care
- Acute onset
- Anemia
- Body image
- Bone metastasis
- Chimeric antigen receptor T-cell therapy
- Chronic onset
- Cytokine release syndrome
- Delirium
- Graft-versus-host disease
- Immune effector cell-associated neurotoxicity syndrome
- Infection
- Intensive care unit
- Multidisciplinary care team
- Neutropenia
- Neutropenic fever
- Palliative rehabilitation
- Postintensive care syndrome
- Postintensive care syndrome–family
- Restorative rehabilitation
- Sepsis
- Septic shock
- Subacute onset
- Supportive rehabilitation
- Thrombocytopenia
- Venous thromboembolism

INTRODUCTION

The demand for high-quality cancer rehabilitation in acute and medically complex settings increases in association with advances in cancer treatment and improvement in survivorship trends. *Acute care* is an inpatient hospital setting where the cancer survivor is admitted because of a serious episode of illness related to the cancer or cancer treatment (e.g., surgery, chemotherapy, immunotherapy, cellular therapy, combination therapy). Admission to a medically complex setting such as the *intensive care unit* (ICU) may be necessary if the condition is critical and requires life-support measures.

A growing body of evidence suggests that improvement in the management of critical illness also increases the survival trends of critically ill cancer survivors (Mokart et al., 2014). This rise in the survival rates observed in the ICU, the hospital, and the first year after cancer diagnosis also increases the prevalence of cancer survivors living with *postintensive care syndrome* (PICS), a term coined in recent years describing new or worsening impairments in mental health status and cognitive and physical function after critical illness (Shimabukuro-Vornhagen et al., 2016). A greater emphasis on and demand for early and aggressive rehabilitative intervention is noted as the medical community recognizes the sequelae associated with critical illness, cancer, and its treatment.

Therefore, cancer critical care rehabilitation is a growing area of practice within cancer rehabilitation as a result of contemporary care initiatives such as early mobilization programs. Overall, the role of occupational therapy practitioners continues to expand in acute and medically complex settings because of greater involvement in performance and quality improvement initiatives to enhance care.

Many of the rehabilitation treatment concepts and approaches used in non-cancer populations may be applicable to cancer survivors in this stage of care. However, it is important to note the difference in the rehabilitation course for cancer survivors because of cancer's dynamic nature and its treatments, which result in fluctuations in occupational performance in the acute phase of care. This chapter discusses clinically relevant factors in providing occupational therapy services for cancer survivors in acute and medically complex settings.

DEFINING FEATURES OF ACUTE AND MEDICALLY COMPLEX SETTINGS AND THE CANCER CARE CONTINUUM

Cancer acute and complex settings are characterized by several care teams interacting with cancer survivors on a regular basis to coordinate and deliver the best course of care. Care takes place in the acute setting to potentially span from inpatient rehabilitation-like settings to the ICU. The specific structural alignment of individual teams may vary among institutions. The ***multidisciplinary care team*** may include and is not limited to:

- Primary medical team (e.g., physician, advanced practice providers [APPs] such as advance practice nurses or physician assistants)
- Consulting medical teams (e.g., critical care, cardiology, endocrine, pulmonary, physical medicine and rehabilitation) also comprised of physicians and APPs
- Nursing
- Rehabilitation services (e.g., occupational therapy, physical therapy, speech–language pathology)
- Clinical pharmacy
- Social work
- Case management
- Chaplaincy
- Nutrition services (e.g., dietitian)
- Child, adolescent young adult care team.

Similar to non-cancer acute care settings, the overall goal of these medical settings is to treat and stabilize the immediate medical or surgical issue to prepare cancer survivors for the transition to home or other care settings such as an acute or subacute rehabilitation setting, a long-term acute care facility, or a skilled nursing facility.

Cancer survivors encountered in acute and medically complex settings may be in the restorative, supportive, or palliative stage of cancer rehabilitation. ***Restorative rehabilitation*** is intended to assist survivors in returning to their prior performance status. ***Supportive rehabilitation*** uses adaptive techniques and therapeutic interventions to allow a patient to reach certain levels of improvement or independence. ***Palliative rehabilitation*** focuses on minimizing or eliminating complications from advanced disease with the goal of improving quality of life (QoL; Silver et al., 2018). The clinical picture of cancer survivors in the acute and medically complex setting is typically evolving because of medical complexity secondary to diagnosis and novel treatments (e.g., immunotherapy) with limited understanding of long-term systemic side effects and comorbidities associated with therapies. Therefore, occupational therapy services may be recommended as part of the care plan in this acute phase of care.

Holistic approaches combined with individualized occupational-based interventions are the gold standard to address diverse needs of cancer survivors. This approach is essential because each cancer survivor may experience different challenges and limitations to roles and occupations, depending on the type of cancer and specific cancer treatments.

COMMON CHALLENGES EXPERIENCED IN ACUTE AND MEDICALLY COMPLEX SETTINGS

Cancer and its treatment can pose a number of physical, emotional, cognitive, and social challenges to patients in acute and medically complex settings; these are listed in Table 9.1. These challenges can vary across cancer type, stage, treatment approach, prognosis, comorbidities, and other personal factors. The first appearance of a sign or symptom of a condition can be acute, subacute, or chronic:

- ***Acute onset*** refers to sudden or rapid presentation of signs or symptoms. It generally takes place over a short course of time and does not indicate the severity of illness.
- ***Subacute onset*** refers to signs or symptoms that develop less rapidly than the acute process.
- ***Chronic onset*** refers to signs or symptoms that are ongoing with a general time frame of 3 months or greater. The presentation may not persist at all times.

Depending on the underlying cause or condition, these onsets can result in secondary conditions. They can also progress to emergent presentations with life-threatening conditions. Some challenges can resolve or improve over time after the treatment is complete, while other challenges are long lasting and can result in long-term effects. These physical, emotional, cognitive, and social challenges can be observed concurrently in this acute phase of care to increase the complexity of the overall clinical picture. Although cancer survivors may face similar challenges to patients without cancer in acute and medically complex settings, there are a number of differences, which are highlighted in the following sections.

Physical Challenges

An established body of evidence confirms that common physical challenges shared by many cancer patients include

- Fatigue,
- Weakness,
- Pain,
- Nausea and vomiting,
- Neuropathy,
- Cachexia,
- Diarrhea or constipation,
- Skin impairments,
- Cardiopulmonary impairments, and
- Toxicities (Naughton & Weaver, 2014).

Please see other chapters of this text for detailed discussions on fatigue, pain, and neuropathy. Specific physical challenges faced by cancer survivors in the acute and medical complex settings are further expanded next.

Hematological considerations

Hematological abnormalities such as thrombocytopenia, anemia, and neutropenia are common and can be brought on by cancer and its treatments (American Cancer Society, 2019). Cancer treatment modalities such as chemotherapy and radiation therapy are generally myelosuppressive therapies that aim to kill cancer cells and in turn also slow down production of platelets, red blood cells (RBCs), and white blood cells (WBCs) in the bone marrow. It is essential for occupational therapy practitioners to understand, check, and follow the trends of clinically relevant lab values before every session to ensure appropriateness and safety of therapeutic interventions.

Thrombocytopenia, or low blood platelet count, is a common hematological abnormality in cancer survivors undergoing active treatment (MD Anderson Cancer Center, 2019a). Because platelets, or thrombocytes, have an essential role in blood clotting, patients with thrombocytopenia are at risk for bleeding. The bleeding can be mild and manifest as bruises,

TABLE 9.1. Challenges Experienced by Patients With Cancer in Acute and Medically Complex Settings

PHYSICAL	EMOTIONAL	COGNITIVE	SOCIAL

■ Fatigue
■ Pain
■ Weakness
■ Nausea or vomiting
■ Diarrhea or constipation
■ Cachexia
■ Skin impairments
■ Edema and lymphedema
■ Sexuality
  • Desire
  • Arousal
  • Orgasm
  • Resolution
■ Infertility
■ Steroid myopathy
■ Neuropathy
■ Toxicities
■ Hematological abnormalities
  • Thrombocytopenia
  • Anemia
  • Neutropenia
■ Neutropenic fever
■ Infection
  • Sepsis
  • Septic shock
■ GVHD
■ Graft failure
■ Bony metastasis
■ Cardiopulmonary considerations
■ LMD
■ Oncologic emergencies
■ Paraneoplastic syndrome
■ Critical illness
■ PICS
	■ Anger
	■ Fear
	■ Anxiety
	■ Depression
	■ PTSD
	■ Body image anxiety
		■ Chemo-induced cognitive impairment
		■ Delirium
		■ Poor orientation
		■ Difficulty following commands
		■ Lack of attention
		■ Poor processing skills
		■ Poor memory
		■ Poor insight
		■ Lack of safety awareness
			■ Financial implications
			  • Treatment and medication costs
			  • Job loss
			  • Job lock (i.e., the inability to leave a job because doing so would result in the loss of benefits, including health insurance)
			■ Issues of dependence, independence, and interruptions in age-related social roles in adolescents and young adults
			■ Loss or shift of roles

Note. GVHD = graft-versus-host disease; LMD = leptomeningeal disease; PICS = postintensive care syndrome; PTSD = posttraumatic stress disorder.

gum bleeds, nosebleeds, blood in urine, blood in stool, or vaginal spotting or unusually heavy menstrual flow in females. Platelet transfusion is used to treat thrombocytopenia. In some cases, *refractory thrombocytopenia,* or persistent thrombocytopenia despite platelet transfusions secondary to condition or immune mediated response, can occur, leading to life-threatening bleeding complications. Platelet count threshold for bleeding concerns occurs at <20 x 10⁹/L (Piel-Julian et al., 2018). Severe complications of thrombocytopenia can be massive gastrointestinal bleeding, urinary tract bleeding, or intracranial hemorrhage (ICH). Emergency management of these critical clinical evolvements often warrants admission to the ICU for close hemodynamic and neurologic monitoring and medical management.

The specific workflow for working with patients with complications of thrombocytopenia when admitted to the ICU may vary among institutions and whether evidence-based intervention protocols such as early mobilization algorithms or monitoring guidelines during activities are present to steer clinical decisions. Cancer survivors often have orders to remain on bedrest to prevent any exacerbation of the bleeding event. Once the clinical picture stabilizes, the activity restrictions may be lifted to allow the survivor to participate with therapy corresponding with the clinical presentation. In these clinical situations, close blood pressure monitoring is necessary during therapy sessions to prevent exacerbation of the bleed. In addition, close neurologic monitoring should be used if ICH is present. The blood pressure goal is often defined by the medical team and is a good objective measure to monitor activity tolerance during the session.

Cancer survivors with hematological cancers are often prescribed an individualized home exercise regimen for health maintenance because of the well-documented benefits of gentle exercise. However, resistive exercises will often be deferred when platelets are <20 x 10⁹/L because of concerns for bleeding (Mohammed et al., 2019). Activities are modified to low intensity with a focus on function. Emphasis is placed on fall prevention and strategies to improve safety during participation of ADLs and IADLs, functional transfers required for participation, setup and navigation of the environment, and caregiver training because of significant concerns for bleeding.

Anemia occurs when RBCs, or the red, iron-based pigment hemoglobin that carries oxygen to organs and tissues, is low. Anemia can be caused by bleeding and renal dysfunction secondary to cancer treatment or renal cancer (MD Anderson Cancer Center, 2019b). Cancer survivors can present with a pale complexion and may report experiencing fatigue, shortness of breath, chest pain, dizziness, and headaches. Blood transfusion, an acute management for anemia, and medications such as erythropoiesis-stimulating agents to prompt RBC production are the two main treatments for anemia. Blood transfusion may be considered when hemoglobin is <7.0 g/dL (Carson et al., 2016). Therefore, the medical and rehabilitation services team often agrees to defer a session or group therapy attendance when the lab value is below this level.

Because individual responses and clinical scenarios are unique, occupational therapy practitioners should discuss and collaborate with the medical team to establish physiologic parameters and activity clarifications. For example, a patient of Jehovah's Witnesses faith who is severely anemic and declines blood transfusions will benefit from the practitioner reaching out to the medical team for an open dialogue about physiologic parameters and goals of care when occupational therapy services are part of the survivor's care plan.

Cardiovascular manifestations commonly observed in anemic patients are tachycardia, dyspnea, and hypotension during increased activity demands (e.g., exercise, transfers, functional mobility, self-care tasks requiring more energy expenditure). Patients should be closely monitored for significant fatigue by their rating of perceived exertion and hemodynamic status such as increased heart rate, decreased blood pressure, and decreased in oxygen saturation level during the session to determine activity tolerance and task progression.

Neutropenia occurs when the number of *neutrophils,* a type of WBCs essential in fighting infections, is low. Those with neutropenia are highly susceptible to infections. Cancer survivors are often on a prophylactic pharmacological regimen against common infections. The Infectious Diseases Society of America (IDSA) defines **neutropenic fever** as
- A single oral temperature of ≥38.3°C (101°F) or
- A temperature of ≥38.0°C (100.4°F) sustained over a 1-hour period (Freifeld et al., 2011).

Prompt treatment using broad-spectrum antibiotics remains the IDSA's recommendation in patients with neutropenia and fever (Freifeld et al., 2011).

Neutropenic precautions are observed for those with neutropenia in the hospital setting; precautions require all providers and visitors to complete hand hygiene and don a mask and gloves before entering the room. When the cancer survivor leaves the room, reverse neutropenic precautions are practiced where the survivor dons a mask and gloves. Cancer survivors with neutropenia are advised to not participate in occupations such as gardening and to avoid raw foods. The specific criteria may vary among institutions, age groups, cancer diagnosis, and cancer treatment modality. For example, those who have undergone adult stem cell transplant (SCT) can leave their room to attend group-based therapy sessions while pediatric SCT survivors may be confined to the room.

Cancer survivors in neutropenic state are predisposed to infections. *Infection* is a major life-threatening concern requiring medical treatment and can necessitate hospitalization. Cancer-related neutropenia hospitalizations in the United States consume significant resources and account for a considerable number of inpatient hospital days (Tai et al., 2017). These hospitalizations
- Cost $2.3 billion and $439 million in adult and pediatric populations, respectively;
- Account for 5.2% of all cancer-related hospitalizations and 8.3% of all cancer-related hospitalization costs;
- Result in an average length of stay of 9.6 days and an average hospital cost of $24,770 per stay for adult patients; and
- Result in an average length of stay of 8.5 days and an average hospital cost of $26,000 per stay for pediatric patients.

Infections can progress to *sepsis,* a clinical syndrome characterized by systemic inflammatory response resulting in organ dysfunction (Singer et al., 2016). Sepsis can result from an infection from anywhere in the body, such as pneumonia, urinary tract infection, surgical wound, pressure ulcer, or influenza. Bacterial infections are the most common cause of sepsis. Sepsis is the leading cause of death from infection; it can lead to **septic shock**, resulting in severe circulatory, cellular, and metabolic abnormalities. Cancer survivors with septic shock are identified by a vasopressor requirement to maintain a mean arterial pressure of 65 mm Hg or greater as defined by the Third International Consensus Definitions for Sepsis and Septic Shock (Sepsis-3; Singer et al., 2016). Mortality significantly increases as the severity of the disease increases—approximately 10%–20% for sepsis, 20%–40% for severe sepsis, and 40%–80% for septic shock.

It is well documented that survivors of severe sepsis experience new and persistent functional and cognitive impairments for up to 8 years after hospital discharge (Iwashyna et al., 2010). Cancer survivors with severe sepsis or septic shock generally require ICU admission for medical intervention. Occupational therapy may be part of the care plan after the patient's hemodynamic status stabilizes.

Critical illness considerations and postintensive care syndrome

Approximately 1 in 20 cancer survivors develops a life-threatening condition that requires life-support measures and ICU admission (Puxty et al., 2015). Table 9.2 categorizes and lists common reasons for ICU admission in cancer survivors. Critical illness superimposed on a cancer diagnosis significantly increases the clinical complexity. Occupational therapy practitioners must understand these clinical aspects to safely intervene and effectively adjust the intensity of the session when working this complex population.

Historical data indicate that cancer survivors have worse outcomes with complications such as sepsis or septic shock than non–cancer survivors. Contemporary evidence shows trends of improved hospital survival of septic cancer survivors. In neutropenic cancer survivors, hospital mortality decreased from 58.7% in 1998–2003 to 43% in 2004–2008 (Legrand et al., 2012). Continued advances in critical care

TABLE 9.2.   Common Reasons for ICU Admission in Patients With Cancer

REASON FOR ADMISSION	EXAMPLE
Surgery	▪ High-risk surgical approaches ▪ Surgical complications
Infections	▪ Pneumonia ▪ Bloodstream infections ▪ Sepsis ▪ Septic shock
Cardiopulmonary	▪ Respiratory insufficiency ▪ Respiratory failure ▪ Acute coronary syndrome ▪ Arrhythmias ▪ Need for vasoactive medications
Neurological	▪ Seizures ▪ Posterior reversible encephalopathy syndrome
Adverse drug reactions	▪ Anaphylaxis ▪ Immune effector cell-associated neurotoxicity syndrome ▪ Cytokine release syndrome
Oncologic emergencies	▪ Tumor lysis syndrome ▪ Hypercalcemia

Note. ICU = intensive care unit.

medicine show favorable trends in ICU survivorship. Unfortunately, survivors of critical illness have long-term effects in physical, cognitive, and mental functions. *PICS* involves new or worsening impairments arising after critical illness and persisting beyond acute care hospitalization in physical (physical function, neuromuscular, and pulmonary), cognitive (attention, memory, executive function, visual–patial, mental processing speed), or mental health (anxiety or acute stress disorder, depression, posttraumatic stress disorder [PTSD]) status.

Having to make difficult decisions on overwhelming matters while feeling worried and confused about the steps taken to monitor and care for their loved ones can place high mental stress on family members. Consequently, the mental health status of family members of ICU survivors may also be negatively affected. The term *postintensive care syndrome–family* (PICS–F) describes the cluster of mental health complications that family members of ICU survivors may experience such as anxiety, PTSD, depression, and complicated grief (Needham et al., 2012). PICS–F is common, but prevalence of specific mental health complications varies within studies. In adult caregivers, PICS–F can affect caregiving abilities. This is significant because critical illness survivors across all age groups will likely depend on continued support from caregivers long after discharge (Davidson et al., 2012).

Contemporary evidence reports that up to 75% ICU survivors have long-term cognitive impairment and up to 25% of ICU survivors have physical impairment (Rawal et al., 2017). Prevention is key for PICS management. The ***ABCDEF bundle*** (Exhibit 9.1) has been recognized as an evidence-based tool for optimizing care of ICU patients.

Early mobility, aggressive occupational and physical therapy interventions, and sedation management have been cited as the most important preventative strategies in decreasing long-term functional challenges associated with PICS (Rawal et al., 2017). A growing body of evidence confirms the feasibility and safety of early mobilization activities in patients facing critical illness. The occupational therapy practitioner's role is described in the development, implementation, and sustainability of a multidisciplinary team approach to an early mobilization program in an oncological medical and surgical ICU at a leading cancer institution (Nguyen et al., 2014). There are limited occupational therapy–specific resources currently available on the acute and chronic management of this complex syndrome in cancer rehabilitation. The understanding of or studies examining long-term outcomes in cancer ICU survivors remain rare (Schellongowski et al., 2016).

A greater push for early and aggressive rehabilitation interventions in cancer patients facing critical illness has taken place in recent years. This is possibly the result of increasing evidence on the benefits of improving the modifiable risk factors for PICS, such as sedation practices, delirium prevention, and early mobilization activities in critically ill patients. Through multidisciplinary collaboration, occupational therapy practitioners can have significant clinical impact in delirium prevention and management along with

EXHIBIT 9.1.   ABCDEF Bundle

A, B, C	Awakening and Breathing Coordination with sedation interruption and ventilator weaning
D	Delirium monitoring and management
E	Early mobilization activities in the intensive care unit
F	Family empowerment and engagement

Source. Adapted from Pun et al. (2019).

family empowerment and engagement. Case Example 9.1 illustrates a clinical scenario of early and aggressive rehabilitation post-SCT in the acute and medically complex setting.

Other complex physical considerations of cancer and its treament

Venous thromboembolism. Cancer survivors are at high risk for developing thrombosis. Cancer-associated thromboembolic complications is the second leading cause of death in cancer patients (Khorana et al., 2007). *Venous thromboembolism* (VTE) is a blood clot in the vein. Deep vein thrombosis (DVT) and pulmonary embolism (PE) are the two types of VTE (American Heart Association, 2019). Approximately 5%–10% of PEs are life threatening and account for 1%-2% of cancer-related deaths. There are several contributing risk factors to the development of cancer-associated thromboembolic complications. Cancer types such as acute leukemia, glioblastoma, renal, lung, ovary, and pancreatic cancer pose the highest risk to developing VTE. Person-related factors such as advanced age, female gender, decreased functional status, and immobility also increase the risk for VTE. Cancer treatment modalities such as chemotherapy, hormone therapy, surgery, and the presence of central venous catheters are additional risk factors to VTE development (MD Anderson Cancer Center, 2019c).

An anticoagulation agent such as low molecular–weight heparin is one of the main recommended treatment options for cancer-related VTE. Placement of an inferior vena cava (IVC) filter may be indicated for patients with contraindications to anticoagulation therapy. An IVC filter may also be considered as an adjunct to anticoagulation therapy for patients with recurrent VTE or progression of thrombosis (Lyman et al., 2013). In acute care settings, bedrest is often prescribed to manage DVT and PE, although there is limited evidence to support this recommendation. A meta-analysis by Aissaoui and colleagues (2009) concluded that there are no differences in increased incidence of new PE or progression of DVT in cancer survivors who are ambulatory versus cancer survivors who are on bedrest. Recent evidence found once therapeutic anticoagulation levels are achieved, early mobility for those with VTE led to decreased overall mortality, improved pain, and lower incidence of new PEs (Kahn et al., 2012).

Bone metastasis. Development of metastases from the primary cancer to the bone is another major complication of cancer. *Bone metastasis* occurs when cancer cells spread from the original cancer site to the bone. Cancers that arise from organs and commonly spread to the bones are breast, lung, kidney, prostate, and thyroid (Mayo Clinic, 2019). In multiple myeloma, a type of hematologic cancer, the cancer cells produce cytokines, which trigger osteoclasts (i.e., bone cells) to also destroy bones to form osteolytic lesions (MD Anderson Cancer Center, 2019d).

Bone metastasis commonly affects the spine, pelvis, femur, and shoulder. It can cause severe pain, weaken and destroy bone structure, and put cancer survivors at increased risk for skeletal-related events, such as pathological fractures. This can result in substantial negative effects on daily function and QoL. The Spinal Instability Neoplastic Score is a useful tool to assess spinal instability and guide clinical discussions (Versteeg et al., 2016).

Because individual clinical scenarios are complex and unique, the specific workflow and criteria may vary among institutions and providers in determining weight-bearing status, activity restrictions, and bracing versus stabilization surgery. It is best practice for occupational therapy practitioners to recognize these pertinent clinical questions to provide effective education on joint protection, spinal precautions during functional transfers and mobility, ADL modifications, and procurement of durable medical equipment (DME) to promote safety and independence during hospitalization and upon discharge, as needed.

Graft-versus-host disease. Cancer treatment such as allogeneic hematopoietic stem cell transplantation can lead to a serious complication called *graft-versus-host disease (GVHD)*. GVHD is an immune process in which the new stem cells (the graft) see the body (the host) as foreign and attack it. It can affect any organ system. Please refer to Chapter 2, "Cancer Treatment Approaches Across the Lifespan," for a description of signs and symptoms of GVHD. GVHD can be acute (within 100 days after transplantation) or chronic (about 3 months after transplantation) and is graded from mild (I) to severe (IV). Acute GVHD is typically treated with high-dose corticosteroids for immunosuppression that is tapered off over a period of time. Symptoms of chronic GVHD are also managed with a long-term immunosuppression regimen such as a steroid, or a combination of immunosuppressive drugs may be necessary (Leukemia and Lymphoma Society, 2019).

Long-term exposure to steroids can make cancer survivors vulnerable to secondary conditions such as *steroid myopathy,* a condition known to cause weakness in proximal strength. Aggressive rehabilitation may be indicated to promote continued participation in self-care skills, functional independence, and safety throughout course of hospitalization and discharge. Because GVHD can affect any organ, cancer survivors with GVHD can benefit greatly from occupational therapy services to overcome functional challenges that can impact occupational performance.

Immunotherapy toxicity. Cancer immunotherapy is a rapidly emerging and promising therapy for cancer patients in which the immune system is enhanced to fight cancer in different ways. There are several types of immunotherapies, each with distinct side effects. *Chimeric antigen receptor (CAR) T-cell therapy* is a type of adoptive cellular therapy in which genetically altered T cells are delivered in the body to fight the cancer (MD Anderson Cancer Center, 2019e). A number of studies reported remission rates as high as 50%–90% for acute lymphoblastic leukemia and large B-cell lymphomas. These impressive responses correlate with the rapidly growing number of CAR T-cell therapy clinical trials over the past 5 years (Gutierrez et al., 2018). For several refractory malignancies, CAR T-cell therapy is considered a promising treatment option. However, this novel immunotherapy therapy has specific toxicities that, if not recognized and treated, can leading to life-threatening complications in the acute and medically complex settings. CAR T-cell therapy can lead to *cytokine release syndrome* (CRS), an exaggerated systemic inflammatory response in

CASE EXAMPLE 9.1. RICK: COMPLICATIONS POST-STEM CELL TRANSPLANT

Rick is age 31 years, single, and a cancer survivor of relapsed germ cell tumor. Early in the summer, Rick was admitted to the hospital for chemotherapy, and several weeks later, he underwent an autologous stem cell transplant. One week later, he developed sepsis and respiratory failure, followed by cardiac arrest. Rick was intubated, resuscitated, and transferred to the ICU. Occupational therapy services was consulted upon ICU admission for the ICU early mobilization program.

Rick subsequently developed acute renal failure, requiring continuous dialysis, and septic shock, requiring vasopressor medications. His critical illness was significant for recurrent gastrointestinal bleeding, requiring numerous emergent blood transfusions and a gastroduodenal artery embolization. Because of his prolonged intubation and mechanical ventilation, he required a tracheostomy secondary to failure to wean. Rick also received an inferior vena cava filter for a left lower extremity deep vein thrombosis in the early fall. Two months after his ICU admission, Rick transferred to another floor, where he continued to receive occupational therapy. He was later admitted to the inpatient rehabilitation unit and eventually discharged home to another state, where he continued with outpatient occupational and physical therapy services.

At the time of evaluation in the ICU, Rick was aphonic secondary to oral intubation and mechanical ventilation. At his bedside, Rick's parents shared that Rick was working full-time at the race track and enjoyed taking care of the land during the weekends when he was not out with friends. Rick was lightly sedated, restless in his bilateral upper extremities restraints, and able to follow simple one-step commands with moderate facilitation and increased time. He showed trace active movements in large distal muscle groups for bilateral upper and lower extremities. Functionally he required total assistance for all ADLs and mobility skills.

Intervention plan

The Person–Environment–Occupation Model was used to evaluate and form a treatment plan for Rick (Law et al., 1996). The occupational therapist reviewed the medical chart and referenced the MD Anderson Cancer Center ICU Adult Early Mobilization Algorithm (Figure 9.1) to determine whether there were medical contraindications that would exclude Rick from therapy. Per

FIGURE 9.1 ICU adult early mobilization algorithm.

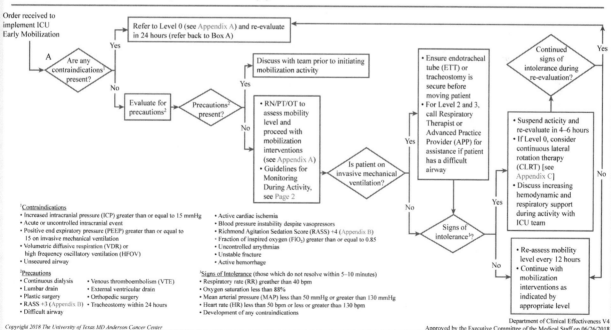

Note. ICU = intensive care unit; OT = occupational therapist; PT = physical therapist; RN = registered nurse.
Source. MD Anderson Cancer Center. Copyright © 2018 The University of Texas MD Anderson Cancer Center. Reprinted with permission.

(Continued)

CASE EXAMPLE 9.1. RICK: COMPLICATIONS POST-STEM CELL TRANSPLANT *(Cont.)*

the algorithm, Rick did not have any medical contraindications to participate in occupational therapy. The Confusion Assessment Method for the ICU, a validated delirium assessment and monitoring tool, showed that Rick was positive for delirium (Ely et al., 2001).

Rick's parents and the medical team hoped that Rick could participate in occupational therapy to improve his delirium and overall functional outcomes. The occupational therapist managed the environment (e.g., mechanical ventilator, arterial line, central lines, Foley catheter, monitoring equipment) to ensure safety while facilitating the highest level of functional participation from the patient. The session goal was for Rick to transfer to the neuro chair to be near the window for improved orientation and wakefulness while promoting cardiopulmonary endurance and sitting tolerance in preparation for ADL and IADL participation.

Intervention implementation

When asked if he would like to sit up on the side of the bed, Rick nodded. The session was coordinated with nursing because of concerns for hemodynamic instability. Physiologic parameters were used to monitor for signs of intolerance during the session (see Figure 9.1). Rick transferred to sit at the edge of bed to participate in facial grooming activities with hand-over-hand assistance. He was dependently transferred to the neuro chair and encouraged to participate in preparatory activities

with the assistance of caregivers. Education on physical and mental strengthening activities and ways to improve delirium were provided to Rick and his caregivers.

Intervention review

Despite being upright, Rick remained fairly drowsy. Further discussion with his nurse and physician allowed for further weaning of his sedation. His mother helped picked out his favorite cap for Rick to don while his father put on his favorite music. Rick smiled several times and began to use the communication board to express his needs and direct his care. His mother was encouraged to place a chair next to Rick and hold his hand so he could have a break from the restraints.

Targeting outcomes

Although Rick's medical status fluctuated significantly, he was followed closely by occupational therapy services. He made gradual and steady functional improvements in self-care and mobility skills from total assistance to minimal assistance. He received intensive therapy on the acute care floor and inpatient rehab unit. Rick's tracheostomy was eventually capped and removed. He was discharged home with 24-hour supervision after more than 4 months of hospitalization. Rick experienced cognitive challenges, sleeping difficulty, neuropathy, right foot drop, and weakness at discharge secondary to PICS.

---

which a large volume of cytokines are produced and released. The most common symptoms of CRS are tachycardia, fever, hypotension, and hypoxemia that can progress to multiorgan failure. CRS usually appears at 7 days but as late as 10–14 days after CAR T-cell infusion (Gutierrez et al., 2018). Early development of CRS is associated with an increased risk of developing severe neurotoxicity (Gust et al., 2018).

Immune effector cell-associated neurotoxicity syndrome (ICANS) is "a disorder characterized by a pathologic process involving the central nervous system following any immune therapy that results in the activation or engagement of endogenous or infused T cells and/or other immune effector cells. Symptoms or signs can be progressive and may include aphasia, altered level of consciousness, impairment of cognitive skills, motor weakness, seizures, and cerebral edema" (Lee et al., 2019, p. 632). Tremors, dysgraphia, mild difficulty with expressive speech (especially in naming objects), impaired attention, apraxia, and mild lethargy are some early symptoms of ICANS. Neelapu et al. in 2018 summarized the grading for ICANS as follows:

- *Mild (Grade 1–2)*: Mild aphasia, mild delirium, decreased attention, tremors and changes in handwriting
- *Moderate (Grade 3)*: Global aphasia, seizures, and obtunded
- *Severe (Grade 4)*: Status epilepticus, cerebral edema, and coma.

In Grade 2 and above, limiting IADLs and ADLs are listed as grading criteria of neurotoxicity. Up to 87% of lymphoma

patients and 60% of B-cell acute lymphoblastic leukemia (B-ALL) patients may experience ICANS with CAR T-cell therapy. Of those lymphoma patients, about 30%–50% are Grade 3 or higher. Similarly, 18% of B-ALL patients also experience ICANS at Grade 3 or higher. The syndrome can progress from mild to severe neurotoxicity in hours to days (Gust et al., 2018). According to Lee et al. (2019), expressive aphasia is a specific symptom of ICANS. Aphasia, starting as

> impaired naming of objects, paraphasic errors, hesitant speech, and verbal perseveration, may progress to global aphasia, characterized by expressive and receptive difficulty. Patients with global aphasia may appear wide awake but are mute and unable to follow commands (akinetic). Many patients have myoclonus or tremor and increased tone. There may be depressed level of consciousness with mild lethargy progressing to obtundation, stupor, or even coma. (Lee et al., 2019, p. 632)

Because of the novelty of CAR T-cell therapy, there is no evidence of the long-term cognitive and functional outcomes related to this treatment modality at this time. Given the projected expansion of this promising cancer treatment in the coming years for both adult and pediatric cancer survivors and its impact on functional status and cognition, occupational therapy practitioners should advocate for intense occupational therapy services in this emerging subset of cancer population.

Emotional Challenges

Nearly all cancer survivors face emotional challenges. Emotions such as fear, anxiety, depression, anger, and loss or grief are acknowledged and well described throughout the literature. Approximately 70% of cancer survivors experience depression, and patients with cancer can experience anxiety and depression at any time throughout their continuum of care (Zeynalova et al., 2019). Cancer patients and caregivers can find themselves facing a host of emotional challenges in acute and medically complex settings. Challenges include facing

- Changes to appearance or body image,
- A serious complication after a surgical or medical treatment for the cancer,
- Changing demands regarding their primary or valued roles during the course of hospitalization, and
- Unfavorable news or needing to make a decision on resuscitative or code status with critical illness.

In a study by Morgan and colleagues (2017), the authors concluded that personality may be associated with physical and psychological symptoms experienced by cancer survivors. When anxiety issues are not effectively managed, progression to severe distress or PTSD is noted. Distress, burnout, and PTSD are prevalent in adult cancer survivors (Pranjic et al., 2016). PTSD is also documented in parents of pediatric cancer survivors, critical illness survivors, and their families. Interestingly, pediatric cancer survivors may experience posttraumatic growth and appear to be resilient (Arpawong et al., 2013). In adult survivors of childhood cancer, hope may be related to posttraumatic growth (Tillery et al., 2016).

Body image, the way the person thinks, perceives, and feels about their body and how it functions, is another important emotional challenge faced by almost all cancer survivors. Cancer and its treatment can alter the body's appearance and function. Therefore, occupational therapy practitioners should initiate a dialogue about body image with all cancer survivors individually; some may experience hair loss, limb loss, incontinence issues, skin changes, sexual dysfunction, or even be in the immediate recovery from plastic and reconstructive surgery in the acute care setting.

Cognitive Challenges

Cancer and its treatment may result in cognitive challenges that impact global or specific mental functions such as

- Consciousness,
- Orientation,
- Attention,
- Memory,
- Sequencing, and
- Higher-level cognitive functions (American Occupational Therapy Association [AOTA], 2014).

Cognitive decline, like cancer, is considered an age-related risk. Authors have suggested that older cancer survivors may experience age-related cognitive declines at a faster pace than non–cancer survivors secondary to cancer and its treatment (Munoz et al., 2015). In cancer survivors, the cause for cognitive challenges can be the result of a primary brain malignancy such as glioblastoma. Cognitive challenges can also be diffused in nature because of secondary malignancies such as leptomeningeal disease (LMD) or metastasis to the leptomeninges (i.e., the lining of the brain and spinal cord). LMD tends to occur in patients with breast cancer, lung cancer, and melanoma because these cancers tend to spread to the central nervous system.

Cognitive challenges can also result from treatment such as whole brain radiation, chemotherapy, and neurological toxicities associated with immunotherapy. In mild (Grade 1–2) ICANS, cognitive challenges such as decreased attention, difficulty concentrating, confusion or delirium, and agitation or somnolence can be observed (Lee et al., 2019). There is limited data on and understanding of cognitive-related outcomes in patients receiving these contemporary immunotherapy treatments. Please refer to Chapter 17, "Cancer-Related Cognitive Impairment," for an in-depth discussion of this topic.

Cognitive challenges can also arise from complex syndromes such as delirium. Cancer survivors facing critical illness are at high risk for developing delirium (Girard et al., 2010). *Delirium* is a brain dysfunction syndrome characterized by

- Changes in cognition (e.g., memory deficit, perceptual disturbance, disorientation);
- Changes in consciousness;
- Decreased ability to focus or sustain attention, or fluctuations in attention over time; and
- Acute development over a short period of time (hours to days; Girard et al., 2008).

Delirium can have a hyperactive, hypoactive, or mixed presentation. Delirium is often underdiagnosed, especially with a hypoactive presentation, and occurs in approximately 7 out of 10 patients receiving mechanical ventilation. Delirium is associated with a multitude of adverse outcomes such as

- Failed extubations,
- Protracted hospital stays,
- Increased cost of care, and
- Increased mortality (Brummel & Girard, 2013).

Delirium is a good prognosticator of long-term cognitive challenges in survivors of critical illness. The syndrome can be quickly and reliably diagnosed with assessment instruments such as the Intensive Care Delirium Screening Checklist (Bergeron et al., 2001) and the Confusion Assessment Method for the ICU (CAM–ICU; Ely et al., 2001), which is often used by occupational therapy practitioners to assess delirium in ICU patients. Prevention of delirium is the best approach for this syndrome. Modifiable risk factors for delirium prevention include sedation management, early mobilization, and sleep hygiene (Brummel & Girard, 2013).

In the acute care setting, occupational therapists frequently assess patients for safety in preparation for discharge. Cognitive challenges affecting performance skills such as attention, memory, sequencing, generalization, or insight can pose safety concerns. This is especially relevant for survivors who have undergone a surgery for which strict postsurgical precautions must be adhered to or who require physical assistance for functional mobility or transfers. Therefore, cognitive challenges can affect discharge dispositions in patients with limited social support. Safety and cognitive assessments through relevant functional tasks are often used by occupational therapy practitioners to recommend one discharge disposition over another.

Social Challenges

Many cancer survivors encounter social challenges in acute and medically complex settings. Social demands may vary among age groups. In adults, many survivors experience social challenges such as those with

- Finances (e.g., cost of care, loss of wages),
- Employment (e.g., loss of job, job lock [i.e., a person must stay with their current employer to have health insurance]),
- Time (e.g., intensity and frequency of treatment),
- Leisure occupations (e.g., loss or limited participation in leisure occupations), and
- Family life and relationships (e.g., shift or loss of roles and change in relationship dynamics).

Results from a study of cancer-related social challenges of survivors and their spouses found that survivors had a higher difficulty score. However, young female spouses (age ≤39) score as high as the cancer survivor on many categories (Takeuchi et al., 2018). In addition, social challenges experienced by adult caregivers are not well understood (Takeuchi et al., 2018). Please see Chapter 27, "Caregiving," for a detailed discussion of this topic.

IMPORTANCE OF CONTEXT AND ENVIRONMENT IN ACUTE AND MEDICALLY COMPLEX SETTINGS

Physical Environment

It is important for occupational therapy practitioners to use elements of the physical environment to promote improved occupational performance for cancer survivors in acute and medically complex settings. Recognizing restrictions faced by survivors in these specific physical environments can help them explore ways to achieve and individualize goals. Cancer survivors are typically placed in private rooms. Adult survivors with hematological cancers undergoing SCT may have to remain in a protective environment room for several weeks. In these instances, survivors cannot have in-person visits with their family and friends in their room. Instead, visitors enter an anteroom and communicate with the cancer survivor using a two-way phone while looking through a large window. To maintain physical function and promote wellness, the patient's room is equipped with exercise equipment and other personal items for comfort.

The physical environment of the ICU can discourage participation in meaningful occupations because of the presence of extensive monitoring and life-support equipment. Elements within the ICU environment can be safely managed to promote participation. For example, the mechanical ventilator and monitors can be arranged to accommodate the bed or specialty chair so it can be placed near the window. Being able to see natural light can improve cognitive status and mood and prevent delirium. Caregivers are encouraged to bring in pictures, music, or familiar objects to individualize the space. These items also help providers see the survivor's identity beyond their role as a patient. Survivors with functional challenges can also be assisted to participate in meaningful ADLs as tolerated with incorporation of specialty DME as needed.

Effective management of the physical environment can afford survivors the opportunity to participate in self-care tasks such as shaving or applying makeup. Although these tasks may seem trivial, they provide great satisfaction to the survivor and caregivers. In addition to ADLs, the environment can be managed to allow patients to be outside of the room for a wide variety of therapeutic activities. Functional activities can include patients playing the guitar for staff, attending a musical event in the waiting room, playing miniature golf in the hallway, going to the barber shop for haircut, going to an indoor observation deck that overlooks the city to visit with family, or going to the chapel to pray with one's spouse. When patients value these functional tasks, improved attention, engagement, functional endurance, and posture are often observed. It is important to note that appropriate monitoring, personnel, and equipment are used to ensure the safety of the session when a critically ill patient leaves the room or unit.

In acute care units outside of the ICU, occupational therapy practitioners routinely use elements of context and the environment to individualize and promote improved occupational performance. For example, an occupational therapist at the MD Anderson Cancer Center coordinated a session for an adult cancer survivor who self-identifies as a chef to prepare a meal in the room for his family. This is an occupation he loves and values; the ingredients and tools he needed were delivered by the hospital kitchen staff. This is an example of how a limited hospital environment can be used to promote the highest level of participation, function, and safety.

The physical environment for pediatric patients is often adorned with colorful decorations and age-appropriate toys to support play exploration. The rooms are often set up with a comfortable space for caregivers. A child-friendly gym or open space for play is sometimes available. Electronic gaming consoles may be available for pediatric and adolescent patients to keep in the room. Life-support devices and monitoring equipment are also set up and managed to promote safety and participation. Children in the pediatric ICU may require specialty seating equipment to participate in activities out of the bed or out of the room.

For adolescent and young adult cancer survivors in the acute care setting, a separate lounge or gaming center may be available. Occupational therapy practitioners can provide adaptations to equipment and clothing and incorporate age-appropriate tasks into interventions. Life tasks, such as preparing to attend meaningful events such as prom, birthdays, celebrations, and graduation events, are creative examples of including occupations in treatment. Case Example 9.2 illustrates clinical treatment of complications after surgery.

Social Environment

Many adult cancer survivors in acute and medically complex settings say they feel "uncomfortable" and "embarrassed" that the hospital room now serves as their living room to meet with providers and visitors, their bedroom to rest, and their bathroom. Individuals with limited functional mobility to complete self-care tasks in the bathroom environment may find themselves feeling more helpless as their most private self-care routines may have to take place in an unfamiliar environment.

CASE EXAMPLE 9.2. WALTER: COMPLICATIONS POSTSURGERY

Walter is age 59 years and married to his college sweetheart. They have two adult children. He worked full-time as an engineer and loves to spend time with his family and watch sports, especially football. He is a survivor of esophageal adenocarcinoma status postresection. In the postoperative period, he developed atrial fibrillation with rapid ventricular response; respiratory distress requiring intubation; and severe multiorgan failure to include ischemic fingers, toes, and bowels requiring multiple surgeries. Walter's course of care was extremely protracted for him to remain in the ICU. Walter developed acute liver failure and continued to require mechanical ventilation.

Intervention

Walter and his wife expressed the desire to visit the chapel together for psychological benefits. Clearance with the primary team was obtained by the primary service. The ICU Adult Early Mobilization Program Guidelines for Monitoring During Activity was used to monitor activity tolerance and progression (MD Anderson Cancer Center, 2018; see Figure 9.2).

Intervention implementation

Because of Walter's limited functional endurance secondary to severe debility, he was dependently transferred to the neuro chair and positioned comfortably. Increased time was required for equipment setup and care coordination because of medical complexity, frequent rest breaks were required because of poor endurance, and an increased need for physical assistance was required because of poor functional status.

Intervention review

Coordinated by the occupational therapist, the respiratory therapist helped transition Walter to the portable ventilator, and the nurse gathered essential emergency medications to accompany Walter and his wife to the chapel for prayers with the chaplain. Upon entry to the chapel, Walter's spouse was tearful and expressed gratitude and appreciation for being able to participate in this meaningful occupation shared between them. Walter also demonstrated improved posture, visual attention, and participation with the people in the environment.

Targeting outcomes

Walter's occupational priorities and needs were assessed and considered in the preparation and coordination to support this meaningful occupation for Walter and his wife. The activity aimed to improve Walter and his spouse's psychological benefits. One day later, Walter was transitioned to end-of-life care because of further significant clinical decline.

FIGURE 9.2 ICU adult early mobilization guidelines for monitoring during activity.

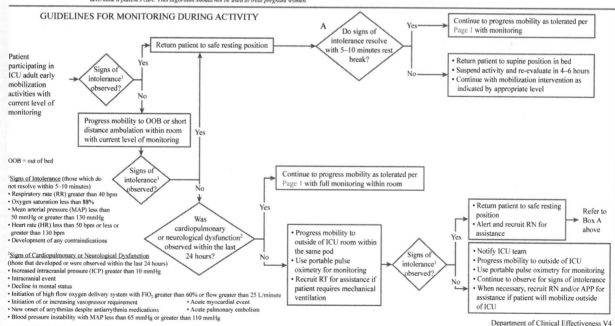

Adult cancer survivors with an extended hospitalization who are parents of young children may feel isolated from their children and experience a disruption in their parent role when young children are not allowed to visit in certain areas of the hospital. This is particularly true in ICUs, where there are restrictions for visitors who are under the age of 13 years. Approval from the medical team and a visit with the social worker is often required before young children can visit family members.

Despite being hospitalized, some adult patients may still work remotely. Cancer survivors may defer or postpone care to host virtual meetings, make phone calls, or want to work with minimal distractions. This can pose unique demands to care coordination and care participation from the patient. Pediatric and adolescent survivors may continue their student role by attending school virtually or in a classroom setting at the hospital.

Cultural Context

Activity patterns and behavioral standards of cancer survivors across the lifespan may be affected in acute and medically complex settings. The degree of impact may vary on an individual level and may be more pronounced when the activity pattern or standards conflict with procedures in these settings. For example, caregivers from certain cultures are more likely to assist patients with self-care tasks as a sign of care than encourage patients to complete the task themselves.

Occupational therapy practitioners may facilitate culturally significant activities such as making ornaments, decorating a miniature Christmas tree with a patient, making a mask with a child in preparation for Halloween, making a hand- or fingerprinting craft for an end-of-life keepsake, or encouraging journaling to help the patient prepare for big events such as anniversaries or even their own funeral.

Personal Context

Maintaining a meaningful personal context in acute and medically complex settings can be challenging. Occupational therapy practitioners understand the importance of helping survivors resume a familiar personal context

---

CASE EXAMPLE 9.3. MAGGIE: POST NEUROSURGERY COMPLICATIONS

Maggie is 36-year-old cancer survivor. She is a wife and a "super mom" to her 4- and 6-year-old sons, and she has very supportive parents. Maggie runs three miles several times a week, practices yoga, loves to read, and embraces full-time care of her children. She is well groomed and highly values her independence. Maggie was admitted to the hospital for resection of her pineal tumor via suprasellar infratentorial approach.

Maggie's hospital course of care was complicated by altered mental status requiring intubation and mechanical ventilation. Occupational therapy was consulted upon ICU admission for the ICU early mobilization program. Maggie presented with right hemiparesis. Postoperatively, Maggie awoke with both eyes fixed into downward gaze and medially deviated. She also developed difficulties in tracking in all directions, diplopia, and nystagmus. She was extubated on post-op Day 5.

Intervention Plan
Maggie agreed to participate in grooming while standing at the sink in the bathroom environment. She had difficulty navigating the door space, and loss of balance was observed. She requested to don an undergarment while sitting at the edge of the bed. Maggie kept her eyes closed 90% of the time. She cited headache and light sensitivity. When Maggie attempted to focus her gaze on the clothing article to ensure she put it on correctly, severe nystagmus was observed in both eyes. Maggie's goals were to be independent with self-care skills, apply her makeup, and read to her children.

Intervention Implementation
Maggie agreed to complete a portion of the Brain Injury Visual Assessment for Adults (Warren, 2006) in a quiet, nondistracting environment to further assess her visual impairments because she continued to experience visual challenges that affected her self-care and functional tasks. Oculomotor function assessments indicated significant visual impairments, including poor visual acuity, diplopia, and impaired eye movements for smooth pursuits (right eye primarily in down gaze and able to achieve primary gaze with maximal effort for 1–2 seconds; left eye primarily in diagonal lower right gaze; both eyes unable to track together in any pursuit). Maggie was noted to have greater control in bringing her right eye to midline, pursuit, and tracking. With corrective lenses, patching of her left eye was initiated during self-care, while practicing household mobility, and when navigating narrow spaces.

Intervention Review
Maggie responded well to the patching of her nondominant eye for time-sensitive or physically demanding tasks in novel environments to improve her safety. She was coached on alternating the patching with periods of rest and was given oculomotor exercises for strengthening and improving the posture of her eyes for improved vision. Maggie was referred to the neuroopthalmology clinic for further medical recommendations and interventions.

Targeting Outcomes
With the interventions and modification in Maggie's corrective lenses, she was able to read a little each day. She practiced reading short sentences to gradually complete an entire book to read to her children. Maggie was admitted to the inpatient rehabilitation unit and then discharged home with 24-hour supervision and outpatient occupational therapy services for vision therapy. Upon discharge, she practiced walking to the mailbox daily, then progressed to walking her 6-year-old to the bus stop. She continued to read short passages and was able to read bedtime stories to her children several months after the initial surgery.

through occupations. Through self-care tasks such as applying their "signature" shade of lipstick, trimming their facial hair a specific way, or donning their favorite football team's jersey during the playoffs, a portion of their self-identity is regained. The personal context can give relevance to functional tasks and goals in preparation for discharge. Practitioners can use countless strategies to promote and restore the personal context of cancer survivors. Case Example 9.3 illustrates personal context and its relation to approaches to intervention in the acute and medically complex setting.

Temporal Context

Cancer survivors can experience major disruptions in the temporal aspects of occupation in acute and medically complex settings. Occupational routines are disrupted, and activities either no longer occur at their usual time or take place at random times of the day. This disruption in routines, in conjunction with poor sleep hygiene and sleep quality, can increase the risk for survivors to develop cognitive challenges such as delirium. Occupational therapy practitioners can collaborate with survivors to set activity goals to be accomplished at a certain frequency or time to promote wellness and normalize day and night cycles. A survivor who is unable to sleep at night will have daytime fatigue and somnolence that affects participation. Restoring temporal context through routines of familiar tasks and grouping of care at night may be possible.

Virtual Context

The virtual context has expanded significantly over the past several years for most people in industrialized countries. Technology intertwines with people across the lifespan through the use of smartphones, tablets, and laptops. In certain age groups, the use of technology is deeply embedded in habits and routines. The virtual context gives cancer survivors a channel to connect with other cancer survivors via blogs, social media, chats, or texting. For younger generations, texting has evolved to be the preferred mode of communication. Occupational therapy practitioners can encourage patients to use applications on smart devices to engage in short meditation sessions, monitor activity, set daily goals, manage medications, and stay organized with appointments.

APPROACHES TO INTERVENTION IN ACUTE AND MEDICALLY COMPLEX SETTINGS

Occupational Profile

The development of the occupational profile gives insight about the cancer survivor's occupational history, patterns and demands of daily living, experiences, values, needs, and priorities. Strengths and challenges related to occupational performance of daily life activities, supports, barriers, and potential occupational disruptions are also identified in building the occupational profile. The approach to gathering information may vary depending on the clinical

situation, personal factors, and environment (e.g., ICU vs. pediatric vs. inpatient rehab vs. acute care floor). Guiding questions related to areas of occupation useful to practitioners may include:

- What are the goals of care for the cancer survivor?
- What are the cancer survivor's desired occupations and occupational priorities at this current phase of care?
- Are occupation-focused goals and a time frame incorporated into the care plan?
- Are surgical or medical-related precautions considered in the determination of occupational demands?
- Are potential discharge needs considered in the recommendation of the discharge disposition?
- What barriers may affect the cancer survivor's occupational performance or participation?

AOTA (2017) has developed a template that can be used as a guide for developing an occupational profile.

SUMMARY

Cancer survivors admitted to acute and medically complex settings can face myriad challenges related to their cancer and its treatment. Some of these challenges can be life-threatening, and other challenges can cause significant disruption in occupational performance.

The physical, social, cultural, personal, temporal, and virtual contexts of an individual's life can be dramatically affected by admission to an acute or medically complex setting. Routines, roles, and common rituals can be disrupted, and there are multiple challenges to occupational performance. Occupational therapy practitioners can play a key role in making adaptations to these contexts to minimize the disruption of roles and routines and to promote occupational performance. This is true even for cancer survivors with significant limitations such as those on mechanical ventilation, in the ICU, or in strict isolation.

REFERENCES

Aissaoui, N., Martins, E., Mouly, S., Weber, S., & Meune, C. (2009). A meta-analysis of bed rest versus early ambulation in the management of pulmonary embolism, deep vein thrombosis, or both. *International Journal of Cardiology, 137,* 37–41. https://doi.org/10.1016/j.ijcard.2008.06.020

American Cancer Society. (2019). *Low blood counts.* Retrieved from https://www.cancer.org/treatment/treatments-and-side-effects/physical-side-effects/low-blood-counts.html

American Heart Association. (2019). *What is venous thromboembolism (VTE)?* Retrieved from https://www.heart.org/en/health-topics/venous-thromboembolism/what-is-venous-thromboembolism-vte.html

American Occupational Therapy Association. (2014). Occupational therapy practice framework: Domain and process (3rd ed.). *American Journal of Occupational Therapy, 68*(Suppl. 1), S1–S48. https://doi.org/10.5014/ajot.2014.682006

American Occupational Therapy Association. (2017). AOTA occupational profile template. *American Journal of Occupational Therapy, 71,* 7112420030. https://doi.org/10.5014/ajot.2017.716S12

Arpawong, T. E., Oland, A., Milam, J. E., Ruccione, K., & Meeske, K. A. (2013). Post-traumatic growth among an ethnically diverse sample of adolescent and young adult cancer survivors. *Psycho-Oncology, 22,* 2235–2244. https://doi.org/10.1002/pon.3286

Bergeron, N., Dubois, M., Dumont, M., Dial, S., & Skrobik, Y. (2001). Intensive Care Delirium Screening Checklist: Evaluation of a new screening tool. *Intensive Care Medicine, 27,* 859–864. https://doi.org/10.1007/s001340100909

Brummel, N. E., & Girard, T. D. (2013). Preventing delirium in the intensive care unit. *Critical Care Clinics, 29,* 51–65. https://doi.org/10.1016/j.ccc.2012.10.007

Carson, J. L., Guyatt, G., Heddle, N. M., Grossman, B. J., Cohn, C. S., Fung, M. K., . . . Tobian, A. A. (2016). Clinical practice guidelines from the AABB: Red blood cell transfusion thresholds and storage. *Journal of the American Medical Association, 316*(19), 2025–2035. https://doi.org/10.1001/jama.2016.9185

Davidson, J. E., Jones, C., & Bienvenu, J. (2012). Family response to critical illness: Postintensive care syndrome–family. *Critical Care Medicine, 40,* 618–624. https://doi.org/10.1097/CCM.0b013e318236ebf9

Ely, E. W., Inouye, S. K., Bernard, G. R., Gordon, S., Francis, J., May, L., . . . Dittus, R. (2001). Delirium in mechanically ventilated patients: Validity and reliability of the Confusion Assessment Method for the Intensive Care Unit (CAM-ICU). *Journal of the American Medical Association, 286,* 2703–2710. https://doi.org/10.1001/jama.208.21.2703

Freifeld, A. G., Bow, E. J., Sepkowitz, K. A., Boeckh, M. J., Ito, J. I., Mullen, C. A., . . . Wingard, J. R. (2011). Clinical practice guideline for the use of antimicrobial agents in neutropenic patients with cancer: 2010 update by the Infectious Diseases Society of America. *Clinical Infectious Diseases, 52*(4), e56–e93. https://doi.org/10.1093/cid/cir073

Girard, T. D., Jackson, J. C., Pandharipande, P. P., Pun, B. T., Thompson, J. L., Shintani, A. K., . . . Ely, E.W. (2010). Delirium as a predictor of long-term cognitive impairment in survivors of critical illness. *Critical Care Medicine, 38,* 1513–1520. https://doi.org/10.1097/CCM.0b013e3181e47be1

Girard, T. D., Pandharipande, P. P., & Ely, E. W. (2008). Delirium in the intensive care unit. *Critical Care, 12*(Suppl 3), S3. https://doi.org/10.1186/cc6149

Gust, J., Hay, K. A., Hanafi, L. A., Li, D., Myerson, D., Gonzalez-Cuyar, L. F., . . . Turtle, C. J. (2018). Endothelial activation and blood-brain barrier disruption in neurotoxicity after adoptive immunotherapy with CD19 CAR-T cells. *Cancer Discovery, 7,* 1404–1419. https://doi.org/10.1158/2159-8290.CD-17-0698

Gutierrez, C., McEvoy, C., Mead, E., Stephens, R. S., Munshi, L., Detsky, M. E., . . . Nates, J. L. (2018). Management of the critically ill adult chimeric antigen receptor-T cell therapy patient: A critical care perspective. *Critical Care Medicine, 46,* 1402–1410. https://doi.org/10.1097/CCM.0000000000003258

Iwashyna, T. J., Ely, E. W., Smith, D. M., & Langa, K. M. (2010). Long-term cognitive impairment and functional disability among survivors of severe sepsis. *Journal of the American Medical Association, 304,* 1787–1794. https://doi.org/10.1001/jama.2010.1553

Kahn, S. R., Lim, W., Dunn, A. S., Cushman, M., Dentali, F., Aki, E. A., . . . Hassan Murad, M. (2012). Prevention of VTE in nonsurgical patients. *Chest, 141*(2 Suppl), e195S–e226S. https://doi.org/10.1378/chest.11-2296

Khorana, A. A., Francis, C. W., Culakova, E., Kuderer, N. M., & Lyman, G. H. (2007). Thromboembolism is a leading cause of death in cancer patients receiving outpatient chemotherapy.

Journal of Thrombosis and Haemostasis, 5, 632–634. https://doi.org/10.1111/j.1538-7836.2007.02374.x

Law, M., Cooper, B., Strong, S., Stewart, D., Rigby, P., & Letts, L. (1996). The Person-Environment-Occupation Model: A transactive approach to occupational performance. *Canadian Journal of Occupational Therapy, 63,* 9–23. https://doi.org/10.1177/000841749606300103

Lee, D. W., Santomasso, B. D., Locke, F. L., Ghobadi, A., Turtle, C. J., Brudno, J. N., . . . Neelapu, S. S. (2019). ASTCT consensus grading for cytokine release syndrome and neurologic toxicity associated with immune effector cells. *Biology of Blood and Marrow Transplantation, 25,* 625–638. https://doi.org/10.1016/j.bbmt.2018.12.758

Legrand, M., Max, A., Peigne, V., Mariotte, E., Canet, E., Debrumetz, A., . . . Azoulay, E. (2012). Survival in neutropenic patients with severe sepsis or septic shock. *Critical Care Medicine, 40,* 43–49. https://doi.org/10.1097/CCM.0b013e31822b50c2

Leukemia and Lymphoma Society. (2019). *Graft-versus-host disease.* Retrieved from https://www.lls.org/treatment/types-of-treatment/stem-cell-transplantation/graft-versus-host-disease

Lyman, G. H., Khorana, A. A., Kuderer, N. M., Lee, A. Y., Arcelus, J. I., Balaban, E. P., . . . Falanga, A. (2013). Venous thromboembolism prophylaxis and treatment in patients with cancer: American Society of Clinical Oncology clinical practice guideline update. *Journal of Clinical Oncology, 31,* 2189–2204. https://doi.org/10.1200/JCO.2013.49.1118

Mayo Clinic. (2019). *Bone metastasis.* Retrieved from https://www.mayoclinic.org/diseases-conditions/bone-metastasis/symptoms-causes/syc-20370191

MD Anderson Cancer Center. (2018). *ICU Adult Early Mobilization* (Version 4). Retrieved from https://www.mdanderson.org/content/dam/mdanderson/documents/for-physicians/algorithms/clinical-management/clin-management-icu-adult-early-mobilization-web-algorithm.pdf

MD Anderson Cancer Center. (2019a). *Anemia and cancer.* Retrieved from https://www.mdanderson.org/patients-family/diagnosis-treatment/emotional-physical-effects/anemia-cancer.html

MD Anderson Cancer Center. (2019b). *Bleeding and bruising in cancer patients.* Retrieved from https://www.mdanderson.org/patients-family/diagnosis-treatment/emotional-physical-effects/bleeding-bruising-cancer.html

MD Anderson Cancer Center. (2019c). *Cancer and pulmonary embolism development.* Retrieved from https://www.mdanderson.org/patients-family/diagnosis-treatment/emotional-physical-effects/pulmonary-embolism-cancer.html

MD Anderson Cancer Center. (2019d). *Immunotherapy.* Retrieved from https://www.mdanderson.org/treatment-options/immunotherapy.html

MD Anderson Cancer Center. (2019e). *Multiple myeloma symptoms.* Retrieved from https://www.mdanderson.org/cancer-types/multiple-myeloma/multiple-myeloma-symptoms.html

Mohammed, J., Aljurf, M., Althumayri, A., Almansour, M., Alghamdi, A., Hamidieh, A., . . . Hashmi, S. (2019). Physical therapy pathway and protocol for patients undergoing hematopoietic stem cell transplantation: Recommendations from the Eastern Mediterranean Blood and Marrow Transplantation (EMBMT) Group. *Hematology/Oncology and Stem Cell Therapy, 12,* 127–132. https://doi.org/10.1016/j.hemonc.2018.12.003

Mokart, D., Pastores, S., & Darmon, M. (2014). Has survival increased in cancer patients admitted to the ICU?

Yes. *Intensive Care Medicine, 40,* 1570–1572. https://doi.org/10.1007/s00134-014-3433-2

Morgan, S., Cooper, B., Paul, S., Hammer, M. J., Conley, Y. P., Levine, J. D., . . . Dunn, L. B. (2017). Association of personality profiles with depressive, anxiety, and cancer-related symptoms in patients undergoing chemotherapy. *Personality and Individual Differences, 117,* 130–138. https://doi.org/10.1016/j.paid.2017.05.039

Munoz, A., Campbell, A., & Bowyer, A. (2015). The role of occupational therapy in older adults with cognitive impairments and an oncology diagnosis. *Topics in Geriatric Rehabilitation, 31,* 281–286. https://doi.org/10.1097/TGR.0000000000000078

Naughton, M., & Weaver, K. (2014). Physical and mental health among cancer survivors considerations for long-term care and quality of life. *North Carolina Medical Journal, 75,* 283–286. https://doi.org/10.18043/ncm.75.4.283

Needham, D., Davidson, J., Cohen, H., Hopkins, R., Weinert, C., Wunsch, H., . . . Harvey, M. (2012). Improving long-term outcomes after discharge from intensive care unit: Report from a stakeholders' conference. *Critical Care Medicine, 40,* 502–509. https://doi.org/10.1097/CCM.0b013e318232da75

Neelapu, S. S., Tummala, S., Kebriaei, P., Wierda, W., Gutierrez, C., Locke, F. L., . . . Shpall, E. J. (2018). Chimeric antigen receptor T-cell therapy—Assessment and management of toxicities. *Nature Reviews Clinical Oncology, 15,* 47–62. https://doi.org/10.1038/nrclinonc.2017.148

Nguyen, V., Thao-Houane, T., & Warren, M. L. (2014). Early mobilization: Occupational therapy within the multidisciplinary team approach. *OT Practice, 19*(16), 15–19.

Piel-Julian, M. L., Mahévas, M., Germain, J., Languille, L., Comont, T., Lapeyre-Mestre, M., . . . Moulis, G. (2018). Risk factors for bleeding, including platelet count threshold, in newly diagnosed immune thrombocytopenia adults. *Journal of Thrombosis and Haemostasis, 16,* 1830–1842. https://doi.org/10.1111/jth.14227

Pranjic, N., Bajraktarevic, A., & Ramic, E. (2016). Distress and PTSD in patients with cancer: Cohort study case. *Materia Socio-Medica, 28,* 12–16. https://doi.org/10.5455/msm.2016.28.12-16

Pun, B. T., Balas, M. C., Barnes-Daly, M. A., Thompson, J. L., Aldrich, J. M., Barr, J., . . . Ely, E. W. (2019). Caring for critically ill patients with the ABCDEF Bundle: Results of the ICU Liberation Collaborative in over 15,000 Adults. *Critical Care Medicine, 47,* 3–14. https://doi.org/10.1097/CCM.0000000000003482

Puxty, K., McLoone, P., Quasim, T., Sloan, B., Kinsella, J., & Morrison, D. S. (2015). Risk of critical illness among patients with solid cancers: A population-based observational study. *JAMA Oncology, 1,* 1078–1085. https://doi.org/10.1001/jamaoncol.2015.2855

Rawal, G., Yadav, S., & Kumar, S. (2017). Post-intensive care syndrome: An overview. *Journal of Translational Internal Medicine, 5,* 90–92. https://doi.org/10.1515/jtim-2016-0016

Schellongowski, P., Sperr, W. R., Wohlfarth, P., Knoebl, P., Rabitsch, W., Watzke, H. H., Staudinger, T. (2016). Critically ill patients with cancer: Chances and limitations of intensive care medicine—A narrative review. *ESMO Open, 1*(5), e000018. https://doi.org/10.1136/esmoopen-2015-000018

Shimabukuro-Vornhagen, A., Boll, B., Kochanek, M., Azoulay, E., & von Bergwelt-Baildon, M. (2016). Critical care of patients with cancer. *CA: A Cancer Journal for Clinicians, 66,* 496–517. https://doi.org/10.3322/caac.21351

Silver, J. K., Raj, V. S., & Wisotzky, E. M. (2018). Oncology rehabilitation. In P. Hopewood & M. J. Milroy (Eds.), *Quality cancer care* (pp. 119–147). Cham, Switzerland: Springer. https://doi.org/10.1007/978-3-319-78649-0_9

Singer, M., Deutschman, C., Seymour, C., Shankar-Hari, M., Annane, D., Bauer, M., . . . Angus, D. (2016). The Third International Consensus Definitions for Sepsis and Septic Shock (Sepsis-3). *Journal of the American Medical Association, 315,* 801–810. https://doi.org/10.1001/jama.2016.0287

Tai, E., Guy, G. P., Dunbar, A., & Richardson, L. C. (2017). Cost of cancer-related neutropenia or fever hospitalizations, United States, 2012. *Journal of Oncology Practice, 1,* e552–e561. https://doi.org/10.1200/JOP.2016.019588

Takeuchi, H., Taki, Y., Nouchi, R., Yokoyama, R., Kotozaki, Y., Nakagawa, S., . . . Kawashima, R. (2018). The effects of family socioeconomic status on psychological and neural mechanisms as well as their sex differences. *Frontiers in Human Neuroscience, 12,* 543, 1–18. https://doi.org/10.3389/fnhum.2018.00543

Tillery, R., Howard-Sharp, K. M., Okado, Y., Long, A., & Phipps, S. (2016). Profiles of resilience and growth in youth with cancer and healthy comparisons. *Journal of Pediatric Psychology, 41,* 290–297. https://doi.org/10.1093/jpepsy/jsv091

Versteeg, A. L., van der Velden, J. M., Verkooijen, H. M., van Vulpen, M., Oner, F. C., Fisher, C. G., & Verlaan, J. J. (2016). The effect of introducing the Spinal Instability Neoplastic Score in routine clinical practice for patients with spinal metastases. *Oncologist, 21,* 95–101. https://doi.org/10.1634/theoncologist.2015-0266

Warren, M. (2006). *Brain injury visual assessment battery for adults: Test manual.* Birmingham, AL: visAbilities Rehab Services.

Zeynalova, N., Schimpf, S., Setter, C., Yahiaou Doktora, M., Zeynalova, S., Lordick, F., . . . Hinz, A. (2019). The association between an anxiety disorder and cancer in medical history. *Journal of Affective Disorders, 246,* 640–642. https://doi.org/10.1016/j.jad.2018.12.019

Prehabilitation

Brent Braveman, OTR, PhD, FAOTA; Latoya Adekoya, OTR, MOT; and Courtland Lee, OTR, MOT

10

LEARNING OBJECTIVES

After completing this chapter, readers should be able to
- Describe and explain the purpose of enhanced recovery programs,
- Define and explain the purpose of prehabilitation for cancer survivors, and
- Describe the occupational therapy process as applied to prehabilitation for cancer survivors.

KEY TERMS AND CONCEPTS

- DREAMS (drinking, eating, analgesia, mobilization, and sleep)
- Enhanced recovery
- Interprofessional team
- Outcomes

- Palliative rehabilitation
- Prehabilitation
- Preventative rehabilitation
- Restorative rehabilitation

- RIOT (Return to Intended Oncologic Therapy)
- Social cognitive theory
- Supportive rehabilitation

INTRODUCTION

Increasingly, it is being recognized that postsurgical or post-procedural effects and complications can slow recovery. New functional problems may arise, and existing functional problems may be exacerbated by surgery or other forms of treatment. As is highlighted throughout this text, cancer survivors face myriad functional impairments, such as cancer-related fatigue (CRF), chemotherapy-induced peripheral neuropathy (CIPN), cancer-related cognitive impairment (CRCI), pain, lymphedema, and others caused by the cancer itself or as sequelae of the cancer treatments. This chapter describes occupational therapy services provided in prehabilitation programs designed to limit the postsurgical or post-procedural problems encountered by cancer survivors. ***Prehabilitation*** is defined as

> a process on the cancer continuum of care that occurs between the time of cancer diagnosis and the beginning of acute treatment and includes physical and psychological assessments that establish a baseline functional level, identify impairments, and provide interventions that promote physical and psychological health to reduce the incidence and/or severity of future impairments. (Silver, 2015, p. 14)

Because other chapters in the book go in to depth on approaches to clinical intervention (see Section IV, "Sequelae of Cancer and Interventions Across the Lifespan"), this chapter focuses on describing the types of services provided to

cancer survivors in prehabilitation and outlining some of the challenges and opportunities in these settings but does not go in to detail on specific intervention strategies.

To date, prehabilitation services have focused primarily on adult and older adult cancer survivors because a primary objective is to address limitations in mobility, nutrition, and physical stamina before surgery or procedure, and these challenges are more widely recognized and often more pronounced in adults and older adults. More limited prehabilitation services are provided for adolescents and young adults (AYAs), but there is an opportunity for developing these services.

REVIEW OF THE CANCER CARE CONTINUUM AND REHABILITATION FOR CANCER SURVIVORS

Rehabilitative services, including occupational therapy, are provided in various settings (e.g., acute care hospitals, acute inpatient rehabilitation units and hospitals, skilled nursing facilities, long-term care hospitals, home health care, outpatient ambulatory settings, hospice). A review of these settings is useful in understanding prehabilitation in context. Table 10.1 provides a brief description of the type of rehabilitative services provided in these varied settings.

Thinking about cancer rehabilitation along a continuum is not new, and in fact, J. Herbert Dietz, an oncologist at the Institute of Rehabilitation Medicine, New York University Hospital and Memorial Hospital for Cancer and Allied Diseases, described four stages of rehabilitation with cancer

TABLE 10.1. Description of Rehabilitation Settings Along a Continuum of Care

TYPE OF REHABILITATION SETTING	DESCRIPTION OF REHABILITATION SETTING
Acute care hospitalization	Rehabilitation for cancer survivors includes OT and PT and, less commonly, SLP. Services focus on safety, early mobilization, and basic ADLs. The focus of rehabilitation is preparation for discharge home or to the next step in the medical continuum of care. Services are typically initiated by an oncologist, a midlevel provider, a hospitalist, or a general physician.
Acute inpatient rehabilitation	Rehabilitation for cancer survivors may include OT, PT, SLP, nursing, psychology, social work, nutrition, case management, and other services. Services are typically coordinated by a physiatrist. Services are described as "intensive," and patients must tolerate at least 3 hours of treatment each day. The focus of rehabilitation is to maximize independence and function to promote discharge to the home, community, or least-care-intense setting possible.
Post-acute skilled nursing facility	Rehabilitation for cancer survivors may include OT, PT, SLP, nursing, nutrition, and case management. Depending on the payer and terms of admission, there may be varied expectations for the intensity and duration of rehabilitative care, but daily services up to 1 hour from each discipline may be required.
Post-acute long-term care	Rehabilitation for cancer survivors may include OT, PT, SLP, nursing, nutrition, and case management. Because patients stay on average 25 days or more, the intensity of services is lower than inpatient rehabilitation or a stay in a skilled nursing facility for rehabilitation.
Hospice	Rehabilitation for cancer survivors may include OT, PT, nursing, nutrition social work, and case management. Because curative treatment for cancer has been stopped, services are limited to promoting function, the alleviation of pain, and other palliative efforts.
Home care	Rehabilitation for cancer survivors may include OT, PT, and SLP in addition to nursing and medical care. Services focus on safety, mobility, and ADLs/IADLs, and the intensity and duration are typically limited. Hospice services may also be provided in the home setting.
Outpatient ambulatory care	Rehabilitation for cancer survivors may include OT, PT, and SLP. The frequency and duration of services may vary a great deal on the basis of the patient's needs and their physical, medical, and psychological impairments. Intensive services may be provided as often as 3 times per week for several weeks or more. Because cancer survivors may experience multiple hospital admissions, they may also be referred to outpatient ambulatory care multiple times.

Note. ADLs = activities of daily living; IADLs = instrumental activities of daily living; OT = occupational therapy; PT = physical therapy; SLP = speech–language pathology.

survivors in 1969 that remains relevant today (Silver et al., 2018):

1. Preventative
2. Restorative
3. Supportive
4. Palliative.

In *preventative rehabilitation,* the goal is to prevent decreases in function before and during active treatment. *Restorative rehabilitation* is intended to assist survivors to return to their prior performance status. *Supportive rehabilitation* employs adaptive techniques and therapeutic interventions to allow a patient to reach certain levels of improvement or independence. *Palliative rehabilitation* focuses on minimizing or eliminating complications from advanced disease with the goal being to improve quality of life (QoL).

ENHANCED RECOVERY PROGRAMS

Barriers to efficient and effective medical care without complications while achieving desired outcomes are receiving increased attention. Particular attention is being given to complicating factors that can occur during medical and surgical interventions; strategies to limit the negative effect that pain, fatigue, decreased mobility, poor

nutritional intake, cognitive or processing impairment, and other postsurgical or post-procedural problems create are also being identified. One global strategy that is increasingly being implemented is *enhanced recovery* programs, which are sets of standardized protocols used before, during, and after a procedure to ensure the best possible outcomes (Kim & Aloia, 2018; Kim et al., 2016). These protocols include strategies such as:

- Preoperative patient education and prehabilitation
- Multimodal opioid-sparing analgesia
- Minimally invasive surgical techniques and limited use of tubes and drains
- Early postoperative mobilization
- Early enteral nutrition (Teeter et al., 2019).

There is much interest in prehabilitation in enhanced recovery programs because improving patients' physical function and minimizing impairment may facilitate postoperative recovery. Moreover, the term *RIOT* (*Return to Intended Oncologic Therapy*) has been used in enhanced recovery literature, indicating that optimization of perioperative care of patients may lead to improved recovery so patients may receive postoperative cancer treatment sooner.

Although enhanced recovery strategies are most commonly applied to surgical procedures, they are now being adopted by other teams, including those providing stem cell transplants (SCTs; Szewczyk et al., 2019). As described by a member of the Enhanced Recovery-Stem Cell Transplant team caring for the hematopoietic stem cell transplant (HSCT) population at MD Anderson Cancer Center,

> the team applied the principles of Enhanced Recovery After Surgery (ERAS) programs which have shown to impact outcomes related to decreased opiate use and pain levels, shortened average length of stay, increased patient satisfaction, and reduce cost. Literature is limited for enhanced recovery pathway within the HSCT population. The program utilized similar approaches of ERAS. This includes evaluation by Prehabilitation (Physical Therapist [PT], Occupational Therapist [OT] and Rehabilitation MD evaluation), Gerontologist, Clinical Nutritionist, clinical pharmacist, and by our Advanced Practice Providers (APPs) and nursing coordinators. (Szewczyk et al., 2019, para. 2)

For more information on SCTs, see Chapter 2, "Cancer Treatment Approaches Across the Lifespan."

The specific components included in enhanced recovery programs can vary, but in general the acronym **DREAMS,** which stands for *d*rinking, *e*ating, *a*nalgesia, *m*obilization, and *s*leep, is useful (Moonesinghe et al., 2017). These provide several opportunities for occupational therapy practitioners to participate in enhanced recovery programming before, during, and after hospitalization or significant procedures. One such opportunity is prehabilitation.

PREHABILITATION

Prehabilitation, often referred to as *prehab,* has been identified and defined as a distinct stage in the cancer rehabilitation process. Chen et al. (2017) noted that the value of prehabilitation with cancer survivors is to address barriers to rehabilitation at a more optimal time than the postoperative period. These barriers include patient factors (e.g., fatigue, pain, poor endurance, limited mobility) as well as factors relating to health care access and health care providers. The goals and benefits of prehabilitation are wide and varied and include

- Improving physical functioning,
- Improving psychological functioning,
- Reducing treatment-related impairments such as fatigue or CIPN,
- Reducing risks for comorbidities,
- Improving health outcomes,
- Improving health-related QoL, and
- Decreasing health care costs (Silver & Baima, 2013).

There is an evolving body of evidence on prehabilitation, but not all of the literature directly addresses occupational therapy, and to some extent, the involvement of occupational therapy in prehab interventions is more recent. For example, Carli and Zavorsky (2005) described the role of exercise, nutrition, and stress reduction but did not describe ADLs or interventions central to occupational therapy's role. Chen et al. (2017) reported that patients in prehabilitation significantly increased the amount of moderate and vigorous intensity physical activities they performed. These same groups of patients also demonstrated

greater improvement in a 6-minute walk test compared to subjects in a control group. Moreover, at the time of surgery, a greater proportion of patients in the prehab group met physical activity guidelines.

Carli and Zavorsky (2005) described the impact of increasing functional reserve in the preoperative period through prehabilitation on accelerating postoperative functional recovery. The goals of prehabilitation are to prevent complications, achieve faster return to baseline function, decrease length of hospital stay, and reduce admissions to rehabilitation facilities postoperatively. This should result in lower health care system costs, improved quality of care, and enhanced patient satisfaction. The value of including prehabilitation is to improve physical capacity and occupational performance before a surgery or procedure and in turn limit the negative impact of the inpatient stay and promote faster recovery to baseline performance.

Prehabilitation Across the Lifespan

Prehabilitation is a relatively new intervention, and services have been more focused on adults and older adults, but some interventions have been developed specifically for AYAs. The effectiveness of prehabilitation for children is increasingly being investigated. For example, Corr et al. (2017) carried out a pilot program to determine the feasibility and functional outcomes of adding prehabilitation during the 10- to 12-week period before a planned surgery to remove a lower extremity sarcoma in children and adolescents and found significant differences in outcomes on a functional mobility assessment.

As with adults and older adults, AYAs are not always physically and psychologically prepared to undergo surgery, SCT, or other difficult cancer treatments. Despite the increased need for adequate exercise, a significant proportion of AYAs with a history of cancer do not meet the Centers for Disease Control and Prevention's recommended weekly minimum of 150 minutes of moderate to vigorous intensity exercise (Rock et al., 2012). Barnes et al. (2016) noted that "while evidence exists supporting interventions delivered at any time point in the cancer journey, the most effective interventions may be those implemented prior to the onset of late effects or noted declines in key health behaviors" (p. 22).

Interprofessional Care

A hallmark of effective prehabilitation is the involvement of an ***interprofessional team***. The primary purpose of prehab is to better prepare the cancer survivor for impending intervention and to decrease the negative effects on postoperative or post-procedural function (i.e., improve occupational performance), which is best accomplished through a comprehensive assessment and prehab intervention and requires the expertise of multiple disciplines. In addition to occupational therapy, prehab teams often include any combination of physical therapy; exercise physiology or kinesiology; nursing; pharmacy; nutrition; case management; and an oncologist, physiatrist, and gerontologist.

The specific composition of the team may vary depending on the program, and occupational therapy may not be involved in all programs. For example, at MD Anderson

Cancer Center, occupational therapy is an integral part of the established Enhanced Recovery Stem Cell Transplant program and an evolving spinal pain program. However, occupational therapy does not see surgical prehab patients. Decisions about the services involved in each prehab effort can be driven by issues of reimbursement, timing of the visit in relationship to the procedure, the length of time that a patient may reasonably be asked to commit to a clinic visit, and the impact that the procedure may have on the survivor's functioning.

Occupations

Like other cancer rehabilitation, prehabilitation focuses on aiding the cancer survivor to return to their home or pre-admission environment as soon as possible with the least negative impact on function as possible. Given this focus, intervention by the occupational therapy practitioner is naturally occupation based. Although some limitations may be inherent in reimbursement guidelines (e.g., Medicare does not pay for return-to-work–related or leisure-based interventions in hospital-based services), the full range of occupation may be considered to some extent (e.g., ADLs, IADLs, rest and sleep, education, work, play, leisure, social participation). With children, it is easier to incorporate play activities because play is recognized as a developmentally appropriate occupation.

In prehab, occupations are considered in the context of a survivor's performance at the time of the visit (i.e., before the surgery or procedure), anticipating performance during an upcoming inpatient admission and postdischarge after the surgery or procedure is complete. Occupational therapy practitioners need to help cancer survivors anticipate how the impending surgery or procedure may affect their ability to participate in valued occupations. For example, a practitioner might address social participation by suggesting to a prehab client that they plan for strategies to maintain familial or social contacts while in isolation during a long hospitalization for an SCT. The use of a smartphone or tablet to video chat may be commonplace for younger survivors but may not be an automatic choice for all survivors.

Strategies provided by the prehab team help the survivor continue or return to daily routines and occupations to the largest extent possible. Interruptions to school, work, parenting, and other roles are common, and occupational

therapy practitioners play a critical role in helping survivors prepare for these interruptions and minimize negative effects.

Client Factors

Values and beliefs can greatly influence the course of prehabilitation because it is important that cancer survivors believe that they can influence the course and outcomes of their cancer treatment through their own health behaviors. Survivors must not only believe that exercise, improved sleep, good nutrition, and other strategies (e.g., fatigue management) can improve QoL and better prepare them for surgery, SCT, or other procedures; they must also believe in their own self-efficacy.

Occupational therapy practitioners can use several models to design and deliver occupational therapy interventions to promote success. Braveman (2016) reviewed the use of models, including the Health Belief Model, Social Cognitive Theory, and the Transtheoretical Stages of Change, to develop occupational therapy programming; these models can be useful in considering and promoting self-efficacy in cancer survivors in prehab and other phases of rehabilitation (Prochaska & DiClemente, 1993; Rosenstock, 1974; Rosenstock et al., 1988). The use of *social cognitive theory* to guide prehabilitation programs is well documented (Allen et al., 2018; Barnes et al., 2016; Levett & Grimmett, 2019).

Braveman (2016) explained that

social cognitive theory holds that behavior is determined by expectancies and incentives. Expectancies can be divided into three types: (1) expectancies about environmental cues, which are called environmental expectancies; (2) expectancies about the consequences of one's own behavior, which are called outcome expectancies; and (3) expectancies about one's competence to perform a behavior necessary to achieve a particular outcome, which are called efficacy expectations. Incentives (or reinforcements) are the value that an individual places on particular outcomes. (p. 388)

Table 10.2 provides examples of social cognitive theory applied to the health behavior of incorporating energy conservation strategies in home management occupations.

TABLE 10.2.   Social Cognitive Theory Applied to Incorporation of Energy Conservation Strategies in Home Management Occupations

TYPES OF EXPECTANCIES AND INCENTIVES	BELIEFS AND LEVEL OF VALUE THAT DRIVES HEALTH BEHAVIORS
Environmental expectancies (what leads to what?)	Belief that continuing the current pattern of behavior contributes to increased levels of fatigue
Outcome expectancies (how behavior is likely to influence outcomes)	Belief that incorporating energy conservation strategies decreases fatigue and increases satisfaction with the ability to perform cherished home management occupations such as baking
Efficacy expectancies (confidence in the ability to perform a behavior)	Belief that one is capable of successfully incorporating energy conservation strategies into daily routines
Incentives (value of an outcome)	Highly valuing the sense of accomplishment and enjoyment from participating in cherished home management occupations such as baking

Performance Skills

Performance skills, including motor skills, cognitive and process skills, and social interaction skills, may be assessed during prehabilitation to help determine the current level of function and to prognosticate the impact of a surgery or procedure on occupational performance and participation and the capacity of the cancer survivor to respond. Early and continued postsurgical mobilization through completion of ADLs, early ambulation, and spending time out of the hospital bed is critical to a cancer survivor's returning to presurgical or pre-procedural levels of function. This can be complicated by pain, fatigue, slowed processing, and other challenges. Beyond the physical capacity to perform self-care and other mobilization activities, the occupational therapy practitioner must assess the survivor's capacity for processing information and unfamiliar situations.

Although a prehab visit occurs before an upcoming surgery or procedure, many cancer survivors have had cancer treatments, sometimes for years, before prehab. The challenge of prehab may be building a survivor's capacity to exercise, ambulate, and perform daily occupations in the face of preexisting CRF, CRCI, or other symptoms. Cancer survivors can be given an overwhelming amount of information in a short time during prehab, and the occupational therapy practitioner's evaluation should include assessment of the survivor's processing and comprehension skills. Survivors benefit from the presentation of educational material in written form in addition to verbal presentation; the information should be written in clear, concise language at a lower level of complexity to make it easy for survivors to understand.

Performance Patterns

As in any other area of occupational therapy intervention, occupational therapy practitioners in prehabilitation seek to understand their clients' habits, routines, rituals, and roles to guide interventions. A challenge to doing this in prehab is the brevity of the initial evaluation. Prehab sometimes consists of a single visit during which the cancer survivor may need to meet with practitioners from multiple disciplines (e.g., occupational therapy, physical therapy, nutrition, pharmacy, nursing, medicine). Each discipline must streamline their assessment process to optimize time spent with each survivor while accomplishing their goals. Coming to a deep appreciation of any cancer survivor's habits, routines, rituals, and roles is difficult, and using common observational assessments that might be administered in other settings is not practical. Instead, occupational therapy practitioners must rely on self-report or the report of family or caregivers attending the prehab visit; they may also administer brief assessments that take little time and directly observe the cancer survivor during the prehab visit (e.g., Does the survivor have any difficulty with ambulation in the clinic hallways? Does the survivor have difficulty with directions or memory during the evaluation?). Asking the survivor to arrive early to complete some self-reported assessments in the waiting room is a helpful strategy.

Context and Environment

As with other areas that require assessment, assessing the impact of cultural, personal, physical, social, temporal, and virtual contexts and environments in prehabilitation is difficult. Occupational therapy practitioners must consider context and environment in two ways during prehab. First, the home or preadmission setting must be considered because this is where the cancer survivor will carry out any recommendations given during prehab before inpatient admission. Second, the hospital setting must be considered because this is where the cancer survivor will be postsurgery or post-procedure. This postintervention period (i.e., inpatient hospitalization) may range from a few days for surgical patients to 3 or 4 weeks for patients undergoing stem cell transplantation.

Strategies for assessing context and environment may include asking the patient to fill out a bulleted list questionnaire regarding ADL or IADL independence level and obtaining a detailed occupational profile via an interview. In the case of young cancer patients, collaborating with their parents to help them understand the hospital environment and plan for an extended stay while adhering to infection control guidelines is helpful. Providing information on what can and cannot be brought into hospital spaces can lessen stress and worry after their child is admitted.

Occupational Performance and Participation

The ultimate objective of occupational therapy intervention is to support participation in social roles and society. However, as with many settings in which occupational therapy practitioners work, the short-term focus may be on occupational performance. Cancer survivors faced with sometimes life-threatening surgeries or with arduous procedures such as SCT may have difficulty thinking about the future and their return to full participation in family, school, work, or leisure roles. Occupational therapy practitioners must balance focus on the immediate (i.e., how can the survivor participate in bathing or dressing or eating meals out of bed) with the long-term goal of returning to full participation.

Strategies can include assisting the survivor in identifying daily routines and meaningful activities that they are currently involved in or want to return to or exploring new leisure interests and activities. Other strategies include the occupational therapy practitioner collaborating with the survivor and caregivers to construct a daily schedule that simulates their daily routine in addition to the consideration and inclusion of activities and protocols of the hospital setting (e.g., adhering to infection control policies of bringing items that are easily sanitized and accommodating for limited space).

OCCUPATIONAL THERAPY PROCESS AND PREHABILITATION

Evaluation

In prehab, initial evaluation and the administration of assessments to help determine goals is typically completed in one visit that may last no more than 60 minutes. Additional visits may occur in some instances, but sometimes cancer survivors have traveled to the site from long distances for prehab and other preadmission testing, or assessment

TABLE 10.3. Sample Assessments for Prehabilitation With Cancer Survivors	
ASSESSMENT	**DESCRIPTION**
Brief Fatigue Inventory (Mendoza et al., 1999)	Short assessment of the severity of fatigue experienced over the past 24 hours and its impact on function
Pain visual analog scale	Visual or spoken scales for rating pain (e.g., 0 = *no pain* to 10 = *worst pain imaginable,* Wong–Baker FACES Scale that uses pictures to express *no hurt* to *worst hurt*)
Activity Measure for Post-Acute Care Short Forms for Inpatient and Outpatient Settings (Jette et al., 2015)	Examines activity limitations in functional activities likely encountered every day
Pittsburgh Sleep Quality Index (PSQI; Buysse et al., 1989)	Measures the quality and patterns of the patient's sleep within the last month
Functional Assessment of Cancer Therapy-Cognitive (FACIT.org, 2019; Wagner et al., 2009)	Assessment designed to assess perceived cognitive function and impact on quality of life in cancer patients

and the prehab visit may be the only time with the survivor before the surgery or procedure. For this reason, the evaluation process must be laser focused, and assessments must be chosen with the brevity of the visit in mind. A sample list of assessments that can be used by occupational therapy practitioners during prehabilitation with cancer survivors is included in Table 10.3.

Occupational profile

Development of a detailed occupational profile is difficult because of the brevity of the typical prehab visit. However, the more the occupational therapy practitioner can learn about the occupational identity of the cancer survivor, the more successful they will be in intervening in ways perceived relevant by the cancer survivor. This can be accomplished by asking direct, specific questions to make sure that examples used apply to the survivor. Simple checklists or self-report assessments that may be completed by the survivor or parents or caregivers in the waiting room before the start of the prehab session are helpful as is a review of medical records. The American Occupational Therapy Association (AOTA) has developed an occupational profile template for documentation, which is a helpful resource (AOTA, 2017).

Analysis of occupational performance

Because prehab may consist of a single preadmission visit, it may be impossible to directly observe and analyze most areas of occupational performance. For this reason, much of the analysis must rely on patient self-reported measures along with input from family or caregivers who may attend the prehab visit with the cancer survivor. Examples of such self-reported measures appropriate for use during cancer prehabilitation include the

- Brief Fatigue Inventory (BFI; Mendoza et al., 1999),
- Activity Measure for Post-Acute Care (AM-PAC; Jette et al., 2015),
- Pittsburgh Sleep Quality Index (PSQI; Buysee et al., 1989), and
- Functional Assessment of Cancer Therapy-Cognitive (FACT-Cog) Version 3 (Wagner et al., 2009).

Ideally, data and information obtained during the prehab evaluation will be available to the team that provides interventions during the inpatient admission when direct observation of occupational performance is more realistic. Areas of daily performance that focus on occupations, sleep hygiene, fatigue levels, ADL and IADL participation, and leisure interests are examined during collaboration to develop strategies to continue engagement in a normalized routine throughout the patient's SCT or other treatments and minimize disruption.

Intervention

Prehabilitation intervention comes primarily in the form of education for the cancer survivor and caregivers and recommendations for steps to be taken between the prehab visit and the inpatient admission. Education may include strategies to address the common symptoms of cancer and its treatments (e.g., CRF, pain, CRCI, CIPN, disturbed sleep) as well as preparation for admission. The education provided depends on the surgery or procedure to be performed, the length of the inpatient admission, and expectations for postsurgical or post-procedure challenges and complications.

Cancer survivors may be given educational materials on strategies to practice at home before inpatient admission. They may also be guided to perform self-assessments such as thinking about their daily routines and roles and identifying aspects of occupational performance they may worry about. Given the seriousness of what many survivors are facing, they may not consider simple familiar occupations such as who will change the cat litter or how meals will be prepared. Alternatively, occupational therapy practitioners should not discount survivor experiences and should ask the survivor how they have faced challenges during earlier treatments and interventions; practitioners should also promote continued problem solving and self-sufficiency.

Targeting Outcomes

According to the *Occupational Therapy Practice Framework: Domain and Process* (3rd ed.), **outcomes** are "the end result of the occupational therapy process; they describe

CASE EXAMPLE 10.1. VINCENZA: PREHABILITATION

Vincenza is a 68-year-old grandmother with three adult children and four grandchildren. She has been diagnosed with acute myeloid leukemia (AML). She is being seen in the Enhanced Recovery for Stem Cell Transplant program at MD Anderson Cancer Center for prehabilitation, and an inpatient admission is planned in 3 weeks with an estimated length of stay of 20–30 days. Her husband, **Carlos,** attends the prehabilitation session with the occupational therapist.

Vincenza has been treated for her AML with multiple rounds of chemotherapy in preparation for her upcoming stem cell transplant (SCT). During her evaluation by an occupational therapist, she immediately reports being anxious about her SCT and is nervous about being in the hospital for so long. She mentions the central role

that she has played in providing care for her grandchildren and is worried about being away from them for so long; she wants to know if she will be able to return to her cherished role of Grandma. She mentions that she has struggled with cancer-related fatigue (CRF) and mild cancer-related cognitive impairment (CRCI), which makes her worry about her grandchildren's safety when they are in her care. She has had multiple inpatient admissions and has received occupational therapy at MD Anderson before.

The occupational therapist begins by developing a brief occupational profile and administering a limited number of assessments to obtain baseline data (see Table 10.4 for a list of assessments used and the foci of information gleaned from each assessment).

TABLE 10.4. Sample Assessments Used in Prehabilitation and Assessment Data for Vincenza

ASSESSMENT	DESCRIPTION	SUMMARY OF RESULTS FOR VINCENZA
Brief Fatigue Inventory (Mendoza et al., 1999)	Short assessment of the severity of fatigue experienced over the past 24 hours and its impact on function	Global average fatigue of 4/10 over the past 24 hours. She rates her fatigue as mildly interfering with her mood and relations with other people but as significantly interfering with normal activities and somewhat interfering with her enjoyment of life (e.g., 5/10).
Pain visual analog scale	Visual or spoken scales for rating pain (e.g., 0 = *no pain* to 10 = *worst pain imaginable,* Wong–Baker FACES Scale that uses pictures to express *no hurt* to *worst hurt*)	0 /10, reporting no pain.
Activity Measure for Post-Acute Care Short Forms for Inpatient and Outpatient Settings (Jette et al., 2015)	Examines activity limitations in functional activities likely encountered every day	Raw score is 45, *t*-scale score 55.43. Vincenza reported she would have a little difficulty performing these tasks as a result of fatigue, weakness, and tremors: sewing on a button, using a hammer to pound a nail in to hang a picture, manipulating small parts with only her hands, cutting her toenails, moving her sofa to clean under it, and lifting a 25-pound object from the floor to a table. She would be unable to lift 100 pounds or perform 5 push-ups without stopping.
Pittsburgh Sleep Quality Index (Buysee et al., 1989)	Self-report questionnaire of sleep quality over the past 30 days	Global score is an 8 (a global score of 5 or greater is indicative of poor sleep quality). Vincenza reports that anxiety about her upcoming SCT admission, getting up frequently each night to use the restroom, and having difficulty falling asleep within 30 minutes each night have affected her overall sleep quality.

(Continued)

(Continued)

CASE EXAMPLE 10.1. VINCENZA: PREHABILITATION *(Cont.)*

TABLE 10.4.   Sample Assessments Used in Prehabilitation and Assessment Data for Vincenza *(Cont.)*

ASSESSMENT	DESCRIPTION	SUMMARY OF RESULTS FOR VINCENZA
Functional Assessment of Cancer Therapy-Cognitive Function (Wagner et al., 2009)	Assessment designed to assess perceived cognitive function and impact on quality of life in cancer patients	Scoring indicates that Vincenza perceives difficulty with cognitive issues several times each week.
Self-reported assessment of ADLs and IADLs	Assessment through self-report of occupational performance in ADLs and IADLs	Vincenza reports being independent in all ADLs most of the time, but after completing her last round of chemotherapy, she has noticed intention tremors that have affected her ability to feed herself at times and prepare her meals. She also reports that while she completes most IADLs independently, she struggles with fatigue, weakness, and tremors and has some difficulty processing. She notes concerns over the quality of her performance and the safety of her grandchildren when they are in her care. She describes altering habits and routines such as giving the children cereal for breakfast instead of preparing a hot meal.
Durable medical equipment assessment	Assessment of equipment needs for mobility, ADLs, and IADLs, prognosticating needs based on self-report and description of the home environment	Potential needs identified as likely including: • Shower chair • Long-handled sponge • Weighted eating utensils

Note. ADLs = activities of daily living; IADLs = instrumental activities of daily living; SCT = stem cell transplant.

Vincenza complains of significant fatigue and mild cognitive deficits, including slowed processing, forgetfulness, and difficulty with complex problem solving in novel situations. The primary problem list identified by the occupational therapy team in conjunction with Vincenza and her husband includes

- Decreased performance in IADLs, including meal preparation, housekeeping, grocery shopping, and activities associated with providing care for her four grandchildren;
- CRF;
- Impaired sleep hygiene;
- Impaired memory and concentration; and
- Slowed processing and difficulty problem solving in novel situations.

The occupational therapist collaborates with Vincenza and Carlos, and together they identify the following goals to achieve before her upcoming inpatient admission:

- Implement sleep hygiene and coping strategies into her daily sleep routine and demonstrate an improved Pittsburgh Sleep Quality Index score to 5 or lower.
- Implement compensatory strategies to assist with problem solving, attention, organization, and functional memory.

- Implement fatigue management/energy conservation strategies into IADL tasks and demonstrate an improved Brief Fatigue Inventory score of 2/10 or better.
- Prepare a hot meal for her grandchildren with modified independence, incorporating compensatory strategies to assist with attention, organization, and memory without assistance.
- Verbalize at least three routine practices to be initiated in preparation for SCT admission to work toward independent health management and maintenance (i.e., develop daily routine and schedule for hospital admission; identify items from home to bring to hospital to help with coping for prolonged stay; use fatigue management strategies, coping strategies, and fall prevention strategies; develop exercise routine).

During the session, the occupational therapist provides Vincenza with educational materials on CRF, CRCI, strategies for improved sleep, strategies to compensate for impaired memory and organization (e.g., using lists, automated reminders), strategies to manage and cope with stress (e.g., relaxation techniques, chair yoga, consistent physical exercise or activity, journaling, meditation), and basic work simplification and energy conservation techniques. As each of these materials is presented, the

(Continued)

CASE EXAMPLE 10.1. VINCENZA: PREHABILITATION *(Cont.)*

therapist continues to develop the occupational profile by learning more about Vincenza and her habits, routines, and roles. The therapist encourages Carlos's active participation in the session because his support before, during, and after Vincenza's SCT is critical to her success.

Much of the prehabilitation session is focused on preparing Vincenza for her upcoming hospitalization. To achieve this, the occupational therapy practitioner addresses the following:

- Incorporation of Vincenza's daily routines experienced at home into a closely comparable routine within the hospital environment;
- Objects that Vincenza may consider bringing with her to promote performance of familiar occupations including hobbies or leisure activities;
- Strategies for promoting socialization and preventing depression, including maintaining contact with her grandchildren and circle of friends (e.g., learning to use video chat features on a tablet), participating in SCT group exercise class, attending the occupational

therapy ACT (*a*ppearances, *c*hanges, *t*ransitions) group, and playing bingo;
- Establishment of effective bedtime routines to promote quality sleep;
- Assertive communication strategies to use during hospitalization to request clustering of care overnight and limit interruptions to sleep;
- Strategies to promote improved coping and to decrease anxiety; and
- Provision of weighted utensils to help improve function with cooking and eating because of occasional intention tremors.

At the conclusion of the prehab visit, the occupational therapist recommends that Vincenza continue outpatient occupational therapy to address current functional impairments to prepare her for her upcoming SCT admission. The therapist communicates the results of the occupational therapy evaluation and request for continued outpatient occupational therapy before admission to the rest of the prehab team.

---

what clients can achieve through occupational therapy intervention" (AOTA, 2014, p. S16). Although the purpose of prehab is to affect the postsurgical or post-procedural outcomes, the outcomes of prehab itself must be more proximal. In fact, the specific outcomes of prehabilitation may be difficult to measure because there is often no contact between the cancer survivor and the occupational therapy practitioner after the prehab evaluation until the time of inpatient admission. For this reason, all reasonable attempts to assess the cancer survivor's understanding of recommendations and educational materials must be made before completion of the prehab session.

Survivors who demonstrate difficulty within the areas assessed, such as proficiency with ADLs, impaired cognition, severe fatigue, sleep hygiene, and activity tolerance with their daily routines, may be recommended to receive intensive occupational therapy to improve functional performance before their surgery or procedure. Case Example 10.1 provides an example of a cancer survivor who received prehabilitation.

SUMMARY

Cancer survivors may benefit from prehabilitation if their treatment includes a procedure such as a surgery or a stem cell transplantation that puts them at risk for new or worsened functional deficits. The goal of prehabilitation is to prevent complications, achieve faster return to baseline function, decrease length of hospital stay, and reduce admissions to rehabilitation facilities postoperatively. Occupational therapy practitioners function as part of an interprofessional prehabilitation team but make distinct contributions toward improving the health, function, well-being, and participation of cancer survivors. Although much of prehabilitation may focus on occupational

performance, practitioners can influence the participation of cancer survivors in their existing social roles by connecting survivors with resources in the community and through interventions to address the full range of challenges experienced by survivors.

REFERENCES

Allen, S., Brown, V., Prabhu, P., Scott, M., Rockall, T., Preston, S., & Sultan, J. (2018). A randomised controlled trial to assess whether prehabilitation improves fitness in patients undergoing neoadjuvant treatment prior to oesophagogastric cancer surgery: Study protocol. *BMJ Open, 8*(12), e023190. https://doi.org/10.1136/bmjopen-2018-023190

American Occupational Therapy Association. (2014). Occupational therapy practice framework: Domain and process (3rd ed.). *American Journal of Occupational Therapy, 68*(Suppl. 1), S1–S48. http://doi.org/10.5014/ajot.2014.682006

American Occupational Therapy Association. (2017). AOTA occupational profile template. *American Journal of Occupational Therapy, 71,* 7112420030. https://doi.org/10.5014/ajot.2017.716S12

Barnes, M., Plaisance, E., Hanks, L., & Casazza, K. (2016). Prehabilitation-promoting exercise in adolescent and young adult cancer survivors for improving lifelong health—A narrative review. *Cancer Research Frontiers, 2*(1), 22–32. https://doi.org/10.17980/2016.22

Braveman, B. (2016). Developing evidence-based occupational therapy programming. In B. Braveman (Ed.), *Leading & managing occupational therapy services: An evidence-based approach* (pp. 375–410). Philadelphia: F. A. Davis.

Buysse, D. J., Reynolds, C. F., Monk, T. H., Berman, S. R., & Kupfer, D. J. (1989). The Pittsburgh Sleep Quality Index (PSQI): A new instrument for psychiatric research and practice. *Psychiatry Research, 28,* 193–213. https://doi.org/10.1016/0165-1781(89)90047-4

Carli, F., & Zavorsky, G. S. (2005). Optimizing functional exercise capacity in the elderly surgical population. *Current Opinion in Clinical Nutrition & Metabolic Care, 8*(1), 23–32. https://doi.org/10.1097/00075197-200501000-00005

Chen, B. P., Awasthi, R., Sweet, S. N., Minnella, E. M., Bergdahl, A., Santa Mina, D., . . . Scheede-Bergdahl, C. (2017). Four-week prehabilitation program is sufficient to modify exercise behaviors and improve preoperative functional walking capacity in patients with colorectal cancer. *Supportive Care in Cancer, 25*(1), 33–40. https://doi.org/10.1007/s00520-016-3379-8

Corr, A. M., Liu, W., Bishop, M., Pappo, A., Srivastava, D. K., Neel, M., . . . Ness, K. K. (2017). Feasibility and functional outcomes of children and adolescents undergoing preoperative chemotherapy prior to a limb-sparing procedure or amputation. *Rehabilitation Oncology (American Physical Therapy Association. Oncology Section), 35*(1), 38–45.

Dietz, J. H. Jr. (1969). Rehabilitation of the cancer patient. *Medical Clinics of North America, 53*, 607–624. https://doi.org/10.1016/S0025-7125(16)32757-2

FACIT.org. (2019). *Questionnaires.* Retrieved from https://www.facit.org/FACITOrg/Questionnaires

Jette, A., Haley, S. M., Coster, W., & Ni, P. S. (2015). *AM-PAC Short Forms for Inpatient and Outpatient Settings: Instruction manual.* Boston: Boston University.

Kim, B. J., & Aloia, T. A. (2018). What is "enhanced recovery," and how can I do it? *Journal of Gastrointestinal Surgery, 22*, 164–171. https://doi.org/10.1007/s11605-017-3605-9

Kim, B. J., Caudle, A. S., Gottumukkala, V., & Aloia, T. A. (2016). The impact of postoperative complications on a timely Return to Intended Oncologic Therapy (RIOT): The role of enhanced recovery in the cancer journey. *International Anesthesiology Clinics, 54*(4), e33–e46. https://doi.org/10.1097/AIA.0000000000000113

Levett, D. Z. H., & Grimmett, C. (2019). Psychological factors, prehabilitation and surgical outcomes: Evidence and future directions. *Anaesthesia, 74*, 36–42. https://doi.org/10.1111/anae.14507

Mendoza, T. R., Wang, X. S., Cleeland, C. S., Morrissey, M., Johnson, B. A., Wendt, J. K., & Huber, S. L. (1999). The rapid assessment of fatigue severity in cancer patients: Use of the Brief Fatigue Inventory. *Cancer, 85*, 1186–1196. https://doi.org/10.1002/(SICI)1097-0142(19990301)85:5<1186::AID-CNCR24>3.0.CO;2-N

Moonesinghe, S. R., Grocott, M. P., Bennett-Guerrero, E., Bergamaschi, R., Gottumukkala, V., Hopkins, T. J., . . . Miller, T. E. (2017). American Society for Enhanced Recovery (ASER) and Perioperative Quality Initiative (POQI) joint consensus statement on measurement to maintain and improve quality of enhanced recovery pathways for elective colorectal surgery. *Perioperative Medicine, 6*(1), 6. https://doi.org/10.1186/s13741-017-0062-7

Prochaska, J. O., & DiClemente, J. C. (1993). In search of how people change: Applications to addictive behavior. *American Psychologist, 47*, 1102–1114. https://doi.org/10.1037/0003-066x.47.9.1102

Rock, C. L., Doyle, C., Demark-Wahnefried, W., Meyerhardt, J., Courneya, K. S., Schwartz, A. L., . . . Gansler, T. (2012). Nutrition and physical activity guidelines for cancer survivors. *CA: Cancer Journal for Clinicians, 62*, 243–274. https://doi.org/10.3322/caac.21142

Rosenstock, I. M. (1974). Historical origins of the health belief model. *Health Education Monographs, 2*, 328–335. https://doi.org/10.1177/109019817400200403

Rosenstock, I. M., Strecher, V. J. & Becker, M. H. (1988). Social learning theory and the Health Belief Model. *Health Education Quarterly, 15*, 175–183. https://doi.org/10.1177/109019818801500203

Silver, J. K. (2015). Cancer prehabilitation and its role in improving health outcomes and reducing health care costs. *Seminars in Oncology Nursing, 31*(1), 13–30. https://doi.org/10.1016/j.soncn.2014.11.003

Silver, J. K. & Baima, J. (2013). Cancer prehabilitation: An opportunity to decrease treatment-related morbidity, increase cancer treatment options and improve physical and psychological health outcomes. *American Journal of Physical Medicine & Rehabilitation, 92*, 715–727. https://doi.org/10.1097/PHM.0b013e31829b4afe

Silver, J. K., Baima, J., & Mayer, R. S. (2013). Impairment-driven cancer rehabilitation: An essential component of quality care and survivorship. *CA: A Cancer Journal for Clinicians, 63*, 295–317. https://doi.org/10.3322/caac.21186

Silver, J. K., Raj, V. S., & Wisotzky, E. M. (2018). Oncology rehabilitation. In P. Hopewood & M. Milroy (Eds.), *Quality cancer care* (pp. 119–147). Cham, Switzerland: Springer International. https://doi.org/10.1007/978-3-319-78649-0_9

Szewczyk, N., Neumann, J. L., Kruse, B., Pang, L., Ngo-Huang, A., Ferguson, J., . . . Popat, U. R. (2019). Experience with applying and improving feasibility of an enhanced recovery model for allogenic stem cell transplant patients aged 65 and older. *Biology of Blood and Marrow Transplantation, 25*(3), S432. https://doi.org/10.1016/j.bbmt.2018.12.497

Teeter, E. G., Mena, G. E., Lasala, J. D., & Kolarczyk, L. M. (2019). Enhanced Recovery After Surgery (ERAS) for thoracic surgery. In P. Slinger (Ed.), *Principles and practice of anesthesia for thoracic surgery* (2nd ed., pp. 873–884). Cham, Switzerland: Springer International.

Wagner, L., Sweet, J., Butt, Z., Lai, J., & Cella, D. (2009). Measuring patient self-reported cognitive function: Development of the Functional Assessment of Cancer Therapy–Cognitive function instrument. *Journal of Supportive Oncology, 7*, W32–W39.

Acute Inpatient Rehabilitation

Brent Braveman, OTR, PhD, FAOTA

11

LEARNING OBJECTIVES

After completing this chapter, readers should be able to
- Define and explain the purpose of acute inpatient rehabilitation for cancer survivors and
- Describe the occupational therapy process as applied to acute inpatient rehabilitation for cancer survivors.

KEY TERMS AND CONCEPTS

- Acute inpatient rehabilitation
- Cancer rehabilitation
- Comprehensive cancer rehabilitation
- Habits
- Inpatient rehabilitation facilities
- Interprofessional team
- Motor skills
- Occupational profile
- Process skills
- Social interaction skills

INTRODUCTION

Many cancer survivors who would benefit from comprehensive oncology rehabilitation services do not receive them despite the fact that oncology survivors can suffer from a number of debilitating impairments that have functional implications that make discharge home from acute care unsafe (Fu et al., 2017). There are only a few acute inpatient rehabilitation units specifically for cancer survivors in the United States, and although survivors may be admitted to noncancer-specific programs, there are challenges, which are be described later in this chapter. Most of the cancer-specific acute rehabilitation units are focused on adults. Pediatric cancer survivors may receive acute inpatient rehabilitation at organizations that provide services to clients with a range of diagnoses.

Acute inpatient rehabilitation may be provided on rehabilitation units located in a larger hospital or in inpatient rehabilitation facilities (IRFs), which are hospitals focused solely on rehabilitation services. In addition, inpatient services may be provided in skilled nursing facilities (SNFs) and long-term acute care hospitals (LTACHs). This chapter describes occupational services provided in acute inpatient rehabilitation settings. Because other chapters in this text go into depth on approaches to clinical intervention, this chapter describes the types of services provided to cancer survivors in acute inpatient rehabilitation settings and some of the challenges and opportunities in these settings but does not go into detail on specific intervention strategies.

WHAT IS ACUTE INPATIENT REHABILITATION?

Acute inpatient rehabilitation is a phase of care provided along the rehabilitation continuum that is commonly recognized as distinct from general acute medical care or long-term care provided in an SNF or LTACH. Acute inpatient rehabilitation is typically provided in an IRF or on an acute rehabilitation unit in a larger hospital or organization. The Centers for Medicare and Medicaid Services (2012) defines *inpatient rehabilitation facilities* as "free-standing rehabilitation hospitals and rehabilitation units in acute care hospitals. They provide an intensive rehabilitation program and patients who are admitted must be able to tolerate 3 hours of intense rehabilitation services per day" (para. 2).

What Is Cancer Rehabilitation?

Cancer rehabilitation is becoming more prevalent and accessible; however, there can be great variation in the types of rehabilitative services available to cancer survivors. It is helpful for occupational therapy practitioners to be aware of these variations and to appreciate what is included in comprehensive care. *Comprehensive cancer rehabilitation* is

a multi-disciplinary effort to optimize quality of life and functioning in physical, social, and vocational domains. The occupational therapist works with patients to maximize the ability to fulfill social roles and perform personally relevant basic and instrumental ADLs, despite challenges created by cancer, its treatment, or other co-morbidities. The physical therapist specializes in reducing musculoskeletal impairment and works on improving mobility and muscle strength, flexibility, balance and endurance needed to be mobile. Speech and language pathologists work on skills needed for communication, production of words, and pronunciations as well as swallowing, and swallowing techniques. The physiatrist is a physician specializing in rehabilitation medicine who uses medication and physical modalities to address pain and musculoskeletal impairments. (Pergolotti et al., 2018, p. 544)

Silver et al. (2015) proposed the following definition of *cancer rehabilitation:*

Cancer rehabilitation is medical care that should be integrated throughout the oncology care continuum and delivered by trained rehabilitation professionals who have it within their scope of practice to diagnose and treat patients' physical, psychological and cognitive impairments in an effort to maintain or restore function, reduce symptom burden, maximize independence and improve quality of life in this medically complex population. (p. 3636)

Who Benefits From Inpatient Cancer Rehabilitation?

Not all cancer survivors are suited for acute inpatient cancer rehabilitation. Payers require that patients admitted to inpatient rehabilitation need 3 hours of intensive rehabilitation services per day. Many cancer survivors can maintain independence in basic ADLs and IADLs during and after active treatment even if they experience significant challenges such as cancer-related fatigue (CRF), cancer-related cognitive impairment (CRCI), and chemotherapy-induced peripheral neuropathy (CIPN). However, some survivors experience significant challenges to daily function and independence that warrant an inpatient admission, such as those experiencing primary brain cancer; metastasis to bone or brain; cancerous tumors of the spine or metastasis causing spinal cord injury; those having hemipelvectomy for sarcoma; and complex bone cancer, including orthopedic surgeries (Fu et al., 2017). The approaches to and strategies for providing these patients acute inpatient rehabilitation have much in common with others admitted to similar settings, but what sets them apart are the complications that come with having cancer.

One potential barrier for admission to inpatient rehabilitation is that inpatient rehabilitation programs that participate in Medicare are required to document that no less than 60% of patients are consistent with 1 of 13 specific conditions. Cancer is not technically included within these diagnoses, although several cancer conditions can be categorized as compliant with Medicare regulations (Silver et al., 2018). Cancer survivors may also be admitted if they meet other requirements for inpatient rehabilitation as long as the organization remains compliant with the 60% rule.

Cancer survivors who are admitted for acute inpatient rehabilitation must meet several criteria that are applied to any acute inpatient rehabilitation candidate (Fu et al., 2017):

- Care must be reasonable and necessary.
- Care must be provided by multiple disciplines, and one must be occupational therapy or physical therapy.
- Care must be intensive (at least 3 hours per day and at least 5 days per week).
- The rehabilitation patient must actively participate, and significant benefit must be anticipated.
- Care must be provided in a coordinated interprofessional team approach.
- A rehabilitation physician must supervise care at least 3 days per week.

Interprofessional Care

As in prehabilitation and other comprehensive rehabilitation programs, acute inpatient rehabilitation requires a broad *interprofessional team.* In addition to occupational therapy practitioners, team members include physical therapists, nurses, pharmacists, nutritionists, case managers, and an oncologist, physiatrist, or a gerontologist (similar to prehabilitation). In addition, inpatient acute rehabilitation settings may offer social work services, psychological treatment, counseling, and spiritual care.

Interventions are typically offered on a one-on-one basis, but unlike prehabilitation and many acute care settings, group therapy services are often provided. Because payers have specific requirements for acute inpatient rehabilitation, an interprofessional plan of care including interprofessional goals may be required. Although collaboration between professions is common in many settings, there is often the explicit expectation that it will occur and be documented as such in acute inpatient rehabilitation.

Occupations

Inherent in the purpose of acute inpatient rehabilitation is the promotion of return to preadmission occupational performance and participation to the fullest extent possible. This means heavy reliance on occupation-based intervention. Areas of ADLs, IADLs, and rest and sleep are typically emphasized in goals and interprofessional care plans for adults. Time is often spent on bathing, dressing, grooming, bed and wheelchair mobility, meal preparation, laundry, medication management, and other areas of self-care and home management.

Education, work, play, leisure, and social participation are also typically addressed; however, because some payers do not directly reimburse for services in medical model settings (e.g., acute inpatient rehabilitation) that emphasize returning cancer survivors to the workplace, schools, or leisure roles, these occupations may not be the expressed focus of intervention. In acute inpatient rehabilitation for children, age-appropriate play occupations are chosen to promote mobility, learn problem-solving skills, and strengthen body systems and structures. Children may also receive additional support from a child-life specialist to promote continued involvement in educational activities (Child Life Council & Committee on Hospital Care, 2006).

Client Factors

A cancer survivor's values, beliefs, and spirituality, including their perceived self-efficacy, can heavily influence the outcome of rehabilitation. It is critically important that occupational therapy practitioners learn what is most important to our clients and understand how the course of their cancer journey has affected these beliefs. Practitioners can incorporate assessments that focus on values and beliefs and employ approaches to client interaction that promote the sharing of life narratives to further understand what is most important to cancer survivors and their caregivers.

Occupational therapy practitioners must recognize the critical interchange among client factors and performance skills, performance patterns, contexts and environments, and occupational performance and participation. Although changes in body functions (e.g., sensory, musculoskeletal, mental, cardiovascular, respiratory, endocrine) and body structures (e.g., those of the eyes, ears, voice, skin, and nervous, cardiovascular, respiratory, digestive, metabolic, reproductive systems) do not automatically mean there will be changes in performance, such changes are common.

Performance Skills

Cancer and its treatments can have a great negative effect on performance skills, including motor skills, process skills, and social interaction skills. *Motor skills* are defined as "occupational performance skills observed as the person interacts with and moves task objects and self around the task environment" (e.g., ADL motor skills, school motor skills; Boyt Schell et al., 2014a, p. 1237). *Process skills* are defined as "occupational performance skills [e.g., ADL process skills, school process skills] observed as a person (1) selects, interacts with, and uses task tools and materials; (2) carries out individual actions and steps; and (3) modifies performance when problems are encountered" (Boyt Schell et al., 2014, p. 1239). *Social interaction skills* are defined as "occupational performance skills observed during the ongoing stream of a social exchange" (Boyt Schell et al., 2014, p. 1241).

Depending on the cancer's location and staging, motor and process skills can be affected if structures and functions of the brain, nervous system, eyes, or ears are affected. Cancer treatments, including chemotherapy, radiation, and others, can also cause problems such as CIPN that can affect motor skills or CRCI that can affect cognitive and process skills. Challenges in body image, sense of self-efficacy, or identity may affect social skills. Occupational therapy intervention in cancer rehabilitation may seek to establish and restore motor, process, and social interaction skills, or modify occupations, their contexts and environments, or their task demands to promote improved performance through adaptation or compensation (American Occupational Therapy Association [AOTA], 2014).

Performance Patterns

Examination of a cancer survivor's habits, routines, rituals, and roles is central to occupational therapy intervention in acute inpatient rehabilitation, as it should be in any setting.

Habits are automatic behaviors performed repeatedly that can support or interfere with occupational performance. Occupational therapy practitioners can promote the adoption of new habits to promote safety, such as consistently locking and checking wheelchair brakes before the initiation of a transfer or checking one's skin each morning and evening during ADLs for early signs of skin breakdown.

Daily routines may require alteration, and understanding the cancer process and the impact of cancer treatments helps practitioners in acute inpatient rehabilitation settings provide intervention that specifically addresses the needs of cancer survivors. For example, alterations in ADL routines such as showering at the end of the day instead of the beginning may lessen the negative impact of CRF.

New routines may be anticipated postdischarge if the cancer survivor must continue with active cancer treatment. Children can experience significant disruption of daily routines because their treatment may require prolonged absences from school or limited social contact as a result of concerns over infections and compromised immune systems. Occupational therapy practitioners can assist survivors and caregivers in preparing for the demands of these routines. In this way, acute inpatient rehabilitation for cancer survivors may be similar to rehabilitation for other populations of patients with chronic illnesses.

To some extent, occupational therapy practitioners can assume that the examination of roles is inherent in the occupational therapy process, including development of the occupational profile. However, a challenge in acute inpatient rehabilitation is that because of limitations placed by payers and reimbursement sources, all roles of the cancer survivor may not receive the same level of attention. Payment for acute inpatient rehabilitation focuses heavily on ADLs, IADLs, and interventions designed to promote increased independence, allowing discharge to the least restrictive environment possible (e.g., home rather than long-term care). This means that roles highly important to an individual cancer survivor, such as student, worker, grandparent, pet owner, or artist, may not be emphasized in rehabilitative goals if addressed at all.

Creative intervention may allow occupational therapy practitioners to incorporate these roles, such as using pet care to apply energy conservation and work simplification techniques for a survivor learning strategies to combat CRF. Addressing roles such as that of worker may be indicative of clear gaps in rehabilitative care that need continued exploration (see Chapter 25, "Work," for more information on work).

Context and Environment

As with any inpatient setting, occupational therapy practitioners in acute inpatient rehabilitation must consider the cultural, personal, physical, social, temporal, and virtual contexts and environments of both the hospital setting and the discharge setting (e.g., home, a long-term care setting). Most acute inpatient rehabilitation settings have understandable limitations to providing contextually and environmentally valid occupational therapy intervention. Although many facilities have functioning ovens, stovetops, dishwashers, and washers and dryers, it is impossible to replicate everyone's home. Limitations in the number, shape, size, weight, and color of objects used in ADLs, IADLs, play, and other areas of occupation are also to be expected. Still, even in the smallest or most resource-challenged organization, occupational therapy practitioners can alter the context and environment to some extent to simulate the discharge location to provide occupation-based interventions. The social environment in the inpatient setting is dramatically different because contact with family and friends may be limited and socialization may be entrenched in medical procedures and with medical caregivers. Use of the virtual environment is one primary strategy for helping cancer survivors maintain social contacts.

Assessing the home environment is challenging without the ability to conduct an onsite home evaluation. However, virtual home visits using a range of applications available on smartphones and tablets or having caregivers provide pictures of the home environment can help occupational therapy practitioners gain a clearer picture of the home or discharge setting. Exploring cultural and personal contexts and social environments for postdischarge occupational performance with cancer survivors and their caregivers helps promote carryover of strategies learned in the inpatient setting.

Occupational Performance and Participation

Although the primary goal of acute inpatient rehabilitation is to promote both improved occupational performance and participation, intervention in acute inpatient rehabilitation may favor a focus on occupational performance. However, practitioners must remember that improving occupational performance as evidenced by improved ability to perform ADLs or IADLs does not automatically translate to fuller participation. Full participation in social roles such as worker or parent is complex, and many cancer survivors will experience treatment-related sequela well after treatment stops. Ness et al. (2006) conducted one of the largest population-based studies on this topic and found that 31% of both recent (<5 years postdiagnosis) and long-term cancer survivors reported restrictions in their ability to participate in roles and life situations. Influencing full participation may be difficult, given the relatively short lengths of stay—typically less than 2 weeks—for cancer survivors in acute inpatient rehabilitation (Gallegos-Kearin et al., 2018). Connecting cancer survivors to community-based resources, including survivorship programs and outpatient rehabilitation programs, can help move survivors toward fuller participation.

Occupational Therapy Process in Inpatient Rehabilitation

Evaluation

Acute inpatient rehabilitation stays are marked by an intensive evaluation process resulting in an interprofessional plan of care. Occupational therapy evaluations typically focus on ADLs, IADLs, body systems, and body structures as they relate to function, the need for assistive and adaptive equipment, and the common effects of cancer and its treatments on functional independence. All areas of function are typically screened, and then discrete assessment approaches are used to gather more detailed information on areas where there are suspected deficits.

For example, an occupational therapist may screen a cancer survivor for cognitive deficits using a tool such as the Functional Assessment of Cancer Therapy–Cognitive (FACT–Cog) Version 3 (Wagner et al., 2009), but if no deficits are reported, a more formal assessment may be forgone (Cella, 2016). However, if deficits are suspected, assessments such as the Executive Function Performance Test (Baum et al., 2003), the Multiple Errands Test (Knight et al., 2002), or the Children's Kitchen Task Assessment (Rocke et al., 2008) may be used. Similarly, most survivors are screened for sensory and motor changes. If a screen of sensation appears within normal limits and full active range of motion is present, formal sensory testing or manual muscle testing may not be necessary. If sensory, motor, or neurological deficits are present, then formal testing may be implemented.

Over the past few decades, the lengths of stay for acute inpatient rehabilitation have decreased; the average stay for cancer survivors is just under 2 weeks. For this reason, the evaluation process and intervention implementation are often blended from the first session because there is not time to spend several days focused only on evaluation. Initial treatment plans and interprofessional goals are normally completed within the first 72 hours after admission. The pressure from short lengths of stay has helped promote adoption of more occupation- and functional-based evaluation; for example, sessions focused on bathing, dressing, grooming, or bed mobility and transfers are used for both baseline assessment and introduction of adaptive techniques or assistive devices as intervention.

Occupational profile

Developing a clear occupational profile and understanding the occupational roles that a cancer survivor performs out of the hospital are critical for choosing occupations for use in interventions that hold both meaning and purpose for the survivor. The *occupational profile* also calls for an understanding of "patterns of daily living, interests, values and needs" (AOTA, 2014, p. S10). The cancer survivor's reason for seeking services, strength and concerns in relation to performing occupations and daily life activities, areas of potential occupational disruption, supports and barriers, and priorities are also identified.

Because of relatively short lengths of stay, wise choices must be made about how to spend time in assessment, but use of strategies such as the Revised Role Checklist (Scott et al., 2019), the Occupational Self-Assessment (Baron et al., 2006), or elements of narrative interviewing can be incorporated in early sessions and can facilitate an understanding of the survivor's life outside of the hospital. It is important to include the survivor's caregivers in the assessment process to understand their concerns and priorities. Tools such as the AOTA Occupational Profile Template can aid efficient documentation of a cancer survivor's occupational profile (AOTA, 2017).

Analysis of occupational performance

A wide range of assessments can be used to assess occupational performance. Such assessments can include observational

CASE EXAMPLE 11.1. DEREK: ADOLESCENT ACUTE INPATIENT REHABILITATION

Derek is a 19-year-old male with a history of glioblastoma multiforme of the brain. This fast-growing glioma develops in the glial cells that support the health of the brain's nerve cells. Before his diagnosis, Derek was a varsity athlete who played soccer, track, football, and baseball. He was highly active and social with friends and family and was preparing to begin a biology degree in hopes of one day becoming an anesthesiologist. Derek lives with his parents, has three dogs that he was responsible for walking, was driving, and helped with chores around the home. He completed whole brain radiation and chemotherapy before referral for occupational therapy as part of acute inpatient rehabilitation. He was seen for his initial evaluation on postoperative Day 1 after a right posterior craniotomy with decompression.

Upon evaluation, Derek presented with left hemiplegia, left inattention, impaired proprioception, significant fatigue, impaired visual acuity (to include double vision), and impaired standing and sitting balance. He had low insight into his impairments, was a high fall risk, and had no history of engagement in occupational therapy. Derek and his parents were highly concerned about Derek safely returning to their home environment. Concern was also expressed surrounding Derek's ability to return to leisure activities without constant supervision. Derek's parents and extended family were very quick to offer aid to Derek in lieu of his performing activities alone.

Occupational therapy intervention began with developing an occupational profile and administering multiple assessments to obtain baseline data for the creation of therapeutic interventions. (See Table 11.1 for a list of assessments used and the foci of information gleaned from each assessment.)

TABLE 11.1. Sample Assessments Used in Inpatient Rehabilitation and Assessment Data for Derek

ASSESSMENT	DESCRIPTION	SUMMARY OF RESULTS FOR DEREK
Functional Independence Measure (Uniform Data System for Medical Rehabilitation, 2012)	An assessment tool containing 18 items (13 motor and 5 cognitive) that provides measures of functional status throughout the rehabilitation process; scored on a scale of 7 (complete independence) to 1 (complete dependence)	Moderate assistance for UB/LB bathing and LB dressing; minimal assistance with grooming and feeding tasks; maximum assistance with toileting
Brief Fatigue Inventory (Mendoza et al., 1999)	Short assessment of the severity of fatigue experienced over the past 24 hours and its impact on function	Global average fatigue of 7/10 over the past 24 hours; fatigue is rated as significantly affecting performance and engagement in normal activities
Wong-Baker FACES Scale (Wong-Baker Faces Foundation, 2016)	Uses pictures to express *no hurt* to *worst hurt*	No pain throughout assessment
Activity Measure for Post-Acute Care Short Forms for Inpatient and Outpatient Settings (Jette et al., 2015)	Examination of activity limitations in functional activities likely encountered every day	Overall score of 14/24 on the Daily Activity Inpatient Short Form, requiring "a lot" of help to complete bathing, toileting, and LB dressing, and "a little" help for grooming
Functional manual muscle testing	Assessment of passive and active range of motion that can be performed on single muscle groups or functionally to assess multiple muscle groups in functional movement	Normal AROM in RUE/LE, normal PROM to LUE/LE, active shoulder flexion to 90° with short ability to maintain statically, 50° of active shoulder abduction
Observational assessment of BADLs, bed mobility, functional mobility, and transfers	Assessment through observation during performance of activities (e.g., rolling from side to side, sitting at the edge of the bed, transferring, performing ADL and IADL tasks in context)	Derek required moderate assistance for LB dressing, bathing, and toileting. Demonstrated grooming with setup. Unable to engage in IADL routine during assessment due to fatigue. He managed bed mobility with moderate assistance and short-distance mobility with minimal assistance within bathroom with cues for scanning of environment.

(Continued)

(Continued)

CASE EXAMPLE 11.1. DEREK: ADOLESCENT ACUTE INPATIENT REHABILITATION *(Cont.)*

TABLE 11.1.   Sample Assessments Used in Inpatient Rehabilitation and Assessment Data for Derek *(Cont.)*

ASSESSMENT	DESCRIPTION	SUMMARY OF RESULTS FOR DEREK
Durable medical equipment assessment	Assessment of equipment needs for mobility, ADLs, and IADLs during performance of functional tasks in an environment that is as similar to the home environment as possible	Initial needs identified included: ▪ Shower chair ▪ Adaptive feeding utensils ▪ Supportive sling for functional use of LUE

Note. ADLs = activities of daily living; AROM = active range of motion; BADLs = basic activities of daily living; IADLs = instrumental activities of daily living; LB = lower body; LE = left extremity; LUE = left upper extremity; PROM = passive range of motion; RUE = right upper extremity; UB = upper body.

Derek's primary complaint was fatigue, and he required increased time for arousal at the start of intervention sessions and throughout task engagement. The occupational therapist noted that he required multiple seated rest periods over the first week of intervention to allow engagement. Derek's family, particularly his mother, was very concerned with his hygiene, and he took daily showers with the assistance of the nursing staff, further adding to his fatigue. This limited his ability to complete therapy. Despite recent surgical intervention, Derek's pain was manageable and continued to improve. The primary problem list identified by the occupational therapy team in conjunction with Derek and his parents included:

▪ Decreased independence in ADLs (i.e., feeding, grooming, toileting, upper- and lower-body dressing, bathing);
▪ Decreased bed, wheelchair, and functional mobility within home, and decreased community mobility;
▪ Cancer-related fatigue (CRF);
▪ Left-side hemiparesis limiting functional ADL engagement; and
▪ Impaired visual acuity and left inattention affecting self-care, mobility, and leisure engagement, and safety.

The occupational therapist met with Derek and his parents, and they identified the following goals for his inpatient stay. At discharge, Derek will demonstrate:

▪ Modified independence in upper extremity/lower extremity (UE/LE) bathing with use of adaptive equipment;
▪ Modified independence with UE/LE dressing in seated position;
▪ Modified independence with functional mobility to include bed, wheelchair, toilet, and shower transfers and home and community mobility with improved safety and scanning of environment for fall prevention;
▪ Modified independence with grooming with improved bimanual integration; and
▪ Modified independence with self-feeding with adaptive equipment and techniques.

Derek participated in occupational therapy daily Monday–Friday for 60 minutes and on Saturdays for 30–45 minutes. In addition, he was seen by physical therapy to address his mobility and fatigue, and speech-language pathology to address cognitive dysfunction related to his cancer and his surgery. Derek was followed closely by his neuro-oncologist, and a physiatrist coordinated his rehabilitative care. He also received care from a case manager, who helped order and arrange insurance coverage for durable medical equipment, and a social worker, who provided Derek and his family psychosocial support.

Derek tolerated therapy sessions well and made great gains, qualifying him for an inpatient rehabilitation stay. Derek was transferred to an acute rehabilitation floor for further focus on meeting his goals through three 1-hour therapy sessions daily after 10 days on his acute surgical unit. During his rehabilitation, Derek and his parents further focused their efforts on safe patient handling, adaptive equipment usage, dynamic balance for safety in the home, and visual scanning for ease of mobility at both the wheelchair and ambulatory level.

Derek was discharged home after an additional week's stay at inpatient rehabilitation, having reached his goals for discharge. He was referred for occupational therapy and physical therapy on an outpatient basis. In addition, the occupational therapist provided Derek and his family the following recommendations:

▪ Continued supervision when ambulating in home for fall prevention;
▪ Consistent use of energy conservation and fatigue management techniques to assist with sleep–wake cycles, CRF, and decreased endurance; and
▪ Use of adaptive equipment in the home for safety and fall prevention, including:
  □ Wheelchair with 2-inch foam cushion,
  □ Tub transfer bench, long-handled sponge,
  □ Built-up utensils, and
  □ Dressing equipment (e.g., dressing stick, sock aid, elastic shoelaces, shoehorn, reacher).

Acknowledgment given to Donna Kelly for contribution to this case.

CASE EXAMPLE 11.2. WALTER: INPATIENT REHABILITATION

Walter is a 52-year-old father of three children, ages 12, 9, and 5 years, who was admitted to the acute inpatient rehabilitation unit with a diagnosis of an intramedullary spinal cord tumor at the T5 level. He was admitted after a 5-day stay on an acute medical surgical unit where he underwent resection of the tumor. His cancer is being treated with chemotherapy, and he and his neurological oncology team are assessing whether to also treat him with radiation. Walter was admitted for intensive acute inpatient rehabilitation with an estimated length of stay of 10 days.

Walter presents with paraplegia with greatly reduced active range of motion in both lower extremities (LEs) and complains of some upper-extremity (UE) weakness as well, although he reports being able to complete his normal occupations that require only UEs such as feeding and grooming. Walter is familiar with rehabilitative services and is eager to participate. He has collaborated with the rehabilitation team to develop his goals and interprofessional plan of care. He has also been participating in occupational therapy and physical therapy on the acute care unit and has been making slow but steady progress on goals for mobility and self-care.

The occupational therapist begins by developing an occupational profile and administering a range of assessments to obtain baseline data (see Table 11.2 for a list of assessments used and the foci of information gleaned from each assessment).

Walter complains of significant fatigue and of spinal pain and pain down his left leg; he also notes that pain increases with movement. He can control his hospital bed independently and manages sheets and blankets using a reacher and dressing stick given to him on the acute care unit, but the occupational therapist and occupational therapy assistant working with Walter note that he fatigues quickly and needs multiple short breaks.

TABLE 11.2. Sample Assessments Used in Inpatient Rehabilitation and Assessment Data for Walter

ASSESSMENT	DESCRIPTION	SUMMARY OF RESULTS FOR WALTER
Functional Independence Measure (Uniform Data System for Medical Rehabilitation, 2012)	An assessment tool containing 18 items (13 motor and 5 cognitive) that provides measures of functional status throughout the rehabilitation process; scored on a scale of 7 (complete independence) to 1 (complete dependence)	Modified independence on eating and grooming; moderate assistance on bathing and LE dressing; minimal assistance on UE dressing
Brief Fatigue Inventory (Mendoza et al., 1999)	Short assessment of the severity of fatigue experienced over the past 24 hours and its impact on function	Global average fatigue of 3/10 over the past 24 hours. He rates his fatigue as having little interference with his mood and relations with other people but as significantly interfering with normal activities and somewhat interfering with his enjoyment of life (e.g., 4/10).
Visual analog scale for pain	Visual or spoken scales for rating pain (e.g., 0 = *no pain* to 10 = *worst pain imaginable*; Wong–Baker FACES Scale [Wong-Baker FACES Foundation, 2016] that uses pictures to express *no hurt* to *worst hurt*)	3/10 at rest, and 6/10 during active movement such as transfers
Activity Measure for Post-Acute Care Short Forms for Inpatient and Outpatient Settings (Jette et al., 2015)	Examines activity limitations in functional activities likely encountered every day	Overall score of 17/24 on the Daily Activity Inpatient Short Form, requiring "a lot" of help to don and doff LB clothing and for bathing and toileting; "a little" for donning and doffing UB clothing; and "none" for grooming and eating meals
Functional manual muscle testing	Assessment of PROM and AROM that can be performed on single muscle groups or functionally to assess multiple muscle groups in functional movement (e.g., Can you raise your arms above your head like you are putting on a shirt?)	Normal PROM in UE and LE. No AROM in bilateral LEs. Score 4 of 5 in both UE for all AROM with full range of movement noted but strength is slightly less than normal limits for his age.

(Continued)

(Continued)

CASE EXAMPLE 11.2. WALTER: INPATIENT REHABILITATION *(Cont.)*

TABLE 11.2.   Sample Assessments Used in Inpatient Rehabilitation and Assessment Data for Walter *(Cont.)*

ASSESSMENT	DESCRIPTION	SUMMARY OF RESULTS FOR WALTER
Observational assessment of BADLs, bed mobility, and transfers	Assessment through observation during performance of activities (e.g., rolling from side to side in bed, sitting at the edge of the bed, transferring, bathing, dressing, completing IADL tasks in context)	Manages bed sheets independently and is independent in feeding, grooming, and UE bathing and dressing. Needs moderate assistance with LE bathing and dressing using equipment. Demonstrates good problem solving in IADLs (laundry and basic meal prep) with adaptive equipment. Moderate assistance with transfers with sliding board. Fatigues quickly and complains of pain. Complains of feeling "foggy" and forgetful, sometimes momentarily forgetting how to perform familiar activities.
DME assessment	Assessment of equipment needs for mobility, ADLs, and IADLs during performance of functional tasks in an environment that is as similar to the home environment as possible	Initial needs identified: ▪ Lightweight manual wheelchair ▪ Wheelchair cushion ▪ Sliding board ▪ Tub bench ▪ Bedside commode (for use until planned bathroom renovations are completed)

Note. ADLs = activities of daily living; AROM = active range of motion; BADLs = basic activities of daily living; DME = durable medical equipment; IADLs = instrumental activities of daily living; LB = lower body; LE = lower extremity; PROM = passive range of motion; UB = upper body; UE = upper extremity.

Intervention begins immediately and is combined with ongoing assessment over the first 2 days of stay. The primary problems identified by the occupational therapy team in conjunction with Walter includes

- Decreased independence in ADLs (UE and LE bathing and dressing) and IADLs (Walter is an active father who shares child care and household responsibilities with his wife, including grocery shopping, meal preparation, laundry, cleaning, pet care);
- Decreased bed, wheelchair, and community mobility;
- Cancer-related fatigue (CRF); and
- Pain (rated 3 out of 10 at rest and 6 out of 10 during active movement such as transfers).

The occupational therapist meets with Walter and his wife, and together they identify the following goals for his inpatient stay. At discharge, Walter will demonstrate

- Modified independence in upper extremity/lower extremity (UE/LE) bathing, including wheelchair-to-tub-bench transfers;
- Modified independence in UE/LE dressing at bed level;
- Independence in bed-to-wheelchair/wheelchair-to-bed and wheelchair-to-tub-bench/tub-bench-to-wheelchair transfers;
- Needing minimal assistance with wheelchair-to-car/car-to-wheelchair transfers using a sliding board;
- Needing minimal assistance with simple meal preparation and laundry from the wheelchair; and

- Application of energy conservation and work simplification strategies to BADLs with cueing.

Walter is in occupational therapy treatment for 60–90 minutes Monday through Friday and for 60 minutes on Saturday and Sunday. In addition, he is seen daily by physical therapy to address his mobility, fatigue, and pain, and by speech–language pathology to address symptoms of chemotherapy-induced cognitive impairment. He is followed closely by his neuro-oncologist, and his rehabilitative care is coordinated by a physiatrist. He also receives care from a case manager who helps order and arrange insurance coverage for durable medical equipment (DME), a social worker who provides Walter and his wife psychosocial support and helps with resources for child care and transportation, and a nutritionist who works with Walter to find foods that he enjoys and can tolerate because he is developing some mucositis as a side effect of his chemotherapy.

In many regards, Walter's occupational therapy intervention on the inpatient rehabilitation unit is much like the intervention that anyone with functional paraplegia would receive on any inpatient rehabilitation unit. His occupational therapy intervention is heavily focused on improving independence in ADLs by using adaptive equipment and DME (e.g., wheelchair, sliding board, reacher, sock assist, dressing stick, long-handled sponge, tub bench). Walter and his wife receive education and training on assistive equipment use and

(Continued)

CASE EXAMPLE 11.2. WALTER: INPATIENT REHABILITATION *(Cont.)*

adaptive techniques for ADLs and IADLs. They learn strategies to manage Walter's CRF and are introduced to energy-conservation and work-simplification techniques. Walter's wife uses a tablet to record a tour of their home; the occupational therapy assistant uses the video to suggest strategies for CRF and pain management when Walter returns to their home. The occupational therapy team completes a full DME assessment in collaboration with Walter, his wife, and the rest of the rehabilitation team, and initial recommendations are provided. Walter agrees that a lightweight manual wheelchair and gel skin protective cushion are appropriate, and orders are placed for this equipment along with a sliding board.

Walter's care continues as expected with one complication. On Day 8 of Walter's stay, he complains of significantly increased spinal and LE pain that he describes as a 9 out of 10 during bed-to-wheelchair transfers, and he notes that the pain continues at a lesser level for at least 1 hour after strong exertion. The neuro-oncologist and physiatrist receive a consultation from the pain team, and some adjustments to Walter's medications are made. However, Walter finds transfers more difficult and at times is hesitant to get out of bed to participate in therapy. The team, including Walter and his spouse, agree that his

stay will be extended for 2 days. Moreover, as part of the standard process of intervention review, the occupational therapy team, Walter, and his wife decide to revise the goals for discharge to include requiring minimal assistance for all LE ADLs and transfers. Although frustrated by the need for physical assistance, Walter finds that he experiences less pain when he accepts assistance with LE ADLs and transfers, and in turn, he has less fatigue and a lower level of enduring pain as he proceeds with his day.

Walter is discharged on Day 12, having reached his modified goals for discharge. He and his spouse receive the following recommendations:

- Outpatient occupational therapy, physical therapy, and speech–language pathology three times per week for 3 weeks;
- Continued education and training in strategies for CRF, pain reduction, work simplification, energy conservation, and compensatory strategies for cognitive dysfunction; and
- Development of a home program to promote and maintain UE/LE strength and range of motion.

Acknowledgment given to Sandra Beals for contribution to this case.

---

assessment during ADLs or IADLs, or administration of standardized and nonstandardized assessments. The two case studies in this chapter include tables highlighting a few commonly used assessments in acute inpatient rehabilitation.

A commonly used assessment in acute inpatient rehabilitation is the Functional Independence Measure (FIM; Uniform Data System for Medical Rehabilitation, 2012). The FIM assesses the burden of care because the use of any form of assistive or adaptive equipment lowers the score from 7 (independent) to 6 (modified independence). The FIM is a reliable and valid 18-item observational sheet and interview schedule for collecting data on the patients' degree of functional independence in various areas of everyday life (Uniform Data System for Medical Rehabilitation, 2012). Each of the patient's activities (eating, grooming, bladder management, social interaction, etc.) is rated between 1 (totally dependent) and 7 (fully independent; Valach & Selz, 2017, p. 173). The FIM is often used to justify admission to an acute inpatient rehabilitation program and is also used to measure the outcomes, effectiveness, and efficiency of rehabilitation programs (Cournan, 2011). The FIM is commonly used in acute inpatient rehabilitation with cancer survivors (Brunello et al., 2018; Pergolotti et al., 2016; Saotome et al., 2015).

On July 31, 2018, the Centers for Medicare and Medicaid Services (CMS) issued a final rule outlining changes on how Medicare reimburses inpatient rehabilitation facilities (IRFs). The rule resulted in removal of the FIM and associated function modifiers from the Inpatient Rehabilitation Patient Assessment Instrument (IRF–PAI; AOTA, 2018; CMS, n.d.). This change was made because CMS began collecting new quality indicator data elements in the IRF–PAI. Some of these elements duplicated elements of the FIM and

associated function modifiers. For discharges after October 1, 2019 the FIM is no longer required. Despite this, the FIM continues to be a widely used functional outcome assessment and is stilled required by some payers to justify admission to an acute inpatient rehabilitation unit or facility.

Intervention

Intervention for cancer survivors in acute inpatient rehabilitation is similar to intervention for most any other population. Although each population has specific needs, acute inpatient rehabilitation focuses on improving function in mobility (e.g., bed mobility, transfers, ambulation if appropriate), self-care, and other areas of occupation to allow survivors to return to their home or the community. Specific interventions for cancer survivors may include those outlined in depth in Section IV of this text, "Sequelae of Cancer and Intervention Across the Lifespan." These include interventions for pain; fatigue; chemotherapy-induced cognitive dysfunction; lymphedema; CIPN; and psychosocial issues, including depression, anxiety, and body image.

Targeting Outcomes

Targeting outcomes involves "selecting types of outcomes and measures, including but not limited to related to occupational performance, prevention, health and wellness, quality of life, participation, role competence, well-being, and occupational justice" (AOTA, 2014, p. S16). As you might imagine from earlier discussion, the targeted outcomes in acute inpatient rehabilitation are typically focused on role competence (e.g., occupational performance) to meet payers' expectations. However, inclusion of measures related to quality of life and participation are highly encouraged because these outcomes and measures best reflect the important and distinct value of occupational therapy practitioners as members of the cancer rehabilitation team. Case Example 11.1 describes the inpatient rehabilitation process with a young adult with glioblastoma multiforme of the brain and Case Example 11.2 describes the rehabilitation process with an adult with a spinal cord tumor.

SUMMARY

Cancer survivors experiencing functional deficits and decreased occupational performance and participation because of cancer or its treatments may benefit from acute inpatient rehabilitation. Occupational therapy practitioners function as part of an interprofessional team but make distinct contributions toward improving the health, function, well-being, and participation of cancer survivors.

Although much of prehabilitation and acute inpatient rehabilitation may focus on occupational performance, occupational therapy practitioners have opportunities to influence the participation of cancer survivors in their existing social roles by connecting survivors with resources in the community and through intervention to address the full range of challenges experienced by survivors.

REFERENCES

American Occupational Therapy Association. (2014). Occupational therapy practice framework: Domain and process (3rd ed.). *American Journal of Occupational Therapy, 68*(Suppl.1), S1–S48. http://doi.org/10.5014/ajot.2014.682006

American Occupational Therapy Association. (2017). Occupational profile template. *American Journal of Occupational Therapy, 71,* 7112420030. https://doi.org/10.5014/ajot.2017.716S12

American Occupational Therapy Association. (2018). *CMS releases FY 2019 inpatient rehabilitation facility final rule.* Retrieved from https://www.aota.org/Advocacy-Policy/Federal-Reg-Affairs/News/2018/CMS-FY-2019-Inpatient-Rehabilitation-Facility-Final-Rule.aspx

Baron, K., Kielhofner, G., Iyenger, A., Goldhammer, V., & Wolenski, J. (2006). *The Occupational Self-Assessment (version 2.2).* Chicago: Model of Human Occupation Clearinghouse, Department of Occupational Therapy, College of Applied Health Sciences, University of Illinois at Chicago.

Baum, C. M., Morrison, T., Hahn, M., & Edwards, D. F. (2003). *Test manual: Executive Function Performance Test.* St. Louis: Washington University.

Boyt Schell, B. A., Gillen, G., & Scaffa, M. (2014). Glossary. In B. A. Boyt Schell, G. Gillen, & M. Scaffa (Eds.), *Willard and Spackman's occupational therapy* (12th ed., pp. 1229–1243). Philadelphia: Lippincott Williams & Wilkins.

Brunello, A., Lombardi, G., & Zagonel, V. (2018). Rehabilitation treatment in older cancer patients. In S. Masiero & U. Carraro (Eds.), *Rehabilitation medicine for elderly patients* (pp. 503–510). Cham, Switzerland: Springer. https://doi.org/10.1007/978-3-319-57406-6_51

Cella, D. (2016). *Functional Assessment of Cancer Therapy: Cognitive Version.* Retrieved from https://www.facit.org/FACITOrg/Questionnaires

Centers for Medicare & Medicaid Services. (n.d.). *Inpatient Rehabilitation Facility–Patient Assessment Instrument.* Retrieved from https://www.cms.gov/Medicare/CMS-Forms/CMS-Forms/Downloads/CMS10036.pdf

Centers for Medicare & Medicaid Services. (2012). *Inpatient rehabilitation facilities.* Retrieved from https://www.cms.gov/Medicare/Provider-Enrollment-and-Certification/CertificationandComplianc/InpatientRehab.html

Child Life Council & Committee on Hospital Care. (2006). Child life services. *Pediatrics, 118,* 1757–1763. https://doi.org/10.1542/peds.2006-1941

Cournan, M. (2011). Use of the Functional Independence Measure for outcomes measurement in acute inpatient rehabilitation. *Rehabilitation Nursing, 36,* 111–117. https://doi.org/10.1002/j.2048-7940.2011.tb00075.x

Fu, J. B., Raj, V. S., & Guo, Y. (2017). A guide to inpatient cancer rehabilitation: Focusing on patient selection and evidence-based outcomes. *PM&R, 9,* S324–S334. https://doi.org/10.1016/j.pmrj.2017.04.017

Gallegos-Kearin, V., Knowlton, S. E., Goldstein, R., Mix, J., Zafonte, R., Kwan, M., . . . Schneider, J. C. (2018). Outcome trends of adult cancer patients receiving inpatient rehabilitation: A 13-year review. *American Journal of Physical Medicine and Rehabilitation, 97,* 514–522. https://doi.org/10.1097/PHM.0000000000000911

Jette, D. U., Stilphen, M., Ranganathan, V. K., Passek, S., Frost, F. S., & Jette, A. M. (2015). Interrater reliability of AM–PAC "6-Clicks" basic mobility and daily activity short forms. *Physical Therapy, 95,* 758–766.

Knight, C., Alderman, N., & Burgess, P. W. (2002). Development of a simplified version of the multiple errands test for use in hospital settings. *Neuropsychological Rehabilitation, 12,* 231–255. https://doi.org/10.1080/09602010244000039

Mendoza, T. R., Wang, X. S., Cleeland, C. S., Morrissey, M., Johnson, B. A., Wendt, J. K., & Huber, S. L. (1999). The rapid assessment of fatigue severity in cancer patients: Use of the Brief Fatigue Inventory. *Cancer, 85,* 1186–1196. https://doi.org/10.1002/(sici)1097-0142(19990301)85:5<1186::aid-cncr24>3.0.co;2-n

Ness, K. K., Wall, M. M., Oakes, J. M., Robison, L. L., & Gurney, J. G. (2006). Physical performance limitations and participation restrictions among cancer survivors: A population-based study. *Annals of Epidemiology, 16,* 197–205. https://doi.org/10.1016/j.annepidem.2005.01.009

Pergolotti, M., Lyons, K. D., & Williams, G. R. (2018). Moving beyond symptom management towards cancer rehabilitation for older adults: Answering the 5W's. *Journal of Geriatric Oncology, 9,* 543–549. https://doi.org/10.1016/j.jgo.2017.11.009

Pergolotti, M., Williams, G. R., Campbell, C., Munoz, L. A., & Muss, H. B. (2016). Occupational therapy for adults with cancer: Why it matters. *Oncologist, 21,* 314–319. https://doi.org/10.1634/theoncologist.2015-0335

Rocke, K., Hays, P., Edwards, D., & Berg, C. (2008). Development of a performance assessment of executive function: The Children's Kitchen Task Assessment. *American Journal of Occupational Therapy, 62,* 528–537. https://doi.org/10.5014/ajot.62.5.528

Saotome, T., Klein, L., & Faux, S. (2015). Cancer rehabilitation: A barometer for survival? *Supportive Care in Cancer, 23,* 3033–3041. https://doi.org/10.1007/s00520-015-2673-1

Scott, P. J., McKinney, K. G., Perron, J. M., Ruff, E. G., & Smiley, J. L. (2019). The Revised Role Checklist: Improved utility, feasibility, and reliability. *OTJR: Occupation, Participation and Health, 39*, 56–63. https://doi.org/10.1177/1539449218780618

Silver, J. K., Raj, V. S., Fu, J. B., Wisotzky, E. M., Smith, S. R., & Kirch, R. A. (2015). Cancer rehabilitation and palliative care: Critical components in the delivery of high-quality oncology services. *Supportive Care in Cancer, 23*, 3633–3643. https://doi.org/10.1007/s00520-015-2916-1

Silver, J. K., Raj, V. S., & Wisotzky, E. M. (2018). Oncology rehabilitation. In P. Hopewood & M. Milroy (Eds.), *Quality cancer care* (pp. 119–147). Cham, Switzerland: Springer International. https://doi.org/10.1007/978-3-319-78649-0_9

Uniform Data System for Medical Rehabilitation. (2012). *The FIM® Instrument: Its background, structure, and usefulness.* Buffalo: Author.

Valach, L. K., & Selz, B. (2017). Rehabilitation programs monitored by Functional Independence Measure: An observational study. *International Physical Medicine & Rehabilitation Journal, 2*, 173–178. https://doi.org/10.15406/ipmrj.2017.02.00039

Wong-Baker FACES Foundation. (2016). *Wong-Baker FACES history.* Retrieved from https://wongbakerfaces.org/us/wong-baker-faces-history/

12

Survivorship

Robin Newman, OTD, OT, OTR, CLT, FAOTA, and Elizabeth G. Hunter, PhD, OTR/L

LEARNING OBJECTIVES

After completing this chapter, readers should be able to
- Understand the importance of posttreatment as a distinct phase of the cancer continuum;
- Comprehend the role of occupational therapy in cancer survivorship, starting with posttreatment;
- Develop a list of challenges commonly faced by cancer survivors after treatment across the lifespan; and
- Comprehend the impact of common survivorship challenges on occupational performance and engagement in occupations across the lifespan.

KEY TERMS AND CONCEPTS

- Acute stage
- Cancer survivor
- Cancer survivorship care plans
- Extended stage
- Financial toxicity
- Late effects
- Long-term side effects
- Permanent stage
- Posttraumatic growth
- Survivorship
- Survivorship care

INTRODUCTION

Cancer survivorship is complex and involves many aspects of care from prevention to screening and rehabilitation (Ferrell et al., 2003). In the United States over the past 3 decades, the 5-year relative survival rate for all cancers combined increased 20 percentage points for Whites, to 68%, and 24 percentage points for Blacks, to 61% (American Cancer Society [ACS], 2017). The number of cancer survivors around the globe is growing substantially. Researchers have estimated that by 2024, there will be 22 million cancer survivors in the United States (ACS, 2019).

Estimates also showed that in 2020, there would be more than 1.8 million new cases of cancer in the United States and more than 600,000 cancer deaths (ACS, 2020). Worldwide, about 1 in 7 seven deaths can be attributed to cancer (ACS, 2019). By 2040, there will be an estimated 27.5 million new cancer cases worldwide and 6.3 million cancer deaths as a result of increased population growth and aging populations (ACS, 2018). National expenditures for cancer care in the United States totaled nearly $147.3 billion in 2017 and could reach $156 billion in 2020 (National Cancer Institute [NCI], 2019a).

There are multiple definitions of **cancer survivor,** but individuals most commonly are considered cancer survivors from the time of diagnosis through the balance of their life (Commission on Cancer [CoC], 2012; Institute of Medicine [IOM] & National Research Council of the National Academies [NRC], 2006). For this reason, we have chosen to use the terms *cancer survivor* and *survivor* throughout this text.

Survivorship is a three-stage process: (1) acute, (2) extended, and (3) permanent. There is no specific timeframe for the stages (Decker et al., 2007; Mullan, 1985). The ***acute stage*** of survivorship is the time surrounding the initial diagnosis, when decisions are made about staging and treatments are initiated (Itano & Taoka, 2005). The ***extended stage*** follows completion of intense treatment and includes possible remission (Itano & Taoka, 2005). The ***permanent stage*** is defined as the achievement of cure or of extended or long-term survival (Decker et al., 2007; Mullan, 1985). This chapter focuses on the extended stage and discusses the needs of survivors as they move from treatment and across the extended survivorship process.

Cancer survivorship can encompass a long time, and if one's quality of life (QoL) is good, it can also be a productive time. However, impaired function and participation will negatively affect QoL and health care costs. Individuals with a history of cancer have higher rates of limitations in ADLs, functional impairment (e.g., mobility), and disability than their peers without a cancer history, according to population-based surveys (Fialka-Moser et al., 2003; Hewitt et al., 2003; Keating et al., 2005). One way to lessen those problems is to connect cancer survivors to rehabilitation when appropriate.

The IOM and NRC (2006) strongly suggest that cancer survivor research should include expanded exploration of alternative models of ***survivorship care,*** such as supportive care and rehabilitation programs. Occupational therapy is a health care discipline that is well suited to survivorship care (Hwang et al., 2015). The profession can help address physical, cognitive, and emotional sequelae of cancer to enhance participation and a full return to life for cancer survivors. Cancer survivorship care is a growing area for occupational therapy. Occupational therapy practitioners may work with this population across all settings on the health care continuum from acute care to the community.

DEFINING FEATURES OF SURVIVORSHIP AND THE CANCER CARE CONTINUUM

Cancer survivors face many serious issues, including physical late effects, lack of consistent long-term medical follow up, psychosocial concerns, employment and insurance problems, and discrimination (Hewitt & Ganz, 2007). With an aging population and longer life expectancy for cancer survivors, it is important to develop a model of care delivery to maximize the health and well-being of survivors of cancer, focusing on effective symptom management, prevention of late effects, and health promotion (Alfano et al., 2012).

The IOM and NRC (2006) highlighted an opportunity to increase the linkage between oncology care and rehabilitation care when they published their report *From Cancer Patient to Cancer Survivor: Lost in Transition*. The report highlighted the importance of care programs specifically tailored for cancer survivors. As the IOM and NRC (2006) report described, survivorship care ideally includes many factors, such as

- Interventions for illnesses secondary to cancer and cancer treatment, including physical consequences of symptoms such as pain and fatigue;
- Psychological distress experienced by cancer survivors and their caregivers; and
- Concerns related to employment, insurance, and disability.

In 2012, the CoC mandated that accredited cancer programs begin to include *cancer survivorship care plans* (CSCPs), with all eligible patients having plans by 2019. In particular, the CSCP needs to address the survivor's long-term care, considering the type of cancer, treatments received, potential side effects, and recommendations for follow up supported by evidence-based guidelines. In addition, CSCPs should encompass preventive practices, how to maintain health and well-being, information on legal protections regarding employment and health insurance, and psychosocial support services that are available in the community (Hewitt & Ganz, 2007). Much of the work and design of care plans was based on guidelines developed by the Children's Oncology Group Nursing Discipline (Hewitt & Ganz, 2007) for survivors of childhood, adolescent, and young adult cancers (Morgan, 2009).

CSCPs have the potential to be strong connectors between cancer survivors and rehabilitation services. Rehabilitation professionals as a whole and occupational therapy practitioners specifically are optimal additions to the cancer care team and offer expertise in functional assessment, morbidity management, and disability prevention (Silver et al., 2015). Post-acute cancer rehabilitation is provided from inpatient rehabilitation facilities, skilled nursing facilities, long-term care hospitals, and hospice facilities as well as through home care and outpatient care (Stout et al., 2016). Multidisciplinary rehabilitation programs strive to address both the physical and the emotional needs of the cancer survivor. CSCPs outline the critical components of cancer care that should be documented and provided to the survivor and health care team (IOM & NRC, 2006).

OVERVIEW OF OCCUPATIONAL THERAPY'S ROLE IN SURVIVORSHIP AFTER CANCER TREATMENT

Cancer survivorship begins at the time of diagnosis (CoC, 2012; IOM & NRC, 2006). This chapter focuses on survivorship from completion of treatment through long-term survivorship. During this time, occupational therapy practitioners may see cancer survivors directly for their rehabilitation needs resulting from cancer and its treatment. Practitioners also may see survivors for a different diagnosis altogether and in a variety of settings, including home health care, skilled nursing facilities, and the community. Regardless, it is important to understand factors related to the type of cancer and treatment a client has had and use that information in clinical decision making. This includes understanding the potential long-term side effects and late effects of treatment that cancer survivors face. *Long-term side effects* are problems that are caused by the cancer or treatment of the cancer and may continue for months or years. Potential long-term side effects of cancer may include problems with body systems such as the heart, lungs, kidneys, or gastrointestinal tract or with client factors such as pain, neuropathy, fatigue, cognitive impairment, and lymphedema (NCI, 2019b). *Late effects* of cancer are health problems that occur months or years after cancer has been diagnosed or after cancer treatment has ended. Late effects may be caused by cancer or cancer treatments and may include physical, psychological, and social problems or second cancers (NCI, 2019c).

The transition from thinking of oneself as a cancer patient to a cancer survivor after completion of treatment can be a stressful time (IOM & NRC, 2006). Coping with anxiety related to relapse, developing ways to pick up the pieces of one's life, and moving from being well embedded in the health care system to being more self-directed can leave cancer survivors feeling adrift. During this transition, the survivor moves from a more medical role back to their personal roles, which might not be the same as before their cancer diagnosis and treatment. This is an important time and one that is well suited to receiving occupational therapy services.

Survivorship does not occur in a vacuum. This time of transition for the cancer survivor also is a time of change for their care partners, family, and social and community networks. During this transition, much of the responsibility of navigating health and wellness, including occupational engagement, is carried by the survivor. Although many survivors continue to engage in occupations throughout the continuum of cancer care, survivorship may also be a time marked by reengagement in valued occupations or engagement in new occupations. Occupational therapy practitioners can support survivors in the development

EXHIBIT 12.1.	Self-Management and Cancer Survivorship

- Tailor interventions to the needs, characteristics, and life circumstances of the survivor.
- Facilitate mastery and self-efficacy to enable the survivor to manage daily occupations.
- Support development and practice problem-solving skills to address barriers to occupational performance and participation.
- Facilitate uptake of occupations through goal setting and action planning.
- Support survivors in developing effective skills to communicate with family, employers, and social networks about occupational performance.

Note. Adapted from Howell et al. (2017).

and continuation of roles, habits, and routines that support occupational engagement throughout the lifespan.

Additionally, helping clients problem solve solutions to perceived barriers, such as stepping back into roles such as employee, homemaker, and student, can be daunting, particularly if clients also are coping with anxiety, fatigue, or pain. Occupational therapy can facilitate role resumption as well as help support self-management and lifestyle redesign as needed. Exhibit 12.1 provides examples of typical interventions occupational therapists might address when focusing on client self-management skills.

COMMON CHALLENGES EXPERIENCED IN SURVIVORSHIP

Cancer survivorship can be looked at as a chronic condition; cancer and cancer treatment can result in changes in function for survivors, including participation in valued roles and daily occupations (Baxter et al., 2017). Survivors may experience challenges with reengagement in personal, professional, and social roles following treatment, including those of family member, student, employee, community member, or friend (Philip & Merluzzi, 2016). Survivors may experience multiple medical conditions or sequelae that are often related to their cancer treatment long into survivorship. Common sequelae include cancer-related fatigue, lymphedema, cancer-related cognitive impairment, chemotherapy-induced peripheral neuropathy, and psychosocial distress (Burkhardt & Schultz-Krohn, 2013). These sequelae may affect physical, psychological, emotional, social, spiritual, and financial well-being.

The experience of cancer can affect one's sense of self (Smith et al., 2016). A survivor's sense of well-being and their ability to carry out previously held roles and responsibilities can be shaped by their experience with their diagnosis, treatment, and the long-term and late effects of cancer and cancer treatment (Zebrack, 2000). Stressors associated with cancer, such as challenges with occupational performance and participation in life roles, can challenge or alter existing identities of survivors, such as family, professional, and social identities (Surbone et al., 2013). Understanding how survivors view themselves in relation to their cancer experience and how this may develop and change over time are important for delivering occupational therapy services

that are individually tailored and occupation focused (IOM & NRC, 2006).

The impact of cancer and cancer treatment on the financial well-being of survivors has become a topic of major concern in recent years (Knight et al., 2018). The financial burden of cancer may lead to medical debt and a decline in financial resources long after the completion of acute cancer treatment (Altice et al., 2017). The term *financial toxicity* is used to describe the financial distress or hardship associated with cancer and cancer treatment (Altice et al., 2017; Yabroff et al., 2004). Rates of financial toxicity after cancer vary widely across survivors, but the risk of bankruptcy is 2.5–5 times higher than those with no history of cancer (Banegas et al., 2016). A recent systematic review found that 12%–62% of cancer survivors reported debt resulting from treatment, while 47%–49% reported some level of cancer-related financial distress (Altice et al., 2017). Further, financial toxicity may interfere with the cancer survivors' ability to cope with symptoms and follow-up care and contribute to poorer health-related QoL and health outcomes (Carrera et al., 2018). As a result, financial toxicity may significantly affect occupational performance across the lifespan and subsequently affect full participation in family, school, community, work, and social roles well into survivorship.

There is no doubt that survivors may experience a variety of stressors. However, it is important for clinicians to understand that although a significant number of survivors may experience posttraumatic stress disorder or posttraumatic stress symptoms resulting from their cancer experience, the experience of cancer may also lead to *posttraumatic growth,* which is the positive psychological changes resulting from trauma related to the cancer experience (Tedeschi & Calhoun, 1995). According to Tedeschi and Calhoun's (1995) paradigm of posttraumatic growth, such growth may include a greater appreciation of life and changed priorities, more intimate relationships with others, a greater sense of personal strength, recognition of new possibilities in one's life, and spiritual development. The opportunity for posttraumatic growth can be a helpful tool for clinicians working with survivors.

Table 12.1 highlights the potential challenges within the domains of well-being that cancer survivors may face across their life course from childhood through old age.

IMPORTANCE OF CONTEXT AND ENVIRONMENT IN SURVIVORSHIP

As survivors are living longer with cancer as a chronic condition throughout the life course, occupational therapy practitioners may encounter cancer survivors months, years, or decades after curative treatment. Past experiences may influence or shape survivors' responses to new health care encounters, occupations, or life roles. Context and environmental factors are extremely important to consider, because survivorship, although individualized, is situated in a cultural context. The following questions may assist occupational therapy practitioners in understanding the meaning of the context and environment to survivors.

Cultural Context

- What is the meaning of survivorship to the client?

TABLE 12.1. Domains of Well-Being in Survivorship

DOMAINS OF WELL-BEING IN SURVIVORSHIP	EXAMPLES OF POTENTIAL CHALLENGES
Physical	■ Management of late effects and long-term effects of cancer treatment ■ Sexual health and fertility ■ Childhood and adolescent growth and development
Psychological or emotional	■ Psychological adjustment to cancer survivorship ■ Loneliness ■ Cognitive functioning ■ Altered sense of self ■ Uncertainty about the future ■ Posttraumatic stress
Social	■ Partnership and relationships ■ Social isolation ■ Community integration ■ Discrimination
Spiritual or existential	■ Living with meaning and hope for the future ■ Feeling a sense of worth ■ Feeling a sense of purpose ■ Feeling connected
Financial	■ Medical debt ■ Decline in financial resources due to cancer, including missed time from work ■ Health care access, including insurance coverage

Sources. Deckx et al., 2014; Hydeman et al., 2019; Kline et al., 2018; Nathan et al., 2011; Peteet & Balboni, 2013; Philip & Merluzzi, 2016.

■ What cultural value does the survivor place on the illness and recovery experience?
■ How do the client's customs and beliefs influence the therapeutic interaction and engagement in the goal-setting process?

Personal Context

■ What are the survivor's educational status and literacy level?
■ What is the survivor's socioeconomic status, and how might this support or inhibit access to resources?
■ How does the client's identity influence their activity choices and group memberships?

Temporal Context

■ What is the life stage of the survivor (e.g., pediatric, adolescent, adult, older adult)?
■ Are late effects of cancer influenced by time of day (e.g., fatigue, pain, depression, anxiety, cognitive dysfunction)?
■ Is participation in occupation influenced by geographical location, time of day, or season?

Virtual Context

■ Does the cancer survivor have access to technology to support health and well-being with health providers, support groups, friends, and families?
■ Do those who provide care for the survivor have access to technology to support their health and well-being as care providers?

APPROACHES TO INTERVENTION IN SURVIVORSHIP

The end of active cancer treatment is often a time to celebrate; however, it can take time to recover from the cancer experience. Survivors and the individuals with whom they interact, such as significant others, family members, friends, and coworkers, may be unprepared for the time that recovery takes.

Survivorship is a time of returning to, continuing, and adopting new roles, habits, and routines. For children, it may be a time of returning to school or play activities. For adolescents and young adults, it may be a time to establish relationships and pursue academic or work experiences. For adults, it may be a time to raise a family or advance in a career, and for older adults, it may be a time to focus on work, volunteer activity, or social participation. As a result, several treatment approaches and approaches to intervention may be suitable for the survivor of cancer. Table 12.2 provides examples of the role of occupational therapy throughout the lifespan, Table 12.3 provides examples of types of occupational therapy interventions, and Table 12.4 provides examples of approaches to interventions.

Case Examples 12.1, 12.2, and 12.3 illustrate salient issues survivors may face across the lifespan. Consider how the role of occupational therapy, including occupational therapy interventions and approaches to intervention, may support occupational performance and participation in the desired occupations.

It is critical that occupational therapy practitioners be aware of the often unmet needs of cancer survivors and proactively assess potential need for enhanced functional

TABLE 12.2.   Examples of the Occupational Therapy Practitioner's Role

STAGES	ROLE OF THE OCCUPATIONAL THERAPY PRACTITIONER
Pediatric	Support involvement in self-care, play, school, social participation
Adolescent and young adult	Support involvement in IADLs, school, social participation, work, driving
Adult	Support involvement in work, school, leisure, IADLs, family, caregiving, sexual activity, health management, driving, social participation
Older adult	Support involvement in work, volunteer, leisure, social participation, IADLs, sexual activity, home management, driving, retirement planning

Note. IADLs = instrumental activities of daily living.

TABLE 12.3.   Examples of Occupational Therapy Interventions

TYPE OF OCCUPATIONAL THERAPY INTERVENTION	EXAMPLES
Occupations and activities	▪ Medication management, home management, driving, education, work
Preparatory methods and tasks	▪ Physical agent modalities for pain management, splints management, assistive technology (e.g., smartphone use, electronic pillbox) ▪ Wheeled mobility ▪ Visual imagery to promote rest and relaxation ▪ Hand-strengthening exercises with therapy putty exercise bands and other tools ▪ Home-based exercise program for lymphedema management
Education and training	▪ Education about the late effects or long-term effects of cancer and cancer treatment and their effects on occupational performance ▪ Education on health promotion and wellness ▪ Training in assistive technology to manage daily routines and occupations (e.g., medication management, use of electronic day planner) ▪ Training with adaptive equipment (e.g., adaptive mirrors, hand controls) to support driving and community mobility ▪ Home and activity modifications
Advocacy	▪ Collaborate with a person to procure reasonable accommodations at a work site as a result of late effects of treatment ▪ Collaborate with parents and schools to request reasonable accommodations as a result of late effects of treatment
Groups	▪ Self-management groups that focus on goal setting, action planning, and problem solving daily life challenges ▪ Psychosocial support, including management of emotional well-being after cancer treatment

TABLE 12.4.   Examples of Approaches to Occupational Therapy Intervention

APPROACHES TO INTERVENTION	EXAMPLES
Establish or restore	▪ Collaborate with a client to help establish morning routines needed to arrive at school or work on time ▪ Collaborate with client to establish a sleep and rest routine ▪ Restore a client's upper extremity movement to support return to driving
Modify	▪ Reduce fatigue by modifying work schedule ▪ Reduce fatigue in the school by adapting classroom environment and daily routines ▪ Simplify task sequences to support morning routines to minimize effects of fatigue ▪ Provide adaptive equipment to support driving (e.g., adaptive mirrors)
Prevent	▪ Prevent social isolation ▪ Prevent loss or reduction of employment ▪ Promote positive health behaviors and engagement in routine cancer screenings

CASE EXAMPLE 12.1. SAM: SUPPORTING ACADEMIC PERFORMANCE IN SURVIVORSHIP

Sam is a 17-year-old survivor of childhood acute lymphoblastic leukemia (ALL). He lives with his family, including his parents, grandmother, and two younger sisters, in a suburban neighborhood 20 miles from the cancer center where he received treatment. He attends the local high school, where he is in his senior year and approaching graduation. He was first diagnosed with ALL when he was 8 years old and underwent central nervous system–directed therapy, including chemotherapy and radiation. Over the years, he has gradually experienced the onset of several late effects of treatment, including obesity, diabetes, and neurocognitive deficits.

He has been receiving occupational therapy in the school district for the past several years as part of his individualized education program to address his academic performance, and he most recently has focused on transition to postsecondary education. Outside of school, he is taking a more active role in his health maintenance and is aware that he is having difficulty managing his medication for his diabetes and keeping track of his follow-up care, including doctor appointments.

In preparation for the college transition away from home, he would like to be able to independently manage his health-related needs. He is seeking outpatient occupational therapy to address self-management skills for health management and maintenance as he transitions to college.

CASE STUDY 12.2. NANCY: SUPPORTING ENGAGEMENT IN DAILY ACTIVITIES

Nancy is a 65-year-old survivor of non-Hodgkin's lymphoma. She lives with her husband in an apartment in an urban area close to the medical center where she received her cancer care. She completed treatment 3 months ago and returned to work as a receptionist on a full-time basis immediately after completion of active treatment. She is the proud grandmother of three young children and was actively involved in their care until her cancer diagnosis, including regular babysitting on the weekends. Her husband is very supportive and has assumed responsibility for home and community activities, such as preparing meals, cleaning, shopping, and scheduling activities and medical appointments. Her employer is very accommodating of her need to flex her schedule to attend to her medical needs.

Nancy is experiencing numerous late effects of her cancer and cancer treatment, including cognitive difficulties with memory and attention, fatigue, a resting tremor in her upper extremities, neuropathy in her hands and feet, and resulting distress about her current situation. These late effects have influenced her sleep and her ability to work, engage in home and community activities, and provide care for her grandchildren.

Nancy is referred to occupational therapy to address the late effects of cancer treatment. She reports that she is upset and wants to reclaim her independence. Her daughter will not let her participate in the care of her grandchildren because she "does not trust" Nancy given her fatigue, attention problems, and numbness in her hands and feet, and her husband has "taken over" things she used to do in the house. Meanwhile, Nancy is struggling to perform her essential job functions now that she has returned to work full-time.

She would like to work with an occupational therapy practitioner to problem solve how to communicate with her family and employer to get the support she needs but also advocate for what she can do without assistance. In addition, occupational therapy can help her incorporate energy conservation strategies, cognitive strategies, and fall prevention strategies into her daily routine as well as assist her in planning ways to safely provide care for her grandchildren.

and QoL outcomes. These often unmet needs might include issues such as financial burden from their cancer experience, identity maintenance or reinvention, and uncertainty for the future and their health. Occupational therapy needs to go beyond physical needs and address issues that may emerge more strongly at the point of transitioning from cancer care to living as a cancer survivor.

SUMMARY

Cancer survivorship is a complex concept and starts from the time of diagnosis. This chapter focused on the survivorship experience after the completion of treatment. This time encompasses the important transition of the cancer patient's focus from medical back to daily life and can be a stressful time for survivors. As this chapter highlighted, there are many ways occupational therapy can benefit people at this stage in their cancer continuum. Clinicians need to be aware of cancer survivorship challenges and to factor the client's experience with cancer into any evaluation and treatment. Survivors often do not receive this care after they transition from being active cancer patients embedded in the health care system.

Clinicians need to keep in mind that they likely will see cancer survivors for secondary diagnosis not related to their cancer. It is still important to factor the cancer

CASE EXAMPLE 12.3. MARIA: SUPPORTING ENGAGEMENT IN COMMUNITY MOBILITY

Maria is a 40-year-old survivor of head and neck cancer who completed cancer treatment 3 months ago. She lives with her partner and their three adolescent children in a ranch-style home in a rural area. Before her cancer diagnosis, Maria was employed as a chef in a restaurant in town. She took a medical leave from her job during her treatment and is planning to return to work. To do so, Maria wants to be able to drive herself to work so that she is not reliant on her partner or children for transportation. Currently, Maria is experiencing a range of effects of her treatment, including restricted neck mobility, pain, and lymphedema of the head and neck. Her lymphedema is well controlled with complete decongestive therapy.

During active treatment, Maria's family drove her to all appointments and family functions. Now that treatment is over, Maria wants to resume this occupation to minimize the burden on her family for transportation. After discussing this goal with her oncologist, Maria is referred to an occupational therapy program for a driver evaluation to assess her driving capacity and potential vehicle modifications to support safe and independent driving.

During the driver evaluation, the occupational therapist creates a thorough occupational profile to better understand the meaning of driving for Maria in terms of its importance both for return to work and for her to assist with family needs. The comprehensive driver evaluation reveals that Maria is a candidate for training in the use of adaptive mirrors to compensate for her potentially permanently restricted cervical range of motion. She participates in an on-road evaluation and training session with the use of the adaptive mirrors, and it is determined that Maria is safe to return to driving with the necessary modification to her vehicle.

---

treatment and potential long-term risks into the plan of care for the new health condition. For example, having had a mastectomy may influence how a woman should be transferred during her inpatient stay for a stroke. The key point to remember about posttreatment cancer survivorship is that occupational therapy practitioners need to support cancer survivors in reengaging in the activities and occupations they valued before their cancer diagnosis as well as in exploring new activities and occupations they would like to become involved in.

REFERENCES

Alfano, C. M., Ganz, P. A., Rowland, J. H., & Hahn, E. E. (2012). Cancer survivorship and cancer rehabilitation: Revitalizing the link. *Journal of Clinical Oncology, 30*, 904–906. https://doi.org/10.1200/JCO.2011.37.1674

Altice, C. K., Banegas, M. P., Tucker-Seeley, R. D., & Yabroff, K. R. (2017). Financial hardships experienced by cancer survivors: A systematic review. *Journal of the National Cancer Institute, 109*(2), 1–17. https://doi.org/10.1093/jnci/djw205

American Cancer Society. (2017). *Cancer facts & figures 2017.* Retrieved from https://www.cancer.org/content/dam/cancer-org/research/cancer-facts-and-statistics/annual-cancer-facts-and-figures/2017/cancer-facts-and-figures-2017.pdf

American Cancer Society. (2018). *Global facts & figures* (4th ed.). Retrieved from https://www.cancer.org/content/dam/cancer-org/research/cancer-facts-and-statistics/global-cancer-facts-and-figures/global-cancer-facts-and-figures-4th-edition.pdf

American Cancer Society. (2019). *Cancer facts & figures 2019.* Retrieved from https://www.cancer.org/content/dam/cancer-org/research/cancer-facts-and-statistics/annual-cancer-facts-and-figures/2019/cancer-facts-and-figures-2019.pdf

American Cancer Society. (2020). *Cancer facts & figures 2020.* Retrieved from https://www.cancer.org/research/cancer-facts-statistics/all-cancer-facts-figures/cancer-facts-figures-2020.html

Banegas, M. P., Guy, G. P. Jr., de Moor, J. S., Ekwueme, D. U., Virgo, K. S., Kent, . . . Yabroff, K. R. (2016). For working-age cancer survivors, medical debt and bankruptcy create financial hardships. *Health Affairs, 35*, 54–61. https://doi.org/10.1377/hlthaff.2015.0830

Baxter, M. F., Newman, R., Longpre, S. M., & Polo, K. M. (2017). Occupational therapy's role in cancer survivorship as a chronic condition. *American Journal of Occupational Therapy, 71*, 7103090010. https://doi.org/10.5014/ajot.2017.713001

Burkhardt, A., & Schultz-Krohn, W. (2013). Oncology. In H. M. Pendleton & W. Schultz-Krohn (Eds.), *Pedretti's occupational therapy: Practice skills for physical dysfunction* (7th ed., pp. 1215–1227). St. Louis: Mosby.

Carrera, P. M., Kantarjian, H. M., & Blinder, V. S. (2018). The financial burden and distress of patients with cancer: Understanding and stepping-up action on the financial toxicity of cancer treatment. *CA: A Cancer Journal for Clinicians, 68*, 153–165. https://doi.org/10.3322/caac.21443

Commission on Cancer. (2012). *Cancer program standards 2012: Ensuring patient-centered care.* Chicago: American College of Surgeons. Available at https://www.facs.org/~/media/files/quality%20programs/cancer/coc/programstandards2012.ashx

Decker, C., Haase, J., & Bell, C. (2007). Uncertainty in adolescents and young adults with cancer. *Oncology Nursing Forum, 34*, 681–688. https://doi.org/10.1188/07.ONF.681-688

Deckx, L., van den Akker, M., & Buntinx F. (2014). Risk factors for loneliness in patients with cancer: A systematic literature review and meta-analysis. *European Journal of Oncology Nursing, 18*, 466–477. https://doi.org/10.1016/j.ejon.2014.05.002

Ferrell, B. R., Virani, R., Smith, S., & Juarez, G.; National Cancer Policy Board and Institute of Medicine. (2003). The role of oncology nursing to ensure quality care for cancer survivors: A report commissioned by the National Cancer Policy Board and Institute of Medicine. *Oncology Nursing Forum, 30*(1), E1–E11. https://doi.org/10.1188/03.ONF.E1-E11

Fialka-Moser, V., Crevenna, R., Korpan, M., & Quittan, M. (2003). Cancer rehabilitation: Particularly with aspects of physical impairments. *Journal of Rehabilitation Medicine, 35*, 153–162. https://doi.org/10.1080/16501970306129

Hewitt, M., & Ganz, P. (2007). *Implementing cancer survivorship care planning: Workshop summary.* Washington, DC: National Academies Press.

Hewitt, M., Rowland, J. H., & Yancik, R. (2003). Cancer survivors in the US: Age, health, and disability. *Journals of Gerontology: Series A, 58,* 82–91. https://doi.org/10.1093/gerona/58.1.m82

Howell, D., Harth, T., Brown, J., Bennett, C., & Boyko, S. (2017). Self-management education interventions for patients with cancer: A systematic review. *Supportive Care in Cancer, 25,* 1323–1355. https://doi.org/10.1007/s00520-016-3500-z

Hwang, E. J., Lokietz, N. C., Lozano, R. L., & Parke, M. A. (2015). Functional deficits and quality of life among cancer survivors: Implications for occupational therapy in cancer survivorship care. *American Journal of Occupational Therapy, 69,* 6906290010. https://doi.org/10.5014/ajot.2015.015974

Hydeman, J. A., Uwazurike, O. D., Adeyemi, E. I., & Beaupin, L. K. (2019). Survivorship needs of adolescent and young adult cancer survivors: A concept mapping analysis. *Journal of Cancer Survivorship, 13,* 34–42. https://doi.org/10.1007/s11764-018-0725-5

Institute of Medicine & National Research Council of the National Academics. (2006). *From cancer patient to cancer survivor: Lost in transition.* Washington, DC: National Academies Press. https://doi.org/10.17226/11468

Itano, J., & Taoko, K. (2005). *Core curriculum for oncology nursing* (4th ed.). St. Louis: Elsevier Sanders.

Keating, N. L., Norredam, M., Landrum, M. B., Huskamp, H. A., & Meara, E. (2005). Physical and mental health status of older long-term cancer survivors. *Journal of the American Geriatrics Society, 53,* 2145–2152. https://doi.org/10.1111/j.1532.5415.2005.00507.x

Kline, R. M., Arora, N. K., Bradley, C. J., Brauer, E. R., Graves, D. L., Lunsford, . . . Ganz, P. A. (2018). Long-term survivorship care after cancer treatment: Summary of a 2017 national cancer policy forum workshop. *Journal of the National Cancer Institute, 110,* 1300–1310. https://doi.org/10.1093/jcni/djy176

Knight, T. G., Deal, A. M., Dusetzina, S. B., Muss, H. B., Choi, S. K., Bensen, J. T., & Williams, G. R. (2018). Financial toxicity in adults with cancer: Adverse outcomes and noncompliance. *Journal of Oncology Practice, 14,* 3665–3673. https://doi.org/10.1200/JOP.18.00120

Morgan, M. (2009). Cancer survivorship: History, quality of life issues, and the evolving multidisciplinary approach to implementation of cancer survivorship care plans. *Oncology Nursing Forum, 36,* 429–436.

Mullan, F. (1985). Seasons of survival: Reflections of a physician with cancer. *New England Journal of Medicine, 313,* 270–273. https://doi.org/10.1056/NEJM198507253130421

Nathan, P. C., Hayes-Lattin, B., Sisler, J. J., & Hudson, M. M. (2011). Critical issues in transition and survivorship for adolescents and young adults with cancer. *Cancer, 117*(Suppl. 10), 2335–2341. https://doi.org/10.1002/cncr.26042

National Cancer Institute. (2019a). *Cancer trends progress report: Prevention.* Retrieved from https://progressreport.cancer.gov/prevention

National Cancer Institute. (2019b). Late effect. *National Cancer Institute Dictionary of Cancer Terms.* Retrieved from: https://www.cancer.gov/publications/dictionaries/cancer-terms/def/late-effect

National Cancer Institute. (2019c). Long-term side effect. *National Cancer Institute Dictionary of Cancer Terms.* Retrieved from: https://www.cancer.gov/publications/dictionaries/cancer-terms/def/long-term-side-effect

Peteet, J. R., & Balboni, M. J. (2013). Spirituality and religion in oncology. *CA: A Cancer Journal for Clinicians, 63,* 280–289. https://doi.org/10.1002/caac.21187

Philip, E. J., & Merluzzi, T. V. (2016). Psychosocial issues in post-treatment cancer survivors: Desire for support and challenges in identifying individuals in need. *Journal of Psychosocial Oncology, 34,* 223–239. https://10.1080/07347332.2016.1157716

Silver, J. K., Raj, V. S., Fu, J. B., Wisotzky, E. M., Smith, S. R., & Kirch, R. A. (2015). Cancer rehabilitation and palliative care: Critical components in the delivery of high-quality oncology services. *Supportive Care Cancer, 23,* 3633–3643. https://doi.org/10.1007/s00520-015-2916-1

Smith, K. C., Klassen, A. C., Coa, K. I., & Hannum, S. M. (2016). The salience of cancer and the "survivor" identity for people who have completed acute cancer treatment: A qualitative study. *Journal of Cancer Survivorship, 10,* 457–466. https://doi.org/10.1007/s11764-015-0489-0

Stout, N. L., Silver, J. K., Raj, V. S., Rowland, J., Gerber, L., Cheville, A., . . . Chan, L. (2016). Toward a national initiative in cancer rehabilitation: Recommendations from a subject matter expert group. *Archives of Physical Medicine and Rehabilitation, 97,* 2006–2015. https://doi.org/10.1016/j.apmr.2016.05.002

Surbone, A., Anmuziata, M. A., Santoro, A., Tirelli, U., & Tralongo, P. (2013). Cancer patients and survivors: Changing words or changing culture? *Annals of Oncology, 24,* 2468–2471. https://doi.org/10.1093/annonc/mdt229

Tedeschi, R. G., & Calhoun, L. G. (1995). *Trauma and transformation: Growing in the aftermath of suffering.* Thousand Oaks, CA: Sage.

Yabroff, K. R., Lawrence, W. F., Clauser, S., Davis, W. W., & Brown, M. L. (2004). Burden of illness in cancer survivors: Findings from a population-based national sample. *Journal of the National Cancer Institute, 96,* 1322–1330. https://doi.org/10.1093/jnci/djh255

Zebrack, B. (2000). Cancer survivor identity and quality of life. *Cancer Practice, 8,* 238–242. https://doi.org/10.1046/j.1523-5394.2000.85004.x

Palliative Care and Hospice

Mack Ivy, OTR, PhD

LEARNING OBJECTIVES

After completing this chapter, readers should be able to
- Understand the role of palliative care and hospice care along the cancer care continuum,
- Distinguish the similarities and differences between palliative care and hospice care,
- Explain the distinct value that occupational therapy adds to end-of-life care, and
- Apply strategies that can enable occupational performance and participation for patients receiving palliative and hospice care.

KEY TERMS AND OBJECTIVES

- Caregiving
- Client-centered care
- Hospice
- Interprofessional team
- Legacy project
- Palliative care
- Quality of life
- Spirituality
- Symptom control

INTRODUCTION

The demand for palliative care is increasing as more people realize that it can help control a wide variety of symptoms. *Palliative care* addresses the physical, cognitive, and psychosocial needs of the patient and caregivers to provide holistic *symptom control*. Physical symptoms can include opiod-induced constipation, delirium, dyspnea, fatigue, and pain. Psychosocial needs can include the emotional impact of serious illness that affects spiritual, existential, and self-image issues. Palliative care involves an *interprofessional team* and can be initiated at any time during the cancer care continuum while the primary team continues to concurrently address curative treatments. A variety of medical, psychological, and spiritual professionals are usually members of this team, although occupational therapy practitioners are often not included (Russell et al., 2016).

Palliative care and hospice provide similar holistic care, but *hospice* is reserved for the terminal stage of the client's condition, when curative treatments are no longer beneficial and the client likely has 6 months or less to live. The occupational therapy profession focuses on holistic, client-centered practice addressing physical and psychological well-being through occupational performance, which makes occupational therapy a natural fit with the philosophy and approach of palliative care (Pearson et al., 2007).

Survivors of cancer often discontinue participation in the activities most meaningful to them because of a decline in functional performance due to cancer-related fatigue from the disease process and curative treatments, including chemotherapy, radiation, and surgery. Occupational therapy practitioners provide skilled intervention to optimize *quality of life* (QoL), which includes resuming valued roles, routines, autonomy, and dignity by enabling clients to engage in ADLs and valued occupations throughout the entire lifespan, including when one's prognosis is less than 6 months to live. Participation in meaningful activities or occupations continues to be as important at the end of life as it is at earlier stages (American Occupational Therapy Association [AOTA], 2016). Occupational therapy practitioners working with patients in palliative care can maximize patients' performance and ability to participate to help them make the most of the remainder of their life (Badger et al., 2016). Working with patients facing the end of life can be very challenging as well as very rewarding. Our own individual life experiences can help us navigate and handle the death process of the patients we serve and how we face our own inevitable death.

This chapter provides highlights on the evolution of hospice and palliative care. Case examples illustrate how occupational therapy can help manage symptoms and provide strategies to optimize the QoL for patients facing the end of life.

HISTORY OF HOSPICE AND PALLIATIVE CARE

"You matter because you are you, and you matter to the end of your life. We will do all we can not only to help

you die peacefully, but also to live until you die." —Dame Cicely Saunders (Crossroads Hospice and Palliative Care [CHPC], 2017, p. 1)

Origin of Hospice

Cicely Saunders founded the first modern hospice and, more than anybody else, was responsible for establishing the discipline and the culture of palliative care. She introduced effective pain management and insisted that dying people need dignity, compassion, and respect as well as rigorous scientific methodology in the testing of treatments. She abolished the prevailing ethic that patients must be cured, that those who could not be cured were a sign of failure, and that it was acceptable and even desirable to lie to patients about a poor prognosis (Richmond, 2005).

Saunders was enrolled at Oxford University to study politics but transferred to London's St. Thomas Hospital to study nursing when World War II began. She cared for injured servicemen until a back injury sent her back to Oxford to train as a social worker, also known as a *hospital almoner* in Britain. Saunders met several patients facing the end of life and decided to focus on how she could help terminally ill patients (CHPC, 2017). She supplemented her almoner work by serving as a volunteer sister at St. Luke's Hospital in north London.

Saunders wanted to have more patient contact and asked her orthopedic surgeon whether she could work as a night nurse at his facility. She reasoned that most of the lifting of patients is done during the day so working at night would put less strain on her back. The doctor believed that people would not listen to Saunders as a nurse or social worker, that doctors are the ones who abandon the dying, and that she could best help dying patients by becoming a medical doctor. Saunders was accepted as a medical student at St. Thomas in 1951 at age of 33 years (Richmond, 2005).

Dr. Saunders earned her medical degree in 1957 and became the first modern doctor to devote her career to dying patients. Over the years, she developed a systematic approach to manage physical pain.

She developed an innovative record-keeping system, using punch cards to track the 1,100 patients being cared for at St. Joseph's. Saunders' approach gave full attention to a patient's needs in terms of physical, social, emotional and spiritual components. She called this a "total pain" perspective. The idea was to focus on the care of the whole person and [embrace] the patient's family and friends as part of that care. Saunders' approach helped guide the development of palliative care, and modern hospice philosophy. (CHPC, 2017, p. 1)

In 1967, Dr. Saunders opened St. Christopher's Hospice, designed to feel like a home with expert pain and symptom control. She died of cancer on July 14, 2005, at 87 years old, at the hospice she founded (CHPC, 2017; Richmond, 2005). A history of hospice care has been provided by the National Hospice and Palliative Care Organization (NHPCO; 2018a) and is included in Appendix 13.A.

The following statements were originally published in the preamble to the NHPCO's 2000 *Standards of Practice for Hospice Programs,* reaffirmed in the 2010 update, and are reflected in the core components in the 2018 update (NHPCO, 2010, 2018b):

Hospice affirms the concept of palliative care as an intensive program that enhances comfort and promotes the quality of life for individuals and their families. When cure is no longer possible, hospice recognizes that a peaceful and comfortable death is an essential goal of health care. Hospice believes that death is an integral part of the life cycle and that intensive palliative care focuses on pain relief, comfort and enhanced quality of life as appropriate goals for the terminally ill. Hospice also recognizes the potential for growth that often exists within the dying experience for the individual and his/her family and seeks to protect and nurture this potential. (NHPCO, 2010, p. 1)

The following hospice philosophy statement is located in the *Standards of Practice for Hospice Programs*:

Hospice provides support and care for persons in the last phases of an incurable disease so that they may live as fully and as comfortable as possible. Hospice recognizes that the dying process is a part of the normal process of living and focuses on enhancing the quality of remaining life. Hospice affirms life and neither hastens nor postpones death. Hospice exists in the hope and belief that through appropriate care, and the promotion of a caring community sensitive to their needs that individuals and their families may be free to attain a degree of satisfaction in preparation for death. Hospice recognizes that human growth and development can be a lifelong process. Hospice seeks to preserve and promote the inherent potential for growth within individuals and families during the last phase of life. (NHPCO, 2010, p. 1)

In the United States, health care insurance tends to follow the direction of the Medicare policy that states that "hospice care is a benefit under the hospital insurance program. To be eligible to elect hospice under Medicare, an individual must be entitled to Part A of Medicare and certified as being terminally ill. An individual is considered to be terminally ill if the medical prognosis is that the individual's life expectancy is 6 months or less if the illness runs its normal course" by a medical doctor or a doctor of osteopathy (Centers for Medicare and Medicaid Services [CMS], 2018, 20.1, p. 4).

The *Medicare Benefit Policy Manual* Section 40.1.8 states that "physical therapy, occupational therapy, and speech–language pathology services *may* be provided for purposes of symptom control or *to enable the individual to maintain activities of daily living and basic functional skills.* Also, see Section 40.5 regarding waivers under certain conditions for provision of these services" (CMS, 2018, p. 27; *italics* added). Although hospice benefits mention occupational therapy, it is often not provided because it is not reimbursed separately with an extra fee for the service but instead is included in a daily flat rate for all hospice services regardless of the number of services provided. Unfortunately, the "*may*" has led decision makers to not include occupational therapy as a service mandated by this document; however, when Section 40.5 states that "in addition to the hospice core services (physician services, nursing services, medical social services and counseling), *the following must be provided by the hospice,* either directly or under arrangements, to meet the needs of the patient and family: Physical and occupational therapy and speech–language pathology services" (CMS, 2018, p. 36; *italics* added). The phrase "*the following must be provided by the hospice*" is a strong statement of support but has not resulted in a wider inclusion of physical therapy, occupational therapy, or speech–language pathology services by hospice agencies because of reimbursement limitations.

It is hoped that by increasing awareness of this mandate, occupational therapy practitioners and others will pressure the decision makers to include occupational therapy more often to "meet the needs of the patient and family" to "enable the individual to maintain activities of daily living and basic functional skills," which occupational therapy practitioners are distinctly able to address.

In addition to the services provided by hospice, occupational therapy services can be provided as home health (CMS, 2019a) and as palliative care and reimbursed with a physician's order
- As a home health benefit under Medicare Part B,
- As an inpatient hospital benefit under Medicare Part A, and
- Under Medicaid and private insurance (CMS, 2018, 2019a, 2019b).

Origin of Palliative Care

Dr. Balfour Mount practiced as a cancer surgeon at the Royal Victoria Hospital in Montreal and visited with Dr. Saunders. He wanted to bring the ideas of the hospice movement to Canada. However, to his patients in Quebec, who spoke French, the term *hospice* was associated with a place of last resort for the poor and derelict, which made its global use difficult. Because of this unfortunate translation, Dr. Mount sought another term. In 1974, Dr. Mount proposed the term *palliative,* from the Latin word *palliare* ("to cloak"; Higginson, 2011).

Although originally intended to be synonymous with the term *hospice,* the latter term has been used by reimbursement decision makers in the United States to define care in the last 6 months of expected life. In contrast, *palliative care* can address symptom management while curative options are beneficial. *Palliative care* is an appropriate term because the focus is not to cure a disease but to cloak, cover up, or shelter the patient by controlling symptoms and improving QoL even if the patient is not yet ready for hospice. Emphasis on management of pain and other symptoms—physical, emotional, and spiritual—for individuals with life-limiting conditions is the nexus of palliative care (World Health Organization [WHO], 2002).

WHO (n.d., 2002) recognized that palliative care is a specialty in the health care domain and defined it as

> an approach that improves the quality of life of patients and their families facing the problem[s] associated with

life-threatening illness, through the prevention and relief of suffering by means of early identification and impeccable assessment and treatment of pain and other problems, physical, psychosocial and spiritual. (WHO, 2002, p. 84)

This definition has not been changed since 2002 and also contains nine additional goals. Goal 5 is of particular interest to occupational therapy because it states that palliative care also "offers a support system to help patients live as actively as possible until death:

- Provides relief from pain and other distressing symptoms;
- Affirms life and regards dying as a normal process;
- Intends neither to hasten nor postpone death;
- Integrates the psychological and spiritual aspects of patient care;
- Offers a support system to help patients live as actively as possible until death;
- Offers a support system to help the family cope during the patient's illness and in their own bereavement;
- Uses a team approach to address the needs of patients and their families, including bereavement counseling, if indicated;
- Will enhance quality of life and may also positively influence the course of illness;
- Is applicable early in the course of illness, in conjunction with other therapies that are intended to prolong life, such as chemotherapy or radiation therapy, and includes those investigations needed to better understand and manage distressing clinical complications." (WHO, n.d.; WHO, 2002, p. 84)

The decision makers in palliative care are to be commended for acknowledging in this document that keeping a person active is a positive goal; however, it has not been made clear how to enable palliative patients to achieve this goal.

Another guide from WHO (2007) on palliative care states that "health-care providers involved in palliative care may include physicians, nurses, social workers, psychologists, spiritual counselors, volunteers, pharmacists and traditional healers" (p. 27). Although this list of interprofessional team members is impressive, it does not include occupational therapy practitioners or any other health profession that specializes in helping "patients live as actively as possible until death" (WHO, 2002, p. 84).

The WHO Global Atlas (WHO, 2014) adopted the 2002 WHO definition of *palliative care* and added further explanation of medical, psychological, and spiritual services, but it did not mention occupational therapy. It is important for occupational therapy practitioners desiring to work with palliative care patients to understand that physicians and other members of the interprofessional team may not be aware of the benefits of occupation. "Therefore, occupational therapists need to take it upon themselves to promote an understanding of the importance and benefits of occupation and choice to their patients" (Badger et al., 2016, p. 230).

OCCUPATIONAL THERAPY'S ROLE IN PALLIATIVE CARE AND HOSPICE ACROSS THE CANCER CARE CONTINUUM

Working With Interprofessional Teams

Ferris et al. (2009) found that palliative cancer care requires an interprofessional team to address the multiple issues that cause suffering for patients and their families and affect their QoL. Pizzi's (2014) study interviewing occupational therapists, physical therapists, social workers, and registered nurses reported "that each discipline, as an interdisciplinary team member, recognized the value of the other team members and that quality of life, health, and well-being until death were the ultimate goals in end-of-life care" (p. 219). Occupational therapy has not been fully used in palliative care interprofessional teams, even though WHO (n.d., 2002) has acknowledged that helping a person stay active until death increases their QoL.

Although WHO's goal is "to help patients live as actively as possible until death", it is important to acknowledge that being active just for its own sake can be viewed as tedious busywork. Including an occupational therapy practitioner on the team not only helps patients stay active but also provides active participation in meaningful activities that maximize the patient's QoL. If occupational therapy practitioners continue to be omitted from the palliative care team, it will "limit the breadth of support care, which in turn may perpetuate physical, cognitive, and emotional issues for clients while limiting function, participation, and quality of life" (Sleight & Duker, 2016, p. 6).

Improving QoL

Occupational therapy practitioners provide skilled intervention to improve QoL by facilitating engagement in daily life occupations throughout the entire lifespan, including the time when one is approaching the end of life (AOTA, 2016). However, the importance of remaining occupied and engaged in meaningful activity continues to be overlooked in provision of care for the terminally ill. In their study, Keesing and Rosenwax (2011) identified four themes that affected people who were dying and their caregivers:

> Ongoing disengagement from usual activities with resultant occupational deprivation; disempowerment of both people who are dying and their carers within palliative care services; "occupation" not being addressed adequately in palliative care[;] and occupational therapists experienc[ing] frustration with limited opportunities to contribute to the care of people who are dying. (p. 329)

A common perception is that few, if any, improvements in function can be achieved while a patient is in palliative care. However, it is important to remember that autonomy and maintenance of independence are highly valued by clients diagnosed with terminal illness (Coyle, 2006). Also, the ability to participate in meaningful occupations in "the face of imminent death—is an option that all people should be allowing to choose if they so desire" (Marcil, 2006, p. 27).

Palliative care recognizes that "whatever the disease, however advanced it is, whatever treatments have already been given, there is always something that can be done to improve the quality of the life remaining to the patient" (Woodruff, 2004, p. 1). Kaye (2006) affirmed that QoL can always be improved: "Loss of independence and role can result in social death prior to biological death. Occupational therapy can help a person to adopt new and appropriate functions and roles and to maintain self-esteem" (p. 214). Some patients may discontinue efforts to participate in important roles and routines once they are not performed at previous levels of independence. Occupational therapy practitioners can normalize this human behavior and then provide strategies to help patients resume participation with some adaptive strategies.

Egan and DeLaat (1997) illustrated how occupation can help one resume roles and relationships to avoid this premature social death, arguing that "it is through our occupations that we live out the relationships that bring meaning to our lives" (p. 116). Prominent palliative care physicians also acknowledge that "palliative cancer care aims to give patients and their families the capacity to realize their full potential, when their cancer is curable as well as when the end of life is near" (Ferris et al., 2009, p. 3055). Occupational therapy practitioners can help explore which occupations and relationships are most meaningful and provide strategies and adaptations to help the patients resume these valued roles, routines, and activities.

Pizzi (1984) wrote that "occupational therapists can emphasize that the dying are still living persons, with feelings, abilities, hopes, and dreams. Our professional calling is to promote maximal adaptation and to maximize occupational roles in accordance with the needs and desires of our terminal patients" (p. 257). Pizzi (1992) added that QoL "is not simply about pain control and keeping people comfortable—it is about enhancing the ability to perform activity important to the person and family system . . . creating opportunities to live fully and productively until death" (p. 1). Pizzi (2014) maintained that even when working with patients at the end of life, occupational therapy practitioners can always promote health, wellness, and QoL. Patients receiving "comfort care" often think that this means being bedridden. Occupational therapy practitioners can help patients focus on which activities they can continue to participate in, with adaptations if needed, instead of just focusing on which activities are now too challenging.

Patients may choose to allow caregivers to perform ADLs, such as donning grip socks, but they may need skilled intervention to continue performing valued occupations, such as applying makeup in their own way. Penfold (1996) stated that in treatment of cancer patients, "the primary drive and focus of the occupational therapist is to facilitate and enable an individual patient to achieve maximum functional performance, both physically and psychologically, in everyday living skills regardless of his or her life expectancy" (p. 75). Patients are often aware of their physical changes and how this affects function but may not be aware of how changes in cognitive and psychosocial skills can effect function and safety.

Patients and caregivers moving to a hospice setting have reported that they perceived "occupational therapy as a practical support that assisted them in preparing for and adapting to discharge from an inpatient palliative care setting" (Marston et al., 2015, p. 694). The occupational therapy literature suggests that occupations are central to a person's identity and competence, determine how one spends time, and influence how one makes decisions (AOTA, 2014). Therapeutic use of occupations can empower a terminally ill patient with a renewed sense of control by helping the patient adapt to physical, cognitive, and psychosocial changes that occur rapidly. Occupational therapy practitioners must share the profession's research and role with other members of the interdisciplinary team who may not be aware of the distinct value of occupational therapy.

Coping With Dying

Corr (1992) proposed a task-based approach for coping with dying that addresses four primary dimensions: (1) physical, (2) psychological, (3) social, and (4) spiritual. Occupation can be a primary source of purpose and meaning in one's daily life, which can include preparation for death (Hasselkus, 2002).

AOTA (1998) also discussed the importance of occupation to enable patients to gain control of themselves and engage in meaningful occupations while also planning for a possible decline in function and eventual death. Occupational therapy practitioners can empower patients with the knowledge and skills needed to adapt and function, which can increase their sense of control over symptoms and situations that seem out of control.

COMMON CHALLENGES IN PALLIATIVE CARE AND HOSPICE

Physical Challenges

Common late and long-term effects of cancer and cancer treatment include overall weakness, pain, fatigue, shortness of breath, and delirium. The medications that bring pain relief to the patient can also cause cognitive changes and constipation. Curative chemotherapy and radiation can create overwhelming fatigue, fragile tissues, and a mental fog or "chemo brain" (i.e., chemotherapy-induced cognitive impairment; see Chapter 17, "Cancer-Related Cognitive Impairment").

Cardiopulmonary concerns are common, along with various other organ failures. Palliative care physicians are highly skilled at managing symptoms by rotating opioids and adjusting medications while using a variety of methods to reduce symptom burden. It is not unusual for a patient to arrive on a palliative care unit unable to tolerate an occupational therapy session because of symptom burden. However, in a few days, once curative treatments are withdrawn and symptom management is the primary focus, the patient may be able to tolerate getting out of bed and going outside with occupational therapy for a community reintegration session. Of course, the opposite is also common: Patients experience functional decline with disease progression. It is important for occupational therapy practitioners working on a palliative care inpatient unit to be flexible because a treatment opportunity window may only be open for a few hours.

A common challenge on the palliative care unit involves transferring patients out of bed and onto a bedside commode or wheelchair after prolonged time in bed. When symptoms are managed and patients feel better, getting out of bed becomes easier. Challenges for functional transfer can include spinal precautions because of bone metastasis, ergonomic adaptations because of general weakness, and pursed-lip breathing techniques before and during functional transfers.

Fatigue is common among all cancer patients, but cancer-related fatigue often increases as the end of life approaches (see Chapter 15, "Cancer-Related Fatigue"). It is counterintuitive, but some palliative care patients report having less fatigue during and after an occupational therapy session, so it is important to explore each patient's individual needs and activity goals.

Client-centered care is important because if the goal is to facilitate function, participation, and performance, it is important to know what the client's priorities are. Occupational therapy practitioners understand that a person who is intrinsically motivated to participate in an activity often can gather the needed reserves of energy to accomplish a highly valued task, whereas performing activities the patient does not view as being meaningful is more difficult (Yoder et al., 1989). Occupational therapy can "increase the awareness that some activities may be more beneficial than others, because there is a significant difference between just being active, and actively doing things that are personally meaningful and purposeful, in other words, through occupation" (Nelson, 1997, p. 11).

Having choices about participating in a meaningful activity is important for any population but is even more critical for patients in palliative care because of their limited time and activity tolerance as they approach the end of their life. In its position statement, the World Federation of Occupational Therapists (WFOT; 2016) noted that "occupational therapists recognize that personal growth and development can occur even in the last phase of life and that participation in occupation can be transformational especially for those approaching the end of life" (p. 2).

Emotional Challenges

Palliative and hospice care professionals willingly walk into an environment of emotional pain, existential suffering, and grief. Patients often report that they have been focusing on curative cancer treatment and only hearing positive news until "someone comes in and gives the hospice talk." This change can happen quickly once curative treatment is no longer beneficial and may in fact be causing harm. This life-limiting news takes time to absorb, and it is important for all of the interprofessional team to be on the same page to help patients and families process the new situation. Patients have reported being told they "failed chemo." This can be distressing; patients should not be told that they failed when in reality the curative treatments "failed them" by not being effective.

Pain can have emotional connotations. It is usually thought of as a physical sensation; however, for cancer patients and especially for patients facing the end of life, the pain caused with movement is not just a nuisance but an existential threat: It reminds them of the cancer that may eventually cause death and separation from loved ones.

Patients often have valid existential grief when they realize that they may not see their children or grandchildren grow up and will miss important milestones and when they think of how their family will cope without them. This is an opportunity to introduce legacy projects and explore strategies on how best to share thoughts with family, such as writing and recording messages to be delivered on important milestones; these strategies are discussed later in this chapter.

Cognitive Challenges

Curative treatments, including whole-brain radiation and chemotherapy, can lead to cognitive changes. (Chemotherapy-induced cognitive impairment is discussed in depth in Chapter 17.) Progressive disease and opioid toxicity may also lead to sedation, neuroexcitation, inhibition, and agitated delirium, which can be very distressful to the patient and family. Delirium is prevalent especially in the last few weeks of life but can be a preterminal event. The etiologies include infection, organ failure, and adverse medication effects (Friedlander et al., 2004, p. 1541).

Social Challenges

Spirituality

Patients facing the end of life have reported a desire to focus on growing spiritually; for example, a home hospice patient reported, "I have spent my life doing my own thing, but now I want to learn more about God since I will be seeing him soon." Some palliative care patients report growing stronger spiritually once their sense of control and physical strength decreases. *Spirituality* is "the aspect of humanity that refers to the way individuals seek and express meaning and purpose and the way they experience their connectedness to the moment, to self, to others, to nature, and to the significant or sacred" (Puchalski et al., 2009, p. 887). A person's faith may be a source of hope or comfort when they are faced with the end of life. This hope could be in life after death, the possibility of healing, spiritual meaning for suffering, acceptance of impermanence, or other understanding (Humbert, 2016). This is why most palliative and hospice interprofessional teams include a chaplain, although each team member can encourage patients to grow spiritually.

Faith traditions can also bring about negative emotions when a person is no longer able to perform certain rituals or travel to a sacred place or when healing does not occur. Well-meaning visitors may try to help the patient by stating a spiritual platitude. Such platitudes may be unhelpful; patients may wonder why others have been healed but they have not, and they may worry their own faith is lacking.

Although occupational therapy practitioners understand spirituality to be an important client factor, few address it in practice (McColl, 2016). Practitioners can explore barriers that inhibit spiritual expression and provide strategies to

overcome these barriers. McColl (2016) recommended that occupational therapists do the following when engaging in client-centered care and spirituality:
- Be clear about what is meant by both *client-centered practice* and *spirituality*;
- Be prepared to take time to move beyond superficial relationships with clients;
- Acknowledge that spirituality and autonomy are present in all clients, not just those who are emotionally or intellectually intact;
- Let go of the need to be in charge and acknowledge that the process is at least 50% owned by the client;
- Embrace a service approach rather than a helping approach or a fixing approach; and
- Acknowledge the reciprocity in the therapeutic relationship and the rich opportunity to continue to learn from clients throughout one's entire career (p. 172).

Social expectations

People are often uncomfortable talking to a person who is facing the end of life and may state a well-meaning platitude or cliché that may unintentionally make the patient feel worse or feel that their grief is not valid. People may tell the patient, "Everything is going to be okay" or "I know how you feel," although they have never faced a similar end-of-life situation themselves. Depending on a patient's social role, they may feel obligated to suppress their emotions because they are expected to stay strong in front of others; for example, a father may not want to cry in front of his children. Relatedly, patients might accept social interaction they do not want or struggle to tolerate out of politeness. Some patients choose to post updates on the social media sites that they have been using, while others create a new account with sites such as CaringBridge (https://www.caringbridge.org/). Patients can post as much or as little as they want so that they don't feel that they need to answer every phone call or email about the current situation. Occupational therapy practitioners can suggest this and provide strategies to the patients or caregivers on how to post.

Many patients facing the end of life have become less social and feel isolated by feeling bedridden and that they are passive recipients of comfort care while family assists with all activities. Occupational therapy practitioners can help palliative patients spend the remainder of their life actively participating in social activities, even if a Hoyer lift to a reclining-back wheelchair is needed. Patients can become empowered and overcome challenges that limit social participation while achieving activity goals that can restore dignity and individuality and resuming cherished roles with an improved self-image (AOTA, 2016).

Caregiving

Caregiving is a co-occupation that is intrinsically social. When the patient is transitioning from hospital care and the care team is planning for what will be needed for home hospice, it is understandable why caregivers tend to be overwhelmed and concerned about being the primary caregiver. Family and caregivers often ask more questions than patients about equipment use and options available from a home hospice agency. Primary caregivers also tend to ask for more education on transfer training from bed to the bedside commode or wheelchair because they will be the ones increasingly assisting the patient at home as the patient's function declines. Therefore, it is best to plan occupational therapy sessions when family and caregivers are available.

It is important to provide patient and family education so that caregivers may feel confident in considering discharging the patient home with hospice as an achievable option and goal. The family is often a primary component of the discharge environment, and the importance of educating caregivers is supported in the nursing literature, which notes that although family caregivers are depended on to provide care, they receive little education and support despite the stressful nature of the work (Reinhard et al., 2008).

CONTEXT AND ENVIRONMENT IN PALLIATIVE CARE AND HOSPICE

Physical Environment

Occupational therapy practitioners can use the physical environment to help patients achieve their individual activity goals by changing the room or transporting the patient out of the room. Some palliative care units do not accept patients younger than 18 years, and pediatric patients may remain on the pediatric unit before transitioning home. Children tend to be more comfortable in a child-friendly environment that facilitates play exploration with fun, colorful, and interactive toys. Adolescents may not want a childish or homelike environment, so some hospitals have an area set apart for adolescents and young adults to play video games and listen to music with peers.

Adults and older adults tend to prefer returning home, if possible, to resume cherished garden, garage, kitchen, or other activities, using adaptations and equipment as needed. Being home, surrounded by familiar objects, can also help a mildly confused patient optimize orientation and continue their familiar routines. Patients often request to leave the unit to sit in a garden, pray in the chapel, purchase an item at the gift shop, get a haircut, play a piano, or visit other destinations of interest to "feel like a person again, not just a patient."

Social Environment

As previously described, patients in palliative care and hospice may feel obligated to allow friends to visit and then entertain them. The family and patient should know that it is okay to limit visitation times and let friends know if it is not a good time to visit.

However, it is important for family and significant others to be allowed by staff to be present, if possible. This is true for all patients but especially important for patients facing the end of life. There are exceptions, but, as a general rule, family members can help orient a patient, decrease confusion, and bring calm to an unfamiliar situation by knowing the patient's personality and preferences. Having family present is helpful with patient care. When the patient wants to interact, family or close friends can provide emotional comfort. For family and others, witnessing the last moments of life, if they desire, can help with emotional healing and closure.

Closure is often important for patients facing the end of life, and occupational therapy practitioners can provide adaptations and equipment to allow some important social milestones to occur. Occupational therapy practitioners have helped provide adaptations and equipment to enable patients to participate in weddings, anniversaries, birthdays, and retirement parties in large community rooms when the patient's hospital room would have been too small for the event (AOTA, 2011).

Cultural Context

Cultural context can vary among family members, and it can vary even more for people whose cultural heritage originated around the globe. Because of this variety, it is best to ask each patient if they have any cultural traditions that they would like for the interprofessional team to be aware of. Parents tend to be more lenient with their children or adolescents who are facing the end of life. This is understandable, but it can be confusing to siblings and other family members. Adolescents and young adults usually expect more privacy, which occupational therapy practitioners can help facilitate.

Spiritual and cultural traditions are important throughout the lifespan, but they tend to be more of a priority among adults and older adults. Culturally significant activities facilitated by occupational therapy include patients recording family stories as a legacy, a mother from Japan wanting to sit up and teach her children origami, and a grandmother wanting to teach her granddaughter how to make her famous "Mexican wedding cookies, just in case I'm not here to make them for your wedding." Case Example 13.1 illustrates how a mother was able to teach her daughters how to perform a ceremony that was important to her ancestors.

Personal Context

Occupational therapy practitioners can help patients resume their personal context, which can include gender identity, age-appropriate activities, group affiliation with peers, and cherished familiar roles. For example, a palliative care patient, Mrs. Aguilar, received word that she had qualified to receive her doctorate; however, she was not able to tolerate leaving her hospital room for graduation.

Instead, the occupational therapist helped Mrs. Aguilar don the graduation gown and doctoral cap as the university faculty and family gathered outside the room. Mrs. Aguilar required maximal assistance with bed mobility because of fatigue, but she reported that the chair position of the bed, with tilt forward and raised height, "allowed me to look at everyone eye to eye without them looking down at me." This was an important personal milestone for the patient, who was now known as Dr. Aguilar. This skilled intervention was also timely, because she died in that room a few days later.

Temporal Context

The temporal context includes the duration of activity, which often requires skilled intervention to optimize

CASE EXAMPLE 13.1. MIAKODA THE SHAMANESS

Miakoda was a descendent of the Cherokee Nation and a patient on the palliative care unit. She wanted to perform a smudging ceremony to bless her family one last time. She was the shamaness, or spiritual leader, of her family, and the smudging ritual had been a family tradition since before history was recorded. The ceremony involves lighting sacred herbs, then blowing the flame out to allow the holy smoke to drive evil spirits away from loved ones.

Because flames and smoke were not allowed in the hospital, the palliative care team had to overcome several challenges for Miakoda to tolerate going outside. The occupational therapist provided a special cushion and reclining-back wheelchair to optimize sitting tolerance because Miakoda had spinal pain when sitting upright. The therapist was able to hold the oxygen mask while the patient lit the herbs and blew out the flames before handing the bundle of herbs to her daughters. Miakoda instructed her daughters how to hold the smoking herbs with various motions to cover each other with this cleansing incense. She reported being pleased to resume this cherished cultural role and teaching her daughters how to perform the smudging ceremony to pass down to future generations.

sitting tolerance and fatigue management. Temporal context includes the time of day because familiar daily routines can provide a sense of control and dignity. Many patients have morning routines, scheduled activities during the day, and rituals before going to sleep. One's stage of life is also a temporal context, including when one believes that one's time on this earth seems to be running out. Facing the end of life can create a sense of urgency, with a desire to "get one's house in order" by finishing personal projects, completing financial and legal documents, and creating a legacy project. Occupational therapy practitioners can help normalize these desires, explore what activities are most meaningful, and provide strategies to enable the patient to perform and participate in the activities they deem most important to complete.

Leaving a legacy can take a lifetime, but leaving a legacy project can be as simple as recording a message for one's descendants to hear. It can be about learning from one's life, applying lessons to the present, and enabling a better future for those who come after. Bosak (2018) noted that

> the idea of legacy may remind us of death, but it's not about death. Being reminded of death is actually a good thing, because death informs life. It gives you a perspective on what's important. But legacy is really about life and living. It helps us decide on the kind of life we want to live and the kind of world we want to live in. (p. 1)

A *legacy project* can be any way of communicating to those who come after us about what was most important about a person's life, wisdom gleaned from lived experiences, and life lessons. These can take many forms and connect lived experiences separated by time by sharing lessons learned from one's elders, who shared their cultural heritage and family history. Patients can share lessons learned from others and combine them with their own to inform future generations about the things in life that truly matter. Patients may choose to record these messages on paper, audio, or video as an activity goal; occupational therapy practitioners can facilitate by providing strategies and adaptations to make this meaningful occupation achievable.

Legacy projects can help the patient review the course of their life, appreciate their experiences, and bring them closure in a positive way. Legacy projects can be therapeutic for the patient but also for the friends and family who love them; such projects share a tangible, life-changing message for future generations as a reminder of their own mortality and to make the most out of life.

Virtual Context

Advances in technology, such as smartphones and tablets, have created more portable opportunities for social interactions, including video conferencing, virtual chat rooms, email, and video games that can be played with peers. Virtual realities can stimulate the senses and serve as a distraction from pain. Social media facilitates patients' inclusion in the daily events of loved ones by allowing blogs and updates between patient and family members, despite their distance. Group forums and chat rooms allow patients to stay connected to like-minded peer groups.

For example, Carlos was a patient on the palliative care unit and reported that he had not seen his brother in more than 50 years. This was before restrictions for traveling to Cuba were reduced and when smartphones were relatively new. A family member in Cuba was able to borrow a smartphone, and the brothers had a virtual face-to-face meeting. The occupational therapist was able to transfer Carlos from the bed to the chair and helped him perform self-grooming using the mirror in the tray table. The two brothers kept talking about how each of them looked like their father, and they were able to catch up with each other as family members listened and laughed in the background.

INTERVENTION APPROACHES IN PALLIATIVE CARE AND HOSPICE

Occupational Profile

When exploring which occupations and activities a patient reports are most meaningful, it may be best to keep the discussion informal and conversational when asking guiding questions. Patients may feel more relaxed while exploring which factors are inhibiting the performance of their activity goals if they do not feel that they are "playing a game of 20 questions."

It is important to mirror the mood of the patient and caregivers before attempting to elevate the patient's perspective. For example, one patient had refused to work

CASE EXAMPLE 13.2. HOW CAN SHE DRAW A PICTURE IF SHE CAN'T HOLD A PEN?

Analysis of occupational performance

Banu, a cancer survivor, developed a spinal tumor that caused incomplete quadriplegia. She presented to the palliative care unit bedbound and unable to verbalize because she did not have a Passy-Muir speaking valve for her tracheostomy. She was not able to write down or indicate her needs. Banu demonstrated right upper extremity (RUE) shoulder and elbow active range of motion with gravity eliminated, but she could not demonstrate wrist or hand movement. Banu's sister reported that Banu was an artist originally from Iran.

Intervention plan

Banu indicated that she was anxious because the only way she could communicate her needs was if others could read her lips. The occupational therapist problem solved and planned various strategies that would allow Banu to communicate with others. They made a secondary plan to allow Banu to resume her valued role and self-identity as an artist. Other plans included asking the attending doctor to write an order to assess the possibility of providing a speaking valve to the patient and getting her into a neurochair to go outside.

Intervention implementation

The occupational therapy team repositioned Banu by adjusting the hospital bed into the chair position and tilted forward in space to optimize her bilateral upper extremity function and lung capacity. An individualized communication sheet was created so that Banu could point at squares labeled with needs, such as suctioning of her tracheostomy, pain medication, repositioning in bed, a damp spongette for her mouth, and calling her sister.

Intervention review

Despite her improved position, Banu was not able to move her RUE enough to point at the desired square, and she seemed frustrated. The occupational therapist put a towel under Banu's right forearm on the tray table to reduce friction. With this, Banu was able to point her finger and touch the desired square indicating a need.

Banu's sister was pleased with this accomplishment and asked whether Banu could put a pen intertwined between her fingers. Banu's lips indicated that if she could hold a pen, then she could draw again. However, Banu was not able to hold the pen in her fingers after repeated attempts with near success. Banu's sister had been verbally encouraging her to try holding the pen another way. When the pen dropped again, Banu's sister asked, "How can she draw a picture if she can't hold a pen?"

The occupational therapist briefly left the room to retrieve a universal cuff, which is an elastic band attached to a small sleeve on the palm to allow patients hold an object without needing to grasp or flex their fingers. The occupational therapist inserted a pen into the universal cuff, and Banu was able to write messages for the first time since experiencing incomplete quadriplegia. The occupational therapist thought that Banu was practicing letters and would throw away the practice paper as discussed. However, Banu was very persistent; she looked up and turned the page to show what she had written. Banu had quoted what the occupational therapist had stated earlier in the session: "Be a person, not a patient." She had written this in English and then in Persian.

Targeting outcomes

Banu was pleased with this accomplishment, and her sister held down and stabilized another sheet of paper while the occupational therapist went to get colorful markers. Banu had met her primary outcome goal of being able to communicate her needs. The team could now address her next goal: to see whether it would be possible to draw pictures again.

The occupational therapist returned with a set of colored markers that would fit in the universal cuff. Banu wrote, "What should I draw?" The occupational therapist replied, "Whatever you want to draw," and the patient seemed perplexed. The occupational therapist encouraged Banu to draw the most beautiful thing she had ever seen.

Banu indicated that she wanted blue, brown, yellow, and green colored markers. With renewed energy, she was able to draw a sailboat with yellow and green striped sails gliding through the blue water. She indicated that she had seen this image decades before while in her home country, Iran. Banu drew other pictures, and these were taped to the wall along with the sailboat drawing. Staff complimented her on the pictures, and she seemed pleased to have resumed her valued role as an artist.

Banu achieved other outcome goals, including demonstrating increased lung capacity while in the chair position of the bed, which allowed her to qualify for a speaking valve. Banu was able to verbalize her needs while enjoying an outing in the neurochair with her family. Occupational therapy provided skilled intervention to help Banu participate in this community reintegration activity because of her fragile condition. The occupational therapist was also required to navigate the neurochair, three oxygen tanks, and IV pole around obstacles, including several elevators and unlevel sidewalks outside. Although an inpatient hospice transfer was planned, Banu's condition changed the week after her goals were met, and she died comfortably on the palliative care unit.

CASE EXAMPLE 13.3. "I COULDN'T BREATHE WHEN I TRIED TO GET OUT OF BED, SO I DON'T WANT TO GET OUT OF BED AGAIN"

Analysis of occupational performance

Sonia had a negative experience becoming short of breath while transferring out of bed before moving to the palliative care unit. Because of this, she reported that she never wanted to feel that way again and that she had chosen to remain in bed. Sonia's choice was to restrict herself to bedrest, which she later commented would have been her "death bed." This comfort zone had become the barrier that kept her from resuming roles and routines that were important to her and her husband.

Intervention plan

An introduction to the occupational therapist's role on the palliative care unit was provided, along with strategies for pursed-lip breathing and positioning that had helped similar patients resume getting out of bed. Sonia agreed that getting out of bed was her goal as long as she "never felt like a fish out of water again." The occupational therapist had measured Sonia's oxygen saturation (SpO_2) during bed mobility, and it remained within normal limits, although she reported slight shortness of breath. The occupational therapist planned to use the pulse oximeter during the intervention to monitor the level of oxygen in Sonia's blood.

Intervention implementation

A pulse and oxygen sensor is not commonly used for palliative care patients because the focus is on how a patient feels or symptom management, such as dyspnea, not on SpO_2 saturation and other data. However, for Sonia, it was a useful tool to help increase her confidence in her newly discovered pursed-lip breathing techniques, and her SpO_2 always remained above 95%. With her new education and confidence, Sonia agreed to attempt more extensive bed mobility and try sitting at the edge of bed. She demonstrated this with modified independence, along with verbal cues not to hold her breath and to "smell the roses and blow out the candles." With renewed confidence, she agreed to attempt standing, which she did at the same level of independence.

Intervention review

Sonia reported being happy achieving her primary activity goal of standing up to get out of bed without becoming short of breath. With this success, she wanted to repeat the sit-to-stand transfer several times. This would be a good next step, given the effectiveness of repetitive therapeutic activity.

However, the occupational therapist remembered that when they were exploring what activities were most meaningful to Sonia, she had mentioned that she most enjoyed slow dancing with her husband. When the occupational therapist reminded her of this, Sonia disclosed which song she most enjoyed dancing to, and the therapist asked whether she would like to attempt a slow dance with her husband. This seemed to startle them both because Sonia had already taken such a big step just to stand again. However, a secondary goal from slow dancing was that the husband and wife would become more comfortable working as a team, with cues for breathing and getting out of bed, in the future for home hospice.

Targeting outcomes

Sonia had met her primary goal of standing up without dyspnea; however, she also reported a meaningful activity goal of slow dancing with her husband. Now that Sonia had demonstrated the ability to stand, slow dancing became an achievable activity goal. A smartphone played the couple's favorite song as they slow danced together, with her husband reminding her to breathe, and eventually Sonia leaned her head on her husband's shoulder with confidence and peace.

The couple's own words are testimony to the value of occupational therapy. Sonia's husband stated in a written survey that they "learned new ways to cope, the dancing was awesome!" Sonia also wrote that this intervention "made me feel good having my husband dance with me. I felt the spiritual closeness between us." With the occupational therapist's skilled intervention, Sonia was able to discharge home with hospice.

This case example supports holistic interventions suggested by Corr (2008), who noted that "the key point was refocusing attention on patients as persons. Not just on their diseases and not merely on what could or could not be done for them or on what resources were or were not available at the time. But on these people as vital human beings in all their physical, psychological, social, and spiritual dimensions" (p. 112).

---

with a particular therapist "because she was too perky and positive. I wasn't ready for that when I just heard some bad news."

Occupational therapy practitioners should review the chart for notes about involved family members, the location of home, and other clues about previous activities. This information is often found on notes written when the patient was first admitted to the hospital. Electronic medical records have made locating these early notes much easier and often mention vocations, previous level of function, and activities that are important to the patient. It is also good to have ideas to suggest in case a patient cannot think of a meaningful activity.

Common activity goals for patients in palliative care include preserving their legacy using audio or video recordings, writing letters, and choosing photos to show at their funeral. If a legacy activity appeals to a patient, occupational therapy practitioners can help the patient create powerful, tangible finished products that future generations can cherish. However, if the patient does not wish to pursue this, move on and explore other meaningful activities. One patient commented when alone with the occupational therapist, "My family is making me feel guilty about not recording something for them; the last thing I need is another thing on my to-do list."

Patients facing the end of life may not have enough energy to fully explore activity options, so listen carefully to them and note what they are saying as well as what they do not talk about. Not all parents want to reconnect with children or return home; occupational profiles and activity preferences are very individualized. Occupational therapy practitioners should have an open mind and not guide the exploration too quickly, or an activity full of meaning may be left hidden.

Sally was a patient on the palliative care unit who could not think of an activity. She had just received news that her life might be ending more quickly than she had planned. After exploring meaningful activities she had done in the past, Sally reported that she unfortunately had to plan her son's funeral when he died in an accident. She decided that she wanted to plan her own funeral and life celebration during the occupational therapy session.

Sally reported that she had not been able to emotionally bear listening to her son's favorite song since it was played at his funeral. After Sally picked out some of her favorite songs, the occupational therapist asked her whether, now planning her own funeral, she felt comfortable listening to her son's favorite song again. She emphatically replied, "You know, I think I want to since I will be seeing him again soon!"

The occupational therapist found the song on his smartphone, with the lyrics, and Sally belted out the chorus with visible emotion. She reported, "I should have done that a long time ago, but no one asked." Sally decided to play this song at her funeral along with the other songs that held meaning in her life. Case Examples 13.2 and 13.3 illustrate how patients can resume valued roles and routines.

SUMMARY

Occupational therapy practitioners understand that participation in meaningful activities can be especially important for patients nearing the end of life; however, occupational therapy practitioners are not always included in the palliative care team. It is important to remember that when we provide evidence and education to demonstrate the distinct value of occupational therapy, the true beneficiaries of this advocacy are the patients, who will be offered a service that they might not have known would benefit them.

The palliative care literature indicates that it is beneficial to assist patients with remaining active as long as they are alive. However, the literature does not detail how this goal of staying active can be achieved. Occupational therapy practitioners are ideal health care professionals not only to help a patient stay active but also to assist with engaging in those activities that provide the most meaning.

Occupational therapy practitioners address the expected declines in function often experienced by patients nearing the end of life by modifying activities and the environment to overcome barriers to function. Occupational therapy

interventions can support a person's ability to maintain important roles and routines and to engage in the activities that are most meaningful to them so that the patient may live each day to its fullest. "Regardless of a clients' life expectancy, occupational therapists provide a unique service that enables function, comfort, safety, autonomy, dignity and social participation through engagement in occupation" (WFOT, 2016, p. 1).

REFERENCES

American Occupational Therapy Association. (1998). Occupational therapy and hospice (statement). *American Journal of Occupational Therapy, 52*, 872–873. https://doi.org/10.5014/ajot.52.10.872

American Occupational Therapy Association. (2011). Role of occupational therapy in end-of-life care. *American Journal of Occupational Therapy, 65*(Suppl. 6), S66–S75. https://doi.org/10.5014/ajot.2011.65S66

American Occupational Therapy Association. (2014). Occupational therapy practice framework: Domain and process (3rd ed.). *American Journal of Occupational Therapy, 68*(Suppl. 1), S1–S48. https://doi.org/10.5014/ajot.2014.682006

American Occupational Therapy Association. (2016). Role of occupational therapy in end-of-life care. *American Journal of Occupational Therapy, 70*(Suppl. 2), 7012410075. https://doi.org/10.5014/ajot.2016.706S17

Badger, S., Macleod, R., & Honey, A. (2016). "It's not about treatment, it's how to improve your life": The lived experience of occupational therapy in palliative care. *Palliative & Supportive Care, 14*, 225–231. https://doi.org/10.1017/S1478951515000826

Bosak, S. (2018). *What is legacy?* Retrieved from https://legacyproject.org/guides/whatislegacy.html

Centers for Medicare and Medicaid Services. (2018). Coverage of hospice services under hospital insurance. In *Medicare benefit policy manual* (rev. ed.). Retrieved from https://www.cms.gov/Regulations-and-Guidance/Guidance/Manuals/Downloads/bp102c09.pdf

Centers for Medicare and Medicaid Services. (2019a). Home health services. In *Medicare benefit policy manual* (rev. ed.). Retrieved from https://www.cms.gov/Regulations-and-Guidance/Guidance/Manuals/Downloads/bp102c07.pdf

Centers for Medicare and Medicaid Services. (2019b). *Physical therapy/occupational therapy/speech-language pathology services.* Retrieved from https://www.cms.gov/Regulations-and-Guidance/Guidance/Manuals/Downloads/bp102c09.pdf

Crossroads Hospice and Palliative Care. (2017). *Remembering Dame Cicely Saunders: Founder of hospice.* Retrieved from https://www.crossroadshospice.com/family-caregivers-blog/2017/july/13/remembering-dame-cicely-saunders-founder-of-hospice/

Corr, C. A. (1992). A task-based approach to coping with dying. *Omega, 24*, 81–94. https://doi.org/10.2190/CNNF-CX1P-BFXU-GGN4

Corr, C. A. (2008). Hospice: Achievements, legacies, and challenges. *Omega, 56*, 111–120. https://doi.org/10.2190/OM.56.1.j

Coyle, N. (2006). The hard work of living in the face of death. *Journal of Pain and Symptom Management, 32*, 266–274. https://doi.org/10.1016/j.jpainsymman.2006.04.003

Egan, M., & DeLaat, M. (1997). The implicit spirituality of occupational therapy practice. *Canadian Journal of Occupational Therapy, 64*, 115–121. https://doi.org/10.1177/000841749706400307

Ferris, F. D. F., Bruera, E., Cherny, N., Cummings, C., Currow, D., Dudgeon, D., . . . Von Roenn, J. H. (2009). Palliative cancer care a decade later: Accomplishments, the need, next steps—From the American Society of Clinical Oncology. *Journal of Clinical Oncology, 27*, 3052–3058. https://doi.org/10.1200/JCO.2008.20.1558

Friedlander, M. M., Brayman, Y., & Breitbart, W. S. (2004). Delirium in palliative care. *Oncology, 18*, 1541–1553.

Hasselkus, B. R. (2002). *The meaning of everyday occupation.* Thorofare, NJ: Slack.

Higginson, I. J. (2011). Dying matters. *Public Service Review: European Science and Technology, 11*, 384–385.

Humbert, T. K. (Ed.). (2016). *Spirituality and occupational therapy. A model for practice and research.* Bethesda, MD: AOTA Press.

Kaye, P. (2006). *Notes on symptom control in hospice and palliative care.* Machiasport, ME: Hospice Education Institute.

Keesing, S., & Rosenwax, L. (2011). Is occupation missing from occupational therapy in palliative care? *Australian Occupational Therapy Journal, 58*, 329–336. https://doi.org/10.1111/j.1440-1630.2011.00958.x

Kübler-Ross, E. (1969). *On death and dying.* New York: Macmillan.

Marcil, W. M. (2006). The hospice nurse and occupational therapy: A marriage of expedience. *Home Health Care Management and Practice, 19*, 26–30. https://doi.org/10.1177/1084822306292514

Marston, C., Agar, M., & Brown, T. (2015). Patients' and caregivers' perceptions of occupational therapy and adapting to discharge home from an inpatient palliative care setting. *British Journal of Occupational Therapy, 78*, 688–696. https://doi.org/10.1177/0308022615586417

McColl, M. (2016). Client-centered care and spirituality. In T. K. Humbert (Ed.), *Spirituality and occupational therapy: A model for practice and research* (pp. 167–174). Bethesda, MD: AOTA Press.

National Hospice and Palliative Care Organization. (2010). *Data analysis and reporting tools. Standards of practice for hospice programs.* Retrieved from https://dart.nhpco.org/ethical-and-position-statements/preamble-and-philosophy

National Hospice and Palliative Care Organization. (2018a). *History of hospice.* Retrieved from https://www.nhpco.org/hospice-care-overview/history-of-hospice/

National Hospice and Palliative Care Organization. (2018b). *Standards of practice for hospice programs.* Retrieved from https://www.nhpco.org/wp-content/uploads/2019/04/Standards_Hospice_2018.pdf

Nelson, D. L. (1997). Why the profession of occupational therapy will flourish in the 21st century (Eleanor Clarke Slagle Lecture). *American Journal of Occupational Therapy, 51*, 11–24. https://doi.org/10.5014/ajot.51.1.11

Pearson, E. J., Todd, J. G., & Futcher, J. M. (2007). How can occupational therapists measure outcomes in palliative care? *Palliative Medicine, 21*, 477–485. https://doi.org/10.1177/0269216307081941

Penfold, S. L. (1996). The role of the occupational therapist in oncology. *Cancer Treatment Reviews, 22*, 75–81. https://doi.org/10.1016/S0305-7372(96)90016-X

Pizzi, M. A. (1984). Occupational therapy in hospice care. *American Journal of Occupational Therapy, 38*, 252–257. https://doi.org/10.5014/ajot.38.4.252

Pizzi, M. (1992). Hospice: The creation of meaning for people with life-threatening illnesses. *Occupational Therapy Practice, 4*(1), 1–7.

Pizzi, M. A. (2014). Promoting health, wellness, and quality of life at the end of life: Hospice interdisciplinary perspectives on creating a good death. *Journal of Allied Health, 43*, 212–220.

Puchalski, C., Ferrell, B., Virani, R., Otis-Green, S., Baird, P., Bull, J., . . . Sulmasy, D. (2009). Improving the quality of spiritual care as a dimension of palliative care: The report of the Consensus Conference. *Journal of Palliative Medicine, 12*, 885–904. https://doi.org/10.1089/jpm.2009.0142

Reinhard, S. C., Given, B., & Bemis, A. (2008). Supporting family caregivers in providing care. In R. G. Hughes (Ed.), *Patient safety and quality: An evidence based handbook of nurses* (Ch. 14). Rockville, MD: Agency for Healthcare Research and Quality. Retrieved from https://archive.ahrq.gov/professionals/clinicians-providers/resources/nursing/resources/nurseshdbk/nurseshdbk.pdf

Richmond, C. (2005). *Dame Cicely Saunders, founder of the modern hospice movement, dies.* Retrieved from: http://www.bmj.com/content/suppl/2005/07/18/331.7509.DC1

Russell, M., & Bahle-Lampe, A. (2016). The Care for the Dying: A critical historical analysis of occupational therapy in hospice. *Open Journal of Occupational Therapy, 4*(2), Article 12. https://doi.org/10.15453/2168-6408.1216

Sleight, A. G., & Duker, L. I. S. (2016). Toward a broader role for occupational therapy in supportive oncology care. *American Journal of Occupational Therapy, 70*, 7004360030. https://doi.org/10.5014/ajot.2016.018101

Tax Equity and Fiscal Responsibility Act of 1982. Pub.L. 94–248.

Woodruff, R. (2004). Palliative care: Basic principles. In E. Bruera, L. De Lima, R. Wenk, & W. Farr (Eds.), *Palliative care in the developing world: Principles and practice* (pp. 1–2). Houston: University of Texas Printing Services.

World Federation of Occupational Therapists. (2016). *Occupational therapy in end life care* (position statement). Retrieved from https://www.wfot.org/resources/occupational-therapy-in-end-of-life-care

World Health Organization. (n.d.). *Definition of palliative care.* Retrieved from http://www.who.int/cancer/palliative/definition/en/

World Health Organization. (2002). *National cancer control programmes: Policies and managerial guidelines* (2nd ed.). Geneva: Author.

World Health Organization. (2007). *Cancer control: Knowledge into action (WHO guide for effective programs): Palliative care.* Retrieved from http://www.who.int/cancer/media/FINAL-Palliative%20Care%20Module.pdf

World Health Organization. (2014). *WHO Global Atlas on palliative care at the end of life.* Retrieved from https://www.who.int/nmh/Global_Atlas_of_Palliative_Care.pdf

Yoder, R. M., Nelson, D. L., & Smith, D. A. (1989). Added-purpose versus rote exercise in female nursing home residents. *American Journal of Occupational Therapy, 43*, 581–586. https://doi.org/10.5014/ajot.43.9.581

APPENDIX 13.A.   History of Hospice Care

The term *hospice* (from the same linguistic root as *hospitality*) can be traced back to medieval times, when it referred to a place of shelter and rest for weary or ill travelers on a long journey. The name was first applied to specialized care for dying patients by physician Dame Cicely Saunders, who began her work with terminally ill patients in 1948 and eventually created the first modern hospice—St. Christopher's Hospice—in a residential suburb of London.

Saunders introduced the idea of specialized care for the dying to the United States during a 1963 visit to Yale University. Her lecture, given to medical students, nurses, social workers, and chaplains about the concept of holistic hospice care, included photos of terminally ill cancer patients and their families, showing the dramatic differences before and after the symptom control care. This lecture launched the following chain of events, which resulted in the development of hospice care as we know it today.

1965: Florence Wald, then dean of the Yale School of Nursing, invited Dame Cicely Saunders to become a visiting faculty member of the school for the spring term.

1967: Saunders created St. Christopher's Hospice in the United Kingdom.

1968: Wald took a sabbatical from Yale to work at St. Christopher's and learn all she could about hospice.

1969: Dr. Elisabeth Kübler-Ross (1969) published a book based on more than 500 interviews with dying patients, titled *On Death and Dying*. The book identified the five stages through which many terminally ill patients progress. It became an internationally known best seller. In it, Kübler-Ross made a plea for home care, as opposed to treatment in an institutional setting, and argued that patients should have a choice and the ability to participate in the decisions that affect their destiny.

1972: Kübler-Ross testified at the first national hearings on the subject of death with dignity, which were conducted by the U.S. Senate Special Committee on Aging. In her testimony, Kübler-Ross stated, "We live in a very particular death-denying society. We isolate both the dying and the old, and it serves a purpose. They are reminders of our own mortality. We should not institutionalize people. We can give families more help with home care and visiting nurses, giving the families and the patients the spiritual, emotional, and financial help in order to facilitate the final care at home."

1974: Wald, along with two pediatricians and a chaplain, founded Connecticut Hospice in Branford, Connecticut.

1974: The first hospice legislation was introduced by Senators Frank Church and Frank E. Moss to provide federal funds for hospice programs. The legislation was not enacted.

1978: A U.S. Department of Health, Education, and Welfare task force reported that "the hospice movement as a concept for the care of the terminally ill and their families is a viable concept and one which holds out a means of providing more humane care for Americans dying of terminal illness while possibly reducing costs. As such, it is the proper subject of federal support."

1979: The Health Care Financing Administration initiated demonstration programs at 26 hospices across the country to assess the cost-effectiveness of hospice care and to help determine what a hospice is and what it should provide.

1980: The W. K. Kellogg Foundation awarded a grant to the Joint Commission on Accreditation of Hospitals to investigate the status of hospice and to develop standards for hospice accreditation.

1982: Congress included a provision to create a Medicare hospice benefit in the Tax Equity and Fiscal Responsibility Act of 1982, with a 1986 sunset provision.

1984: The Joint Commission on Accreditation of Hospitals initiated hospice accreditation.

1986: The Medicare Hospice Benefit was made permanent by Congress and hospices given a 10% increase in reimbursement rates. States were given the option of including hospice in their Medicaid programs. Hospice care is now available to terminally ill nursing home residents.

Source. Adapted from "History of Hospice," by the National Hospice and Palliative Care Organization, 2018. Adapted with permission.

Home Health and the Community

Suzänne (Taylor) Zeta, PhD, MBA, OTR/L

LEARNING OBJECTIVES

After completing this chapter, readers should be able to
- Understand the role of home health and community-based care along the cancer care continuum,
- Identify the similarities and differences between home health care and home care,
- Explain the distinct value that occupational therapy adds to home health care and community-based care for cancer survivors, and
- Apply strategies that enable occupational performance and participation for cancer survivors receiving home health care and community-based care.

KEY TERMS AND CONCEPTS

- Acute survivorship
- Advanced-stage disease
- Community-based practice
- Cultural context
- Extended survivorship
- Home care
- Home health care
- Interdisciplinary teams
- Performance scales
- Performance status
- Permanent survivorship
- Personal context
- Physical environment
- Psychosocial disruption
- Social environment
- Survivorship
- Survivorship care plan
- Symptom burden
- Temporal context
- Virtual context

INTRODUCTION

Advancements in cancer treatments and improved survival rates have led to increasing numbers of cancer survivors. In addition, there is increased awareness of late, long-term, and persistent side effects associated with cancer itself and its medical treatments, which in turn has increased the demand for rehabilitative services. Research suggests that upward of 90% of individuals who are currently undergoing or have recently completed cancer treatments have one or more impairments that indicate the need for rehabilitation (Alfano et al., 2012; Thorsen et al., 2011). This need, along with the delivery of cancer treatments occurring beyond traditional acute care and hospital settings, has facilitated the extension of the cancer care continuum into a variety of settings, including home health and community-based practice, at all phases of survivorship.

Survivorship refers to living with, through, and beyond cancer and the associated medical treatments. Survivorship begins on the day of diagnosis. It is sometimes categorized in three survivorship phases (American Society of Clinical Oncology [ASCO], 2018):
1. *Acute survivorship* begins at the diagnosis and continues through initial medical treatment. The primary medical focus is treatment of the cancer.

2. *Extended survivorship* starts at the end of initial medical treatment and continues through the months following. The primary focus is to mitigate the effects of the cancer itself and the side effects of the medical treatments.
3. *Permanent survivorship* refers to the period of time (years) since the medical cancer treatments ended when recurrence is less likely. The primary focus is addressing the long-term effects of the cancer itself and the side effects of the medical treatments.

Although none of these phases specifically includes recurrence of cancer, once an individual begins undergoing active cancer treatments, they are considered to be in the acute survivorship phase.

Note that none of these phases directly includes Stage IV or *advanced-stage disease,* which refers to cancer that has spread, or become metastatic, and usually cannot be cured or controlled with treatment. In advanced-stage disease, the individual may still undergo cancer treatments, with a goal of controlling progression or reducing the cancer burden. Cancer treatments may also be used as a palliative approach to reduce symptom burden or improve quality of life (QoL).

It is also important to remember that individuals who have advanced-stage disease more than likely already have undergone multiple cancer treatments. Therefore, they may be experiencing side effects from prior cancer treatments that are compounded by the impact of advanced-stage disease. An exception is for those individuals who were initially diagnosed with cancer at Stage IV (with metastatic disease). As noted, the medical treatment plan for individuals with advanced-stage disease may still have a primary focus on treating the cancer (i.e., acute survivorship), or it may focus on mitigating the effects of cancer and treatments (i.e., extended survivorship).

Regardless of survivorship phase, recognizing the rehabilitative needs and extension of the cancer care continuum into home health care and community-based practice provides occupational therapy practitioners opportunities (Coninck et al., 2017). These include the opportunity to

- Help decrease the effects of cancer treatments and optimize performance status;
- Mitigate side effects and optimize functional performance, performance status, and activity engagement;
- Develop community-based programming to help mitigate lingering and persistent side effects, educate about self-management, and organize support groups; and
- Raise the bar of expectations that survivors reach the levels of functional performance and activity engagement they had before being diagnosed with cancer.

FEATURES OF HOME HEALTH CARE AND COMMUNITY-BASED PRACTICE AND THE CANCER CARE CONTINUUM

The primary defining feature of both home health care and community-based settings is that the clients receive care within their environment rather than in a structured or institutionalized setting (American Occupational Therapy Association [AOTA], 2013). This unique aspect allows occupational therapy practitioners to work directly with cancer survivors as they engage within their actual environmental, temporal, and social contexts. The benefits include the ability to highly personalize the occupational therapy evaluation, interventions, recommendations, and education (Coninck et al., 2017).

Home Health Occupational Therapy and the Cancer Care Continuum

Home health care refers to receiving skilled clinical services in the home, prescribed by a physician and as part of a plan of care, typically after a hospitalization. Home health care is not to be confused with *home care,* which refers to care provided by home care aides, generally as part of a routine to assist with ADLs or to provide companionship. Home care is nonclinical and is often considered personal or companion care. In home health care, the clinical and skilled services provided may include nursing, rehabilitation, and patient education.

In the home health care practice setting, the provider travels to the home to provide services. This naturally results in a great variety of locations and types of homes in which services may be provided. Homes may be rural or urban, single family, part of an apartment complex, or an assisted living or independent living community. Regardless of this diversity, the primary benefit of practice in home health care is the ability to work directly with clients in their personal environment.

Services are provided by *interdisciplinary teams*, including, among others, nursing, occupational therapy, physical therapy, and social work. Although there are a variety of methods to maintain interdisciplinary communication, the actual delivery of each discipline's services generally occurs independently from the others. Medicare and many third-party payers provide coverage for home health occupational therapy services, provided qualifying criteria are met:

- The plan of care is prescribed and certified by a physician,
- The client is considered homebound, and
- The services provided are medically necessary and reasonable for an intermittent period of time.

Occupational therapy services in the home health care setting may be required for individuals who are in the acute phase of survivorship and undergoing active cancer treatment, are in the extended phase of survivorship and have recently completed cancer treatment, or have advanced-stage cancer (AOTA, 2013; Braveman & Hunter, 2017; Coninck et al., 2017).

Community-Based Occupational Therapy and the Cancer Care Continuum

Community-based practice occurs outside of the medical model and includes a focus on the collective health needs of the community to enable independence and engagement of the people. This is why community-based practices are unique to the occupational therapy practitioner and the programs are unique to each community. Rather than working solely with individual clients, community-based practitioners also work with organizations and populations on a wide range of health-related areas, including acute and chronic medical care, health disparities, and health promotion.

Community-based practice may occur in a variety of settings, including community mental health, nonprofit organizations, adult day care, supported employment, supervised housing, wellness centers, and continuing-care retirement communities, and involves a variety of team members. Because community-based practice is outside of the medical model, services are not reimbursed through health insurance policies. Funding for this setting may be supported through businesses, community organizations, nonprofit organizations, and grants. Occupational therapy services and programs in a community-based practice setting may be established for individuals who have been diagnosed with cancer, and their family and caregivers, across all stages of cancer and survivorship phases (O'Brien et al., 2014; Polo & Smith, 2017).

OVERVIEW OF OCCUPATIONAL THERAPY'S ROLE IN HOME HEALTH CARE AND THE COMMUNITY ACROSS THE CANCER CARE CONTINUUM

Occupational therapy's core purpose is to facilitate daily engagement in meaningful activities at an optimal level of performance, which is why occupational therapy plays a significant role in cancer care across the cancer care continuum. *Performance status* refers to how much time during waking hours the individual is "up" (i.e., out of bed, not lying on the couch or sedentary in a chair) and whether they are able to complete self-care and basic home management activities. Performance status is a key factor in cancer care and is used to determine cancer treatment options, as an indicator of how well cancer treatments are tolerated, to decide whether to continue cancer treatments, and as an understanding of overall prognosis.

Oncologists commonly determine performance status through use of *performance scales,* such as the Eastern Cooperative Oncology Group Scale of Performance Status (Oken et al., 1982) and the Karnofsky Performance Scale (Karnofsky & Burchenal, 1949). Because the cancer itself and associated medical treatments have been shown to negatively affect literally every aspect of the cancer survivor, including their physical, cognitive, and emotional abilities (Hwang et al., 2015; Neo et al., 2017; Taylor, 2017; Thorsen et al., 2011), there is a significant risk of decreased ability to engage in activities, leading to a lower performance status (Saotome et al., 2015). Occupational therapy practitioners are uniquely skilled to provide interventions and develop programs designed to facilitate functional performance in home health care and community-based practice settings.

Occupational Therapy in Home Health Care

Although the overall role of occupational therapy for cancer survivors in the home health care setting is to facilitate engagement in meaningful activities (AOTA, 2013; Vance, 2016), the focus should vary according to where the individual is on the cancer care continuum. In the home health setting, there are three primary points during the acute and extended survivorship phases:

1. Individuals who are actively undergoing cancer treatments or have precautions associated with cancer treatments that limit their ability to be in public settings, such as after high-dose chemotherapy treatment;
2. Individuals who recently underwent a cancer treatment that limited their functional abilities, such as after a surgical intervention; and
3. Individuals who have advanced disease and impaired functional abilities, who may still be undergoing cancer treatment; their diagnosis is often complicated with symptom burdens such as pain, fatigue, nausea, and difficulty breathing.

Occupational therapy in home health care during active cancer treatments

Occupational therapy has a unique role in home health care for individuals who are undergoing active cancer treatment or have precautions associated with cancer treatments that limit their ability to be in public settings. For these survivors, occupational therapy practitioners can work to understand how the individual may be affected by the cancer and treatments and how their lifestyle and individual factors may influence their ability to remain engaged in daily activities.

Occupational therapy interventions should have a focus that considers precautions and physiological tolerance, with overarching goals to facilitate the client's ability to remain engaged in daily activities and prevent further loss of functional abilities. Emphasis should be placed on the importance of attempting daily activity, even when the client is experiencing side effects of the cancer treatments. Recommendations should include how and when to incorporate principles of energy conservation and task simplification to remain engaged in daily activity.

It is also important to educate cancer survivors on anticipated changes in function, precautions associated with cancer treatments, and how these might affect the survivor's performance abilities. Risk factors that may lead to decreased function include the following:

- *Disease related:* Primary and metastatic cancer obstructing the normal functioning of the body's structures and organ systems
- *Treatment related:* Surgery, chemotherapy, radiation, hormonal therapy, bone marrow transplant, and secondary medications
- *Lifestyle related:* Sedentary versus active lifestyle, health behaviors
- *Individual factors:* Mood, coping skills, emotional responses, internal or external locus of control.

Education for family or caregivers should include how to provide assistance only to the level needed rather than assisting by completing the full task and inadvertently rendering the cancer survivor dependent during that activity (AOTA, 2013).

Occupational therapy in home health care after cancer treatments

In the months after cancer treatments end, the expectation is for symptoms to begin resolving. Levels of pain, fatigue, and cognitive impairment should lessen, and physiological tolerance for activity should improve. The overall focus of occupational therapy at this point is rehabilitative in nature and centers on improving strength, cognition, and ability to engage in daily activities at prediagnosis levels.

Interventions should also include education in self-management, including signs and symptoms of risks specific to the cancer and its treatments. For example, occupational therapy practitioners should provide education on the signs and symptoms of lymphedema for an individual after mastectomy, removal of lymph nodes, and radiation treatment across the region.

Occupational therapy in home health care and advanced-stage disease

Occupational therapy's role in home health care for individuals with advanced-stage disease is to maximize their ability to engage in meaningful activities primarily through compensating for areas of lost function. For cancer survivors with advanced-stage disease and symptom burden, occupational therapy interventions should be designed with a compensatory approach and include environmental modifications and caregiver education to facilitate continued engagement with meaningful activities and an overall improved QoL.

Occupational therapy interventions must be congruent with the medical plan of care; overall prognosis; and considerations for how well the individual, their family, and their caregivers understand the situation. It is important for occupational therapy practitioners to know the answers to the following questions:

- Will there be continued medical treatments for the cancer? If so, what is the goal?
- What is the overall prognosis?
- How well does the individual understand the diagnosis and prognosis?
- How well does the family understand the diagnosis and prognosis?
- If palliative cancer treatments are recommended, does the individual understand the purpose as palliative or as another line of treatment for a potential cure?

Symptom burden is one of the primary factors that causes impaired functional abilities and an inability to engage in meaningful activities (Brandt et al., 2016; Lipson et al., 2017; Taylor, 2017). Symptoms of pain, lingering fatigue, difficulty breathing, and poor activity tolerance are commonly reported in advanced disease. With an understanding that achieving full resolution of symptom burden may not be possible and that there may be continued progression of the cancer, occupational therapy interventions should focus on mitigating the effects of symptoms while facilitating the client's ability to engage in meaningful activities. This may be accomplished through a variety of compensatory interventions and approaches, including:

- Education on how to most effectively use the client's current tolerance for activities to balance activity engagement with appropriate periods of rest, according to symptom burden, medical plan of care, and what is meaningful for the client;
- Education on the use of compensatory strategies to avoid exacerbation of symptoms;
- Graded tasks and activities to levels that are within tolerance;
- Recommendations for environmental modifications and adaptive aids to reduce effort and improve safety;
- Education to further modify environments and grade activities as needed to continue activity engagement; and
- Training for family and caregivers on how to safely provide physical assistance for the client's current functional abilities and for lower functional abilities.

It may be helpful to explain to the individual and their family and caregivers that there may be days when the symptom burden is worse. Those are the times when more physical assistance may be needed and the environment may need to be adjusted. It is more valuable to be able to participate in a meaningful activity at some level than to avoid the activity because of a lower functional ability.

Occupational Therapy in Community-Based Practice

There are several avenues for occupational therapy services and programming in community-based practice across the cancer care continuum (Blignault et al., 2017; Lauckner et al., 2011; Leclair, 2010; Scaffa, 2001). One avenue is to facilitate survivorship care plans by developing programming

for self-management, support groups, prevention, and wellness (Hwang et al., 2015; Salz et al., 2014).

Another area is to organize and facilitate the integration and communication of oncology resources across institutions, businesses, and organizations to meet the complex needs of survivors. Another area in which occupational therapy practitioners are well suited is developing an oncology community of practice across disciplines and organizations. This helps strengthen the community practitioners' communication while elevating their understanding of occupational therapy's role of increasing survivors' engagement in activity and in the community.

COMMON CHALLENGES EXPERIENCED IN HOME HEALTH AND THE COMMUNITY

The scope of practice for occupational therapy in home health care and community-based practice settings includes addressing those areas that affect the cancer survivor's ability to engage in their roles and responsibilities. These areas include client factors, performance patterns, and performance skills. Research has shown that cancer and cancer treatments may negatively affect physical and physiological functioning, cognitive abilities, emotional abilities, and social interactions.

Physical Challenges

Although the intensity and duration of cancer effects vary and depend on survivors' specific cancer and treatments, a recent study suggested that at least 50% of cancer survivors experience late effects of cancer treatment (Valdivieso et al., 2012). The most common physical challenges are pain and fatigue (Harrington et al., 2010). Pain across all cancers and at all stages is reported by as many as 50% of cancer survivors, with more than one-third rating the pain as moderate or severe (van den Beuken-Everdingen et al., 2017). Up to 10% of cancer survivors have persistent pain for months or years, even when disease free (Glare et al., 2014).

Along with pain caused by the cancer, pain may develop after survivors undergo surgery, radiation therapy, chemotherapy, and other cancer treatments (Taylor, 2017; Zucca et al., 2012). Late effects of cancer treatments include radiation necrosis, axillary web syndrome, and chemotherapy-induced peripheral neuropathy. Fatigue has been shown to affect as many as 80%–90% of cancer survivors who have undergone chemotherapy or radiation and nearly 100% of those who have undergone a combination of cancer treatments (Ebede et al., 2017; Zucca et al., 2012). Feelings of fatigue may lead to self-restriction of daily activities and inactivity, which has been shown to contribute to decreased functioning and a lower performance status. Cancer survivors may also experience changes in physiological functioning, leading to cardiotoxicity and cardiovascular disease, lymphedema, or secondary cancers.

Cognitive Challenges

Research shows that upward of 75% of cancer survivors experience cognitive dysfunction, and nearly one-third of these individuals continue to experience cognitive impairments for months to years after cancer treatments, even when disease free (Janelsins et al., 2011; Williams et al., 2016). The most commonly described cognitive difficulties are with attention and concentration, short-term memory, verbal memory, and visual–perceptual abilities, all of which contribute to executive functioning. Difficulties in these cognitive processes may negatively affect performance in activities such as medication management, financial management, planning, and problem solving.

Emotional Challenges

Cancer survivors have an increased risk of mood disorders and have been shown to have greater rates of clinical anxiety and depression than the general population without cancer (Linden et al., 2012; Yi & Syrjala, 2017). Unfortunately, the incidence of suicide among patients with cancer has been shown as nearly twice that of the general population (Kendal, 2007; Miller et al., 2008; Misono et al., 2008).

Social Challenges

As a survivor's journey progresses from receiving a diagnosis of cancer through treatments and into remission, there may be continued changes in their own beliefs, values, coping skills, mood, and emotions. The impact of cancer has also been shown to extend beyond the cancer survivor to the cosurvivor (e.g., spouse, partner) and family unit (Carmack et al., 2011; Hoffman et al., 2009; Taylor, 2017).

Likewise, family members and social supports may have changes in their roles, including moving into and out of being a caregiver. These changes place the cancer survivor and the survivor's family and support system at risk for a cycle of increased stress for those involved, leading to *psychosocial disruption,* which occurs when there is a disturbance or situation that negatively affects the interrelationship of the individual and their social environment. If not addressed, this disruption can progress to psychosocial impairment, which has been shown to have negative effects on health (Carmack et al., 2011). Individual factors that influence psychosocial well-being include personal beliefs, emotions, and mood. Social factors that influence psychosocial well-being include family structure, the individual's social supports, and their work environment.

IMPORTANCE OF CONTEXT AND ENVIRONMENT IN HOME HEALTH AND THE COMMUNITY

The context and environment in which the individual performs activities play an important role in the success of activity engagement. To effectively meet the needs of clients who have cancer or have undergone cancer treatments, occupational therapy practitioners must embrace this concept and incorporate interventions as needed to modify, enhance, or educate, with an understanding of the interplay between the individual and their contexts and environments.

Physical Environment

The *physical environment* includes all of the areas in which the client performs activities, from where they sleep and complete self-care through where they perform daily activities, the vehicle in which they ride, and the sidewalks and buildings where they conduct business. As noted previously, one of the benefits of providing occupational therapy services in home health care is the ability to work with cancer survivors in their environment. Occupational therapy practitioners can work directly with the physical environment to facilitate engagement in daily activity by considering the following:

- *Is this person undergoing active cancer treatments?* If so, encourage continued engagement in the usual physical environments but educate on options for rearranging and modifying heights of furniture if needed. It is important to continue daily activity, even at a modified or reduced level, rather than to become sedentary.
- *Has this person completed cancer treatments?* If so, encourage return to the usual physical environments, including at community levels.
- *Does this person have advanced disease or symptom burden?* If so, arrange placement and modify heights of items, including the bed, chair, and commode, to decrease the impact of symptom burden. Incorporate the use of adaptive equipment and durable medical equipment to facilitate engagement in meaningful activities.

Social Environment

The *social environment*—that is, the cancer survivor's relationships with and expectations of people with whom they interact—plays a role in the ability to remain engaged in daily activities. When appropriate, occupational therapy sessions should include the significant other, family, or caregivers. Points to consider in the home health care and community-based practice settings include the following:

- Does the cancer survivor require physical assistance? If so, who provides this care? If it is their significant other, how has the role of caregiver affected the couple's relationship and intimacy?
- What is the expectation of the client's social environment so they can continue performing activities associated with their roles? How does this affect the client's ability to modify their daily routine or activities?

Cultural Context

As explained in the *Occupational Therapy Practice Framework: Domain and Process* (3rd ed.; *OTPF;* AOTA, 2014), an individual's **cultural context** influences their identity and activity choices. Occupational therapy practitioners should consider the following questions:

- What are the cancer survivor's beliefs and expectations about the cancer diagnosis, prognosis, treatments, and potential side effects?
- What are the expectations of the survivor to continue performing activities associated with their roles?

Personal Context

The **personal context,** or one's demographics, may play a role in the client's ability to follow through with recommendations. Occupational therapy practitioners should consider the following areas when developing the plan of care and providing interventions in home health care and community-based practice settings:

- Does the client's socioeconomic status, health insurance benefits, or financial resources limit access to equipment or their ability to continue receiving occupational therapy sessions?
- What is the client's educational level? Are the written materials provided at the proper level? How well do the client and their caregivers understand the education provided and the recommendations made?
- What is the client's level of health literacy? How does this affect their overall understanding of the diagnosis, prognosis, and recommendations from various health care team members?

Temporal Context

The *temporal context* refers to when this person is experiencing cancer and cancer treatments, relative to who they are. The following points should be considered:

- What stage of life is this person in, and what are their roles? In which roles does this person wish to engage?
- How long has this person been diagnosed with cancer?
- Have they experienced a loved one having cancer?
- Have they experienced cycles of lowered performance abilities, improved abilities, and lower performance abilities? If so, what is their understanding of the current prognosis and what is their expectation of achieving improved functional abilities?
- If they have a lower performance status, how long has it been since they were able to engage in their usual routines and roles?

Virtual Context

The *virtual context* provides an avenue for individuals to have interactions "in a simulated, real-time, or near-time situation absent of physical contact" (AOTA, 2014, p. S9). This avenue is the basis for telehealth and may be incorporated in outpatient, home health care, and community-based settings. To maintain an individualized approach, the occupational therapy practitioners must consider the following:

- Did this person use technology before receiving a diagnosis of cancer?
- Is this person willing to use technology for reminders?
- Does this person use motivational programs, blogs, or online support groups? If so, does this influence their expectations of prognosis or recovery of functional abilities?

APPROACHES TO INTERVENTION IN HOME HEALTH CARE AND THE COMMUNITY

Occupational therapy interventions in home health care should include educating the cancer survivor on how to remain active each day within physiological tolerance and with considerations for precautions. Emphasize the importance of attempting daily activity, even when the client is experiencing side effects of the cancer treatments.

Recommendations should include how and when to incorporate principles of energy conservation and task simplification to remain engaged in daily activity.

It is also important to educate the cancer survivor on anticipated changes in function, precautions associated with cancer treatments, and how these might affect the survivor's performance abilities. Education for family and caregivers should include how to provide assistance only to the level needed rather than assisting by completing the full task and inadvertently rendering the cancer survivor dependent during that activity.

Although occupational therapy interventions and programming in community-based practice settings may vary widely, the overarching focus should be on facilitating survivorship care plans by developing programming for self-management, support groups, prevention, and wellness. A *survivorship care plan* is an individualized report and plan developed by the oncology team that includes a record of cancer and treatment history as well as guidelines for monitoring and maintaining health and addressing common lingering and persistent side effects associated directly with the cancer and its treatments (ASCO, 2018; Hewitt et al., 2005).

Another focus for occupational therapy programming in community-based practice settings is that of organizing and facilitating the integration and communication of oncology resources across institutions, businesses, and organizations to meet the complex needs of survivors in that community (Leclair, 2010; Polo & Smith, 2017; Scaffa, 2001). This may also be achieved through an oncology community of practice developed across disciplines and organizations. Not only does this serve to strengthen the community practitioners' communication, it provides a platform to elevate their understanding of occupational therapy's role of increasing survivors' engagement in activity and in the community.

For both home health care and community-based practice settings, to be most effective with occupational therapy interventions, practitioners must gain an appreciation for who the client is in terms of their everyday life, how they have been affected by cancer and the treatments, and how they may be further affected. This understanding is gained through an occupational profile and an analysis of the client's occupational performance.

Occupational Profile

A person's occupational profile refers to the roles and responsibilities that they have. Consider the following questions:

- What were the client's roles and responsibilities before being diagnosed with cancer?
- What are their roles and responsibilities now? Is it feasible to continue with these roles and responsibilities?
- If there has been a change in roles and responsibilities, how well has the client adjusted to this change? Do they have support, or has someone else assumed those roles and responsibilities?
- If there has not been a change in roles or responsibilities, is it reasonable to expect that there may need to be a change? If so, does the client have support or someone willing to assist?

Analysis of Occupational Performance

After determining the cancer survivor's occupational profile, the occupational therapy practitioner can determine the survivor's ability to perform the tasks and activities associated with those roles and responsibilities. Unfortunately, for people who have cancer and are undergoing cancer treatments, functional abilities frequently fluctuate, especially if the individual is experiencing side effects of fatigue, pain, cognitive dysfunction, or emotional disturbance.

Case Example 14.1 highlights the importance of determining the occupational profile, completing an analysis of occupational performance, and educating the cancer survivor and their family and caregivers on anticipated fluctuations in their performance abilities.

CASE EXAMPLE 14.1. HOW CAN I TAKE CARE OF THE HOUSE IF I CAN'T BEND OVER?

Responding to the news that she needed to avoid bending forward and lifting, **Monica** questioned, "How can I take care of the house if I can't bend over?" A mother of two sons ages 15 years and 11 years, Monica took pride being able to have her sons and husband come home each day to a homemade dinner in a clean house. She explained that this became very important to her after losing the ability to work as an elementary school teacher a couple of years prior. She resigned from that position after the lingering fatigue and ongoing breast cancer treatments interfered with her physical tolerance for the daily demands of that role. Now, with metastatic disease causing unstable vertebral bodies in the thoracic and cervical regions, Monica was advised to follow back precautions.

Intervention

After the occupational therapist ensured Monica's understanding of back precautions and implications for her daily routine, they spent time discussing the emotional importance of tasks such as baking and laundry, especially in light of Monica's desire to preserve her current occupational profile. Pulling from Monica's previous occupational profile of being an elementary school teacher, coupled with her role as a mother, the occupational therapist incorporated task modification in the context of adjusting Monica's view of her occupational profile.

Intervention plan

The plan for this intervention included task analysis of activities that Monica considered vital to her current occupational profile. These tasks included baking, doing laundry, vacuuming, and changing bed linens. One task in particular, baking, included a high-level component of leisure for Monica.

The intervention plan was to have Monica complete those steps of each task that fell within the back precautions and to encourage Monica to receive help on the remaining steps by considering this as a teaching opportunity for her sons. Reframing tasks into having her sons engage in household tasks on arrival home from school allowed Monica to retain a sense of independence and vitality in her current occupational profile, while also incorporating the primary aspect of her previous occupational profile as an educator.

Intervention implementation

The implementation of this intervention began with client education. Monica was provided education on the back precautions, including what was involved and why. For Monica, it was particularly useful to review the areas of metastatic disease, the structures that were affected, and the potential outcomes of collapsed or shifted vertebral bodies.

Education then progressed to task analysis. The occupational therapist spent time discussing with Monica how each activity is composed of multiple steps, some of which were well within her abilities, and others of which would place her at risk for further injury by violating the back precautions.

After Monica demonstrated understanding of the education, the occupational therapist used the primary benefit of the home health setting by engaging Monica in an activity. Given the importance of baking to Monica, this became the initial activity of focus. As Monica simulated completing the agreed-on portions of baking, the occupational therapist made environmental adjustments to further help Monica succeed in maintaining back precautions. Examples of adjustments included placing commonly used items on the counter to decrease the likelihood of accidentally bending over to lower cabinets and strategically locating a chair and stool in the kitchen for Monica to rest as needed.

Targeting outcomes

As explained in the *OTPF*, *outcome measures* are the objective measures used to analyze the effectiveness of treatment interventions (AOTA, 2014). In this case example, the primary outcome measure is whether Monica is able to engage in daily activities while following back precautions, as measured by having Monica complete

- Verbal repeat-back of back precautions;
- Demonstration of activities that are affected by back precautions;
- Verbal report of how she has educated her sons; and
- A parallel task analysis on a different activity affected by back precautions, having Monica state which portions of the activity she would complete and which portions she would teach her sons.

SUMMARY

The unique aspect of home health care and community-based practice is that occupational therapy practitioners work directly with clients as they engage in their actual environmental, temporal, and social contexts. The benefits include the ability to highly personalize the occupational therapy evaluation, interventions, recommendations, and education.

By facilitating daily engagement in meaningful activities at an optimal level of performance, occupational therapy practitioners play a significant role in cancer care in both the home health care and the community-based practice settings.

Recognizing the rehabilitative needs and extension of the cancer care continuum into home health care and community-based practice provides occupational therapy practitioners opportunities to

- Help decrease the effects of cancer treatments and optimize performance status;
- Mitigate side effects and optimize functional performance, performance status, and activity engagement;
- Develop community-based programming to help mitigate lingering and persistent side effects, educate on self-management, and organize support groups; and
- Raise the bar of expectations that survivors reach the levels of functional performance and activity engagement they had before being diagnosed with cancer.

REFERENCES

Alfano, F. M., Ganz, P. A., Rowland, J. H., & Hahn, E. E. (2012). Cancer survivorship and cancer rehabilitation: Revitalizing the link. *Journal of Clinical Oncology, 30,* 904–906. https://doi.org/10.1200/JCO.2011.37.1674

American Occupational Therapy Association. (2013). *Occupational therapy's role in home health* [Fact sheet]. Retrieved from https://www.aota.org/About-Occupational-Therapy/Professionals/PA/Facts/Home-Health.aspx

American Occupational Therapy Association. (2014). Occupational therapy practice framework: Domain and process (3rd ed.). *American Journal of Occupational Therapy, 68*(Suppl. 1), S1–S48. https://doi.org/10.5014/ajot.2014.682006

American Society of Clinical Oncology. (2018). *What is survivorship?* Retrieved from https://www.cancer.net/survivorship/about-survivorship

Blignault, I., McDonnell, L., Aspinall, D., Yates, R., & Reath, J. (2017). Beyond diagnosis and survivorship: Findings from a mixed-methods study of a community-based cancer support service. *Australian Journal of Primary Health, 23,* 391–396. https://doi.org/10.1071/PY16067

Brandt, Å., Pilegaard, M. S., Oestergaard, L. G., Lindahl-Jacobsen, L., Sørensen, J., Johnsen, A. T., & la Cour, K. (2016). Effectiveness of the "Cancer Home-Life Intervention" on everyday activities and quality of life in people with advanced cancer living at home: A randomised controlled trial and an economic evaluation. *BMC Palliative Care, 15,* Article 10. https://doi.org/10.1186/s12904-016-0084-9

Braveman, B., & Hunter, E. (2017). *Occupational therapy practice guidelines for cancer rehabilitation with adults.* Bethesda, MD: AOTA Press.

Carmack, C. L., Basen-Engquist, K., & Gritz, E. R. (2011). Survivors at higher risk for adverse late outcomes due to psychosocial and behavioral risk factors. *Cancer Epidemiology, Biomarkers & Prevention, 20,* 2068–2077. https://doi.org/10.1158/1055-9965.EPI-11-0627

Coninck, L. D., Bekkering, G. E., Bouckaert, L., Declercq, A., Graff, M. J. L., & Aertgeerts, B. (2017). Home- and community-based occupational therapy improves functioning in frail older people: A systematic review. *Journal of American Geriatrics Society, 65,* 1863–1869. https://doi.org/10.1111/jgs.14889

Ebede, C. C., Jang, Y., & Escalante, L. P. (2017). Cancer-related fatigue in cancer survivorship. *Journal of Medical Clinics of North America, 101,* 1085–1097. https://doi.org/10.1016/j.mcna.2017.06.007

Glare, P. A., Davies, P. S., Finlay, E., Gulati, A., Lemanne, D., Moryl, N., . . . & Syrjala, K. L. (2014). Pain in cancer survivors. *Journal of Clinical Oncology, 32,* 1739–1747. https://doi.org/10.1200/JCO.2013.52.4629

Harrington, C. B., Hansen, J. A., Moskowitz, M., Todd, B. L., & Feuerstein, M. (2010). It's not over when it's over: Long-term symptoms in cancer survivors—A systematic review. *Internal Journal of Psychiatry Medicine, 40,* 163–181. https://doi.org/10.2190/PM.40.2.c

Hewitt, M., Greenfield, S., & Stovall, E. (Eds.). (2005). *From cancer patient to cancer survivor: Lost in translation.* Washington, DC: National Academies Press. Retrieved from https://www.nap.edu/catalog/11468.html

Hoffman, K. E., McCarthy, E. P., Recklitis, C. J., & Ng, A. K. (2009). Psychological distress in long-term survivors of adult-onset cancer: Results from a national survey. *Archives of Internal Medicine, 169,* 1274–1281. https://doi.org/10.1001/archinternmed.2009.179

Hwang, E. J., Lokietz, N. C., Lozano, R. L., & Parke, M. A. (2015). Functional deficits and quality of life among cancer survivors: Implications for occupational therapy in cancer survivorship care. *American Journal of Occupational Therapy, 69,* 6906290010. https://doi.org/10.5014/ajot.2015.015974

Janelsins, M. C., Kohli, S., Mohile, S. G., Usuki, K., Ahles, T. A. & Morrow, G. R. (2011). An update on cancer- and chemotherapy-related cognitive dysfunction: Current status. *Seminars in Oncology, 38,* 431–438. https://doi.org/10.1053/j.seminoncol.2011.03.014

Karnofsky, D. A., & Burchenal, J. H. (1949). The evaluation of chemotherapeutic agents in cancer. In C. M. Macleod (Ed.), *Evaluation chemotherapy agents* (pp. 191–205). New York: Columbia University Press.

Kendal, W. (2007). Suicide and cancer: A gender-comparative study. *Annals of Oncology, 18,* 381–387. https://doi.org/10.1093/annonc/mdl385

Lauckner, H. M., Krupa, T. M., & Paterson, M. L. (2011). Conceptualizing community development: Occupational therapy practice at the intersection of health services and community. *Canadian Journal of Occupational Therapy, 78,* 260–268. https://doi.org/10.2182/cjot.2011.78.4.8

Leclair, L. L. (2010). Re-examining concepts of occupation and occupation-based models: Occupational therapy and community development. *Canadian Journal of Occupational Therapy, 77,* 15–21. https://doi.org/10.2182/cjot.2010.77.1.3

Linden, W., Vodermaier, A., MacKenzie, R., & Greig, D. (2012). Anxiety and depression after cancer diagnosis: Prevalence rates by cancer type, gender, and age. *Journal of Affective Disorders, 142,* 343–351. https://doi.org/10.1016/j.jad.2012.03.025

Lipson, A., Douglas, S., & Daly, B. (2017). Preferences for quality or length of life: An analysis of patients with advanced cancer and their family caregivers prior to death. *Journal of Pain and Symptom Management, 53,* 417–418. https://doi.org/10.1016/j.jpainsymman.2016.12.225

Miller, M., Mogun, H., Azrael, D., Hempstead, K., & Solomon, D. H. (2008). Cancer and the risk of suicide in older Americans. *Journal of Clinical Oncology, 26,* 4720–4724. https://doi.org/10.1200/JCO.2007.14.3990

Misono, S., Weiss, N. S., Fann, J. R., Redman, M., & Yueh, B. (2008). Incidence of suicide in persons with cancer. *Journal of Clinical Oncology, 26,* 4731–4738. https://doi.org/10.1200/JCO.2007.13.8941

Neo, J., Fettes, L., Gao, W., Higginson, I. J., & Maddocks, M. (2017). Disability in activities of daily living among adults with cancer: A systematic review and meta-analysis. *Cancer Treatment Reviews, 61,* 94–106. https://doi.org/10.1016/j.ctrv.2017.10.006

O'Brien, M., Stricker, C. T., Foster, J. D., Ness, K., Arlen, A. G., & Schwartz, R. N. (2014). Navigating the seasons of survivorship in community oncology. *Clinical Journal of Oncology Nursing, 18,* 9–14. https://doi.org/10.1188/14.CJON.S1.9-14

Oken, M. M., Creech, R. H., & Tormey, D. C. (1982). Toxicity and response criteria of the Eastern Cooperative Oncology Group. *American Journal of Clinical Oncology, 5,* 649–655.

Polo, K. M., & Smith, C. (2017). Taking our seat at the table: Community cancer survivorship. *American Journal of Occupational Therapy, 71,* 7102100010. https://doi.org/10.5014/ajot.2017.020693

Salz, T., McCabe, M. S., Onstad, E. E., Baxi, S. S., Deming, R. L., Franco, R. A., . . . & Oeffinger, K. C. (2014). Survivorship care plans: Is there buy-in from community oncology providers? *Cancer, 120,* 722–730. https://doi.org/10.1002/cncr.28472

Saotome, T., Klein, L., & Faux, S. (2015). Cancer rehabilitation: A barometer for survival? *Supportive Cancer Care, 23,* 3033–3041. https://doi.org/10.1007/s00520-015-2673-1

Scaffa, M. E. (2001). *Occupational therapy in community-based practice settings.* Philadelphia: F.A. Davis.

Taylor, S. F. (2017). Cancer. In B. J. Atchison & D. P. Dirette (Eds.), *Conditions in occupational therapy: Effect on occupational performance* (5th ed., pp. 513–539). Philadelphia: Wolters Kluwer.

Thorsen, L., Gjerset, G. M., Loge, J. H., Kiserud, C. E., Skovlund, E., Fløtten, T., & Fossa, S. D. (2011). Cancer patients' needs for rehabilitation services. *Acta Oncologica, 50,* 212–222. https://doi.org/10.3109/0284186X.2010.531050

Valdivieso, M., Kujawa, A. M., Jones, T., & Baker, L. H. (2012). Cancer survivors in the United States: A review of the literature and a call to action. *Internal Journal of Medical Sciences, 9,* 163–173. https://doi.org/10.7150/ijms.3827

Vance, K. (Ed.). (2016). *Home health care: A guide for occupational therapy practice.* Bethesda, MD: AOTA Press.

van den Beuken-van Everdingen, M. H., de Graeff, A., Jongen, J. L., Dijkstra, D., Mostovaya, I., Vissers, K. C., & National Guideline Working Group "Diagnosis Treatment of Cancer Pain." (2017). Pharmacological treatment of pain in cancer patients: The role of adjuvant analgesics, a systematic review. *Pain Practice, 17,* 409–419. https://doi.org/10.1111/papr.12459

Williams, A. M., Janelsins, M. C., & van Wijingarden, E. (2016). Cognitive function in cancer survivors: Analysis of the 1999–2000 National Health and Nutrition Examination Survey. *Supportive Care in Cancer, 24,* 2155–2162. https://doi.org/10.1007/s00520-015-2992-2

Yi, J. C., & Syrjala, K. L. (2017). Anxiety and depression in cancer survivors. *Medical Clinics of North America, 101,* 1099–1113. https://doi.org/10.1016/j.mcna.2017.06.005

Zucca, A. C., Boyes, A. W., Linden, W., & Girgis, A. (2012). All's well that ends well? Quality of life and physical symptom clusters in long-term cancer survivors across all cancer types. *Journal of Pain and Symptom Management, 43,* 720–731. https://doi.org/10.1016/j.jpainsymman.2011.04.023

PART IV.

Sequelae of Cancer and Interventions
Across the Lifespan

Cancer-Related Fatigue

Anissa E. Hill, MOT, OTR/L

LEARNING OBJECTIVES

After completing this chapter, readers should be able to
- Understand occupational therapy's unique contributions in evaluating and treating cancer-related fatigue (CRF) across the lifespan;
- Relate the objective and subjective multidimensional nature, causes, and symptoms of CRF to theory-driven and evidence-based occupational therapy practice;
- Predict the impact of CRF on occupational roles and routines across the lifespan;
- Summarize the tools used to measure the cancer survivor's fatigue experience, including assessments and outcome measurements that identify deficits caused by CRF symptoms across the lifespan; and
- Construct occupation-based interventions for the treatment and management of CRF across the lifespan.

KEY TERMS AND CONCEPTS

- Cancer-related fatigue
- Energy conservation
- Fatigue journal
- Flow
- Pacing
- Permission
- Planning
- Positioning
- Prioritizing
- Psychoneurological cluster

INTRODUCTION

Cancer-related fatigue (CRF) is defined as a "distressing, persistent, subjective sense of physical, emotional and/or cognitive tiredness or exhaustion related to cancer or cancer treatment that is not proportional to recent activity and interferes with usual functioning" (Berger et al., 2015, p. 1012). According to National Comprehensive Cancer Network (NCCN), cancer patients report CRF as more distressing than pain or nausea and vomiting (Berger et al., 2015). Nearly 80% of all cancer survivors who receive chemotherapy or radiation experience CRF, and many experience it well past the cessation of treatment (Berger et al., 2015). Fatigue can be associated with decreased cancer treatment compliance and survival rates (Weis & Horneber, 2015). Occupational therapy practitioners intervene with clients experiencing CRF to improve their occupational performance, participation, and quality and quantity of life.

CRF may adversely affect a cancer survivor's physical, emotional, and cognitive function or well-being, leading to restrictions in participation in meaningful activities. Occupational therapy has a unique holistic perspective that encompasses the interactions of client factors, performance skills, performance patterns, contexts, and environments (American Occupational Therapy Association [AOTA], 2014). Through evaluation of such components,

occupational therapy practitioners guide cancer survivors through an extensive and personalized assessment of CRF to enrich their understanding and teach them strategies to minimize the impact of CRF. This allows survivors to manage their CRF to improve occupational outcomes, fulfill roles and routines, and ultimately improve quality of life (QoL) along the continuum of care and the lifespan. This chapter provides practical options to guide patients and caregivers through self-management of CRF.

DEFINING FEATURES OF CRF ACROSS THE LIFESPAN

CRF has multifactorial causes that amplify negative symptomology associated with cancer and its treatments and thereby create an exponentially profound negative impact on various aspects of life across the continuum of care and the lifespan. CRF includes physical, emotional, and mental or cognitive implications and causes. Table 15.1 shows examples of CRF symptoms cancer survivors have experienced.

Multiple modifiable factors contribute to CRF, such as pain, emotional distress, sleep disturbances, nutritional deficits or imbalances, decreased activity levels, poor blood values, medication side effects, and comorbidities (e.g., unrelated chronic or acute illnesses, injuries, or disorders;

TABLE 15.1.   Cancer-Related Fatigue Symptomology Descriptors

SYMPTOM TYPE	BRIEF DESCRIPTION
Physical	▪ Lack of energy ▪ Exhaustion ▪ Heavy limbs ▪ Tiredness ▪ Difficulty moving ▪ Inability to get out of bed
Emotional	▪ Poor motivation to engage in activities ▪ Decreased self-efficacy with meaningful occupations ▪ Feelings of depression or anxiety ▪ Irritability
Mental and cognitive	▪ Difficulty with concentration ▪ Difficulty with word finding ▪ Poor memory ▪ Difficulty processing information ▪ Confusion

Berger et al., 2015; Pureel et al., 2009). Additionally, psychosocial factors, including depression and anxiety, affect the symptom experience of CRF and occupational performance. Furthermore, sociodemographic factors, such as social support, employment, and education, contribute to a cancer survivor's sensitivity to the impact of CRF.

Occupational therapy practitioners can address the majority of these factors during intervention. However, other factors may require referrals to colleagues such as nutritionists, psychiatrists, social workers, or additional complementary members of the interprofessional team. Factors such as the disease process itself are out of the cancer survivor's control. However, factors such as proper hydration, sleep hygiene, scheduling priorities, and delegation of other commitments are controllable.

Teaching survivors to identify controllable and uncontrollable factors empowers them to manipulate and maneuver contextual factors to provide a sense of control in a conceivably uncontrollable situation. This shift in perspective is therapeutic in itself. These factors influence the survivor's perception of CRF, which, in turn, creates a negative influence on performance areas and QoL. Figure 15.1 illustrates the multidimensional nature of CRF factors.

FIGURE 15.1.   Contributing factors to cancer-related fatigue.

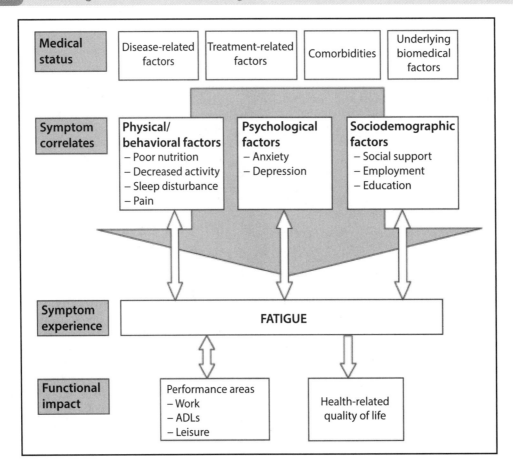

Note. ADLs = activities of daily living.

Source. Reprinted from "Cancer-Related Fatigue: A Review and a Conceptual Framework to Guide Therapists' Understanding," by A. Pureell, J. Fleming, T. Haines, & S. Bennett, 2009, *British Journal of Occupational Therapy, 72,* p. 84. Copyright © 2009 by SAGE Publications. Reprinted by permission of SAGE Publications.

Cancer survivors experience many symptoms associated with their cancer experience. Much of the literature refers to these symptoms in clusters because they frequently present concurrently (Kwekkeboom, 2016). Being familiar with the clusters provides a lens through which clinicians possibly can predict commonly correlated symptoms as well as anticipate implications for participation in occupations.

For example, there is a relationship between increased severity of pain and fatigue because they are both part of the same symptoms cluster known as the ***psychoneurological cluster***. This cluster includes pain, fatigue, insomnia, depression, and cognitive dysfunction (Kim et al., 2012). Other common symptom clusters are the gastrointestinal (e.g., nausea, anorexia, vomiting) and respiratory (e.g., dyspnea, anxiety, cough) clusters, but the most frequently reported symptom cluster is the psychoneurological cluster (Kwekkeboom, 2016).

Occupational therapy practitioners can use this information to guide intervention choices to address symptom clusters. For example, addressing pain can positively affect fatigue because of a correlated symptom presentation relationship. Conversely, depression makes fatigue worse.

Similar to the cluster symptoms, there is a strong correlation between cancer treatment and psychosocial distress (Hwang et al., 2015). CRF is further complicated and exacerbated by psychosocial issues such as stress, isolation, depression, and anxiety (Hwang et al., 2015; Palmadottir, 2009). The all-consuming role of being a patient disrupts participation in and fulfillment of previously meaningful roles and routines (Hwang et al., 2015; Palmadottir, 2009). The role of patient becomes paramount, and remaining roles go unfulfilled or are fulfilled inadequately, which causes additional stress, anxiety, depression, isolation, and fatigue. The mere absence of meaningful roles and routines often results in decreased energy, impaired interest, lack of flow, and poor volition to engage in meaningful occupations, thereby creating a vicious cycle of decreased occupational participation. This cycle may lead to more fatigue and, in turn, further occupational participation restrictions.

Occupational therapy practitioners foster meaningful engagement in occupation to create flow to diminish the negative impact of fatigue. *Flow* is a sense of timelessness and peak performance that results from participation in a meaningful activity that matches a person's current abilities with positive engagement (Csikszentmihalyi, 1990; Nidamboor, 2018). Occupational therapy practitioners treat CRF by facilitating activity engagement to help clients create flow; find balance between rest and activity; and increase occupational engagement, role fulfillment, and energy management. This results in decreased fatigue perception and increased QoL (Hwang et al., 2015; Palmadottir, 2009).

CONSIDERATIONS ACROSS THE LIFESPAN

Although symptomology and interventions for CRF are consistent across the lifespan, there are special considerations for various age-related groups pertaining to the developmental stages associated with each generation. There is a scarcity of adequate research on the growing population of adolescent and young adult (AYA) cancer survivors, despite the more than 80% 5-year survival rate for pediatric cancer survivors (American Cancer Society, 2018). The National Cancer Institute (2006) defines the AYA population as ages 15–39 years. However, Spathis et al. (2015) conducted a systematic literature review and defined AYAs as ages 13–24 years. They found that AYA cancer survivors experienced more severe fatigue compared with younger or healthy counterparts.

Typical teen development, including fluctuating hormones, changing circadian rhythms, and poor sleep habits, coupled with the cancer disease process, creates exponential fatigue factors for this vulnerable population (Spathis et al., 2015). Teenage years are characterized by a high emphasis on social events and building relationships, but fatigue is a barrier to social interactions. These formative years are the foundation for lifelong habits, and fatigue may perpetuate inactivity, further disability, and social isolation (Spathis et al., 2015). Occupational therapy practitioners must be keenly aware of the exponential potential for untreated CRF and its long-lasting implications for this particularly vulnerable population.

Another age group requiring special consideration is the older adult cancer population. The aging process contributes to body decline, including decreased muscle effectiveness in both power and size; circadian disruption; and cytokine dysregulation, which results in inflammation, stress, and susceptibility to fatigue (Giacalone et al., 2013). Occupational therapy practitioners must evaluate and guide older adult cancer survivors through describing their experience of CRF; clients frequently underreport CRF because they believe it to be unavoidable (Giacalone et al., 2013).

Because of this decline in function related to decreased body efficiency, older adults are susceptible to inactivity, which leads to more deconditioning, frailty, and fatigue and creates a cycle of disability. Additionally, this period of life frequently includes loss of friends and loved ones. Therefore, a focus on spiritual and emotional fatigue, grief, and depression can be vital with older adult cancer survivors.

ASSESSING CRF

Intervention for CRF begins with assessment. Effective assessment tools provide language for discussion with loved ones and caregivers, create a platform for collaboration on goals, and offer justification for skilled intervention services. Assessments should be multilayered to illustrate the extensive impact of CRF on occupational performance to increase awareness for the survivor, ultimately improving adherence to intervention. Evaluating the onset, pattern, and duration of CRF aids in early recognition of signs, symptoms, and associated factors (e.g., clumsy walking, increased pain, irritability). Because it may be challenging to accurately assess oneself, caregivers can offer an outside perspective of fatigue signs and how they affect occupational performance.

Early recognition of CRF indicators allows survivors more opportunities to implement strategies. Increased awareness of impending exhaustion allows clients to rebound to higher energy levels instead of overdoing activities and becoming exhausted, which can cause cessation of activities.

Assessments can be unidimensional, with a single question to measure the presence of fatigue, or multidimensional, including the impact of CRF on several domains such as role performance, physical, psychosocial, cognitive, and general QoL. A unidimensional example is a simple interval scale ranging from 0–10.

Occupational therapy practitioners can break down a 0- to 10-point scale of fatigue to identify mild, moderate, and severe fatigue (Berger et al., 2015). *Mild fatigue* is indicated by a score of 1–3, *moderate fatigue* is indicated by a score of 4–6, and *severe fatigue* is indicated by a score of 7–10. A score of 0 represents cancer survivors' baseline function and energy levels when they were fully participating in all meaningful roles and routines. A score of 10 represents the proverbial "crash"—when survivors feel they have to cease involvement in all occupations. This explanation reinforces comparison with previous roles and routines rather than the current role and routines of a patient.

NCCN's *Clinical Practice Guidelines* (Berger et al., 2015) suggest using a slightly different scale with pediatric and adolescent cancer survivors. With children younger than age 5 years, parents or caregivers and clinicians can observe for signs and symptoms of fatigue. With children ages 5–6, the scale anchors should be *tired* and *not tired*.

For improved communication between pediatric cancer survivors and their parents and caregivers, children can learn to use red light, yellow light, and green light indicators. *Red light* means the child is feeling exhausted, has severe fatigue, and should not be pushed. *Yellow light* indicates moderate fatigue; the child would benefit from balance between activity and rest. *Green light* communicates minimal to no fatigue.

When working with children, occupational therapy practitioners also can use emoji faces to represent fatigue levels. This strategy can be used concurrently with other methods. For older children and adolescents ages 7–12 years, use a scale ranging from 1 = *no fatigue* to 5 = *the worst fatigue*.

Although the 0–10 scale can provide some basic information, it excludes quality of fatigue and the impact on participation in occupations. Many other assessments provide a rich understanding beyond a 0–10 scale. Table 15.2 describes various assessments.

Using multiple assessments provides a rich base for a specialized, individualized intervention program to be designed and implemented. Partnering with survivors to synthesize the assessments and devise pertinent treatment plans and goals for each client is paramount to success. This allows occupational therapy practitioners to integrate measurable assessments that are congruent with the survivor's goals and sensitive enough to measure progress.

OVERVIEW OF OCCUPATIONAL THERAPY'S ROLE FOR CRF

Occupational therapy has a unique, holistic perspective that provides comprehensive intervention for CRF. During the occupational profile phase of evaluation, practitioners frequently hear the cancer survivor's narrative as it relates to life

TABLE 15.2.   Cancer-Related Fatigue Assessment Tools and Strategies

ASSESSMENT	DESCRIPTION
Brief Fatigue Inventory (Mendoza et al., 1999)	9 questions answered on 0–10 scale reflecting intensity of fatigue and its impact on function in the past 24 hours
Cancer Fatigue Scale (Okuyama et al., 2000)	15-item self-report including 3 subscales: Physical, Affective, and Cognitive
Functional Assessment of Cancer Therapy: Fatigue (Yellen et al., 1997)	41 questions that include 5 domains of fatigue: physical well-being, social and family well-being, emotional well-being, functional well-being, and fatigue
Model of Human Occupation Screening Tool (Parkinson et al., 2006)	Observational or interview assessment that uses the concept of the Model of Human Occupation (volition, habituation, skills, and environment) to assess what facilitates, allows, inhibits, or restricts participation in meaningful ADLs and IADLs
Multidimensional Fatigue Inventory (Smets et al., 1995)	22-item self-report that measures general fatigue, physical fatigue, mental fatigue, reduced motivation and reduced activity (Smets et al., 1995)
Multidimensional Fatigue Symptom Inventory—Short Form (Stein et al., 2004)	14-item self-report inventory to measure intensity, pattern, and impact of fatigue in the past week
Patient-Reported Outcomes Measurement Information System's Fatigue Item Bank (Cella et al., 2007)	Extensive assessment of fatigue symptoms, available in short form or computerized; options include self-report adult, adult with cancer, pediatric (ages 8–17 years), and parent proxy versions
Piper Fatigue Scale–Revised (Reeve et al., 2012)	22 items answered on a 0–10 scale that are used to calculate 4 subscales: Behavioral, Affect, Sensory, and Cognitive/Mood; assessment includes 5 additional items for qualitative responses
Return to Normal Living Index (Wood-Dauphinee & Williams, 1987)	Measures degree to which a debilitating illness affects reintegration to normal activities, including leisure and productive occupations, movement in the home and community, and engagement with family roles

TABLE 15.3. Intervention Focus Along the Continuum of Care

STAGE OF CARE	TREATMENT FOCUS
Screening or prevention	Provide education on signs and symptoms of CRF, introduce fatigue management. Initiate intervention if more than mild fatigue. Conduct ongoing evaluation or screening.
Active treatment	Self-monitoring, energy conservation strategies, exercise or activity program
Posttreatment	Prevention of overexertion during return to previous roles and routines
Supportive or palliative	Engage in QoL activities, eliminate nonessential activities
End of life	Engage in QoL activities, eliminate nonessential activities, stress importance of meaningful interactions

Note. CRF = cancer-related fatigue; QoL = quality of life.
Source. Care stages and treatment focus adapted from Berger et al. (2015).

outside of the cancer experience, which requires active listening and therapeutic use of self. This begins the first phase of intervention: creating an emotionally safe environment for processing and healing. Validation and normalization of the fatigue experience create rapport between the occupational therapy practitioner and client, thereby beginning the intervention process of guiding survivors toward recognition of and adaptation to the signs and symptoms of CRF.

Interventions for CRF are therapeutic during all stages of the cancer care continuum. Occupational therapy practitioners effectively address CRF during screening, active treatment, and posttreatment in conjunction with palliative treatment, hospice, and end-of-life care. (See Table 15.3 for correlated types of intervention associated with each stage.) During all stages, intervention must include education to reiterate that fatigue is not necessarily an indication of disease progression or treatment intolerance.

Screening for CRF should be frequent and scheduled at regular intervals for all survivors during their cancer experience, including monitoring for indications, signs, or symptoms of CRF. If screening identifies fatigue, general fatigue-management strategies should be introduced as well as education on recognizing and addressing CRF signs and symptoms. Active treatment should include self-monitoring, integrating graded activities in addition to educating on contributing factors, and training in fatigue management strategies. Posttreatment interventions should include all of the above as well as additional training to prevent overexertion, given that increased participation in usual roles and routines may deplete energy levels and decrease engagement.

Implementing ongoing lifestyle modification is an integral part of survivorship after treatment. Although palliative care can be provided concurrently with active treatment or symptom management, it is distinct from end-of-life or hospice care. With end-of-life interventions, training should focus on QoL activities, including eliminating unnecessary activities to ensure the client has substantial energy levels to engage with their most meaningful occupations, roles, and routines. At all points of intervention, it is paramount to provide treatment with the focus of maintaining dignity for all clients.

CRF INTERVENTIONS

A comprehensive review of literature from cancer and rehabilitation organizations, including AOTA, *Journal of Physiotherapy,* and the NCCN (Berger et al., 2015), suggests that the main tenets of intervention to address CRF include the following:

- Education about CRF
- Energy conservation strategies
- Sleep hygiene
- Psychosocial interventions (Hunter et al., 2017)
- Exercise (Meneses-Echávez et al., 2015; Santa Mina et al., 2017).

Sleep hygiene is addressed in Chapter 10, "Prehabilitation," but the remaining concepts are discussed in this section.

Energy Conservation

Tanya Packer et al.'s (1995) original work on fatigue management and energy conservation strategies remains effective today. Packer et al. (1995) discussed an analogy for energy management referred to as *banking and budgeting,* which is a proactive method of saving energy. Similar to a financial budget, one must keep track of debits and expenses. Cancer survivors must be aware of the amount of energy they have and the amount of energy tasks require so they can calculate how much energy they have to spend (Packer et al., 1995).

A specific method of energy budgeting is known as *energy conservation,* which is the "deliberately planned management of one's personal energy resources to prevent their depletion. It encompasses a common-sense approach that helps survivors set realistic expectations, prioritize and pace activities, and delegate less essential activities" (Berger et al., 2015, p. 1025). The principles of energy conservation require attention to habits and routines and the ability to adapt one's usual manner of living.

Training cancer survivors to self-monitor to identify early onset of fatigue signs and symptoms is the primary means of developing an internal locus of control and self-efficacy to implement effective energy conservation strategies. Arranging how to use one's valuable but frequently limited energy involves three steps:
1. Evaluating priorities,
2. Exploring personal standards, and
3. Making decisions about activities that result in the ultimate goal of saving energy on necessary tasks to expend more energy on enjoyable tasks (Packer et al., 1995).

General energy conservation strategies are commonly referred to as the *5 Ps* and are the cornerstone of energy conservation education and strategy use. The 5 Ps are *prioritizing*, *positioning*, *pacing*, *planning*, and *permission* (Dreiling, 2009; Packer et al., 1995).

Prioritizing encompasses evaluating tasks throughout the day and week. Because individuals have different values regarding occupational choice, the process of prioritizing is highly personalized. Appraising which occupations hold value and support independence and which occupations can be delegated or delayed constitutes the initial stage of this strategy (Dreiling, 2009). Priorities frequently shift during the cancer experience. However, despite shifts in priorities, one's habits, roles, and routines may remain stable and require a conscious assessment. Increasing awareness to change habits and routines that reflect a shift in priorities may improve energy levels, perpetuating positivity and increasing occupational performance.

Positioning incorporates concepts of body mechanics and ergonomics to emphasize large muscle groups, align joints for efficiency, and set the environment to minimize energy task demands (Packer et al., 1995). Assessing body mechanics during activity engagement allows clients to maximize their muscle power while minimizing exertion (Dreiling, 2009).

Pacing includes "finding a balance between activity and rest" (Dreiling, 2009, p. 28). Pacing requires supporting survivors to identify natural stopping points of activity performance and making a plan to prevent overexertion.

Planning requires coordinating activities, alternating those with high energy expenditure with activities that require less energy expenditure, and planning for future events with higher energy. It includes planning for extra time to avoid having to rush and waste energy, planning to avoid crowds, and organizing to avoid clutter and maximize efficiency of the environment. Survivors should also plan for visitors and social interactions, because they can demand a lot of energy (Dreiling, 2009).

Permission relates to encouraging personal consent for clients to engage in self-care, despite perceived familial and societal obligations, whether those obligations are imposed by the patient, their culture, or society. Permission involves a self-evaluation of standards and how they affect occupational engagement. Standards relate to priorities in that they have their basis in personal values (Packer et al., 1995).

Clients must ask themselves probing questions to fully assess their standards, to determine the source of those standards and how they affect day-to-day activities, and to decide how their standards can be changed to facilitate an energy surplus. Permission also encourages clients to answer, "How are you?" honestly to authentically communicate their needs. Clients may need permission to communicate the profound impact of the hidden, disabling effects of fatigue. Proper communication allows the client to feel a locus of control, solicit useful support, foster understanding, and decrease isolation (Packer et al., 1995).

The focus of the 5 Ps strategies is to guide patients through "active decision-making to regain control and balance . . . evaluate where you spend your energy [priority] . . . how much energy you want to spend [standards] . . . examine options . . . and do what you want to do" (Packer et al., 1995, p. 99). Table 15.4 provides examples of questions to guide patients through evaluation of priorities and

TABLE 15.4. Probing Questions for Client Self-Evaluation

SELF-EVALUATION CATEGORIES	QUESTIONS
Priorities	▪ What needs to be done? What is necessary for my lifestyle? ▪ What do I like to do? What activities (e.g., hobbies, leisure) bring me enjoyment? ▪ What do others expect me to do? ▪ How much energy do these activities use? ▪ What can I eliminate? ▪ What can I delegate?
Standards	▪ Do my standards affect my activities? ▪ Are they forcing me to expend excessive energy? ▪ Can my standards be changed? ▪ What activities give me pleasure? ▪ What are the most rewarding activities for me? ▪ Are there activities I have given up that I would like to start again?

Source. Questions adapted from Packer et al. (1995).

standards. These energy conservation concepts represent generalized strategies, however; only by guiding patients through self-evaluation of priorities and standards can the occupational therapy practitioner determine the precisely personalized implementation of these principles. See Table 15.5 for specific examples related to case studies.

Exercise Intervention

CRF typically results in decreased activity and deconditioning; however, studies indicate that activity is one of the ultimate strategies to ameliorate CRF. A robust body of research supports that frequent (3–5 times a week) supervised aerobic and resistance exercise at low to moderate intensity is an effective strategy to address CRF (Velthuis et al., 2010). In a recent systematic review, Meneses-Echávez et al. (2015) found that supervised physical activity (including both aerobic and resistive exercises) significantly reduced CRF. Furthermore, Schuler et al. (2017) determined exercise to be most effective with cancer patients who report "severe fatigue" at initial evaluation. The authors defined *physical activity* as "any body movement causing an increase in energy expenditure, and involving a planned or structured movement of the body performed in a systematic manner in terms of frequency, intensity and duration and . . . designed to maintain or enhance health-related outcomes" (p. 4). Physical activity improves CRF, social and emotional well-being, balance, cardiopulmonary function, and QoL during and after treatment (Meneses-Echávez et al., 2015; Santa Mina et al., 2017).

Contraindications and extra caution should be considered when patients have comorbidities of bony metastases; irregular blood values, including thrombocytopenia (i.e., low platelets) or anemia (i.e., low red blood cells); or any indications of active infections (Berger et al., 2015).

TABLE 15.5.   The 5 Ps of Energy Conservation Related to Case Examples

ENERGY CONSERVATION PRINCIPLE	RAJAN	HARLEY	REBECCA
Prioritizing	• Help wife unpack • Engage in woodworking • Work on cars • Choose to prioritize his treatment proximity over tending to his farm	• Participate in her children's events (ballet and soccer) • Return to yoga and running • Return to work • Integrate spirituality back into her life with a God Box • Keep a list of tasks she feels compelled to do independently and what tasks she would feel comfortable delegating	• Dance • Do math • Play with her friends and go to the park
Positioning	• Set up woodshop for proper body mechanics, minimize reaching and bending • Use a shower chair • Sit down at a table to unpack items • Position himself closer to the hospital by moving to a new house	• Do floor stretches instead of standing yoga • Watch sermons online at her house instead of at church • Sit on the sidelines instead of standing at her son's soccer games	• Take seated rest breaks to read or paint her nails
Pacing	• Set alarm for short breaks throughout the day • Take short walks three times a day instead of one long walk	• Coordinate with another parent to bring kids home from activities so she can leave if she feels tired but can still attend the event	• Use "red, yellow, and green" light • Take rest breaks—as encouraged by her mother—with fun activities
Planning	• Plan woodworking on days he is not at the hospital • Coordinate with his sons to assist with unpacking • Plan discussions with family and friends to talk about the impact of fatigue	• Use fatigue journals to predict fatigue levels and plan her schedule to be correlated with high energy levels to avoid overexertion • Plan for one-way transportation of her kids • Hire assistance for cleaning her home	• Follow mother's sleep–wake cycle • Plan activities for each stage ("red," "yellow," and "green")
Permission	• Provide permission to himself to create a new norm with a slower lifestyle but continue to engage in meaningful occupations • Provide permission to cancel plans sometimes when his fatigue levels are high	• Provide permission to delegate some of her responsibilities as she is recovering	• Is able, with her mother's permission, to make her own decisions about her activities within each stage of fatigue

However, aerobic and resistive exercises have been shown to significantly decrease the negative effects of CRF symptoms. Occupational therapy practitioners' clinical expertise in supervising, grading, and adjusting physical activity for maximal therapeutic gains is associated with increased adherence and compliance. Hunter et al. (2017) found that physical activities such as yoga and Qigong had similar effects to aerobic and resistive exercises and proved to be advantageous for improving sleep, reducing CRF, and generally conditioning the body.

Psychosocial Intervention

Fatigue may also be emotional, spiritual, or mental–cognitive in nature. To address these aspects of fatigue, interventions should include psychosocial components such as cognitive–behavioral therapy, including problem solving, supportive and expressive therapies, relaxation strategies, meditation and mindfulness practices, breathing exercises, life review, or exploration of occupations, that create a sense of flow for patients (Ando et al., 2010; Csikszentmihalyi, 1990; Nidamboor, 2018). Psychosocial interventions are more suitable to address emotional, spiritual, and cognitive or mental fatigue for improved occupational outcomes because these are psychosocial manifestations of fatigue (Boggero et al., 2017). Furthermore, fostering expression through participation and engagement in modified occupations or development of new occupations increases patients' self-confidence and well-being (Lyons, 2006). Rajan (Case Example 15.1), Harley (Case Example 15.2), and Rebecca (Case Example 15.3) illustrate integration of these intervention strategies for various types of patients.

CASE EXAMPLE 15.1. RAJAN: IMPROVED FATIGUE, DESPITE PROGRESSIVE DISEASE

Rajan is 76-year-old man who has been married for 54 years. He has 4 children, 7 grandchildren, and 12 great-grandchildren. He retired 16 years ago from his job as a commercial airline pilot. His hobbies include working on antique cars, woodworking, tending to his farm, and spending time with family.

Rajan was diagnosed 10 years ago with renal cell carcinoma, which was treated surgically. Recently, Rajan's carcinoma has spread, with bony metastases throughout his body. Although Rajan has been receiving chemotherapy since his diagnosis, the medical team has changed his chemotherapy to a more aggressive form because of the cancer's progression. After the changes in his treatment, Rajan and his wife decided to move closer to the medical team. In this relocation, the couple left behind most of their support system.

Rajan was referred to occupational therapy because of deconditioning and fatigue. During the occupational therapy evaluation, he reported that fatigue has left him "feeling incompetent" and that he is having difficulty coping with the drastic change in function. On the analysis of occupational performance, Rajan identified his top priorities as being able to help his wife unpack after their move and return to woodworking and his antique cars.

The occupational therapist used the Brief Fatigue Inventory (BFI; Mendoza et al., 1999) and the Model of Human Occupation Screening Tool (MOHOST; Parkinson et al., 2006) to assess Rajan's level of fatigue and its impact on occupational performance and participation. The MOHOST revealed an extensive list of factors that facilitate and allow for occupational participation. Rajan's participation was inhibited by the following factors: routines, adaptability, posture and mobility, strength and effort, physical space (his new home), physical resources (tools), social groups, and occupational demands. Only one factor was identified as restricting Rajan's occupational performance, which was energy. Rajan's initial BFI (Mendoza et al., 1999) score was 7.3 out of 10, indicating severe fatigue with an enormous impact on function.

Using therapeutic use of self, validation, normalization, and active listening, Rajan's occupational therapist began intervention that included general education about CRF and identifying applicable contributing factors. Rajan was trained in energy conservation strategies and environmental adaptations during engagement in meaningful occupations. Specific examples of energy conservation strategies used with Rajan are included in Table 15.5. Additional interventions for Rajan included psychosocial interventions for problem solving to get his house unpacked and coping strategies for his decreased energy levels and change in functional outcomes.

Rajan learned communication skills and terms related to CRF to allow effective discussions with his family and friends regarding his fatigue and limitations. He was trained on a home program for improved posture, which the MOHOST identified as inhibiting his occupational function and performance (Parkinson et al., 2006). Resistive exercises were contraindicated because of the bony metastases; however, his program was focused on aerobic activities, such as walking and stretching for postural correction. Rajan required a general lifestyle modification to improve his occupational outcomes and quality of life. At discharge, despite the fact that none of his medical treatments or conditions had changed, Rajan's BFI score was 2.3 out of 10, indicating a mild fatigue. The MOHOST indicated that nothing was either inhibiting or restricting his occupational participation as a result of the occupational therapy intervention.

OVERVIEW OF OCCUPATIONAL THERAPY'S ROLE IN MANAGING CRF: USING THE *FRAMEWORK*

The *Occupational Therapy Practice Framework: Domain and Process* (*OTPF;* 3rd ed.; AOTA, 2014) provides common language and ideology for the occupational therapy profession. Concepts include an analysis of occupational therapy's domain and process that dictates practice. Below are highlighted dimensions applying CRF to the evaluation process (occupational profile and analysis of performance) and the intervention process. Case Example 15.2 provides further explanation of using the *OTPF* as it relates to a specific case.

Occupational Profile

The experience of CRF is personal and affects each cancer survivor in a unique way. It is important that the occupational profile capture the daily lived experience of the cancer survivor so the intervention plan can be tailored to the survivor's specific needs. The following questions are examples to foster a deeper understanding of the impact of CRF on occupational performance during the occupational profile interview process:

- How is fatigue affecting your abilities to engage in daily life activities?
- What occupations are you not engaging in because you feel too tired?
- How does your environment support you to feel energized, and what about your environment makes you feel drained?
- What concerns do you have about fulfilling your roles?
- What are your values and interests?
- What did your daily life roles entail before your diagnosis?
- How has fatigue changed your engagement in roles?
- What is the first thing you would do if you had enough energy?

Analysis of Occupational Performance

It is critical that occupational therapy practitioners hear a cancer survivor's full story, not just the medical journey.

CASE EXAMPLE 15.2. HARLEY: APPLICATION OF CRF MANAGEMENT RELATED TO THE *OTPF*

The *OTPF* breaks down the process of occupational therapy service into evaluation, intervention, and targeting of outcomes (AOTA, 2014). The evaluation process includes the occupational profile and analysis of occupational performance. The intervention process includes the intervention plan, intervention implementation, and intervention review. The targeting of outcomes includes the outcomes themselves. This case applies the occupational therapy process to a CRF intervention.

Occupational profile

Harley is a 38-year-old married woman with chronic lymphocytic leukemia. She has two children: a daughter age 5 years, and a son age 7 years. She works as a civil engineer and plans to return to her profession as soon as possible. She enjoys yoga and running as hobbies. She is also involved with her children's extracurricular activities, including soccer and ballet.

Harley's treatment plan included a matched, unrelated stem cell transplant. She was referred to occupational therapy for fatigue and reported that she does not have enough energy to rear her children, take care of her home, or return to work. Harley reported that she has a great support system, including her husband, family, friends, church community, and employer. However, she feels decreased efficacy because she needs assistance with her meaningful IADLs and roles and routines such as parenting, home management, and meal preparation. She has a strong faith; however, she has not been practicing her usual spiritual routines because she is too tired to go to church.

Analysis of occupational performance

CRF, decreased efficacy, and reintegration to Harley's normal roles and routines were identified as the focus of occupational therapy intervention. Harley's social interaction skills were identified as impaired performance skills. All of Harley's performance patterns were impaired, including habits, routines, rituals, and roles.

The Piper Fatigue Scale (Reeve et al., 2012) was used for its subscales of Behavioral, Affect, Sensory, and Cognitive–Mood aspects of fatigue. The Return to Normal Living Index (Wood-Dauphinee & Williams, 1987) was used to measure the impact of perceived integration to life. Harley scored 8.73 on the Piper Fatigue Scale, indicating severe fatigue, and scored 29.09% of reintegration on the Return to Normal Living Index on initial evaluation.

Targeted outcomes identified included increased satisfaction with role participation and use of positive coping strategies. Harley's Piper Fatigue Scale results indicated that her mood and behavior were the most negatively affected by fatigue and ultimately were hindering her performance. The focus of intervention was determined to include fatigue management, energy conservation, coping strategies training, and graded engagement in meaningful occupations so that Harley could

significantly increase her participation in meaningful roles and routines.

Goals for intervention included
- Decreased Piper Fatigue Scale score by more than 3 points;
- Return to Normal Living Index percentage improvement to greater than 70%; and
- Independence with health management, including fatigue management, positive coping strategies, and home exercise program.

Potential approaches included a cognitive–behavioral approach, psychosocial interventions and energy conservation strategies for fatigue management, coping strategies, and problem solving.

Intervention process

Intervention began with validation, support, and normalization of Harley's fatigue experiences, enhanced with therapeutic use of self throughout. Education was provided on CRF and its contributing factors, including identification of mental and emotional implications. A fatigue journal was recommended to identify fatigue levels associated with various activities.

Harley was trained in energy conservation strategies, including (see Table 15.5 for specific examples of Harley's strategies)
- Planning energy for high-priority events, such as her children's extracurricular activities;
- Structuring daily routines around her energy levels;
- Graded reintegration to children's events (e.g., planning to attend local games vs. away games, gradually increasing commitments as energy levels allow); and
- Psychosocial interventions, including relaxation strategies, deep breathing, and visualization for coping strategies.

The occupational therapist assisted Harley with finding community resources to help with housecleaning and support through a volunteer group that matches patients to survivors with similar diagnoses. The therapist also guided Harley to integrate her faith into daily practice with prayer and by creating a God Box to represent a physical manifestation of letting go and handing over her worries and problems to her God. Education and training were provided in physical activities (Qigong and light stretching) that Harley could integrate into her routines to bring joy in preparation for returning to running and yoga.

Targeting outcomes

The main outcomes targeted for intervention were improved self-efficacy in role fulfillment, perceived overall well-being, and increased occupational performance. At discharge, the occupational therapist completed a formal reevaluation with the Piper Fatigue Scale on which Harley improved her score from 8.73 to 3.05 and increased her percentage on the Return to Normal Living Index from 29.09% to 89.09% of reintegration.

CASE EXAMPLE 15.3. REBECCA: 7-YEAR-OLD GIRL IN REMISSION

Rebecca is a 7-year-old girl with a history of medulloblastoma who was treated surgically and has completed multiple rounds of chemotherapy. Rebecca is now on a maintenance chemotherapy regimen. She had achieved remission at the time of referral.

Rebecca was referred to occupational therapy for fatigue management because her mom reported Rebecca was "sleeping all day and night." Rebecca's mom had been letting her sleep because she thought that was best for her daughter. However, she became increasingly concerned about Rebecca's lack of participation in activities. In response to focused questions to evaluate her standards and priorities, Rebecca identified dancing, doing math, playing with her friends, and going to the park to get on the swings as her favorite occupations.

At initial evaluation, Rebecca was quite disengaged and even reluctant to play. She frequently placed her head on the table and whined. Rebecca denied pain; she indicated that she was tired but was unable to communicate the intensity of fatigue within the NCCN's guidelines (Berger et al., 2015) recommendation of the 1–5 scale for her age group. Rebecca responded with, "I don't know," accompanied with a sigh when asked to rate her fatigue.

The occupational therapist introduced a visual aid that included red, yellow, and green lights. She explained the indications of each color, with red meaning, "Stop, I feel yucky"; yellow meaning, "Eh, so-so right now"; and green meaning, "I feel good. Let's go play." Rebecca pointed to the red light. The occupational therapist encouraged Rebecca to identify further descriptors with use of emoji correlated with each color to explain to her mom how she was feeling.

Rebecca's extensive sleeping patterns and lack of activity exacerbated her fatigue, so her intervention included guiding Rebecca's mom through planning an appropriate general sleep–wake cycle, including gradually getting her up earlier each morning and allowing just a 30-minute nap if necessary while modifying her activities to correlate with her fatigue levels. The occupational therapist led Rebecca through listing enjoyable activities to plan a schedule that inspired motivation for engagement. Because Rebecca chose her own meaningful activities, she was eager to engage, encouraging maximal participation. The occupational therapist included Rebecca with each decision to encourage her to make choices for herself, thereby facilitating a locus of control, as opposed to the requirements of a patient role in which most decisions were made for her.

Intervention also included guiding Rebecca's mother and Rebecca to make a list of priority activities that Rebecca could participate in when she was feeling "yellow," such as using math flash cards and playing hide-and-seek or house, while encouraging her for pacing and taking seated rest breaks with increased fatigue. Rebecca also identified activities that allowed her to rest when she was feeling "red," such as listening to music, watching videos, coloring, having her favorite book read to her, or painting her nails. Additionally, intervention included integrating physical activities to combat fatigue through use of dance video games and regularly scheduled play dates with her friends. With the use of the "red, yellow, and green light" strategy, Rebecca was able to effectively communicate how she was feeling, and her mother was able to implement energy conservation strategies to maximize Rebecca's functional outcomes and fulfillment of the child role.

Commonly, survivors have poor insight into the impact of fatigue on daily activities because caregivers are performing ADLs and IADLs for them. An activity analysis of participation in activities helps therapists, caregivers, and survivors gain insight.

Intervention Process

Intervention for CRF aims to facilitate engagement in activities as it relates to the survivor's occupational profile, values, priorities, and fulfillment of meaningful roles and routines that have been disrupted. Intervention implementation focuses on several aspects of the domain of occupational therapy, including context, environment, performance patterns, and skills. Implementation review allows for evaluation and reevaluation of strategies as energy and fatigue levels fluctuate and roles and routines evolve.

Subjective and objective components of assessments are addressed throughout the intervention process. This process of intervention review allows for ongoing collaboration with the cancer survivor to ensure targeted outcomes with achievable and meaningful progress and goals as well as any necessary modifications. Using homework

for self-assessment can be a helpful tool to allow the survivor to make necessary adjustments throughout the day as needed to maximize occupational outcomes.

One possible tool to achieve increased awareness of the intervention and implementation review is use of a *fatigue journal*, which includes lists of daily activities and a personal assessment of associated fatigue levels with recorded occupations. Additional notes or personal observations may be included to encourage habits of consistent self-monitoring and identification of activities that require adaptation or modification. A fatigue journal provides an opportunity for ongoing self-evaluation of the client's activities, fatigue levels, and strategies and solutions for ongoing analysis.

SUMMARY

CRF is a destructive force that disrupts engagement with and participation in meaningful roles and routines across the lifespan. CRF is most effectively addressed through the lens of the holistic approach of occupational therapy to accurately assess and intervene in the multicontextual physical, emotional–spiritual, psychosocial, and cognitive–mental implications of fatigue. Frequent evaluation, discussions, and reassessment of CRF and its impact on daily life are required to sufficiently monitor and treat CRF's insidious nature. A thorough client profile matched with specific assessments to capture the impact of CRF on functional outcomes, occupational performance, roles, and routines provides an outline for individualized programs to foster patients' return to meaningful engagement. Addressing all aspects of CRF to foster specialized interventions of education, energy conservation strategies, psychosocial interventions, and exercise results in profoundly improved quality and quantity of life across the lifespan.

REFERENCES

American Cancer Society. (2018). *Key statistics for childhood cancers.* Retrieved from https://www.cancer.org/cancer/cancer-in-children/key-statistics.html

American Occupational Therapy Association. (2014). Occupational therapy practice framework: Domain and process (3rd ed.) *American Journal of Occupational Therapy, 68*(Suppl. 1), S1–S48. https://doi.org/10.5014/ajot.2014.682006

Ando, M., Morita, T., Akechi, T., Okamoto, T., & Japanese Task Force for Spiritual Care. (2010). Efficacy of short-term life-review interviews on the spiritual well-being of terminally ill cancer patients. *Journal of Pain and Symptom Management, 39*(6), 993–1002. https://doi.org/10.1016/j.jpainsymman.2009.11.320

Berger, A. M., Mooney, K., Alvarez-Perez, A., Breitbart, W. S., Carpenter, K. M., Cella, D., . . . Smith, C. (2015). Cancer-Related Fatigue, Version 2.2015. *Journal of the National Comprehensive Cancer Network, 13,* 1012–1039. https://doi.org/10.6004/jnccn.2015.0122

Boggero, I. A., Rojas-Ramirez, M. V., & Carlson, C. R. (2017). All fatigue is not created equal: The association of fatigue and its subtypes on pain interference in orofacial pain. *Clinical Journal of Pain, 33,* 231–237. https://doi.org/10.1097/AJP.0000000000000391

Cella, D., Yount, S., Rothrock, N., Gershon, R., Cook, K., Reeve, B., . . . Rose, M. (2007). The Patient-Reported Outcomes Measurement Information System (PROMIS): Progress of an NIH Roadmap cooperative group during its first two years. *Medical Care, 45*(Suppl. 1), S3–S11. https://doi.org/10.1097/01.mlr.0000258615.42478.55

Csikszentmihalyi, M. (1990). *Flow: The psychology of optimal experience.* New York: Harper Perennial.

Dreiling, D. (2009). Energy conservation. *Home Health Care Management and Practice, 22,* 26–33. https://doi.org/10.1177/1084822309340301

Giacalone, A., Quitadamo, D., Zanet, E., Berretta, M., Spina, M., & Tirelli U. (2013). Cancer-related fatigue in the elderly. *Support Care Cancer, 21*(10), 313–335. https://doi.org/10.3109/07380570903242433

Hunter, E. G., Gibson, R. W., Arbesman, M., & D'Amico, M. (2017). Systematic review of occupational therapy and adult cancer rehabilitation: Part 1. Impact of physical activity and symptom management interventions. *American Journal of Occupational Therapy, 71,* 7102100030. https://doi.org/10.5014/ajot.2017.023564

Hwang, E. J., Lokietz, N. C., Lozano, R. L., & Parke, M. A. (2015). Functional deficits and quality of life among cancer survivors: Implications for occupational therapy in cancer survivorship care. *American Journal of Occupational Therapy, 69,* 6906290010. https://doi.org/10.5014/ajot.2015.015974

Kim, H.-J., Barsevick, A. M., Beck, S. L., & Dudley, W. (2012). Clinical subgroups of a psychoneurologic symptom cluster in women receiving treatment for breast cancer: A secondary analysis. *Oncology Nursing Forum, 39,* E20–E30. https://doi.org/10.1188/12.ONF.E20-E30

Kwekkeboom, K. L. (2016). Cancer symptom cluster management. *Seminars in Oncology Nursing, 32,* 373–382. https://doi.org/10.1016/j.soncn.2016.08.004

Lyons, K. D. (2006). Occupation as a vehicle to surmount the psychosocial challenges of cancer. *Occupational Therapy in Health Care, 20,* 1–16. https://doi.org/10.1080/J003v20n02_01

Mendoza, T. R., Wang, X. S., Cleeland, C. S., Morrissey, M., Johnson, B. A., Wendt, J. K., & Huber, S. L. (1999). The rapid assessment of fatigue severity in cancer patients: Use of the Brief Fatigue Inventory. *Cancer, 85,* 1186–1196. https://doi.org/10.1002/(SICI)1097-0142(19990301)85:5<1186::AID-CNCR24>3.0.CO;2-N

Meneses-Echávez, J. F., González-Jiménez, E., & Ramírez-Vélez, R. (2015). Effects of supervised multimodal exercise interventions on cancer-related fatigue: Systematic review and meta-analysis of randomized controlled trials. *BioMed Research International, 2015,* 328636. https://doi.org/10.1155/2015/328636

National Cancer Institute. (2006). *Closing the gap: Research and care imperatives for adolescents and young adults with cancer: Report of the Adolescent and Young Adult Oncology Progress Review Group.* Retrieved from https://www.cancer.gov/types/aya/research/ayao-august-2006.pdf

Nidamboor, R. (2018). Being in the zone is divine frenzy. *Positive Health Online, 246,* Article 5.

Okuyama, T., Akechi, T., Kugaya, A., Okamura, H., Shima, Y., Maruguchi, M., . . . Uchitomi, Y. (2000). Development and validation of the Cancer Fatigue Scale: A brief, three-dimensional, self-rating scale for assessment of fatigue in cancer patients. *Journal of Pain and Symptom Management, 19,* 5–14. https://doi.org/10.1016/S0885-3924(99)00138-4

Packer, T. L., Brink, N., & Sauriol, A. (1995). *Managing fatigue: A six-week course for energy conservation.* Tucson, AZ: Therapy Skill Builders.

Palmadottir, G. (2009). The road to recovery: Experiences and occupational lives of Icelandic women with breast cancer. *Occupational Therapy in Health Care, 23,* 319–335. http://dx.doi.org/10.3109/07380570903242433

Parkinson, S., Forsyth, K., & Kielhofner, G. (2006). *A user's manual for the Model of Human Occupation Screening Tool (MOHOST).* Chicago: University of Illinois.

Pureell, A., Fleming, J., Haines, T., & Bennett, S. (2009). Cancer-related fatigue: A review and a conceptual framework to guide therapists' understanding. *British Journal of Occupational Therapy, 72,* 79–86. https://doi.org/10.1177/030802260907200205

Reeve, B. B., Stover, A. M., Alfano, C. M., Smith, A. W., Ballard-Barbash, R., Bernstein, L., . . . Piper, B. F. (2012). The Piper Fatigue Scale–12 (PFS-12): Psychometric findings and item reduction in a cohort of breast cancer survivors. *Breast Cancer Research and Treatment, 136,* 9–20. https://doi.org/10.1007/s10549-012-2212-4

Santa Mina, D., Au, D., Brunet, J., Jones, J., Tomlinson, G., Taback, N., . . . Howell, D. (2017). Effects of the community-based Wellspring Cancer Exercise Program on functional and psychosocial outcomes in cancer survivors. *Current Oncology, 24,* 284–294. https://doi.org/10.3747/co.24.3585

Schuler, M. K., Hentschel, L., Kisel, W., Kramer, M., Lenz, F., Hornemann, B., . . . Kroschinsky, F. (2017). Impact of different exercise programs on severe fatigue in patients undergoing anticancer treatment: A randomized controlled trial. *Journal of Pain and Symptom Management, 53,* 57–66. https://doi.org/10.1016/j.jpainsymman.2016.08.014

Smets, E. M., Garssen, B., Bonke, B., & De Haes, J. C. (1995). The Multidimensional Fatigue Inventory (MFI) psychometric qualities of an instrument to assess fatigue. *Journal of Psychosomatic Research, 39,* 315–325. https://doi.org/10.1016/0022-3999(94)00125-O

Spathis, A., Booth, S., Grove, S., Hatcher, H., Kuhn, I., & Barclay, S. (2015). Teenage and young adult cancer-related fatigue is prevalent, distressing, and neglected: It is time to intervene. A systematic literature review and narrative synthesis. *Journal of Adolescent and Young Adult Oncology, 4,* 3–17. https://doi.org/10.1089/jayao.2014.0023

Stein, K. D., Jacobsen, P. B., Blanchard, C. M., & Thors, C. (2004). Further validation of the Multidimensional Fatigue Symptom Inventory—Short Form. *Journal of Pain and Symptom Management, 27,* 14–23. https://doi.org/10.1016/j.jpainsymman.2003.06.003 https://doi.org/10.1046/j.1523-5394.1998.006003143.x

Velthuis, M. J., Agasi-Idenburg, S. C., Aufdemkampe, G., & Wittink, H. M. (2010). The effect of physical exercise on cancer-related fatigue during cancer treatment: A meta-analysis of randomised controlled trials. *Clinical Oncology, 22,* 208–221. https://doi.org/10.1016/j.clon.2009.12.005

Weis, J., & Horneber, M. (2015). Definition and prevalence of cancer-related fatigue. In *Cancer-related fatigue* (pp. 1–8). New York: Springer Healthcare. https://doi.org/10.1007/978-1-907673-76-4_1

Wood-Dauphinee, S., & Williams, J. I. (1987). Reintegration to normal living as a proxy to quality of life. *Journal of Chronic Diseases, 40,* 491–499. https://doi.org/10.1016/0021-9681(87)90005-1

Yellen, S. B., Cella, D. F., Webster, K., Blendowski, C., & Kaplan, E. (1997). Measuring fatigue and other anemia-related symptoms with the Functional Assessment of Cancer Therapy (FACT) measurement system. *Journal of Pain and Symptom Management, 13,* 63–74. https://doi.org/10.1016/S0885-3924(96)00274-6

Cancer-Related Pain

Jennifer Nicholson, OTR, MOT

16

LEARNING OBJECTIVES

After completing this chapter, readers should be able to

- Evaluate typical types of cancer-related pain experienced by cancer survivors across the lifespan,
- Examine cancer-related pain and its relationship to occupational performance and participation across the lifespan,
- Develop treatment approaches in response to a cancer survivor's pain across the lifespan, and
- Apply knowledge of pain in cancer to promote safe engagement in occupational performance across the lifespan.

KEY TERMS AND CONCEPTS

- Assistive devices
- Bone metastases
- Cancer-related pain
- Central sensitization
- Chemotherapy-induced peripheral neuropathy

- Energy conservation
- Ergonomics
- Modification
- Neuropathic pain
- Occupational engagement
- Orthotics

- Pain
- Physical agent modalities
- Plexopathy
- Survivorship
- Therapeutic exercise
- Thrombocytopenia

INTRODUCTION

Cancer-related pain is pain resulting from cancer treatment or the disease process itself. It is a notable and pervasive sequela of cancer and can have a negative impact on occupational engagement at every stage of the lifespan. *Occupational engagement* has been described as "occur[ring] when the individual is ready and interested in taking part in an activity and the opportunity to do so presents itself" (Brown & Kandirikirira, 2007, p. 4). Pain is one of the most common symptoms reported in the cancer literature, along with cancer-related fatigue and breathlessness (Hunter et al., 2017).

With survival rates on the rise, cancer is now regarded as a chronic condition for many (Centers for Disease Control and Prevention & Lance Armstrong Foundation, 2004; Hewitt et al., 2005). As a result of increased *survivorship,* which is defined by the National Cancer Institute (NCI; n.d.-b) as encompassing the period from diagnosis to end of life, clinicians must recognize pain as a symptom that can be persistent throughout the continuum of cancer and occur in any stage of development.

Jibb et al. (2014) estimated that approximately 49%–62% of children and adolescents with cancer experience pain related to the disease or associated invasive procedures and treatments. In fact, children who have chronic pain or are exposed to invasive procedures have been shown to have a greater predisposition for chronic and new types of pain as adults (von Baeyer et al., 2004; Walker et al., 2010). As many as 90% of adults with cancer may have some experience of pain (Bao et al., 2016).

The symptom of *pain* is a mixed mechanism, including both neuropathic and nonneuropathic origins. It involves inflammatory, neuropathic, ischemic, and compression mechanisms at multiple sites. Of key interest to occupational therapy practitioners is the correlation between uncontrolled pain and poor performance in occupations, including ADLs and IADLs (Landi et al., 2009).

Occupational therapy practitioners should also consider psychological consequences, because cancer survivors may experience high levels of distress and mental health disruption as a result of pain, and they may have consequent loss of engagement in valued occupations and performance patterns. Colloca et al. (2015) described *pain* as a sensation in part or parts of the body but also an unpleasant and therefore emotional experience.

This chapter explores typical types of pain that occupational therapy practitioners might encounter when working with the cancer population, including

- Neuropathic, testing, surgical, and procedural pain;
- Radiation therapy–induced pain; and
- Pain from bony metastatic disease and pathological fracture.

Additionally, this chapter addresses considerations for occupational therapy practitioners working with patients with cancer pain across the lifespan as well as pain assessment and interventions supported by the literature.

FEATURES OF CANCER-RELATED PAIN

Cancer pain is a distressing symptom that tends to increase in frequency and intensity as cancer advances. Prevalence of pain among adults living with cancer can be as high as 90%; as many as 75%–90% of people with cancer would describe pain as having a major impact on their daily life (Bao et al., 2016). In the pediatric population, 49% of patients in one study reported pain at diagnosis and during early phases of treatment (Allen et al., 2016).

Occupational therapy practitioners should consider a wide variety of pain concerns when treating clients with cancer, including but not limited to psychiatric comorbidity, reduced quality of life (QoL), impaired sleep, loss of roles, and disruptions to routines. These impairments can present in chronic states, so practitioners should also keep them in mind when working with those who have a history of cancer or a history of anticancer therapies.

TYPES OF CANCER PAIN

Occupational therapy practitioners must be prepared to evaluate and establish treatment plans for cancer survivors experiencing various types of pain. Although this chapter discusses some of the more common pain classifications specific to cancer, cancer survivors may present with one discrete type of pain or several types of pain concurrently. Intervention approaches depend on survivors' presentation of pain and how it affects occupational engagement.

Neuropathic Pain

Neuropathic pain is the result of nerve damage that causes a constellation of symptoms, including pain, numbness, and weakness. Neuropathic pain is triggered by lesions to the somatosensory nervous system, which alter its structure and function. As a consequence, pain occurs spontaneously and responses to noxious and innocuous stimuli are pathologically amplified (Costigan et al., 2009). Neuropathic pain can be a direct consequence of cancer, such as a cancer involving the central nervous system, or a consequence of anticancer therapies, including chemotherapy and radiation.

Unique to the cancer population is *chemotherapy-induced peripheral neuropathy* (CIPN), which is acute and chronic dysfunction or injury to the peripheral nervous system as a result of cancer treatment. Although most of the research regarding CIPN has been conducted among adults, pediatric populations are gaining attention because of increased survivorship over the past 60 years. As Kandula et al. (2016) discussed, peripheral nerve toxicity can be caused by vinca alkaloids, platinum compounds, taxanes, epothilones, bortezomib, and thalidomide. Vinca alkaloids and platinum compounds are the more commonly used agents in childhood cancer. See Chapter 19, "Chemotherapy-Induced Peripheral Neuropathy," for more information on this topic.

Diagnosing peripheral neuropathy in the pediatric cancer population can be challenging because routine neurophysiological assessment is difficult with young children, given the associated discomfort. However, nerve conduction studies, which are also performed with adults, can be helpful in identifying the symptoms (Kandula et al., 2016).

Peripheral neuropathy typically presents with symptoms of paresthesia and numbness; however, some people experience extremely painful symptoms that present as cramping or severe hypersensitivity. Pharmacological interventions may include topical medications, antidepressants, and pain medications. Chemotherapy dose adjustments are also to be considered. It is important to communicate with the primary medical team regarding the impact of these medications on clients' functional performance.

Occupational therapy practitioners also have a role in detecting the onset of symptoms of neuropathy, especially in the setting of pain, and communicating these symptoms to the physician. Depending on the severity of neuropathic pain, occupational therapy practitioners may consider assistive devices, retraining on balance and stability, correction of body posture, and instruction on compensatory patterns of movement.

Radiation Therapy–Induced Pain

Radiation therapy can produce an array of persistent syndromes and negative side effects, including radiation burn; tissue changes; range of motion (ROM) deficits; and, in severe cases, osteoradionecrosis and plexopathies. *Plexopathy* is a disorder that affects a network of nerves, blood vessels, or lymphatic vessels (NCI, n.d.-a). The brachial or lumbosacral plexus may be affected. Clinical signs of plexopathy may include sensory changes, atrophy of muscles, and persistent pain. In cases where radiation is a treatment option, early intervention and detection of negative complications are critical. Tissue fibrosis, which often results in painful movement of extremities, and other complications of radiation may be reduced with intervention in early stages.

Occupational therapy practitioners may address specific deficits through several treatment approaches, including
- Postural exercises to improve strength and stability for occupational engagement,
- Gentle stretching to maintain ROM and reduce painful tightness to promote independence in self-care areas,
- Engagement in routine for oral and skin care, and
- ROM exercise for functional range and reduced pain with functional reach.

Without appropriate intervention, complications may have a compounding effect. A cancer survivor may experience improvement in physical abilities but not occupational performance as a result of fear and anxiety.

Pain Related to Bony Metastatic Disease and Pathological Fracture

Metastasis of cancer to bones is a common and unfortunate consequence of cancer. *Bone metastases* are the most common cause of pain related to cancer, reducing QoL and sometimes threatening life expectancy (Bonetto et al., 2017). Although bone metastasis is clinically plausible in many cancers, certain diagnoses, including breast, lung, and prostate cancers as well multiple myeloma, carry even higher risk of pathological fracture and lytic lesions (Coleman, 2001; Luo et al., 2016; Roodman, 2004).

Occupational therapy practitioners working in oncology must be mindful that bony metastatic disease that has resulted in a fracture cannot always be stabilized because of complicating factors related to surgical stabilization, including abnormal lab values, poor performance status, and organ dysfunction in the setting of cancer. Education and activity modification are key intervention approaches in these scenarios. Cancer survivors must be educated on how to move safely and in a pain-reduced state to optimize function.

Pathological fracture of the spine is one of the more common areas of metastasis and can present with high levels of pain. Education on normal lordotic and kyphotic curve is important for clients experiencing spinal fractures because abnormal curvature can increase pain, disrupt the nervous system, and disrupt blood flow. Further education on spinal precautions, such as avoiding bending, lifting, and twisting, is indicated in the setting of spinal fracture. Occupational therapy practitioners may train survivors in the log roll technique for bed mobility, make recommendations for spinal bracing, issue long-handled equipment and train the client in its use, and promote positioning strategies. Each of these interventions can increase occupational engagement and support performance while protecting the spine.

Pain from pathological fracture or bony metastatic disease in areas outside the spine can be reduced with appropriate orthotic selection and use in the context of daily occupation. This may include splints and upper-extremity braces or slings. Furthermore, education on how to integrate precautions into routine ADLs, such as reduced ROM at a certain joints or weight-bearing restrictions, is also critical. Occupational therapy practitioners are skilled in analyzing performance and providing intervention that ensures good integration of mobility precautions and proper body mechanics during performance of everyday occupations.

Testing, Surgical, and Procedural Pain

Pain related to testing, procedures, and surgeries can be common, given that all people living with cancer begin their cancer journey with diagnostic workup, including procedures such as diagnostic lab draws, biopsies, and lumbar punctures. Surgical resection of solid tumors or lymph nodes, with or without reconstruction, can induce pain and interfere with occupational performance.

Occupational therapy practitioners working in oncology must be aware of precautions and indications of specific tests, procedures, and surgeries. Having knowledge of these, practitioners can then provide education and training around occupational engagement before and after the procedure. For example, in the case of a transverse rectus abdominis flap reconstruction after mastectomy, the occupational therapy practitioner can aid in postoperative pain control by instructing the patient in mobility, transitional movements, and ADLs without causing strain to the abdomen or applying pressure to newly reconstructed breasts. Additionally, in the postsurgical case, it is helpful to provide education on restricting ROM at certain joints, address strict postsurgical postural recommendations, and instruct the client on breathing and pacing strategies to manage pain. See Table 16.1 for distinctions among different types of pain.

CANCER-RELATED PAIN ACROSS THE LIFESPAN

Children

Although pediatric cases make up less than 1% of all cancers diagnosed each year, pain is a lifelong consideration, given that more than 84% of children with cancer now survive 5 years or more (American Cancer Society [ACS], 2020). Acute lymphoblastic leukemia, central nervous

TABLE 16.1. Distinctions Among Types of Cancer-Related Pain	
PAIN TYPE	**DESCRIPTION**
Neuropathic pain	▪ Is the result of nerve damage ▪ Can result in a constellation of symptoms, including pain, numbness, and weakness ▪ Can occur spontaneously, and responses to stimuli are pathologically amplified (Costigan et al., 2009) ▪ Can be the direct consequence of cancer, such as cancer involving the central nervous system ▪ Can be the result of anticancer therapies, including radiation and chemotherapy ▪ Can cause extreme pain, painful hypersensitivity, and cramping in severe cases
Radiation therapy–induced pain	▪ Can occur from radiation therapy causing radiation burn, resulting in painful tissue changes and limitations in range of motion ▪ In severe cases, osteoradionecrosis and plexopathies can occur.
Bony metastatic disease and pathological fracture	▪ Can occur from metastasis of cancer to bones ▪ May result in pathological fracture, which sometimes cannot be surgically stabilized
Testing, procedural, and surgical	▪ Painful diagnostic workup, including biopsies, lumbar punctures, and lab draws ▪ Pain with positioning required for diagnostic imaging (e.g., client with known back pain from pathological fracture lying flat during magnetic resonance imaging study) ▪ Surgical resection of solid tumors or lymph nodes ▪ Reconstructive surgeries

system tumors, and neuroblastoma are the three most common types of pediatric cancers (An et al., 2017). Specific to pediatric cancer survivors, there is the added dimension of assessing pain related to diagnosis and treatment and how that might influence development and long-term emotional functioning. Allen et al. (2016) noted that pediatric pain can negatively affect QoL and emotional functioning and can lead to deconditioning and functional disability. Furthermore, chronic and recurrent pain at this stage have been associated with psychiatric comorbidity in adulthood (Chitkara et al., 2005; Kashikar-Zuck et al., 2014).

Play is the primary occupation of children, and it can be adversely affected by a disease process such as cancer. Mohammadi et al. (2017) discussed the development of sensory, motor, and cognitive processes through play in childhood. Cancer-related pain can create additional barriers to engagement in play, resulting not only in occupational deprivation but also in impairments in these key areas of development. Through play, children develop performance skills, including motor skills such as coordination, functional grip, and manipulation skills. They also form process skills, including task initiation, sequencing, and termination as well as social skills.

Occupational therapy practitioners' role is to reduce obstacles to play and promote play experiences for children living with cancer-related pain. Interventions may be centered around problem-solving types of play that do not exacerbate pain. Occupational therapy practitioners also can, for example, make determinations around positioning needs to reduce pain and incorporate a ROM and stretching program to reduce pain before a child engages in play.

Adolescents

When addressing the adolescent population, occupational therapy practitioners may be guided by developmentally typical occupational engagement for this age group. IADLs (e.g., driving), communication management, sleep participation, leisure exploration, social participation, and educational participation all might be disrupted by cancer-related pain. Approximately 49%–62% of children and adolescents with cancer experience pain related to the disease or associated invasive procedures and treatments (Jibb et al., 2014). With respect to sleep, disruption is common with acute, chronic, and recurrent pain and related to decreased QoL (Butbul Aviel et al., 2011; Kunderman et al., 2004).

Pain can be a disruptive symptom for adolescents and serve as a barrier to their participation in typical roles and related social engagement. Such roles might include student, athlete, sibling, son or daughter, or club member. Research supports that children and adolescents with chronic pain have fewer friends and may be viewed as more isolated and less likable compared with healthy peers (Manworren & Stinson, 2016). Through appropriate analysis of activity and occupational demands for clients in this age group, occupational therapy practitioners can support adolescents and young adults in engaging in meaningful occupations. Case Example 16.1 illustrates how an occupational therapist might consider developmentally typical occupations and use appropriate evaluation tools and intervention strategies to promote engagement in the setting of cancer-related pain.

Adults

As discussed in Case Example 16.2, adults living with cancer-related pain may experience disruption in primary roles identified with this age group such as parent, grandparent, homemaker, spouse, employee, and financial provider. Navigating cancer and cancer-related pain through these major life roles provides additional challenges and stressors. Occupational therapy practitioners working with clients in this age group should explore how pain is affecting clients' job performance and their ability to meet demands relative to household management and familial interaction.

Furthermore, occupational therapy practitioners should consider how cancer-related pain might increase risk for challenges related to psychosocial well-being. According to Eiser et al. (2009) and Zebrack et al. (2009), younger adults may be at risk for developing psychosocial difficulties because the period of young adulthood is marked by increasing autonomy, identity formation, career and family planning, and intimate relationships.

Adults dealing with cancer-related pain may experience a reduced QoL if they are not able to engage in work, a valued occupation for many in this age group. Participation in the labor market, according to Baanders et al. (2002), results not only in material benefits but in the maintenance of preferred occupational identity. Occupational therapy practitioners might address pain management for cancer survivors actively engaged in work as well as those who are returning to work with ongoing pain management concerns.

Older Adults

Older adults make up the largest percentage of new cancer diagnoses, representing two-thirds of all new cases (White et al., 2019). Cancer risk increases with age; the median age of new cancer diagnosis is age 66 years. Older adults (ages 65 years or older) are commonly affected by a cancer diagnosis, and the average age at death from cancer is age 72 years (Guerard & Cleary, 2017). Occupational therapy practitioners working with older adults with a diagnosis of cancer must consider additional complications because of age. These might include increased comorbidities, potential cognitive impairment, and social isolation (Li et al., 2017).

Although some older adults may continue work as an occupation, occupational therapy practitioners are more likely to support engagement in ADLs, IADLs, sleep participation, volunteer exploration, and social participation. Physicians also consider occupational performance, especially in the areas of ADLs and IADLs, when making decisions about anticancer treatments. Older adults who need assistance with ADLs have increased risk of nursing home placement and mortality (Wildes et al., 2015). The complex nature of cancer treatment is challenging for older adults, especially with respect to IADLs, which can include making and following schedules for appointments, managing medication, and performing home management tasks.

Pain can further complicate older adults' participation in these areas of occupation. Occupational therapy practitioners should consider the interaction between the client and their environment when intervening with older adults with cancer-related pain. Activity demands and exacerbating factors of pain may be quite different for an older adult

CASE EXAMPLE 16.1. THOMAS: CANCER-RELATED PAIN IN AN ADOLESCENT

Thomas is a 12-year-old who attends a local elementary school. He is an avid athlete and particularly enjoys soccer. In the second game of the soccer season, Thomas went to his parents about pain in the left femur. Initially, the pain symptoms were dismissed as growing pains; however, the pain persisted. In addition to pain, Thomas complained of persistent swelling and joint mobility limitations at the knee. The persistence of symptoms led Thomas's parents to take him to his primary care physician. After a series of blood tests, imaging studies, and ultimately a biopsy, Thomas was found to have osteosarcoma.

Thomas's treatment was extensive, including radiation and chemotherapy, and resulted in chronic pain. After more conservative treatment approaches were found to be ineffective, the decision was made to complete left lower extremity amputation. Because of the extensiveness of disease, a rotationplasty was not clinically indicated as part of the surgical plan. Occupational therapy was consulted after surgery to address deficits in occupational performance after amputation.

During the evaluation process, Thomas identified his primary roles as student, athlete, friend, and brother to his two younger sisters. In addition to severe postsurgical pain, Thomas was quite distressed and fearful he would never have a normal life again. Thomas worried most about being able to return to playing soccer; moving safely around his school; maintaining privacy from his mother during self-care; and his self-concept and self-image, especially with respect to maintaining interest from girls in his class.

The occupational therapist administered the following assessments to provide objective data regarding Thomas's pain experience: Wong–Baker FACES® Pain Scale (Wong-Baker FACES Foundation, 2016), Neuropathic Pain Scale (Galer & Jensen, 1997), and Adolescent Pediatric Pain Tool (APPT; Jacob et al., 2014; Savedra et al., 1989). On the basis of the assessment, Thomas's pain types were noted to be both acute and neuropathic in nature. Despite pharmacological intervention, Thomas rated his pain as 8, or "hurts whole lot," on the Wong–Baker FACES Pain Scale.

Using the APPT (Jacob et al., 2014; Savedra et al., 1989), Thomas identified the left distal femur surgical site as the site of pain, marking it on the body schematic provided as part of the assessment. Thomas circled the words *miserable, sharp, always,* and *uncontrollable* to describe his pain symptoms. Thomas also described a prickling type of pain, which indicated an additional neuropathic source for pain. Because of the acute nature of the pain and early postoperative status, the occupational therapist cleared with the surgeon before beginning desensitization techniques. Thomas was instructed on initial desensitization techniques to the residual limb, which included gradual and graded introduction of texture and pressure.

An assessment of function resulted in findings of poor sitting balance and transfer performance because of the loss of limb, resulting in loss of independence with ADLs and the secondary consequence of loss of privacy from his mother. Early interventions focused on static sitting balance, progressing to dynamic sitting balance with independent engagement in ADLs, IADLs, and leisure as the outcome. To address this skill, the occupational therapist incorporated play. Because of Thomas's interest in sports, a ball was incorporated for catch-and-release types of activities.

Improvements to balance directly translated to more independent performance with ADLs and IADLs, allowing Thomas to have a greater sense of pride. He also verbally reported satisfaction that his mother was no longer required to provide assistance. Because he had limited acute care hospitalization days, Thomas was referred to another occupational therapist to continue rehabilitation as an outpatient.

---

cancer survivor living alone with limited support than for a survivor in the context of a long-term placement.

HOW IS PAIN MEASURED?

When pain interferes with engagement in meaningful occupations, an occupational therapy assessment is indicated. Correct identification of the dominant type of cancer pain is helpful in promoting wellness and QoL. Pain may be neuropathic, nonneuropathic, or centrally sensitized in its origin. According to Malfliet et al. (2017), **central sensitization** is the general hypersensitivity of the somatosensory system.

The timeline for pain is also an important consideration because cancer-related pain can present in an acute, chronic, or breakthrough state. (See Table 16.2 for a description of these types of pain.) Occupational therapy practitioners must consider all of these factors when treating a cancer survivor with cancer-related pain and should appreciate the possibility of reduced level of occupational engagement because of it.

Both subjective and objective measures of pain are critical to thorough assessment. Attention to the words a survivor uses to describe pain can be helpful. For example, a survivor describing pain that radiates down the limbs might suggest a neuropathic component to the pain. Developing an occupational profile is useful in identifying current concerns relative to engaging in occupations and should be included in formal occupational therapy assessment of pain and its impact on occupational performance.

Assessing pain should begin with a full patient interview as part of the process of constructing the occupational profile. The location, quality, exacerbating factors, alleviating factors, and previous treatments are critical to practitioners understanding patients' pain experience. Assessment of

CASE EXAMPLE 16.2. AVA: CANCER-RELATED PAIN IN AN ADULT

Ava is a 67-year-old grandmother who lives with her adult daughter and three grandchildren. She was diagnosed with multiple myeloma after anemia and severe pain in her middle and low back signaled the need for her to visit her doctor. She was found to have multiple compression deformities and fractures throughout the thoracic and lumbar spine as a consequence of the disease. During the hospital admission, Ava began developing right lower-extremity (LE) weakness. After emergent imaging, she was found to have compression of the spinal cord at L1.

Ava's treatment team consulted occupational therapy while she was an inpatient to provide assessment and treatment for occupational performance deficits, including fatigue, acute back pain, and LE weakness. At the start of the evaluation process, the occupational therapist developed an occupational profile. Ava identified her primary roles and interests as head of household, avid knitter, and caregiver to her three young grandchildren because her daughter was often at work. Ava perceived that her function and engagement in ADLs, IADLs, and leisure were severely disrupted.

Ava also reported psychosocial distress related to high degree of pain and her feared inability to care for herself or uphold her commitment to her daughter and grandchildren. Ava told her occupational therapist, "I am so scared to even move from this bed for fear of pain or injuring myself further."

The occupational therapist administered the following assessments to provide objective data regarding Ava's pain experience: the Roland–Morris Disability Questionnaire (Roland & Morris, 1983), the Visual Analog Scale (McCormack et al., 1988), and the Brief Pain Inventory (Cleeland & Ryan, 1994).

As part of the inpatient mobility assessment, Ava was observed performing bed mobility, functional transfer to a bedside chair, and simulated household tasks, including repositioning a bedside chair, carrying a light object across the room, and picking up an object from floor level. This allowed the occupational therapist to observe Ava's body mechanics and real-time pain response to various types of activities. The occupational therapist noted very poor body mechanics, with observed frequent spinal-twisting compression through extremes of flexion and extension during task completion. Ava was additionally noted to rush through tasks, not allowing herself to rest or attend to good body mechanics, which further worsened pain and resulted in increased risk for safety incidences, especially with known LE weakness.

With the understanding that Ava's pain, now acute, would likely be a chronic condition as she continued with cancer care, intervention implementation focused on promotion of valued activities, modification, and prevention of further injury or pain exacerbation as well as fall prevention in the setting of LE weakness. With this in mind, the occupational therapist focused on correcting body mechanics, providing education on spinal precautions, and monitoring for safe integration of these into ADLs, IADLs, and leisure. The occupational therapist also issued a long-handled reacher for retrieval of floor-level items. Additional education was provided on energy conservation principles for pain management, including breaking up more demanding and pain-provoking tasks, such as washing dishes, with more sedentary, pain-alleviating activities, such as assisting her granddaughters with their homework or knitting, as part of leisure participation.

TABLE 16.2.	Pain Definitions
PAIN TYPE	**DEFINITION**
Chronic pain	▪ Persists past normal healing time and lacks the acute warning function of physiological nociception ▪ No recognizable endpoint ▪ Adverse effects, including depressed mood and fatigue ▪ Often results in physical deconditioning and leads to disability (Chapman & Vierck, 2017)
Acute pain	▪ Unpleasant, complex, and dynamic psychophysiological response ▪ Response to tissue trauma ▪ Provoked by a specific disease or injury (Grichnik & Ferrante, 1991) ▪ Self-limited ▪ Confined to a given period of time ▪ Serves a useful biologic purpose and fosters healing ▪ Rate at which acute pain resolves is a key feature (Chapman & Vierck, 2017)
Breakthrough pain	▪ Erupts while a patient is already medicated with a long-acting painkiller ▪ Transitory increase in pain intensity, either spontaneously or in relation to a trigger ▪ Occurs despite client report of relatively stable and adequate pain control ▪ Frequent complication among patients with advanced cancer (Mercadante et al., 2019)

pain should be frequent and ongoing throughout the intervention process because the subjective experience of pain may change. The change in subjective experience may be the result of alterations in treatment, disease status, or level of activity, among other possible factors. Self-report measures are most common type of pain assessment because pain is considered to be a subjective experience. Standardized assessments can also be helpful in understanding and tracking a survivor's experience of cancer-related pain.

With regard to pediatric assessment, Manworren and Stinson (2016) recommended assessment and reassessment of pain with developmentally age-appropriate assessment tools. The Visual Analog Scale (McCormack et al., 1988), for example, has been adapted for children as young as 3 years. Adequate assessment, sufficient evaluation, and appropriate response are essential because failure to do so can perpetuate poor management of pain.

Occupational therapy practitioners assessing pain in the pediatric cancer population must also make considerations for children who are noncommunicative or nonverbal. Vocalizations, changes to facial expressions, and large body movements (e.g., withdrawal from stimuli) can signal pain. Changes to social behavior or appetite are also helpful in identifying pain among nonverbal pediatric survivors (Manworren & Stinson, 2016). Examples of tools for adult and pediatric pain assessment can be found in Table 16.3.

INTERVENTION FOR CANCER-RELATED PAIN

The level of intervention is often dictated by the type and severity of cancer-related pain; however, approaches to intervention, as discussed in the *Occupational Therapy Practice Framework: Domain and Process* (3rd ed.; *OTPF*; American Occupational Therapy Association [AOTA], 2014), are helpful in making decisions about intervention.

TABLE 16.3. Assessment Tools for Cancer-Related Pain

ASSESSMENT	DESCRIPTION
Adolescent Pediatric Pain Tool (Jacob et al., 2014)	Indicated for children ages 8 years and older and validated to assess pain intensity, pattern or timing, location (using a body drawing), and quality of pain reported by the pediatric client. Child indicates or circles sensory, affective, evaluative, and temporal words. Available in Spanish and English.
Brief Pain Inventory (Cleeland & Ryan, 1994)	Patients rate the severity of their pain and the degree to which their pain interferes with common dimensions of feeling and function.
Children's Hospital of Eastern Ontario Pain Scale (McGrath et al., 1985; Suraseranivongse et al., 2001)	Indicated for children ages 4 months–17 years. Measures the sum of 6 parameters (cry, facial, verbal, torso, touch, legs) for a total score of 4–13. May be used for procedural and postoperative pain assessment.
McGill Pain Questionnaire (Melzack, 1975)	Assesses 3 categories of word descriptors: sensory, affective, and evaluative. Includes a body diagram for patients to identify the area of their pain. Can be used to monitor the quality and quantity of pain, assess changes in pain over time, and determine the effectiveness of any intervention.
Neuropathic Pain Scale (Galer & Jensen, 1997)	Designed to assess distinct pain qualities associated with neuropathic pain.
Numeric Rating Scale (Hartrick et al., 2003)	Segmented numeric version of the Visual Analog Scale (McCormack et al., 1988) in which a respondent selects a whole number (0–10 integers) that best reflects the intensity of their pain. The common format is a horizontal bar or line.
Numerical rating scales	Indicated for assessment of acute, procedural, and postoperative pain. Typically, 0 is least pain, and higher number values indicate higher pain levels.
Oswestry Disability Index (Fairbank & Pynsent, 2000)	Patient-completed questionnaire that gives a subjective percentage score of level of function (disability) in ADLs for clients rehabilitating from low back pain.
Roland–Morris Disability Questionnaire (Roland & Morris, 1983)	24-item self-report questionnaire about how low-back pain affects functional activities.
Varni/Thompson Pediatric Pain Questionnaire (Varni et al., 1987)	Indicated for children 5 years and older and validated to assess chronic pain intensity and location and the sensory, evaluative, and affective qualities of pain. Available in 7 languages.
Visual Analog Scale (McCormack et al., 1988)	Aims to measure a characteristic or attitude that is believed to range across a continuum of values and cannot easily be directly measured. Often used in epidemiologic and clinical research.
West Haven–Yale Multidimensional Pain Inventory (Kerns et al., 1985)	Designed to provide a brief, psychometrically sound, and comprehensive assessment of the important components of the chronic pain experience.
Wong–Baker FACES Pain Rating Scale (Wong-Baker FACES Foundation, 2016)	Self-report measure of pain intensity developed for children. Adapted so that the sensation of pain is rated on the widely accepted 0–10 metric. The scale shows a series of faces ranging from a happy face at 0, which represents "no hurt," to a crying face at 10, which represents "hurts worst."

Note. ADLs = activities of daily living.

Approaches to intervention include creating and promoting (i.e., health promotion), establishing and restoring, maintaining, modifying, and preventing.

In cancer practice, occupational therapy practitioners might expect interventions to occur primarily in the areas of modification and prevention. However, restoration of function, such as improving ROM of a limb, can aid in pain management. Promotion of health is advisable in cases when pain is not yet present but risk factors are high, such as instruction in body mechanics and conditioning programming before surgery when postoperative pain, worsened by poor-quality mobilization, is anticipated.

Table 16.4. Summary of Interventions for Cancer-Related Pain

INTERVENTIONS	CLINICAL APPLICATION
Activity modification	▪ Foundation is in activity analysis ▪ Recommendations on changes to activity and occupational demands, such as required body functions, sequencing and timing, objects used and their properties, space demands (AOTA, 2014) ▪ Typical recommendations for pain management may include alterations to positioning, incorporation of wheelchairs and seating systems, use of long-handled equipment ▪ May include safe integration of body mechanics and ergonomics
Physical agent modalities (PAMs)	▪ Superficial heat or cold ▪ Deep heat ▪ Electrotherapeutic (transcutaneous electrical nerve stimulation) ▪ Desensitization ▪ Mechanical
Therapeutic exercise	▪ A useful intervention, especially when paired with other modalities, such as PAMs ▪ Used to strengthen muscles to increase stability and support around painful areas ▪ Can serve to increase range of motion, improve blood circulation, and reduce painful edema in extremities ▪ Caution should be taken in the case of bony disease or pathological fracture because repetitive stress can result in further injury or pain ▪ Should not be used in isolation but introduced as a means to improve occupational performance and engagement ▪ Should be structured application of specific demands to the body
Cognitive–behavioral, psychosocial, self-management	▪ Education and counseling about the fear of movement, the positive effects of movement, and decatastrophizing of pain (Jay et al., 2016) ▪ Use of guided imagery, deep-breathing techniques, and patient journaling as a means to manage pain (Hunter et al., 2017) ▪ Helps clients to identify and manage persisting symptoms, such as pain (Boland et al., 2017) ▪ Development of personal coping strategies, including terminating unhelpful thought patterns and boosting deficient emotional regulation (Eccleston et al., 2014)
Orthotics	▪ Pain may be reduced with appropriate orthotic selection and use ▪ Spinal, upper extremity, and lower extremity bracing and orthotics are commonly used in cancer practice ▪ Orthotics are a reasonable option to promote safety and reduced pain during occupational engagement until surgical stabilization or natural healing occurs ▪ Consider training in doffing and donning procedures, care and maintenance of the orthotic, and modifying activities to allow for safe integration of orthotics
Assistive devices	▪ Often integrated as a means of reducing activity demands and thereby reducing pain ▪ Can enhance both safety and autonomy of a patient's mobility (Cheville & Basford, 2014) ▪ A painful grasp during feeding can be reduced by use of built-up handles ▪ Wheelchairs, Hoyer lifts, and powered mobility can reduce pain with transfers and locomotion in the home and community ▪ Integration of long-handled equipment, including long-handled sponges, long-handled reachers, sock aids, and shoehorns, may lower incidence of pain by reducing or eliminating bending, twisting, and reaching (Cheville & Basford, 2014) ▪ Tub transfer bench or shower chair during bathing as part of pain management
Energy conservation	▪ Pacing ▪ Positioning ▪ Permission ▪ Planning

Note. Refer to Table 16.5 for more information about PAMs.

Analysis of occupational performance and incorporation of pain assessment tools can aid occupational therapy practitioners in understanding of how clients' pain is affecting their function. When choosing interventions for survivors with cancer-related pain, occupational therapy practitioners appreciate activity demands and client factors and their relationship to the client's therapeutic goals, contexts, and environments (AOTA, 2014). Furthermore, when considering the pain-inducing activity or occupational demands, occupational therapy practitioners are guided by the *OTPF* in determining the relevance and importance to the survivor, the objects used and their properties, space demands, social demands, sequencing and timing, required actions and performance skills, required body functions, and required body structures. See Table 16.4 for a summary of interventions.

Activity Modification

As experts in activity analysis, occupational therapy practitioners are skilled at analyzing occupational performance and making appropriate recommendations for modification that can reduce levels of pain. According to Dunn et al. (1998), *modification,* as an intervention approach, is directed at "finding ways to revise the current context or activity demands to support performance in the natural setting" (p. 588). The detailed and intentional observation of a task or occupation can inform the occupational therapist of pain-aggravating factors.

For example, a patient with chronic pain may be observed retrieving an object from the floor using poor body mechanics or doffing and donning socks and shoes by bending forward to reach their feet as opposed to coming into a figure-of-4 position. The occupational therapy practitioner should educate the cancer survivor on joint protection principles in an attempt to decrease aggravation of pain, discuss incorporation of long-handled equipment for retrieval from low surfaces, and encourage the survivor to ask for assistance from others to retrieve low-level objects or to perform lower-body dressing if these types of activity are not deemed relevant or important.

In clinical practice, activity modification may also include alterations in positioning, and assessment and provision of seating and positioning equipment (e.g., wheelchairs and other seating systems) may positively affect occupational engagement in daily life, which provides people value and meaning. With respect to wheelchair mobility, provision of an adequately wide wheelchair can reduce incidence of shoulder pain, and instruction on good-quality grasp and push stroke can reduce pain from repetitive efforts during wheelchair mobility. Occupational therapy practitioners are skilled at seating and positioning for both pediatric and adult populations.

Additionally, safe integration of body mechanics and *ergonomics,* or the study of efficiency of one's work environment, may be included in the occupational therapy intervention, especially for clients who are living with cancer-related pain and are returning to work. Ergonomic principles can be incorporated to ease musculoskeletal pain as a consequence of cancer. Strategies include adjusting work space heights so that head and neck alignment is neutral and addressing seating needs so that spinal alignment is maintained and upper extremities are in an optimal position per job requirements.

Physical Agent Modalities

Physical agent modalities (PAMs) are defined as interventions and procedures that may be used in a systematic way for the modification of client factors (AOTA, 2008). This could include the use of superficial thermal agents, electrotherapeutic agents, and mechanical devices, incorporated as an adjunct to or in preparation for purposeful activities to manage pain symptoms. It is important to be familiar with and assess the risks associated with each type of PAM because few modalities have been explicitly validated in the cancer setting (Cheville & Basford, 2014). However, clinical effectiveness can be argued by practitioners with "common sense and extensive experience" (Cheville & Basford, 2014, p. 1691).

There are additional considerations for use of PAMs with the cancer population. For example, superficial thermal agents can cause harm to clients with neuropathy, who might not be able to detect tissue damage as a result of heat. Occupational therapy practitioners must also make determinations regarding appropriateness. Superficial thermal agents should be avoided when clients have open tumor-related wounds, and there is a risk of tumor growth with the use of deep heat because growth is related to angiogenesis and blood flow (Loh & Gulati, 2015). See Table 16.5 for descriptions of PAMs and considerations for use with cancer survivors.

Therapeutic Exercise

Therapeutic exercise is the structured application of specific demands to the body and is a useful intervention in the management of pain, especially when paired with other modalities, such as PAMs. Therapeutic exercise can be used to strengthen muscles to increase stability and support around painful areas, such as abdominal strengthening in the setting of spinal pain. Additionally, therapeutic exercise can serve to increase ROM, improve blood circulation, and reduce painful edema in extremities through the mechanical action of muscles to move fluid toward lymph nodes. Caution should be taken in the case of bony disease or pathological fracture because repetitive stress can result in further injury or pain. Occupational therapists should ask the primary team of physicians about restrictions to therapeutic exercise to maintain patient safety.

Occupational therapy practitioners should not use therapeutic exercise in isolation but should introduce it as a means to improve occupational performance and engagement. According to Cheville and Basford (2014), "therapeutic exercise is the cornerstone of all rehabilitative approaches to pain arising from muscles, tendons, and ligaments" (p. 1699). Given the goal of pain management, the role of therapeutic exercise is stabilization of painful body areas and optimization of control of myofascial pain (Cheville & Basford, 2014).

Cognitive–Behavioral, Psychosocial, and Self-Management Interventions

Cognitive–behavioral, psychosocial, and self-management interventions are within the scope of occupational therapy

TABLE 16.5. Physical Agent Modalities and Considerations for Cancer Rehabilitation

MODALITY	MODALITY CHARACTERISTICS	CLINICAL CONSIDERATIONS
Superficial heat and cold	▪ Focuses on the musculoskeletal system ▪ Alters nerve conduction, blood flow, and collagen extensibility ▪ Typically combined with program of exercise and mobilization ▪ Examples of superficial heat include hot packs, fluidotherapy, paraffin baths, contrast baths, whirlpools, and warm water soaks ▪ Examples of superficial cold include cold packs, ice massage, cooling sprays, and ice baths	▪ CIPN and decreased heat and cold sensitivity ▪ Open wounds ▪ Cutaneous disease ▪ Diffuse tumor burden
Deep heat	▪ Goal of enhancing elasticity of tissue ▪ Targets deep tissues, including muscles and joints ▪ Paired with range of motion and fibrous-release techniques (Cheville & Basford, 2014) ▪ Examples of deep heat include ultrasound and phonopheresis	▪ CIPN and decreased heat sensitivity ▪ Abnormal pain response ▪ Open wounds ▪ Cutaneous disease ▪ Controversial because tumor growth is dependent on angiogenesis and blood flow (Loh & Gulati, 2015)
Electrotherapy	▪ Noninvasive means to provide afferent sensory stimuli posited to block nociceptive signals (Chen et al., 1998) ▪ Examples include transcutaneous electrical nerve stimulation, neuromuscular electrical stimulation, iontophoresis, and interferential current	▪ Can contribute to skin irritation and mild discomfort ▪ Consider decreased sensitivity as a result of CIPN ▪ Open wounds ▪ Cutaneous disease ▪ Diffuse tumor burden ▪ Cardiac concerns, such as arrhythmias
Desensitization	▪ Attenuates pain intensity ▪ Builds tolerance for increasingly intense stimuli	▪ Open wounds ▪ Damage to compromised skin if materials are too abrasive ▪ Ongoing monitoring of skin integrity
Mechanical	▪ May include continuous passive motion, whirlpool, and sequential compression pumps for lymphedema	▪ CIPN ▪ Ongoing monitoring of skin integrity

Note. CIPN = chemotherapy-induced neuropathy.

practice and can help cancer survivors identify and manage persisting symptoms such as pain (Boland et al., 2017). These approaches are supported for both adult and pediatric populations (Malfliet et al., 2017). Psychological distress and decreased QoL are associated with unmet functional needs and can result in increased health care use and expense (Akechi et al., 2011; Park & Hwang, 2012). In fact, about one in four people with cancer experience clinical depression (ACS, 2015).

Occupational therapy practitioners are skilled at addressing psychosocial burdens and stressors in the adult population, which may include social isolation, decreased participation, and financial and familial strain (Foster & Fenlon, 2011). Psychosocial burdens and stressors in the pediatric population may include school performance, body image, social strain, and decreased participation in play. Difficulty reengaging in meaningful occupations, such as work, leisure, socialization, sleep, and sexual activity, can be a consequence of lasting psychosocial burden and coexisting late effects of treatment (Breukink & Donovan, 2013; Hwang et al., 2015).

Jay et al. (2016) discussed the importance of educating and counseling clients about the fear of movement, informing them about the positive effects of movement, and decatastrophizing pain. The literature additionally supports use of guided imagery, deep-breathing techniques, and patient journaling as a means to manage pain (Hunter et al., 2017). For pediatric survivors dealing with chronic pain, research from the psychological field supports the use of behavioral or cognitive–behavioral therapy focused on development of personal coping strategies, including terminating unhelpful thought patterns and improving deficient emotional regulation (Eccleston et al., 2014).

Orthotics

Pain as a consequence of pathological fracture can be reduced with selection and use of appropriate *orthotics,* which are "externally applied device(s) used to modify the structural and functional characteristics of the neuromuscular and skeletal systems" (Healy et al., 2018, p. 2). Spinal, upper-extremity, and lower-extremity bracing and orthotics are commonly used in oncology practice. Cancer survivors may have comorbidities and abnormal laboratory values that make them poor candidates for surgical stabilization of a pathological fracture or *lytic lesion,* an area of bone destruction caused by disease.

Barriers to surgery might include poor clotting factor of blood (i.e., ***thrombocytopenia***), immune deficiency, impaired oxygen transport in blood, cardiovascular comorbidities, or other organ deficiency. In these cases, orthotics are a reasonable option to promote safety and reduced pain during occupational engagement until surgical stabilization can be performed or natural healing occurs. Occupational therapy practitioners are skilled not only in selecting appropriate orthotic options but in providing training in doffing and donning procedures, instructing clients in care and maintenance of the orthotic, and modifying activities to allow for safe integration of orthotics.

Assistive Devices

Recommendation and training on use of assistive devices is another key way occupational therapy practitioners can intervene with clients experiencing cancer-related pain. ***Assistive devices*** are tools that aid a person in the completion of a task they would otherwise not be able to perform and are often integrated as a means of reducing activity demands, thereby reducing pain. Devices can enhance both the safety and the autonomy of a patient's mobility (Cheville & Basford, 2014).

A painful grasp during feeding can be reduced by use of built-up handles, and wheelchairs, Hoyer lifts, and powered mobility can reduce pain with transfers and locomotion within the home and community. Additionally, integration of long-handled equipment, including long-handled sponges, long-handled reachers, sock aids, and shoehorns, may lower incidence of pain by reducing or eliminating bending, twisting, and reaching (Cheville & Basford, 2014). Survivors may also be instructed to use a tub transfer bench or shower chair during bathing as part of pain management.

Energy Conservation

Packer et al. (1995) developed the language and strategies to address fatigue management. Although their work was initially focused on fatigue management for adults without a cancer diagnosis, occupational therapy practitioners can certainly expand these strategies to address pain management for cancer survivors. Proposed strategies are modifying the environment, changing standards, setting priorities, analyzing and modifying activity, adhering to ergonomic principles, resting throughout the day, and integrating proper body mechanics.

These strategies also can be used for management of pain. Instruction in ***energy conservation*** and pacing can aid clients in managing pain through balancing rest with activity and understanding limitations in respect to the duration for which they perform an activity. Because of the often chronic nature of cancer and cancer-related pain, these strategies—including but not limited to sitting rather than standing, breaking up activities into manageable parts, giving permission to others to assist with pain-provoking activities, prioritizing activities of greater value over those of lesser value, and balancing more taxing activities with those of lesser pain consequence—may be useful in helping clients perform valued occupations with more quality and for a longer time period across the cancer-care continuum.

SUMMARY

Occupational therapy practitioners working with cancer survivors at any point in the lifespan can encounter the disastrous effects of pain firsthand. Occupational therapy practitioners have a unique perspective and key role in management of pain, which can improve QoL and optimize engagement in valued occupations for clients living with cancer. This chapter has sought to provide a clearer understanding of pain as a symptom that is a largely complex, notable, and pervasive sequela of cancer, and one that can have a negative impact on occupational engagement at every stage of the lifespan.

Pain can be a devastating consequence of cancer or its treatment at any stage of the lifespan and across the cancer care continuum. As a result of advancements in the field of oncology, cancer is considered a chronic rather than fatal condition, so occupational therapy practitioners must consider the impact of pain at any stage of the lifespan. This chapter has explored pain assessment and assessment tools, types of pain commonly treated by occupational therapists working in oncology, and recommendations for interventions.

Assessment of cancer pain is a critical first step because it aids occupational therapy practitioners in making decisions leading to intervention and in evaluating outcomes of intervention. The assessment of pain and intervention is a complex and dynamic process between the cancer survivor and the occupational therapy practitioner. The development of the occupational profile helps create a plan of care that is client centered.

Intervention is often dictated by the type and severity of cancer-related pain. Interventions recommended in this chapter include but are not limited to activity modification, PAMs, therapeutic exercise, orthotics, assistive devices, and energy conservation. Furthermore, occupational therapy practitioners should consider the stage of development and associated occupations, client factors, and performance patterns when choosing interventions.

Occupational therapy practitioners working with cancer survivors have a critical role in optimizing function and promoting QoL in the setting of pain. With occupational therapy's unique, holistic perspective, occupational therapy practitioners may understand and address each survivor's pain experience.

REFERENCES

Akechi, T., Ockuyama, T., Endo, C., Sagawa, R., Uchida, M., Nakaguchi, T., . . . Furkawa, T. A. (2011). Patient's perceived need and psychological distress and/or quality of life in ambulatory breast cancer patients in Japan. *Psycho-Oncology, 20,* 497–505. https://doi.org/10.1002/pon.1757

Allen, J. M., Graef, D. M., Ehrentraut, J. H., Tynes, B. L., & Crabtree, V. M. (2016). Sleep and pain in pediatric illness: A conceptual review. *CNS Neuroscience & Therapeutics, 22,* 880–893. https://doi.org/10.1111/cns.12583

American Cancer Society. (2015). *Treatment and support: Depression.* Retrieved from https://www.cancer.org/treatment/treatments-and-side-effects/physical-side-effects/changes-in-mood-or-thinking/depression.html

American Cancer Society. (2020). *Cancer in children: Key statistics for childhood cancers.* Retrieved from https://www.cancer.org/cancer/cancer-in-children/key-statistics.html

American Occupational Therapy Association. (2008). Physical agent modalities: A position paper. *American Journal of Occupational Therapy, 62,* 691–693. https://doi.org/10.5014/ajot.62.6.691

American Occupational Therapy Association. (2014). Occupational therapy practice framework: Domain and process (3rd ed.). *American Journal of Occupational Therapy, 68*(Suppl. 1), S1–S48. https://doi.org/10.5014/ajot.2014.682006

An, Q., Fan, C. H., & Xu, S. M. (2017). Current views of common pediatric cancers: An update. *European Review for Medical and Pharmacological Sciences, 21*(Suppl. 4), 20–24.

Baanders, N., Rigken, P. M., & Peters, L. (2002). Labour participation of the chronically ill: A profile sketch. *European Journal of Chronic Health, 12,* 124–130. https://doi.org/10.1093/eurpub/12.2.124

Bao, Y. J., Hou, W., Kong, X. Y., Yang, L., Xia, J., Hua, B. J., & Knaggs, R. (2016). Hydromorphone for cancer pain. *Cochrane Database of Systematic Reviews, 2016,* CD011108. https://doi.org/10.1002/14651858.CD011108.pub2

Boland, L., Bennett, K., & Connolly, D. (2017). Self-management intervention for cancer survivors: A systematic review. *Supportive Care in Cancer, 26,* 1585–1595. https://doi.org/10.1007/s00520-017-3999-7

Bonetto, R., Tallet, A., Mélot, A., Calderon, B., & Barlesi, F. (2017). The management of bone metastasis. *Bulletin du Cancer, 104,* 585–592. https://doi.org/10.1016/j.bulcan.2017.02.004

Breukink, S. O., & Donovan, K. A. (2013). Oncology. In H. M. Pendleton & W. Schultz-Krohn (Eds.), *Pedretti's occupational therapy: Practice skills for physical dysfunction* (7th ed., pp. 1215–1227). St. Louis: Mosby.

Brown, W., & Kandirikirira, N. (2007). *Recovering mental health in Scotland. A report on narrative investigation of mental health recovery.* Glasgow: Scottish Recovery Network.

Butbul Aviel, Y., Stremler, R., Benseler, S. M., Cameron, B., Laxer, R. M., Ota, S., . . . Feldman, B. M. (2011). Sleep and fatigue and the relationship to pain, disease activity and quality of life in juvenile idiopathic arthritis and juvenile dermatomyositis. *Rheumatology, 50,* 2051–2060. https://doi.org/10.1093/rheumatology/ker256

Centers for Disease Control and Prevention & Lance Armstrong Foundation. (2004). *A national action plan of cancer survivorship: Advancing public health strategies.* Atlanta: Centers for Disease Control and Prevention.

Chapman, R., & Vierck, C. J. (2017). The transition of acute postoperative pain to chronic pain: An integrative overview of research on mechanisms. *Journal of Pain, 18*(4), 359.e1–359.e38. https://doi.org/10.1016/j.jpain.2016.11.004

Chen, L., Tang, J., White, P. F., Sloninsky, A., Wender, R. H., Naruse, R., & Kariger, R. (1998). The effect of location of transcutaneous electrical nerve stimulation on the postoperative opioid analgesic requirement: Acupoint versus nonacupoint stimulation. *Anesthesia and Analgesia, 87,* 1129–1134. https://doi.org/10.1213/00000539-199811000-00028

Cheville, A. L., & Basford, J. R. (2014). Role of rehabilitation medication and physical agents in the treatment of cancer-associated pain. *Journal of Clinical Oncology, 32,* 1691–1702. https://doi.org/10.1200/JCO.2013.53.6680

Chitkara, D. K., Rawat, D. J., & Talley, N. J. (2005). The epidemiology of childhood recurrent abdominal pain in Western countries: A systematic review. *American Journal of Gastroenterology, 100,* 1868–1875. https://doi.org/10.1111/j.1572-0241.2005.41893.x

Cleeland, C. S., & Ryan, K. M. (1994). Pain assessment: Global use of the Brief Pain Inventory. *Annals of the Academy of Medicine Singapore, 23*(2), 129–138.

Coleman, R. E. (2001). Metastatic bone disease: Clinical features, pathophysiology and treatment strategies. *Cancer Treatment Review, 27,* 165–176. https://doi.org/10.1053/ctrv.2000.0210

Colloca, G., Lattanzio, F., Balducci, L., Onder, G., Ronconi, G., Landi, F., . . . Bernabei, R. (2015). Treating cancer and no-cancer pain in older and oldest old patients. *Current Pharmaceutical Design, 21,* 1706–1714. https://doi.org/10.2174/1381612821666150130124926

Costigan, M., Scholz, J., & Woolf, C. J. (2009). Neuropathic pain: A maladaptive response of the nervous system to damage. *Annual Review of Neuroscience, 32,* 1–32. https://doi.org/10.1146/annurev.neuro.051508.135531

Dunn, W., McClain, L. H., Brown, C., & Youngstrom, M. J. (1998). The ecology of human performance. In M. E. Neistadt & E. B. Crepeau (Eds.), *Willard and Spackman's occupational therapy* (9th ed., pp. 525–535). Philadelphia: Lippincott Williams & Wilkins.

Eccleston, C., Palermo, T. M., Williams, A. C., Lewandowski Holley, A., Morley, S., Fisher, E., & Law, E. (2014). Psychological therapies for the management of chronic and recurrent pain in children and adolescents. *Cochrane Database Systematic Review, 5,* CD003968. https://doi.org/10.1002/14651858.CD003968.pub4

Eiser, C., Penn, A., Katz, E., & Barr, R. (2009). Psychosocial issues and quality of life. *Seminars in Oncology, 36,* 275–280. https://doi.org/10.1053/j.seminoncol.2009.03.005

Fairbank, J., & Pynsent, P. B. (2000). The Oswestry Disability Index. *Spine, 25,* 2940–2953. https://doi.org/10.1097/00007632-200011150-00017

Foster, C., & Fenlon, D. (2011). Recovery and self-management support following primary cancer treatment. *British Journal of Cancer, 105*(Suppl. 1), S21–S28. https://doi.org/10.1038/bjc.2011.419

Galer, B. S., & Jensen, M. P. (1997). Development and preliminary validation of a pain measure specific to neuropathic pain: The Neuropathic Pain Scale. *Neurology, 48,* 332–338. https://doi.org/10.1212/wnl.48.2.332

Grichnik, K. P., & Ferrante, F. M. (1991). The difference between acute and chronic pain. *Mount Sinai Journal of Medicine, 58,* 217–220.

Guerard, E. J., & Cleary, J. (2017). Managing cancer pain in older adults. *Cancer Journal, 23,* 242–245. https://doi.org/10.1097/PPO.0000000000000276

Hartrick, C. T., Kovan, J. P., & Shapiro, S. (2003). The Numeric Rating Scale for clinical pain measurement: A ratio measure? *Pain Practice, 3,* 310–316. https://doi.org/10.1111/j.1530-7085.2003.03034.x

Healy, A., Farmer, S., Pandyan, A., & Chockalingam, N. (2018). A systematic review of randomised controlled trials assessing effectiveness of prosthetic and orthotic interventions. *Public Library of Science One, 13*(3). https://doi.org/10.1371/journal.pone.0192094

Hewitt, M., Greenfield, S., & Stovall, E. (2005). *From cancer patient to cancer survivor: Lost in transition.* Washington, DC: National Academies Press.

Hunter, E. G., Gibson, R. W., Arbesman, M., & D'Amico, M. (2017). Systematic review of occupation therapy and adult cancer rehabilitation: Part 1. Impact of physical activity and symptom management interventions. *American Journal of*

Occupational Therapy, 71, 7102100030. https://doi.org/10.5014/ajot.2017.023564

Hwang, E. J., Lokietz, N. C., Lozano, R. L., & Parke, M. A. (2015). Functional deficits and quality of life among cancer survivors: Implications for occupational therapy in cancer survivorship care. *American Journal of Occupational Therapy, 69*, 6906290010. https://doi.org/10.5014/ajot.2015.015974

Jacob, E., Mack, A. K., Savedra, M., Van Cleve, L., & Wilkie, D. J. (2014). Adolescent Pediatric Pain Tool for multidimensional measurement of pain in children and adolescents. *Pain Management Nursing, 15*, 694–706. https://doi.org/10.1016/j.pmn.2013.03.002

Jay, K., Brandt, M., Jakobsen, M. D., Sundstrup, E., Berthelson, K. G., Schraefel, M. C., . . . Andersen, L. L. (2016). Ten weeks of physical–cognitive–mindfulness training reduces fear-avoidance beliefs about work related activity. *Medicine, 95*, e3945. https://doi.org/10.1097/MD.0000000000003945

Jibb, L. A., Stevens, B. J., Nathan, P. C., Seto, E., Cafazzo, J. A., & Stinson, J. N. (2014). A smartphone-based pain management app for adolescents with cancer: Establishing system requirements and a pain care algorithm based on literature review, interviews, and consensus. *JMIR Research Protocols, 3*(1), e15. https://doi.org/10.2196/resprot.3041

Kandula, T., Park, S., Cohn, R. J., Krishnan, A. V., & Farrar, M. (2016). Pediatric chemotherapy induced peripheral neuropathy: A systematic review of current knowledge. *Cancer Treatment Reviews, 50*, 118–128. https://doi.org/10.1016/j.ctrv.2016.09.005

Kashikar-Zuck, S., Cunningham, N., Sil, S., Bromberg, M. H., Lynch-Jordan, A. M., Strotman, D., . . . Arnold, L. M. (2014). Long-term outcomes of adolescents with juvenile-onset fibromyalgia in early adulthood. *Pediatrics, 133*, e592–e600. https://doi.org/10.1542/peds.2013-2220

Kerns, R. D., Turk, D., & Rudy, T. E. (1985). The West Haven–Yale Multidimensional Pain Inventory (WHYMPI). *Pain, 23*, 345–356. https://doi.org/10.1016/0304-3959(85)90004-1

Kunderman, B., Krieg, C. C., Schreiber, W., & Lautenbacher, S. (2004). The effect of sleep deprivation on pain. *Pain Research and Management, 9*, 25–32. https://doi.org/10.1155/2004/949187

Landi, F., Russo, A., Liperoti, R., Danese, P., Maiorana, E., Pahor, M., . . . Onder, G. (2009). Daily pain and functional decline among old adults living in the community: Results from the ilSIRENTE Study. *Journal of Pain and Symptom Management, 38*, 350–357. https://doi.org/10.1016/j.jpainsymman.2008.10.005

Li, D., Soto-Perez-de-Celis, E., & Hurria, A. (2017). Geriatric assessment and tools for predicting treatment toxicity in older adults with cancer. *Cancer Journal, 23*, 206–210. https://doi.org/10.1097/PPO.0000000000000269

Loh, J., & Gulati, A. (2015). The use of transcutaneous electrical nerve stimulation (TENS) in a major cancer center for the treatment of severe cancer-related pain and associated disability. *Pain Medicine, 16*, 1204–1210. https://doi.org/10.1111/pme.12038

Luo, Q., Xu, Z., Wang, L., Ruan, M., & Jin, G. (2016). Progress in the research on the mechanism of bone metastasis in lung cancer. *Molecular and Clinical Oncology, 5*, 227–235. https://doi.org/10.3892/mco.2016.917

Malfliet, A., Leysen, L., Pas, R., Kuppensb, K., Nijs, J., Van Wilgena, P., . . . Ickmansa, K. (2017). Modern pain neuroscience in clinical practice: Applied to post-cancer, paediatric and sports-related pain. *Brazilian Journal of Physical Therapy, 21*, 225–232. https://doi.org/10.1016/j.bjpt.2017.05.009

Manworren, R., & Stinson, J. (2016). Pediatric pain measurement, assessment and evaluation. *Seminars in Pediatric Neurology, 23*, 189–200. https://doi.org/10.1016/j.spen.2016.10.001

McCormack, H. M., Horne, D. J. L., & Sheather, S. (1988). Clinical applications of visual analogue scales: A critical review. *Psychological Medicine, 18, 1007–1019*. https://doi.org/10.1017/s0033291700009934

McGrath, P. A., Johnson, G., Goodman, J. T., McGrath, P. J., Schillinger, J., Dunn, J., . . . Johnston, G. A. (1985). CHEOPS: A behavioral scale for rating postoperative pain in children. In H. L. Fields, R. Dubner, & F. Cervero (Eds.), *Advances in pain research and therapy* (Vol. 9, pp. 395–402). New York: Raven Press.

Melzack, R. (1975). The McGill Pain Questionnaire: Major properties and scoring methods. *Pain, 1*, 277–299. https://doi.org/10.1016/0304-3959(75)90044-5

Mercadante, S., Adile, C., Masedu, F., Valenti, M., & Aielli, F. (2019). Breakthrough cancer pain in patients with abdominal visceral cancer pain. *Journal of Pain and Symptom Management, 57*, 966–970. https://doi.org/10.1016/j.jpainsymman.2019.02.014

Mohammadi, A., Mehraban, A. H., & Damavandi, S. A. (2017). Effect of play-based occupational therapy on symptoms of hospitalized children with cancer: A single-subject study. *Asia Pacific Journal of Oncology Nursing, 4*, 168–172. https://doi.org/10.4103/apjon.apjon_13_17

National Cancer Institute. (n.d.-a). *NCI dictionary of cancer terms: Plexopathy*. Retrieved from https://www.cancer.gov/publications/dictionaries/cancer-terms/def/plexopathy

National Cancer Institute. (n.d.-b). *NCI dictionary of cancer terms: Survivorship*. Retrieved from https://www.cancer.gov/publications/dictionaries/cancer-terms/def/survivorship

Packer, T. L., Brink, N., & Sauriol, A. (1995). *Managing fatigue: A six-week course for energy conservation*. Tucson, AZ: Therapy Skill Builders.

Park, B. W., & Hwang, S. Y. (2012). Unmet needs and their relationship with quality of life among women with recurrent breast cancer. *Journal of Breast Cancer, 15*, 454–461. https://doi.org/10.4048/jbc.2012.15.4.454

Roland, M., & Morris, R. (1983). A study of the natural history of low-back pain. Part II: Development of guidelines for trials of treatment in primary care. *Pain, 8*, 145–150. https://doi.org/10.1097/00007632-198303000-00005

Roodman, G. D. (2004). Mechanisms of bone metastasis. *New England Journal of Medicine, 350*, 1655–1664. https://doi.org/10.1056/NEJMra030831

Savedra, M. C., Tesler, M., Holzemer, W. L., Wilkie, D. J., & Ward, J. A. (1989). Pain location: Validity and reliability of body outline markings by hospitalized children and adolescents. *Research in Nursing & Health, 12*(5), 307–314. https://doi.org/10.1002/nur.4770120506

Suraseranivongse, S., Santawat, U., Kraiprasit, K., Petcharatana, S., Prakkamodom, S., & Muntraporn, N. (2001). Cross-validation of a composite pain scale for preschool children within 24 hours of surgery. *British Journal of Anaesthesia, 87*, 400–405. https://doi.org/10.1093/bja/87.3.400

Varni, J. W., Thompson, K. L., & Hanson, V. (1987). The Varni/Thompson Pediatric Pain Questionnaire: I. Chronic musculoskeletal pain in juvenile rheumatoid arthritis. *Pain, 28*, 27–38. https://doi.org/10.1016/0304-3959(87)91056-6

von Baeyer, C. L., Marche, T. A., Rocha, E. M., & Salmon, K. (2004). Children's memory for pain: Overview and implications for practice. *Journal of Pain, 5,* 241–249. https://doi.org/10.1016/j.jpain.2004.05.001

Walker, L. S., Dengler-Crish, C. M., Rippel, S., & Bruehl, S. (2010). Functional abdominal pain in childhood and adolescence increases risk for chronic pain in adulthood. *Pain, 150,* 568–572. https://doi.org/10.1016/j.pain.2010.06.018

White, M. C., Holman, D. M., Goodman, R. A., & Richardson, L. C. (2019). Cancer risk among older adults: Time for cancer prevention to go silver. *Gerontologist, 59*(Suppl. 1), S1–S6. https://doi.org/10.1093/geront/gnz038

Wildes, T. M., Dua, P., & Fowler, S. A., Miller, J. P., Carpenter, C. R., Avidan, M. S., & Stark, S. (2015). Systematic review of falls in older adults with cancer. *Journal of Geriatric Oncology, 6,* 70–83. https://doi.org/10.1016/j.jgo.2014.10.003

Wong-Baker FACES Foundation. (2016). *Wong–Baker FACES® Pain Rating Scale.* Retrieved from http://www.WongBakerFACES.org.

Zebrack, B., Hamilton, R., & Smith, A. W. (2009). Psychosocial outcomes and service use among young adults with cancer. *Seminars in Oncology, 36,* 468–477. https://doi.org/10.1053/j.seminoncol.2009.07.003

Cancer-Related Cognitive Impairment

17

Robin Newman, OTD, OT, OTR, CLT, FAOTA

LEARNING OBJECTIVES

After completing this chapter, readers should be able to
- Understand the multidimensional etiology of cancer-related cognitive impairment (CRCI) in cancer survivors across the lifespan,
- Describe a range of occupational performance challenges across the lifespan for survivors living with CRCI,
- Articulate occupational therapy's role in supporting occupational performance and participation for survivors living with CRCI across the lifespan,
- Identify appropriate tools and methods to screen for CRCI in cancer survivors, and
- Articulate the rationale for using select intervention approaches to support occupational engagement and performance in cancer survivors living with CRCI.

KEY TERMS AND CONCEPTS

- Allostatic load
- Cancer-related cognitive impairment
- Central nervous system cancer
- Functional cognition
- Neuroimaging studies
- Neuropsychological testing
- Non-central nervous system cancer
- Self-report

INTRODUCTION

Cognitive function is central to the performance of daily occupations and to a person's identity and social role performance (Henneghan, 2016). However, cancer and cancer treatment may affect survivors' cognitive function and participation in meaningful activities across the lifespan. For years, cancer survivors have reported changes in cognitive function as a result of cancer and cancer treatment, but it was not until the 1980s that the cognitive impairment resulting from cancer was acknowledged by the medical community as a side effect of cancer treatment (Silberfarb et al., 1980). Currently, *cancer-related cognitive impairment* (CRCI) is widely recognized as an ongoing issue before, during, and after cancer treatment (Boykoff et al., 2009; Player et al., 2014; Rust & Davis, 2013; Schmidt et al., 2016).

CRCI is characterized by subtle yet enduring changes in attention and concentration, working memory, executive function, speed of processing, new learning, and word-finding abilities (Ahles & Hurria, 2018; Andreotti et al., 2015). CRCI is often reported in the context of both central nervous system (CNS) and non-central nervous system (non-CNS) cancers. *CNS cancers* include cancers that originate in the brain and spinal cord, and *non-CNS cancers* originate outside of the CNS. Regardless of the etiology of the cognitive impairment, the cognitive changes experienced by cancer survivors can significantly affect a survivors' quality of life (QoL; Ahles & Hurria, 2018; Andreotti et al., 2015) and have been reported by many survivors as the most feared and devastating side effect of cancer treatment (Boykoff et al., 2009). Functionally, CRCI can be debilitating and cause serious disruption in life roles such as work, caring for oneself, or caring for others (Boykoff et al., 2009; Player et al., 2014; Rust & Davis, 2013).

Because CRCI affects survivors across the lifespan and across a variety of cancer types, occupational therapy practitioners have the opportunity to support occupational performance and participation in daily life roles and occupations for a wide range of survivors living with the cognitive effects of cancer and cancer treatments. This chapter focuses on occupational therapy's role in maximizing the occupational performance and participation of cancer survivors living with CRCI across the lifespan by describing the multidimensional etiology of CRCI, lifespan considerations, and an overview of approaches to assessment and intervention.

DEFINING FEATURES OF CRCI

CRCI was initially conceptualized from a pharmacotoxicology perspective. That means individuals diagnosed with cancer were assumed to have normal cognitive function before treatment, and it was believed that exposure to certain chemotherapeutic agents would cause cognitive changes. This gave rise to the term "chemo brain" (Ahles & Hurria, 2018; Silberfarb et al., 1980). However, in recent years, this perspective has been broadened to examine the cognitive impact of cancer, cancer treatments, and factors that increase the risk for cognitive decline (Ahles & Hurria, 2018), giving way to the terminology of CRCI.

CRCI is common in a range of cancers. Exhibit 17.1 highlights non-CNS cancers associated with CRCI. Research on CRCI has largely focused on chemotherapy-related cognitive impairment; however, CRCI has also been documented in the absence of chemotherapy, which may suggest associations with the cancer itself, surgery, or other adjuvant

therapies used to treat the cancer (Janelsins et al., 2014; Joly et al., 2015; Wefel et al., 2015).

The underlying mechanisms that contribute to CRCI are not fully understood; however, many factors may be involved. Potential factors include cancer and cancer treatments; biological, psychological, physiological, and genetic factors; sociodemographic and lifestyle factors; and allostatic load. **Allostatic load** is defined as "the wear and tear on the body and brain resulting from chronic overactivity or inactivity of physiological systems that are normally involved in adaptation to environmental challenge" (McEwen, 1998, p. 6). In a recent review, Ahles and Hurria (2018) highlighted these factors in a comprehensive, multidimensional, and interrelated model that are outlined in Figure 17.1. Of particular interest to occupational therapy practitioners are the potentially modifiable factors that influence CRCI such as psychological (e.g., stress, anxiety, depression, social support), physiological (e.g., fatigue), and lifestyle factors (e.g., smoking, exercise, diet, sleep hygiene).

The severity of CRCI is typically mild to moderate and can persist for months to years after cancer treatment. It is generally milder than the cognitive impairment associated with neurodegenerative diseases and stroke (Wefel et al., 2015); however, for CNS cancer survivors, the cognitive impairments associated with brain tumors may be more severe and are associated with the lesion location in the brain, size, and tumor grade (Ali et al., 2018; Hardy et al., 2018).

Cognitive impairments in survivors of brain tumors have been reported with a high prevalence (Mukand et al., 2001). In a systematic review of cognitive functioning in adult survivors of low-grade gliomas (i.e., tumors that arise from the supportive tissues of the brain; American

EXHIBIT 17.1.	Non-CNS Cancers Associated With CRCI

- Breast
- Head and neck
- Lung
- Multiple myeloma
- Prostate
- Colorectal
- Leukemia
- Lymphoma
- Ovarian
- Testicular

Note. CRCI = cancer-related cognitive impairment.
Source. Adapted from Vannorsdall (2017).

FIGURE 17.1. Conceptual model of factors contributing to cognitive changes in cancer survivors.

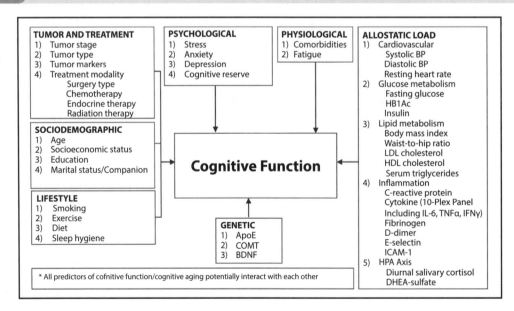

Note. ApoE = apolipoprotein E; BDNF = brain-derived neurotrophic factor; BP = blood pressure; COMT = catechol-O-methyltransferase; DHEA = dehydroepiandrosterone sulphate.
Source. Reprinted from "New Challenges in Psycho-Oncology Research IV: Cognition and Cancer: Conceptual and Methodological Issues and Future Directions," by T. A. Ahles & A. Hurria, 2018, *Psycho-Oncology, 27*(1), 4. Copyright © 2018 by Wiley. Reprinted with permission.

TABLE 17.1. Gliomas and Defining Features

GLIOMAS	DEFINING FEATURES
Astrocytomas	Arise from astrocytes, which are a type of cell that makes up the supportive tissues of the brain
Oligodendrogliomas	Arise from oligodendrocytes, which are a type of cell that makes up the supportive tissues of the brain
Ependymomas	Arise from ependymal cells, which line the ventricles of the brain and the center of the spinal cord
Mixed gliomas	Usually contain a high proportion of one or more types of cell (astrocytes, oligodendrocytes, ependymal cells)

Source. American Brain Tumor Association (2019).

Brain Tumor Association [ABTA], 2019), a range of prevalence (19%–83%) of cognitive impairments was reported (van Loon et al., 2015). Low-grade astrocytomas, such as pilocytic astrocytomas or diffuse astrocytomas, are usually localized and grow slowly, while high-grade astrocytomas, such as anaplastic astrocytomas or glioblastomas, grow at a rapid pace. The majority of astrocytoma tumors in children are low grade, while the majority of astrocytomas in adults are high grade (ABTA, 2019). (See Table 17.1 for a description of defining features of gliomas.) Survivors of high-grade gliomas, however, often demonstrate greater overall cognitive impairments compared to survivors of low-grade gliomas.

For survivors of non-CNS cancers, up to 40% of survivors have reported cognitive changes before any treatment, up to 75% of survivors have reported cognitive changes during treatment, and up to 60% of survivors have reported cognitive changes that persist for months or years after treatment (Andreotti et al., 2015; Wefel et al., 2015). For many survivors of non-CNS cancers, CRCI improves after completion of curative treatment; however, an estimated 20%–30% of survivors who experience CRCI experience only partial recovery of symptoms and may report persistent changes up to 20 years after cancer treatment (Koppelmans et al., 2012).

CONSIDERATIONS ACROSS THE LIFESPAN

Survivors of cancer across the lifespan may experience CRCI. This section briefly highlights salient considerations for survivors at each life stage; however, additional information is provided in chapters related to special considerations across the lifespan for pediatric, adolescent and young adults, adults, and older adults (see Part II, "Impact of Common Forms of Cancer Across the Lifespan").

Childhood Cancer Survivors

Childhood cancer survivors may experience more frequent and more severe forms of cognitive impairment than adult survivors of cancer (Castellino et al., 2014). The cognitive impairment complicating childhood cancers, such as brain cancers and acute lymphoblastic leukemia, may present at diagnosis, soon after diagnosis, or emerge insidiously in the years after treatment and may persist for decades (Castellino et al., 2014). Although most commonly reported in pediatric survivors of CNS cancers, pediatric survivors of non-CNS cancers may also be at risk of developing CRCI (Willard et al., 2017).

An emerging body of literature suggests that young children with cancer may enter preschool at a cognitive and academic disadvantage because prolonged periods of time in a hospital setting may lead to missed opportunities to support cognitive development, such as opportunities for play (Willard et al., 2017). Children who develop neurocognitive problems after cancer diagnosis and treatment may experience an effect on long-term development, including educational attainment, employment, and functional independence (Krull et al., 2018). A recent study of childhood cancer survivors found that children with CNS tumors reported the poorest functioning in all aspects of cognition and showed poorer adaptation to adult life, as demonstrated by lower educational, occupational, and financial attainment and a decreased likelihood of marriage when compared to non-CNS cancer survivors (Castellino et al., 2014).

For some childhood survivors who receive cranial radiation, the impact on academics and global cognitive abilities may not emerge until at least 5 years after diagnosis, with a steady decline in cognitive function over time (Castellino et al., 2014). With regard to school performance, parents and teachers have described children as spending excessive time on homework but having poor acquisition and retention of school subjects, including mathematics, spelling, and reading (Castellino et al., 2014). Exhibit 17.2 highlights common cognitive impairments, academic challenges, and potential effects on occupational performance for childhood cancer survivors.

Adolescent and Young Adults

Adolescents and young adults (AYAs) may demonstrate greater resilience to cognitive impairments compared to adults as a function of greater cognitive reserve and greater neuroplasticity. Despite this, AYA cancer survivors may demonstrate greater impairments in cognitive abilities that peak later in life, such as vocabulary and arithmetic, compared to older cancer survivors (Jim et al., 2018). CRCI may affect a range of daily activities at a time when survivors may be negotiating autonomy in independent living.

Importantly, cognitive demands likely differ between and among younger AYA survivors; some survivors may be more focused on educational attainment and the development of social and romantic relationships, and older AYA survivors may be more focused on work and family responsibilities (Krull et al., 2018). Exhibit 17.3 highlights common cognitive impairments for adult survivors, including AYAs, adults, and older adults, and the potential impact on occupational performance.

Adult and Older Adult Survivors

It is hypothesized that cancer treatments may accelerate the aging process, including cognitive aging (Ahles et al.,

EXHIBIT 17.2.	Common Cognitive Impairments and Potential Impact on Occupational Performance Associated With Treatment Among Childhood Cancer Survivors of ALL and Brain Tumors

COMMON TREATMENT-RELATED COGNITIVE EFFECTS	
CNS-Directed Chemotherapy	**Radiation Therapy To The Brain**
<ul><li>Attention or concentration</li><li>Visual–motor integration</li><li>Visual–spatial awareness</li><li>Working memory</li><li>Executive function</li><li>Speed of information processing</li></ul>	<ul><li>Attention</li><li>Learning</li><li>Working memory</li><li>Information processing speed</li><li>Visual–spatial ability</li><li>Fine motor skills</li></ul>
POTENTIAL IMPACT ON INTELLECTUAL OR ACADEMIC FUNCTIONING	
<ul><li>Learning disabilities</li><li>Declines in math achievement</li><li>Lowered self-esteem</li></ul>	<ul><li>Learning disabilities</li><li>Declines in global cognitive abilities and academics</li><li>Gradual onset of deficits and decline in functions over time</li><li>Lowered self-esteem</li></ul>
POTENTIAL IMPACT ON OCCUPATIONAL PERFORMANCE AND PARTICIPATION	
<ul><li>ADLs</li><li>IADLs</li><li>Education</li><li>Sleep and rest</li><li>Play</li><li>Leisure</li><li>Social participation</li></ul>	

Note. ADLs = activities of daily living; ALL = acute lymphocytic leukemia; CNS = central nervous system; IADLs = instrumental activities of daily living.
Sources. Castellino et al. (2014); Krull et al. (2018); Willard et al. (2017).

EXHIBIT 17.3.	Common Cognitive Impairments and Potential Impact on Occupational Performance Associated With Treatment of Non-CNS Cancers in Young Adults, Adults, and Older Adults

COMMON TREATMENT-RELATED COGNITIVE EFFECTS

- Concentration
- Attention
- Working memory
- Executive function
- Information processing speed
- New learning
- Language (e.g., word-finding difficulties)

POTENTIAL IMPACT ON OCCUPATIONAL PERFORMANCE AND PARTICIPATION

- Sleep and rest
- ADLs
- IADLs
- Education
- Leisure
- Social participation

Note. ADLs = activities of daily living; CNS = central nervous system; IADLs = instrumental activities of daily living.
Sources. Ahles et al. (2012); Ahles & Hurria (2018); Boykoff et al. (2009); Player et al. (2014).

2012). In adulthood, CRCI may significantly affect the daily functioning of survivors across a variety of occupations at a time in their lives when they may be parenting, working, or caregiving (Boykoff et al., 2009; Player et al., 2014). Further, survivorship care and health maintenance activities, such as medication management, adherence to surveillance, and coordination of care across providers, may also be affected by CRCI (Mandelblatt et al., 2016). Given the higher prevalence of preexisting cognitive impairment in older adults, the impact of cancer treatment on older adults may be more significant than in adults (Loh et al., 2016; Mandelblatt et al., 2016) and may require closer monitoring.

HOW IS CRCI MEASURED?

At present, there is no gold standard for how to measure CRCI in cancer survivors or its impact on participation in daily activities. However, several methods are currently used to evaluate how cancer and cancer treatment affect cognitive function. They include

- Neuropsychological testing,
- Neuroimaging studies, and
- Self-report (Asher & Meyers, 2015; Lai et al., 2014; Pullens et al., 2010).

Exhibits 17.4 and 17.5 highlight common assessments and methods used to assess CRCI in adults and children.

EXHIBIT 17.4. Common Assessments Used With Adults With CRCI

SELF-REPORT MEASURES

- Functional Assessment of Cancer Therapy–Cognition (Wagner et al., 2009)
- Cognitive Symptom Checklist–Work 21 (Dorland et al., 2016)
- Patient's Assessment of Own Functioning Inventory (Chelune et al., 1986; Van Dyk et al., 2016)
- Attentional Function Index (Cimprich et al., 2011)
- Cognitive Failures Questionnaire (Broadbent et al., 1982)

OBJECTIVE MEASURES

The International Cognitive and Cancer Task Force (Joly et al., 2015) recommends at least the following:
- Hopkins Verbal Learning Test–Revised (Benedict et al., 1998)
- Trail Making Test (Trites, 1977)
- Controlled Oral Word Association Test of the Multilingual Aphasia Examination (Benton et al., 1994)

OCCUPATION OR ACTIVITY-BASED MEASURES

- Executive Function Performance Test (Baum & Wolf, 2013)
- Weekly Calendar Planning Activity (Toglia, 2015)
- Assessment of Motor and Process Skills (Fisher & Jones, 2012)
- A–ONE (Árnadóttir, 1990)
- Multiple Errands Test (Knight et al., 2002)

CONTRIBUTING FACTORS

Refer to the following chapters for measures related to
- Pain—Chapter 16
- Fatigue—Chapter 15
- Psychosocial function—Chapter 20
- Sleep/rest—Chapter 22

Note. CRCI = cancer-related cognitive impairment.

EXHIBIT 17.5. Common Assessments Used With Children or Adolescents With CRCI

SELF-REPORT

- Behavior Rating Inventory of Executive Function (Strauss et al., 2006)

OBJECTIVE ASSESSMENTS

- Beery–Buktenica Developmental Test of Visual–Motor Integration (Beery et al. 2010)
- Digit Span Test (Wechsler, 1991)
- Verbal Fluency Test (Benton et al., 1983)
- Trail Making Test (Trites, 1977)

OCCUPATION OR ACTIVITY-BASED ASSESSMENT

- Children's Kitchen Task Assessment (Rocke et al., 2008)
- Weekly Calendar Planning Activity (Toglia, 2015)
- A–One (Árnadóttir, 1990)
- Assessment of Motor and Process Skills (Fisher & Jones, 2012)

CONTRIBUTING FACTORS

Refer to the following chapters for measures related to
- Pain—Chapter 16
- Fatigue—Chapter 15
- Psychosocial function—Chapter 20
- Sleep and rest—Chapter 22

Note. CRCI = cancer-related cognitive impairment.

Neuropsychological Testing

Neuropsychological testing requires specialized training and measures cognitive domains such as executive function, processing speed, attention, and working memory. For survivors with CNS cancer, neuropsychological evaluation may help to understand the pattern and degree of neurocognitive strengths and weaknesses and determine the presence of underlying neurologic dysfunction (Noll et al., 2019). For survivors of non-CNS cancers, neuropsychological assessment may help determine whether cognitive changes are consistent with the adverse effects of cancer and cancer treatment, or reflective of other potentially modifiable factors such as pain, fatigue, sleep disturbance, or distress.

Neuropsychological testing may also suggest the need for more monitoring and management of mood in survivors of both CNS and non-CNS cancers (Noll et al., 2018). Referral to neuropsychology may provide valuable information to guide occupational therapy intervention. For some survivors, however, neuropsychological testing may lack sensitivity to capture subtle cognitive changes experienced before, during, or after cancer treatment and may lack ecological validity to simulate real-world situations in which some survivors of cancer must function (Asher & Meyers, 2015).

Despite a range of assessments, no universally accepted battery has been adopted across survivor groups or treatment settings to measure CRCI. In response, the

International Cognition and Cancer Task Force recommended three core tests based on sensitivity in measuring key cognitive domains affected in cancer survivors (Joly et al., 2015): the (1) Hopkins Verbal Learning Test–Revised (Benedict et al., 1998), (2) Trail Making Test (Trites, 1977), and (3) Controlled Oral Word Association Test of the Multilingual Aphasia Examination (Benton et al., 1994).

Neuroimaging Studies

Neuroimaging studies generally include structural magnetic resonance images (MRIs) to measure white and gray matter volume and functional MRIs to measure neural activity (Holohan et al., 2013). Neuroimaging studies indicate that there are changes to the prefrontal cortex and other regions, such as hippocampal structure, in the brains of cancer survivors experiencing CRCI (Ahles & Hurria, 2018; Apple et al., 2018). The National Comprehensive Cancer Network (NCCN) guidelines for cognitive function recommend neuroimaging be restricted to survivors who demonstrate focal deficits or those at high risk for CNS disease (Denlinger et al., 2014; NCCN, 2017).

Self-Report

Self-report, unlike neuropsychological testing, relies on the survivors' perceptions of cognitive decline and is measured through surveys or patient-reported outcome measures (Pullens et al., 2010). There is often little correlation between self-report and neuropsychological testing; however, self-report is an important indicator of the impact of CRCI on daily function and QoL (Asher & Meyers, 2015).

A variety of self-report measures can be used to assess CRCI, including the Attentional Function Index (Cimprich et al., 2011), the Functional Assessment of Cancer Therapy–Cognitive Function (Wagner et al., 2009), the Patient's Assessment of Own Functioning Inventory (Chelune et al., 1986), the Cognitive Symptom Checklist–Work 21 (Dorland et al., 2016), and the Cognitive Failures Questionnaire (Broadbent et al., 1982).

In addition to neuropsychology testing, self-report, and neuroimaging studies, the NCCN (2017) recommends that cancer survivors should be screened for potentially reversible factors that may contribute to cognitive impairment, such as sleep disturbances, depression, and fatigue. This highlights the need for a comprehensive assessment of cognitive, emotional, and physical functioning when determining the extent and severity of CRCI effect on occupational performance.

OVERVIEW OF OCCUPATIONAL THERAPY'S ROLE IN MANAGING CRCI ACROSS THE LIFESPAN

Presently, there is no established, gold standard treatment for CRCI (Ahles & Hurria, 2018). Current approaches to addressing the problem of CRCI focus largely on attempts to reduce the cognitive symptoms that survivors experience through cognitive behavioral techniques, pharmacologic approaches, and mindfulness stress reduction. However, there is no established treatment for CRCI (Treanor et al.,

2016). Compensatory strategies, however, may be more helpful to support participation in meaningful occupations during and after cancer treatment because survivors place high importance on efforts to manage, organize, and structure their daily routine (Von Ah et al., 2013). Current research suggests interventions for cancer survivors may also include modifiable factors, such as lifestyle, physiological, or psychological factors, that may affect CRCI (Henneghan, 2016).

Occupational therapy practitioners can select from a range of interventions to promote occupational performance and participation in life roles and meaningful occupations for cancer survivors. Based on the survivor's specific needs, disease course, severity of cognitive changes, and the developmental stage, the occupational therapy practitioner can select from:

- Education and counseling,
- Cognitive and behavioral techniques,
- Self-management interventions,
- Strategy use (compensatory or meta-cognitive),
- Mindfulness-based interventions,
- Cognitive remediation,
- Physical activity,
- Sleep hygiene,
- Educational interventions and school-based accommodations,
- Workplace accommodations, and
- Habit and routine development.

A review of the current literature supports these interventions falling within the scope of occupational therapy practice (Cifu et al., 2018; Krull et al., 2018; NCCN, 2017; Newman et al., 2019; Sleight, 2016; Treanor et al., 2016; Von Ah et al., 2013; Willard et al., 2017; Wolf et al., 2016).

Recently, NCCN (2017) identified occupational therapy practitioners as first-line intervention in the management

TABLE 17.2. Approaches to Intervention Across the Lifespan	
APPROACHES TO INTERVENTION	**EXAMPLES**
Create/promote (health promotion)	Promotion of healthy habits, including: - Physical activity - Sleep hygiene - Mindfulness-based stress reduction
Establish/restore	- Cognitive remediation - Physical activity - Sleep hygiene - Development of habits and routines to support occupational performance
Modify (compensation/ adaptation)	- Cognitive and behavioral techniques - Self-management strategies - Compensatory or metacognitive strategies - Environmental modifications - Fatigue management
Prevent (disability prevention)	- Social, physical, and psychosocial interventions to reduce social isolation, emotional distress, and physical inactivity

TABLE 17.3.   Occupational Therapy Interventions Across the Lifespan

OCCUPATIONAL THERAPY INTERVENTIONS	EXAMPLES
Occupations and activities	The practitioner ▪ Supports engagement in meaningful occupations that support cognitive health. ▪ Supports habit and routine development to enhance occupational performance and participation in life roles.
Preparatory methods and tasks	The practitioner ▪ Provides opportunities for the survivor to participate in simulated activities, such as communicating needs and wants, to prepare for self-advocacy with family, work, school, and community.
Education and training	The practitioner ▪ Provides education on the multifactorial etiology of CRCI to survivor, family, workplace, school, and community. ▪ Provides education on the importance of access to workplace accommodations to support cognitive performance. ▪ Provides education on the importance of access to academically focused technology to support academic skills. ▪ Provides education on age-appropriate toys that support development and preacademic skills.
Advocacy self-advocacy	The practitioner ▪ Collaborates with clients to procure a reasonable accommodation at a worksite. ▪ Collaborates with clients and their families to procure reasonable accommodations at school. The client ▪ Requests and receives reasonable accommodations in the workplace. ▪ Requests and receives reasonable accommodations in school. ▪ Requests and receives support and assistance from family, friends, and coworkers.
Group interventions	Groups ▪ Participate in occupation-based groups that focus on participation in meaningful occupations.

Note. CRCI = cancer-related cognitive impairment.

CASE EXAMPLE 17.1. LUIS: IMPACT OF CRCI ON WORK

Luis is a 55-year-old survivor of Stage II colon cancer. He is nearing completion of active treatment with one additional cycle of chemotherapy. He lives alone in an apartment in an urban area where he takes public transportation to and from work. He has no family in the area but does have a supportive network of friends and coworkers. He has been working full-time through treatment as an accountant in a small family-owned company.

Luis has been experiencing cognitive symptoms related to his cancer and cancer treatment, such as difficulty with concentration, speed of information processing, and difficulty with multitasking. These symptoms are affecting his ability to perform his essential job functions in his customary manner. Luis is worried that he could lose his job and therefore his health insurance. At a regularly scheduled oncology visit, Luis reports these difficulties to his oncologist. The oncologist provides Luis with a referral to occupational therapy for management of cognitive side effects of cancer treatment and their effects on work performance.

During the occupational therapy evaluation, the occupational therapist engages Luis in creating an occupational profile to better understand how his cognitive symptoms are affecting his work performance. Luis reports that he is falling behind on important work tasks and has difficulty

concentrating on tasks that require attention to detail. He has noticed that he is making mistakes on financial documents and, although he catches most of them, is concerned that he will make a mistake that others will notice. He is concerned about the extra time he needs to complete his work and fears that his clients will complain about his performance. This is causing him significant distress; he does not want others to question his work ability. Work has always been a place of support for Luis, and his coworkers have been very helpful to him during his cancer experience. He does not want to take advantage of their kindness, but he feels that, at times, they are losing patience with him. He recently stopped going to lunch with his colleagues so he could "catch up" on his work. He reports that his goal is to feel in control of his cognitive difficulties in relation to his work responsibilities.

During the occupational therapy evaluation, the occupational therapist administers the Canadian Occupational Performance Measure (COPM; Law et al., 2019) and requests that Luis complete the Functional Assessment of Cancer Therapy–Cognitive (FACT–Cog; Wagner et al., 2009) and the Functional Assessment of Cancer Therapy–General (FACT–G; Cella et al., 1993), which measure social, emotional, physical, and functional well-being.

(Continued)

CASE EXAMPLE 17.1. LUIS: IMPACT OF CRCI ON WORK *(Cont.)*

When asked to describe a typical day, Luis reports that he often wakes up tired as a result of having difficulty with restful sleep. He procrastinates as long as possible and then gets ready for work as quickly as he can and heads to catch the bus for work. He often gets to work right on time; however, he reports that he used to get to work early to settle in before his start time. He works from 9 a.m.–5 p.m. and then heads home. Once home, he reports that he is exhausted, both mentally and physically. He has given up on taking part in social outings with his coworkers and generally makes dinner, watches television, and goes to sleep.

Luis identifies several priority areas to address in occupational therapy, as noted on the COPM (Table 17.4; Law et al., 2019). They include rest and sleep, work, and social and leisure participation, including attending after work outings with his colleagues. He attributed high importance to these activities and overall low performance and satisfaction.

The FACT–Cog and FACT–G scores suggest that Luis is experiencing cognitive difficulties on a daily basis, and these are affecting his ability to work and his overall quality of life.

The occupational therapist begins intervention with education about the multidimensional etiology of CRCI. The therapist continues by examining how the challenges Luis is reporting can affect his ability to work, and she explains the importance of rest and sleep. Luis is reassured because he was not aware that his fatigue and distress could be contributing to his cognitive impairment. She discusses the benefits of establishing some new habits and routines to support his ability to work. Luis expresses interest in developing new routines and is eager to learn strategies to help him be more effective at work.

In the coming week, Luis and the occupational therapist address sleep hygiene. Luis agrees to incorporate several strategies into his evening routine to promote better quality sleep, including setting aside "worry time" before bed, which will provide him time to make a plan for the next day; maintaining a consistent bedtime; and enhancing his sleep environment by keeping his room dark, quiet, and at a comfortable temperature. He anticipates that these strategies will help him not only sleep better, but also reduce his distress and support his ability to work with greater ease.

Upon his return to occupational therapy, Luis reports that he has accomplished his goal and has found the time away from his desk restorative. He feels that he was a little less short with his coworkers and looks forward to incorporating the additional breaks into his work routine moving forward. He agrees to continue this goal for the upcoming week with the goal of doing this every day. (Refer to Chapter 22, "Sleep and Rest," for additional information regarding strategies to support sleep.)

TABLE 17.4. Luis's COPM Results

OCCUPATION	IMPORTANCE	SATISFACTION	PERFORMANCE
Rest and sleep	10	2	3
Work	10	1	4
Social activities	10	1	1

Note. COPM = Canadian Occupational Performance Measure.

---

of CRCI. In turn, occupational therapy practitioners can support survivors of cancer by addressing functional cognition. ***Functional cognition*** is

the interaction of cognitive skills and self-care, and community living skills. It refers to the thinking and processing skills needed to accomplish complex everyday activities such as household and financial management, medication management, volunteer activities, driving, and work. (American Occupational Therapy Association [AOTA], 2017, p. 1)

This appreciation of the relationship among the cancer survivor, their daily occupations or roles, and the context in which the occupation is performed supports occupational therapy practitioners in addressing the cognitive changes that negatively affect participation in life roles and occupations (Newman et al., 2019). The occupational therapy practitioner's role in the management of CRCI, then, is to maximize participation in life roles and occupational performance across the lifespan. Tables 17.2 and

17.3 highlight intervention approaches and approaches to intervention as aligned with the *Occupational Therapy Practice Framework: Domain and Process* (3rd ed.; *OTPF*; AOTA, 2014).

As highlighted throughout this chapter, CRCI is multidimensional in etiology. As a result, a variety of intervention approaches may be helpful to support an occupation-based approach to intervention. Case Example 17.1 highlights approaches to intervention consistent with the *OTPF* as well as occupational therapy interventions.

SUMMARY

CRCI affects survivors of cancer across the lifespan, from children to older adults, and has the potential to affect performance in a range of occupations, from self-care to IADLs to work, education, and social and leisure participation. Survivors report CRCI as one of the most feared side effects of cancer and cancer treatment. Commonly reported cognitive impairments include difficulty with attention, concentration, working memory, executive function, information processing speed, new learning, and word finding.

CRCI is multidimensional. Cancer and cancer treatment, physical, psychological, genetic, and lifestyle factors play important and interrelated roles.

At present, there is no gold standard assessment or intervention for CRCI; however, a variety of methods are currently used to evaluate the impact of cancer and cancer treatment on cognitive function, including self-report, neuropsychological testing, and neuroimaging studies. Survivors may report challenges with cognitive function before, during, and for years after the completion of cancer treatment. As a result, occupational therapy practitioners may support survivors at various points on the cancer care continuum and support survivors living with CRCI by addressing participation in meaningful life roles and occupations across the lifespan.

REFERENCES

Ahles, T. A., & Hurria, A. (2018). New challenges in psycho-oncology research IV: Cognition and cancer: Conceptual and methodological issues and future directions. *Psycho-Oncology, 27*, 3–9. https://doi.org/10.1002/pon.4564

Ahles, T. A., Root, J. C., & Ryan, E. L. (2012). Cancer- and cancer treatment-associated cognitive change: An update on the state of the science. *Journal of Clinical Oncology, 30*, 3675–3686. https://doi.org/10.1200/JCO.2012.43.0116

Ali, F. S., Hussain, M. R., Gutierrez, C., Demireva, P., Ballester, L. Y., Zhu, L. Y., . . . Esquenazi, Y. (2018). Cognitive disability in adult patients with brain tumors. *Cancer Treatment Reviews, 65*, 33–40. https://doi.org/10.1016/j.ctrv.2018.02.007

American Brain Tumor Association. (2019). *Glioma.* Retrieved from abta.org/tumor_types/glioma

American Occupational Therapy Association. (2014). Occupational therapy practice framework: Domain and process (3rd ed.). *American Journal of Occupational Therapy, 68*(Suppl. 1), S1–S48. https://doi.org/10.5014/ajot.2014.682006

American Occupational Therapy Association. (2017). *Occupational therapy's role in adult cognitive disorders* [Fact sheet]. Bethesda, MD: Author. Retrieved from http://www.aota.org/~/media/Corporate/Files/AboutOT/Professionals/WhatIsOT/PA/Facts/Cognition%20fact%20sheet.pdf

Andreotti, C., Root, J. C., Ahles, T. A., McEwen, B. S., & Compas, B. E. (2015). Cancer, coping, and cognition: A model for the role of stress reactivity in cancer-related cognitive decline. *Psycho-Oncology, 24*, 617–623. https://doi.org/10.1002/pon.3683

Apple, A. C., Schroeder, M. P., Ryals, A. J., Wagner, L. I., Cella, D., Shih, P.-A., . . . Wang, L. (2018). Hippocampal function connectivity is related to self-reported cognitive concerns in breast cancer patients undergoing adjuvant therapy. *NeuroImage: Clinical, 20*, 110–118. https://doi.org/10.1016/j.nicl.2018.07.010

Árnadóttir, G. (1990). *The brain and behavior: Assessing cortical dysfunction through activities of daily living.* St. Louis: Mosby.

Asher, A., & Meyers, J. S. (2015). The effect of cancer treatment on cognitive function. *Clinical Advances in Hematology & Oncology, 13*, 441–450.

Baum, C. M., & Wolf, T. J. (2013). *Executive Function Performance Test (EFPT).* St. Louis: Washington University School of Medicine.

Beery, K. E., Buktenica, N. A., & Beery, N. A. (2010). *Beery–Buktenica Developmental Test of Visual–Motor Integration* (6th ed.). New York: Pearson Assessments.

Benedict, R. H. B., Schretlen, D., Groninger, L., & Brandt, J. (1998). Hopkins Verbal Learning Test–Revised: Normative data and analysis of inter-form and test-retest reliability. *Clinical Neuropsychologist, 12*, 43–55. https://doi.org/10.1076/clin.12.1.43.1726

Benton, A. L., Hamsher, K., Rey, G. L., & Sivan, A. B. (1994). *Multilingual Aphasia Examination* (3rd ed.). Iowa City, IA: AJA Associates.

Benton, A. L., Hamsher, K. D., & Sivan, A. (1983). *Multilingual Aphasia Examination* (3rd ed.). Iowa City, IA: AJA Associates.

Boykoff, N., Moieni, M., & Subramanian, S. K. (2009). Confronting chemobrain: An in-depth look at survivors' reports of impact on work, social networks, and health care response. *Journal of Cancer Survivorship, 3*, 223–232. https://doi.org/10.1007/s11764-009-0098-x

Broadbent, D. E., Cooper, P. F., FitzGerald, P., & Parkes, K. R. (1982). The Cognitive Failures Questionnaire (CFQ) and its correlates. *British Journal of Clinical Psychology, 21*, 1–16. https://doi.org/10.1111/j.2044-8260.1982.tb01421.x

Castellino, S. M., Ullrich, N. J., Whelen, M. J., & Lange, B. J. (2014). Developing interventions for cancer-related cognitive dysfunction in childhood cancer survivors. *Journal of the National Cancer Institute, 106*, 186. https://doi.org/10.1093/jnci/dju186

Cella, D. F., Tulsky, D. S., Gray, G., Sarafian, B., Linn, E., Bonomi, A., . . . Brannon, J. (1993). The Functional Assessment of Cancer Therapy scale: Development and validation of the general measure. *Journal of Clinical Oncology, 11*, 570–579. https://doi.org/10.1200/JCO.1993.11.3.570

Chelune, G. J., Heaton, R. K., & Lehman, R. A. (1986). Neuropsychological and personality correlates of patients' complaints of disability. In G. Goldstein & R. Tarter (Eds.), *Advances in Clinical Neuropsychology* (Vol. 3, pp. 95–126). New York: Springer. https://doi.org/10.1007/978-1-4613-2211-5_4

Cifu, G., Power, M. C., Shomstein, S., & Arem, H. (2018). Mindfulness-based interventions and cognitive function among breast cancer survivors: A systematic review. *BMC Cancer, 18*, 1163–1174. https://doi.org/10.1186/s12885-018-5065-3

Cimprich, B., Visovatti, M., & Ronis, D. L. (2011). The Attentional Function Index—A self-report cognitive measure. *Psycho-Oncology, 20*, 194–202. https://doi.org/10.1002/pon.1729

Denlinger, C. S., Ligibel, J. A., Are, M., Baker, K. S., Denmark-Wahrenfried, W., Friedman, D. L., . . . & Freedman-Cass, D. A. (2014). Survivorship: Cognitive Function, Version 1.2014. *Journal of the National Comprehensive Cancer Network, 12*, 976–986. https://doi.org/10.6004/jccn.2014.0094

Dorland, H. F., Abma, F. I., Roelen, C. A. M., Smink, A., Feuerstein, M., Amick, B. C., . . . Bültmann, U. (2016). The Cognitive Symptom Checklist–Work in cancer patients is related with work functioning, fatigue and depressive symptoms: A validation study. *Journal of Cancer Survivorship: Research and Practice, 10*(3), 545–552. https://doi.org/10.1007/s11764-015-0500-9

Fisher, A. G., & Jones, K. B. (2012). *Assessment of Motor and Process Skills: Development, standardizations, and administration manual* (7th ed., rev.). Fort Collins, CO: Three Star Press.

Hardy, S. J., Krull, K. R., Wefel, J. S., & Janelsins, M. (2018). Cognitive changes in cancer survivors. *American Society of Clinical Oncology Educational Book, 38*. https://doi.org/10.1200/EDBK_201179

Henneghan, A. (2016). Modifiable factors and cognitive dysfunction in breast cancer survivors: A mixed-method systematic review. *Supportive Care in Cancer, 24,* 481–497. https://doi.org/10.1007/s00520-015-2927-y

Holohan, K. N., Von Ah, D., McDonald, B. C., & Saykin, A. J. (2013). Neuroimaging, cancer, and cognition: State of the knowledge. *Seminars in Oncology Nursing, 29,* 280–287. https://doi.org/10.1016/j.soncn.2013.08.008

Janelsins, M. C., Kesler, S. R., Ahles, T. A., & Morrow, G. R. (2014). Prevalence, mechanisms, and management of cancer-related cognitive impairment. *International Review of Psychiatry, 26,* 102–113. https://doi.org/10.3109/09540261.2013.864260

Jim, H. S. L., Jennewein, S. L., Quinn, G. P., Reed, D. R., & Small, B. J. (2018). Cognition in adolescent and young adults diagnosed with cancer: An understudied problem. *Journal of Clinical Oncology, 36,* 2752–2754. https://doi.org/10.1200/JCO.2018.78.0627

Joly, F., Giffard, B., Rigal, O., De Ruiter, M. B., Small, B. J., Dubois, M., . . . Castel, H. (2015). Impact of cancer and its treatments on cognitive function: Advances in research from the Paris International Cognition and Cancer Task Force symposium and update since 2012. *Journal of Pain and Symptom Management, 50,* 830–841. https://doi.org/10.1016/j.jpainsymman.2015.06.019

Knight, C., Alderman, N., & Burgess, P. W. (2002). Development of a simplified version of the Multiple Errands Test for use in hospital settings. *Neuropsychological Rehabilitation, 12,* 231–255. https://doi.org/10.1080/09602010244000039

Koppelmans, V., Breteler, M. M., Boogerd, W., Seynaeve, C., Gundy, C., & Schagen, S. B. (2012). Neuropsychological performance in survivors of breast cancer more than 20 years after adjuvant chemotherapy. *Journal of Clinical Oncology, 30,* 1080–1086. https://doi.org/10.1200/JCO.2011.37.0189

Krull, K. R., Hardy, K. K., Kahalley, L. S., Schuitema, I., & Kesler, S. R. (2018). Neurocognitive outcomes and interventions in long-term survivors of childhood cancer. *Journal of Clinical Oncology, 36,* 2181–2189. https://doi.org/10.1200/JCO.2017.76.4696

Lai, J. S., Wagner, L. I., Jacobsen, P. B., & Cella, D. (2014). Self-reported cognitive concerns and abilities: Two sides of one coin? *Psycho-Oncology, 23,* 1133–1141. https://doi.org/10.1002/pon.3522

Law, M., Baptiste, S., Carswell, A., McColl, M., Polatajko, H., & Pollock, N. (2019). *Canadian Occupational Performance Measure* (5th ed., rev.). Altona, Manitoba: COPM Inc.

Loh, P. K., Janelsins, M. C., Mohile, S. G., Holmes, H. M., Hsu, T., Inouye, S. K., . . . Ahles, T. A. (2016). Chemotherapy-related cognitive impairment in older patients with cancer. *Journal of Geriatric Oncology, 7,* 270–280. https://doi.org/10.1016/j.jgo.2016.04.008

Mandelblatt, J. S., Clapp, J. D., Luta, G., Faul, L. A., Tallarico, M. D., McClendon, T. D., . . . Isaacs, C. (2016). Long-term trajectories of self-reported cognitive function in a cohort of older survivors of breast cancer: CALBG 369901 (Alliance). *Cancer, 122,* 3555–3563. https://doi.org/10.1002/cncr.30208

McEwen, B. S. (1998). Stress, adaptation, and disease. Allostasis and allostatic load. *Annals of the New York Academy of Sciences, 840,* 33–44. https://doi.org/10.1111/j.1749-6632.1998.tb09546.x

Mukand, J. A., Blackinton, D. D., Crincoli, M. G., Lee, J. J., & Santos, B. B. (2001). Incidence of neurologic deficits and rehabilitation of patients with brain tumors. *American Journal of Physical Medicine & Rehabilitation, 80,* 346–350. https://doi.org/10.1097/00002060-200105000-00005

National Comprehensive Cancer Network. (2017). *NCCN guidelines for survivorship.* Retrieved from https://www.nccn.org/professionals/physician_gls/pdf/survivorship.pdf

Newman, R., Lyons, K. D., Coster, W. J., Wong, J., Festa, K., & Ko, N. (2019). Feasibility, acceptability and potential effectiveness of an occupation-focused cognitive self-management program for breast cancer survivors. *British Journal of Occupational Therapy, 82,* 604–611. https://doi.org/10.1177/0308022619861893

Noll, K. R., Bradshaw, M. E., Parsons, M. W., Dawson, E. L., Rexer, J., & Wefel, J. S. (2019). Monitoring of neurocognitive function in the care of patients with brain tumors. *Current Treatment Options in Neurology, 21,* 33–46. https://doi.org/10.1007/s11940-019-0573-2

Noll, K. R., Bradshaw, M. E., Rexer, J., & Wefel, J. (2018). Neuropsychological practice in the oncology setting. *Archives of Clinical Neuropsychology, 33,* 344–353. https://doi.org/10.1093/arclin/acx131

Player, L., Mackenzie, L., Willis, K., & Loh, S. Y. (2014). Women's experiences of cognitive changes or "chemobrain" following treatment for breast cancer: A role for occupational therapy? *Australian Occupational Therapy Journal, 61,* 230–240. https://doi.org/10.1111/1440-1630.12113

Pullens, M. J., De Vries, J., & Roukema, J. A. (2010). Subjective cognitive dysfunction in breast cancer patients: A systematic review. *Psycho-Oncology, 19,* 1127–1138. https://doi.org/10.1016/j.ctrv.2012.05.002

Rocke, K., Hays, P., Edwards, D., & Berg, C. (2008). Development of a performance assessment of executive function: The Children's Kitchen Task Assessment. *American Journal of Occupational Therapy, 62,* 528–537. https://doi.org/10.5014/ajot.62.5.528

Rust, C., & Davis, C. (2013). Chemobrain in underserved African American breast cancer survivors: A qualitative study. *Clinical Journal of Oncology Nursing, 17,* E29–E34. https://doi.org/10.1188/13.CJON.E29-E34

Schmidt, J. E., Beckjord, E., Bovbjerg, D. H., Low, C. A., Posluszny, D. M., Lowery, A. E., . . . Rechis, R. (2016). Prevalence of perceived cognitive dysfunction in survivors of a wide range of cancers: Results from the 2010 LIVESTRONG survey. *Journal of Cancer Survivorship, 10,* 302–311. https://doi.org/10.1007/s11764-015-0476-5

Silberfarb, P. M., Philibert, D., & Levine, P. M. (1980). Psychosocial aspects of neoplastic disease: II. Affective and cognitive effects of chemotherapy in cancer patients. *American Journal of Psychiatry, 137,* 597–601. https://doi.org/10.1176/ajp.137.5.597

Sleight, A. (2016). Coping with cancer-related cognitive dysfunction: A scoping review of the literature. *Disability and Rehabilitation, 38,* 400–408. https://doi.org/10.3109/09638288.2015.1038364

Strauss, E., Sherman, E. M. S., & Spreen, O. (2006). *Behavior Rating Inventory of Executive Function (BRIEF). A compendium of neuropsychological tests, administration, norms, and commentary* (3rd ed., pp. 1090–1099). New York: Oxford University Press.

Toglia, J. (2015). *Weekly Calendar Planning Activity: A performance test of executive function.* Bethesda, MD: AOTA Press.

Treanor, C. J., McMenamin, U. C., O'Neill, R. F., Cardwell, C. R., Clarke, M. J., Cantwell, M., & Donnelly, M. (2016). Non-pharmacological interventions for cognitive impairment due to systemic cancer treatment. *Cochrane Database of Systematic*

Reviews, 16(8), CD011325. https://doi.org/10.1002/14651858. CD011325.pub2

Trites, R. L. (1977). *Neuropsychological test manual.* Ottawa, Ontario: Royal Ottawa Hospital.

Van Dyk, K., Ganz, P. A., Ercoli, L., Petersen, L., & Crespi, C. M. (2016). Measuring cognitive complaints in breast cancer survivors: Psychometric properties of the patient's assessment of own functioning inventory. *Supportive Care in Cancer, 24,* 4939–4949. https://doi.org/10.1007/s00520-016-3352-6

van Loon, E. M. P., Heijenbrok-Kal, M. H., van Loon, W. S., van den Bent, M. J., Vincent, A. J. P. E., de Koning, I., & Ribbers, G. M. (2015). Assessment methods and prevalence of cognitive dysfunction in patients with lowgrade glioma: A systematic review. *Journal of Rehabilitation Medicine, 47,* 481–488. https://doi.org/10.2340/16501977-1975

Vannorsdall, T. D. (2017). Cognitive changes related to cancer therapy. *Medical Clinics of North America, 101,* 1115–1134. https://doi.org/10.1016/j.mcna.2017.06.006

Von Ah, D., Storey, S., Jansen, C. E., & Allen, D. H. (2013). Coping strategies and interventions for cognitive changes in patients with cancer. *Seminars in Oncology Nursing, 29,* 288–299. https://doi.org/10.1016/j.soncn.2013.08.009

Wagner, L., Sweet, J., Butt, Z., Lai, J., & Cella, D. (2009). Measuring patient self-reported cognitive function: Development of the Functional Assessment of Cancer Therapy–Cognitive Function Instrument. *Journal of Supportive Oncology, 7,* W32–W39.

Wechsler, D. (1991). *Wechsler Intelligence Scale for Children: Third edition manual.* San Antonio Psychological Corporation.

Wefel, J. S., Kesler, S. R., Noll, N. R., & Schagen, S. B. (2015). Clinical characteristics, pathophysiology, and management of non-central nervous system cancer-related cognitive impairment in adults. *CA: A Cancer Journal for Clinicians, 65,* 123–138. https://doi.org/10.3322/caac.21258

Wefel, J., Patwardhan, S., & Strange, C. (2010). Concurrent and criterion validity related evidence for the neurocognitive function clinical trial battery in brain tumor patients. *Neuro-Oncology, 12,* iv58–iv61.

Willard, V. W., Cox, L. E., Russell, K. M., Kenney, A., Jurbergs, N., Molnar, A. E., Jr., & Harman, J. L. (2017). Cognitive and psychosocial functioning in preschool-aged children with cancer. *Journal of Developmental & Behavioral Pediatrics, 38,* 638–645. https://doi.org/10.1097/DBP.0000000000000512

Wolf, T. J., Doherty, M., Kallogieri, D., Coalson, R., Nicklaus, J., Ma, C. X., . . . Piccirillo, J. (2016). The feasibility of using metacognitive strategy training to improve cognitive performance and neural connectivity in women with chemotherapy-induced cognitive impairment. *Oncology, 91,* 143–152. https://doi.org/10.1159/000447744

18

Lymphedema

Katie M. Polo, DHS, OTR, CLT–LANA

LEARNING OBJECTIVES

After completing this chapter, readers should be able to
- Understand general information regarding the incidence, risk factors, etiological classification, and clinical stages of lymphedema;
- Identify specialized lymphedema symptom intervention and management across the lifespan and appropriate timing of client referral to clinicians with advanced lymphedema certification;
- Select methods for evaluating risk for the early surveillance and detection of secondary lymphedema onset;
- Explain common occupational performance deficits in cancer survivors with lymphedema across the lifespan; and
- Identify interventions to address risk reduction, self-management, and creation of healthy routines in cancer survivors with lymphedema across the lifespan.

KEY TERMS AND CONCEPTS

- Cellulitis
- Complete decongestive therapy
- Compression
- Elephantiasis
- Erysipelas
- Fibrosclerosis
- Fibrosis
- Latency stage
- Lymphatic load
- Lymphedema
- Manual lymphatic drainage
- Primary lymphedema
- Secondary lymphedema
- Self-management
- Skin treatment and care
- Spontaneously irreversible stage
- Spontaneously reversible stage
- Transport capacity

INTRODUCTION

Lymphedema is a chronic inflammatory disease caused by mechanical insufficiency (i.e., failure) of the lymphatic system that leads to an abnormal collection of fluid beneath the skin. Lymphedema can occur in any exterior region of the body such as arms, legs, breast, trunk, head, neck, and genitals (Földi & Földi, 2012). Lymphedema has been described as one of the most significant survivorship issues that may affect roles and participation in daily occupations.

Breast cancer–related lymphedema is one of the most commonly reported types of lymphedema with incidence postmastectomy varying from 8%–56% of patients; reports of time of onset vary from within days to more than 30 years after the treatment of breast cancer (Paskett et al., 2007). A meta-analysis of the literature revealed overall incidence of lymphedema to be 16.3% after melanoma, 10.1% after genitourinary cancers, and 19.6% after gynecologic malignancies; the meta-analysis noted that rates are higher in the lower extremity than the upper extremity (Cormier et al., 2010).

Cormier et al. (2010) also concluded that the wide ranges in incidence are related to the type and extent of cancer treatment, anatomic location of the cancer, the diversity of assessment methods used, and the length of follow-up. The risk of developing lymphedema is lifelong and does not diminish over time (National Lymphedema Network [NLN], 2011a).

Lymphedema can cause a wide range of impairments in the performance of daily activities. The significance of these performance deficits depends on the chronicity and severity of its presentation (Shigaki et al., 2013). Lymphedema can have a negative effect on all areas of occupation, including ADLs, IADLs, rest and sleep, education, work, play, leisure, and social participation (American Occupational Therapy Association [AOTA], 2014). This chapter explores the defining features of lymphedema, specialized interventions for symptomology management, and occupational therapy's role in the management of lymphedema across the lifespan.

ETIOLOGICAL CLASSIFICATION

Primary lymphedema is the result of a developmental defect of the lymph vessels and is present in some congenital and hereditary conditions; it is not related to cancer survivorship. It can be further classified according to age of onset (Földi & Földi, 2012).

Secondary lymphedema can occur at any age and results in lymph vessel damage that can occur as a complication of blockage by a malignant tumor, cancer surgery, radiotherapy, infections, parasites, or trauma (Földi & Földi, 2012; Viehoff et al., 2015). Worldwide, filariasis, not cancer, is the leading cause of lymphedema. *Filariasis* is a condition caused by a parasite native to tropical rain forests; the parasite enters the

FIGURE 18.1	Secondary upper-extremity breast cancer–related lymphedema of the right arm.

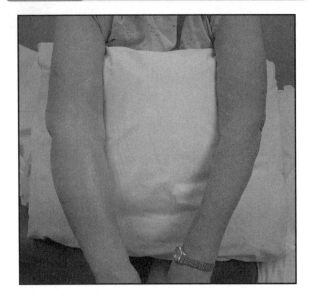

Source. K. M. Polo. Used with permission.

body through a bite from an infected mosquito and causes eventual lymph vessel paralysis (Földi & Földi, 2012). The most common cause of secondary lymphedema in the United States is cancer or treatments used in the management of the disease (Greene, 2015). See Figure 18.1.

DEFINING FEATURES OF LYMPHEDEMA AND CONSIDERATIONS ACROSS THE LIFESPAN

Although the true etiology of secondary lymphedema remains unknown, identified risk factors associated with its development include surgery, lymph node removal, adjuvant treatment such as radiation or chemotherapy, and having an elevated body mass index (Jammallo et al., 2013; McLaughlin, 2012). Veins and lymphatic vessels are responsible for removing waste comprised of water and solid debris from the body. In general, veins remove water waste, and the lymphatic vessels primarily are responsible for removal of the solid debris. ***Lymphatic load*** refers to the volume of lymph waste substances that require removal from the lymph vessels; this can include fluid that is not reabsorbed by the veins (net ultrafiltrate), cells, proteins, and fat (Földi & Földi, 2012). ***Transport capacity*** is the volume of lymph that the lymphatic system can transport per unit of time (Földi & Földi, 2012).

In simple uncomplicated lymphedema, mechanical insufficiency of the lymphatic system occurs, and the transport capacity drops below the lymphatic load (volume of lymph fluid); thus, the removal of the lymphatic load cannot happen appropriately:

- Normal lymph system = transport capacity > lymphatic load
- Insufficient lymph system = lymphatic load > transport capacity.

In secondary lymphedema from cancer, cancer treatments such as surgical resection or radiation, or infections can compromise the pumping mechanisms in the *lymphatic* system and limit the transport capacity's ability to remove the lymphatic load present. Lymphedema can progress if treatment or intervention does not occur in a timely fashion, but the rate of progression through four clinical stages varies.

CLINICAL STAGE CLASSIFICATION

Although lymphedema has no cure, it can be successfully managed when properly diagnosed and treated, especially in earlier stages (NLN, 2011a). *Lymphedema* is often defined as a 2 cm or greater difference in limb girth, a 10% or greater difference in limb volume, or a 200 ml or greater difference in limb volume (Armer & Stewart, 2005). Lymphedema is classified by its clinical stage, regardless of whether it is primary or secondary in

---

TABLE 18.1.   Lymphedema Stages, Signs, and Symptoms

STAGE	SIGNS AND SYMPTOMS
0 Latency	- No visible or palpable edema present - Impaired transport capacity but still sufficient for amount of lymph being removed - Subjective complaints possible (e.g., heaviness, fatigue)
1 Spontaneously reversible	- Accumulation of protein-rich edema - Pitting edema when pressed by fingertip - Reduces with elevation
2 Spontaneously irreversible	- Accumulation of protein-rich edema - Nonpitting edema when pressed by fingertip - Fibrosis is moderate to severe
3 Elephantiasis	- Accumulation of protein-rich edema like Stage 2 but with a degree of severity - Nonpitting edema - Fibrosis and sclerosis are severe - Skin changes

Note. Based on the work of the International Society of Lymphology (2016) and Földi & Földi (2012).

nature. Clinical staging ranges from 0–3 and is defined by the pathology and symptoms that are present (Földi & Földi, 2012).

Stage 0 is also known as the ***latency stage***. Those in this stage might have had an excision of a lymph node, but their transport capacity still exceeds the normal lymphatic load, thus no edema or symptoms are noted (Földi & Földi, 2012).

The ***spontaneously reversible stage,*** or *Stage 1,* is caused by an accumulation of high-protein fluid and fibrosclerotic changes or tissue hardening that may be present only in specific areas (Földi & Földi, 2012). Stage 1 edema is soft, and finger pressure can leave a deep indentation or a "pitting" presence. In this beginning stage, the edema can fully or partially regress when the body part is elevated (Földi & Földi, 2012). In early stages of lymphedema, symptoms include subjective sensations of tightness; many patients report that jewelry or clothes feel uncomfortable or tight on their affected body parts. It is imperative that early diagnosis and treatment occur in this stage when symptoms of lymphedema can be reversed (Silver et al., 2013).

In the absence of treatment, lymphedema can progress into the ***spontaneously irreversible stage,*** or *Stage 2,* and become chronic in nature (Földi & Földi, 2012). Stage 2 lymphedema is associated with extensive fibrosclerosis, or hardening of the tissues. Pressure no longer causes an indentation in the edema, and elevating the limb has no effect on reduction (Földi & Földi, 2012).

Stage 3, or ***elephantiasis,*** has the same features of Stage 2 lymphedema, but the fibrosclerosis is more extensive in nature (Földi & Földi, 2012). See Table 18.1 for lymphedema stages, signs, and symptoms.

LYMPHEDEMA COMPLICATIONS

Some inflammatory complications of lymphedema are more common as a result of mechanical insufficiency of the lymphatics if left untreated over time.

Connective Tissue Proliferation

If lymphedema remains untreated (Stages 2 and 3), connective tissue proliferation can occur and create a hardening of the affected tissues called ***fibrosclerosis*** or ***fibrosis.*** This hardening can cause breaks in the skin, exposing the area to the possibility of infections such as erysipelas and cellulitis (Földi & Földi, 2012). To reduce the risk of developing an infection, those with lymphedema are encouraged to adopt a thorough daily skin hygiene regimen; occupational therapy practitioners can educate and support clients in adopting a regimen into their daily routine.

Erysipelas and Cellulitis

The lymphatic system of those with lymphedema has a lowered ability to remove toxic substances because of mechanical insufficiency. Therefore, bacterial invasion such as erysipelas and cellulitis is more likely to occur (Földi & Földi, 2012).

Erysipelas is an acute superficial form of cellulitis that can involve dermal lymph vessels (Földi & Földi, 2012). ***Cellulitis*** can develop after erysipelas and is an acute, diffuse spreading of inflammation of the subcutaneous tissues

---

EXHIBIT 18.1. Signs and Symptoms of Infection

Signs and symptoms of infection may vary but generally include:
- Pain or tenderness
- Redness
- Rash or red blotchy skin
- Itching of the affected area
- Increased swelling
- Increased temperature of the skin at the site
- Heaviness in the affected limb
- Flulike symptoms
- Sudden onset of high fever or chills.

Source. NLN (2018).

(Földi & Földi, 2012). Both types of infection can cause lymphedema to become worse (Földi & Földi, 2012). Health care providers, including occupational therapy practitioners, and those with lymphedema must provide ongoing surveillance and monitoring for these conditions as well as work to reduce the risk of occurrence with proper skin hygiene regimens. See Exhibit 18.1 for signs and symptoms of infection.

Erysipelas and cellulitis are contraindications for specialized treatment of lymphedema such as complete decongestive therapy (CDT); therefore, medical treatment must take place before the initiation of CDT.

Physical and Psychosocial Effects

Cancer survivors with lymphedema experience a variety of issues, including altered sensation, loss of body confidence and self-image issues, decreased physical activity, fatigue, psychological distress, and overall loss of quality of life (QoL; Merchant & Chen, 2015).

Physical effects of lymphedema can present as limitations in upper-body strength, range of motion (ROM), and grip strength; reduced wrist and shoulder flexion; decreased endurance; and loss of kinesthetic sense of the hand (Hayes et al., 2010; Karadibak & Yavuzsen, 2015; Smoot et al., 2010). The most common self-reported symptoms in those with lower-extremity lymphedema are difficulty with walking, aches, puffiness, and pain (Brown et al., 2013).

The psychosocial effects of lymphedema should not be underestimated. Fu et al. (2013) conducted a systematic review and found that poor psychological and social well-being are common in survivors with lymphedema. They also found that psychological well-being is affected by negative self-identity, emotional disturbance, and psychological distress in those with lymphedema. Social well-being is affected in those with lymphedema by marginalization of health care providers, public insensitivity, financial burden, perceived diminished sexuality, and social isolation (Fu et al., 2013).

OVERVIEW OF MANAGING LYMPHEDEMA ACROSS THE LIFESPAN

Regardless of the type, stage, or severity of lymphedema, most survivors who experience lymphedema, regardless of age, are treated similarly with an evidence-based intervention called **CDT**, which has been found to be effective in reducing lymphedema (Lasinski et al., 2012). CDT for lymphedema volume and symptom management consists of two phases, (1) intensive and (2) maintenance. Both are performed by a certified lymphedema therapist (CLT), who may be an occupational therapy practitioner, a physical therapy practitioner, or massage therapist. See Figure 18.2 for a visual representation of CDT.

See Table 18.2 for objectives and components of Phase I and Phase II CDT.

Skin Care

Meticulous *skin treatment and care* are provided at each session, including washing the affected area, drying it completely to avoid infections, and applying moisturizing lotions that are pH-neutral because patients with

---

FIGURE 18.2 Visual of CDT Phase I and Phase II.

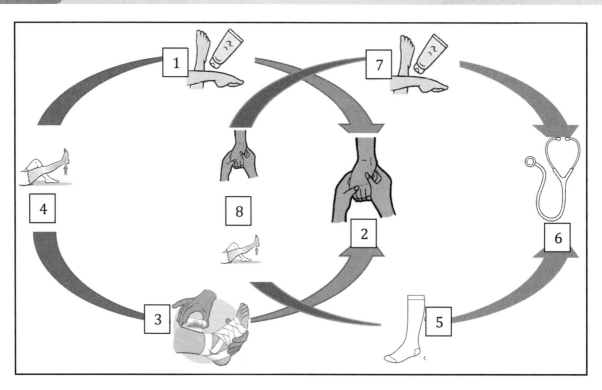

Note. The measures used in the first phase are coordinated with, and transition into, the interventions used in the second phase. In CDT Phase I (blue circle), the interventions consist of (1) skin treatment and care, (2) manual lymph drainage, (3) compression bandages/systems, and (4) movement and exercise. In CDT Phase II (green circle), the interventions consist of (5) compression therapy using compression stockings, (6) regular checkups by the physician, (7) skin care, and (8) manual lymph drainage and exercise. Patient compliance is of utmost importance during both phases.
CDT = complete decongestive therapy.

Source. Based on Asmussen & Strößenreuther (2012, p. 500).

TABLE 18.2. Objectives and Components of Phase I and Phase II CDT

	PHASE I (INTENSIVE PHASE)	PHASE II (MAINTENANCE PHASE)
Objectives	• To reduce volume (i.e., decongestion) • Symptom management	• Preserving results (i.e., maintenance) • Greater responsibility for client's own care (self-management)
Components	• Meticulous skin treatment and care • MLD • Compression bandaging • Movement and exercise	• Meticulous skin treatment and care • MLD • Compression garments • Movement and exercise

Note. CDT = complete decongestive therapy; MLD = manual lymphatic drainage.

FIGURE 18.3   Stage III elephantiasis lymphedema and fibrosis or "tissue hardening" of the lower extremity before and after CDT treatment with focus on skin care and hygiene.

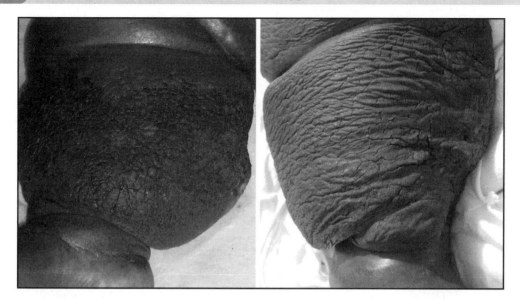

Note. CDT = complete decongestive therapy.
Source. K. M. Polo. Used with permission.

lymphedema have sensitive skin (Asmussen & Strößenreuther, 2012). Skin care is important to avoid cracking and dryness of the skin, which can increase the risk of developing infections, especially in those who have tissue fibrosis (NDN, 2011a). When applying moisturizers in Phase II CDT, all products must be fully absorbed by the skin (approximately 5–10 minutes) before placing on compression garments. This assures proper skin absorption and helps to preserve compression garments for a longer duration (Asmussen & Strößenreuther, 2012). Proper skin care coupled with all components of CDT can decrease fibrosis and improve skin integrity. See Figure 18.3, which shows fibrotic skin before and after CDT treatment.

Manual Lymphatic Drainage

Manual lymphatic drainage (MLD) is a specialized manual technique that stimulates superficial lymphatic vessels and boosts lymphatic transportation and fluid removal to areas of the body where lymphatics are functioning (NLN, 2011a). In Phase I CDT, specialized therapy practitioners perform MLD on patients and teach them the steps for self-performance; in Phase II, it is performed as needed by the patient.

Compression Therapy

Compression is applied during Phase I CDT by using multilayered, short-stretch, compression bandages with limited elasticity. Compression bandages should be changed at least daily and worn 23 hours per day. The bandages are strategically applied to give gradient pressure that steadily decreases swelling in a distal to proximal manner. Patients should be instructed on how to apply the bandages themselves and slowly work toward independently donning as part of self-care during Phase II (Asmussen &

Strößenreuther, 2012). See Figure 18.4, which shows multilayer compression bandaging.

When maximal volume reduction of the affected limb or area has been achieved, the occupational therapy practitioner will measure the area for custom-made medical

FIGURE 18.4   Multilayer compression bandaging of the lower extremity.

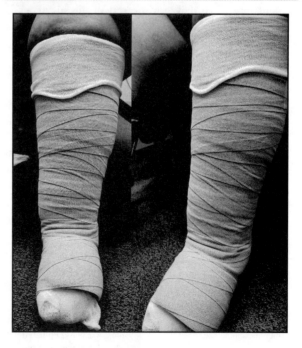

Source. K. M. Polo. Used with permission.

FIGURE 18.5   Custom compression arm garment for right upper-extremity breast cancer–related lymphedema is applied after maximal volume reduction has occurred with compression bandages.

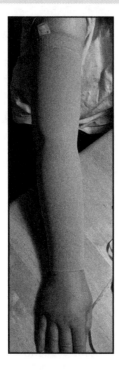

Source. K. M. Polo. Used with permission.

compression garment(s), which are critical for continued compression during Phase II CDT. These compression garments are worn daily for the rest of the survivor's life because lymphedema is a chronic disease (Asmussen & Strößenreuther, 2012).

The short-stretch bandages and garments used with those with lymphedema provide lower pressure when the client is not moving (i.e., resting pressure) and a higher pressure when muscle contraction against the resisting compression occurs (i.e., working pressure; Asmussen & Strößenreuther, 2012; NLN, 2011a). Therefore, the cycling between low-resting pressure and high-working pressure creates a pumping action that encourages movement of the fluid (NLN, 2011a). For this reason, all patients in Phase I CDT are encouraged to wear compression bandages, and those in Phase II are encouraged to wear their compression garments while exercising. See Figure 18.5, which shows a custom compression garment.

Movement and Exercise

Remedial exercises in Phase I CDT should be performed daily while the cancer survivor is in compression bandages. Exercises should progress distal to proximal involving active, repetitive, nonresistive motion to aid in decongestion and reduce the size of the affected area (Asmussen & Strößenreuther, 2012; NLN, 2011a). Remedial exercises can then be transitioned into an individually designed home exercise program in Phase II CDT. Programs can include resistive aerobic or cardiopulmonary exercise, depending on the client's limitations, and should be integrated into daily routines for ongoing self-management.

Assessment

Various methods of assessment are used to provide ongoing monitoring of lymphedema in the affected limb or area. Such assessments not only allow screening and early detection of lymphedema but also are used to identify severity and document outcomes throughout the course of CDT (NLN, 2011c). For all methods of assessment, specific protocols should be defined, including standard positions, measurement locations, and time intervals for these

TABLE 18.3.   Methods of Lymphedema Assessment Within the Literature

METHOD	DESCRIPTION
Tape measurements	■ Taken with a flexible nonelastic tape measure at defined intervals, measurements are used with a geometric formula to calculate a limb volume ■ Most accurate when the same person performs measurement each time
Perometry	■ An infrared optical electronic scanner and computer that calculates volume of the affected limb ■ Requires accurate positioning of the body part the same way with each use and must be calibrated to assure accuracy
Water displacement	■ The affected body part is immersed in water within a large cylinder, and the water pushed out is measured ■ Rarely used because of its inconvenience, messiness with water, and time it takes to perform and clean equipment
Electrical conductance testing or bioimpedance spectroscopy	■ Machine that measures interstitial fluid by using certain electrical current frequencies to determine if more fluid exists as compared to the nonaffected limb ■ Can detect early changes associated with lymphedema

Source. NLN (2011a).

procedures (NLN, 2011c). Table 18.3 illustrates the various methods of assessment within the literature.

LYMPHEDEMA TRAINING FOR OCCUPATIONAL THERAPY PRACTITIONERS

Occupational therapy practitioners are able to provide traditional lymphedema therapy, as previously described, by participating in a lymphedema therapy certification course to fulfill the requirements for becoming a CLT. Practitioners need to have completed a minimum of 135 hours of decongestive therapy coursework that meets certain criteria; provide proof of satisfactory completion of 12 credit hours of college-level human anatomy, physiology, or pathophysiology from an accredited college or university; and have a current unrestricted licensure in a related medical field (e.g., occupational therapists, occupational therapy assistants, physical therapists, physical therapist assistants, massage therapists, speech–language pathologists, registered nurses, medical doctors, doctors of osteopathic medicine, physician assistants, and athletic trainers; NLN, 2010).

When these criteria have been successfully met, the practitioner can add the CLT credentials. This education and certification process is important because clinicians who want to provide traditional CDT treatment to those with lymphedema must understand the indications and contraindications for treatment, dosages, and possible risks for treatment. To ensure these criteria are met, occupational therapy practitioners are encouraged to seek CLT training through an approved education provider from the North American Lymphedema Education Association (NALEA). See Table 18.4 for a list of NALEA-approved certification schools and their contact information.

OVERVIEW OF OCCUPATIONAL THERAPY'S ROLE WITH LYMPHEDEMA ACROSS THE LIFESPAN

Although lymphedema is not a curable condition, when early application of treatment occurs, it can be substantially reversed, especially in the first stages or before a significant volume increase occurs (Silver et al., 2013). Unfortunately, health care professionals often provide limited or conflicting educational resources and support for those with lymphedema, which may delay diagnosis and intervention (Binkley et al., 2012). Occupational therapy practitioners working with cancer survivors need to address ongoing and rigorous lymphedema surveillance, teach self-management and risk reduction practices, establish healthy routines; address occupational performance deficits, provide accurate and timely patient and caregiver education, and make timely referral to a CLT when a lymphedema onset is suspected.

In the pediatric population, secondary lymphedema from cancer or malignant lymphedema is extremely rare, so the following sections on evaluation and treatment are geared heavily toward the adult and older adult populations.

OCCUPATIONAL THERAPY EVALUATION

Cancer survivorship is increasingly viewed as a chronic condition (Baxter et al., 2017), and lymphedema is a sequelae of cancer that is also considered chronic. Occupational therapy practitioners should be an integral part of assessing and providing intervention to support chronic disease management in this population. Occupational therapy practitioners might also encounter those with a history of lymphedema or those at risk of developing lymphedema and need to understand how to properly screen clients for therapy services, provide ongoing surveillance during therapy, and make proper referrals.

A thorough medical history targeted at various known risk factors, objective measurements of the limbs, and symptomology reports can inform an occupational therapy practitioner as to whether a client will need a triage referral to a CLT at the time of assessment because of an onset of lymphedema. This medical history is also important to collect when working with those with a diagnosed history of lymphedema.

Medical History

Surveillance for the signs and symptoms for early detection of lymphedema starts with a thorough medical history regarding swelling of the limb and identification of at-risk areas of the body affected by cancer treatment (Armer et al., 2013). Risk factors associated with lymphedema development will need to be assessed with a thorough review of the survivor's medical history, including but not limited to surgery for removal of cancer, lymph node dissection (i.e., removal of the lymph nodes during surgery), adjuvant treatment such as radiation and chemotherapy, and obesity.

TABLE 18.4. NALEA-Approved Certification Schools to Become a CLT	
APPROVED SCHOOLS	**WEBSITE**
Academy of Lymphatic Studies	https://www.acols.com/
Dr. Vodder School International	https://www.vodderschool.com/
Klose Training and Consulting	https://klosetraining.com/
Norton School of Lymphatic Therapy	http://www.nortonschool.com/index.html

Note. CLT = certified lymphedema therapist; NALEA = North American Lymphedema Education Association.

The practitioner should note if the survivor has previously been diagnosed with lymphedema, in what area of the body swelling is present, and whether it is under control or an exacerbation is suspected.

Occupational Performance Deficits

Occupational therapy practitioners need to establish rapport with cancer survivors by understanding the person and their prior, current, and desired level of performance through development of the occupational profile. Assessment of occupational performance deficits and a focus of sustaining or improving current status are priorities with survivors with or without lymphedema. The type of assessments chosen and length of the evaluation process depend on the survivor's presentation and cognitive status.

The occupational therapy evaluation should include a client interview or occupational profile, clinical observation and occupation-based assessments of occupational performance, assessment of performance patterns, and consideration of other client factors. Practitioners should additionally assess a survivor's self-efficacy, psychosocial concerns, and support systems; developing effective self-management strategies and adopting healthy routines based on these factors lead to improved chronic disease management.

Occupational therapy practitioners should pay special attention to the areas of lymphedema self-management, risk reduction practices, and proper skin hygiene routines during the evaluation process to know whether suggestions for improvements need to be made. Practitioners may also need to incorporate caregivers into the evaluation process because those with a diagnosis of lymphedema may rely on others to perform these routines for them.

Objective Measurements

Objective measurements of the at-risk limb are recommended for prospective monitoring and surveillance for the early detection of lymphedema (NLN, 2011c). Unfortunately, these practices are not standard in clinic settings (Chance-Hetzler et al., 2015). Few survivors are referred to rehabilitation services, and even fewer receive baseline assessments to facilitate early detection of lymphedema (Binkley et al., 2012). Occupational therapy practitioners need to integrate rigorous surveillance and screening methods alongside standard survivorship care for their clients who are at risk for lymphedema.

Circumferential girth measurements of the affected limb are recommended by using a nonstretch flexible tape measure to screen for changes over time. Occupational therapy practitioners can ask survivors if they have recorded baseline measurements in the past for comparative analysis. Measurements should be taken at evaluation for baseline of treatment and shared with the survivor for ongoing self-monitoring within the intervention plan. Practitioners must perform measurements the same way each time, and a standard technique should be adopted across practitioners for improved consistency and reliability. Practicing measurements with feedback from the person who is being measured regarding consistency of tape tension, limb position, and points of measurement have been recommended as ways to improve consistency within clinics (Tidhar et al., 2015).

Measurements in centimeters are taken in a variety of ways using predetermined sites, and it is recommended to include six measurements at minimum (NLN, 2011c). Measurements of the involved limb are then compared to the uninvolved limb to indicate the possibility of an onset of lymphedema; a 2-cm difference in any of the circumference measurements warrants immediate triage to a CLT. Occupational therapy practitioners should use the same method of measurement as prior screenings if the survivor has already been in surveillance care. If surveillance methods have not been adopted, practitioners should administer a standard protocol for baseline and ongoing measurement. Additional training of a caregiver might be necessary for older adults or those who are unable to perform these measurements independently. See Exhibit 18.2 for recommended circumferential measurement methods for upper- and lower-extremity surveillance.

Unfortunately, measurement techniques are not as precise when used on truncal, breast, genital, and head or neck regions. Therefore, patient symptom reports and observation when swelling occurs in these areas are necessary for ongoing surveillance.

Symptoms and Client Factors

Assessing for early symptoms is essential in early detection and surveillance during the occupational therapy process with survivors at risk for lymphedema. Occupational therapists should assess initially and throughout the intervention process for early self-reported signs and symptoms of lymphedema in the affected body part. Signs and symptoms may include

- Jewelry or clothing feeling uncomfortable or tight (e.g., rings, shirt sleeves, socks, shoes);
- Feelings or sensations of heaviness, tightness, fullness, or stiffness;
- Aching; and
- Observations of swelling or increases in circumferential girth measurements.

Triage for further assessment from a CLT is recommended when symptoms (e.g., sensation of heaviness, observed swelling), girth, or volume measures increase (Armer et al., 2013) or an onset of lymphedema or lymphedema exacerbation is suspected.

Additional client factors that might need to be assessed by the occupational therapist are mental functions such as energy levels, drive, and sleep, and include the secondary diagnoses of depression, anxiety, and body image issues; sensitivity to temperature, pressure, and pain; neuromusculoskeletal and movement-related functions such as ROM, strength, and mobility; and skin functions.

OCCUPATIONAL THERAPY INTERVENTION

Occupational Performance Deficits

Occupational therapy intervention is aimed at improving participation during an exacerbation of lymphedema or during the latency stage (Stage 0). Intervention approaches for occupational performance deficits can include restoring, maintaining, or modifying activities and

EXHIBIT 18.2. Circumferential Measurement Methods for Upper- and Lower-Extremity Surveillance

UPPER-EXTREMITY CIRCUMFERENTIAL MEASUREMENT TECHNIQUE

*These measurements should be performed on **both** arms for comparative analysis.*

1.) Mid-hand*

2.) Wrist*

3.) Elbow*

4.) Upper arm just below the axilla

5.) 10 cm distal to and proximal to the lateral epicondyle

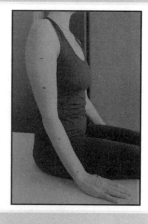

LOWER-EXTREMITY CIRCUMFERENTIAL MEASUREMENT TECHNIQUE

*These measurements should be performed on **both** legs for comparative analysis.*

1.) Mid-foot*

2.) Ankle (2 cm above medial malleolus)

3.) 10 cm above the superior pole of the patella

4.) 10 cm below the inferior pole of the patella

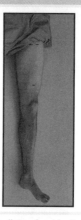

Note. 2-cm change in any of the circumferential measurements in an at-risk limb warrants immediate referral for further evaluation by a trained professional.

*Indicates further clinic consensus and development of precise protocol prior to administration.

Source. Table based on the work of the NLN (2011c) and Lymphoedema Framework (2006). Photos courtesy K. M. Polo. Used with permission.

are accomplished by therapeutic use of occupations and activities as well as education and training. A multifactorial approach needs to be considered because survivors with lymphedema may also present with pain, reduced functional mobility, limited ROM, and fatigue that create occupational performance deficits.

Occupational therapy practitioners may address occupational performance through a modified approach such as introducing adaptive strategies or incorporating adaptive equipment to promote increased performance and engagement; or practitioners may use a self-management approach. For survivors who have a diagnosis of lymphedema, general occupational therapy practitioners need to ensure their clients can perform daily self-management routines that include donning and doffing their compression garment; following a proper skin hygiene regimen; and completing any recommended maintenance strategies, including MLD and compression bandaging at night. Practitioners can make suggestions for adapting, modifying, or improving engagement in these tasks for the client or their caregiver. Table 18.5 includes occupational therapy interventions with this population. Table 18.6 describes the various intervention

approaches occupational therapy practitioners can use while caring for those with or at risk for lymphedema.

Self-Management

Being responsible for one's day-to-day self-care over the length of an illness, or *self-management,* becomes a lifetime task for most people with chronic conditions, including lymphedema (Lorig & Holman, 2003). Self-management is an effective approach to managing chronic health conditions, and occupational therapy practitioners have the skills, knowledge, and capacity to help survivors transform self-management strategies into routine practice for chronic issues such as lymphedema (AOTA, 2015a).

Helping cancer survivors who are at risk for lymphedema, or who have active lymphedema adopt self-management practices, needs to be driven by the client's concerns and problems. Therefore, occupational therapy practitioners need to take a client-centered and collaborative problem-solving approach.

Occupational therapy self-management approaches should integrate ongoing surveillance and monitoring of the affected limb, regardless of whether a survivor has a

TABLE 18.5.   Occupational Therapy Interventions

INTERVENTIONS	EXAMPLES
Occupations and activities	▪ Engagement in meaningful occupations ▪ Development of performance skills and performance patterns to enhance occupational engagements that hold meaning, relevance, and utility for the client ▪ Development and engagement in self-management routines, including a skin hygiene regimen and donning/doffing and caring for compression garments
Education and training	▪ Education on the multifactorial etiology of lymphedema ▪ Education on risk reduction factors related to onset of lymphedema ▪ Self-management training for ongoing surveillance of lymphedema
Advocacy	▪ Communication with health care providers on suspected onsets of lymphedema

TABLE 18.6.   Approaches to Occupational Therapy Intervention

APPROACHES TO INTERVENTION	EXAMPLES

Create/promote (health promotion)	▪ Promotion of healthy habits, including:
	  • Physical activity, exercise
	  • Diet
	  • Self-management strategies and ongoing monitoring or surveillance of edema
	  • Management of functional deficits resulting from comorbidities

Establish/restore	▪ Complete decongestive therapy
Modify (compensation/adaptation)	▪ Problem-solving strategies for continued independence with self-care and self-management strategies ▪ Goal setting and action planning ▪ Coping strategies for dealing with chronic disease
Prevent (disability prevention)	▪ Social, psychosocial, and physical interventions to minimize social isolation, emotional distress or stress, physical inactivity ▪ Incorporation of risk reduction practices into daily routines to minimize possible onset or exacerbation

diagnosis of lymphedema or is considered at risk for developing lymphedema. Education should be provided to the client on how to perform objective circumferential measurements and how to monitor symptoms; they should also understand the need to contact a health care provider immediately if they notice changes indicative of an onset or exacerbation of lymphedema.

Effective self-management for those with lymphedema requires ongoing performance of the steps in Phase II of CDT. This includes meticulous skin and nail care; the ability to routinely self-bandage the affected limb; the ability to care for and replace compression garments and independently don and doff them daily; and the ability to integrate risk reduction practices and exercise into daily routines. Occupational therapy practitioners should provide self-management interventions to survivors with or at risk of lymphedema and integrate them into the survivor's daily routines to promote effective long-term chronic disease management (see Figure 18.6).

Occupational therapy practitioners should address self-management strategies in regard to general skin care recommendations during and after the radiation process to ensure adequate healing and avoidance of infection that can cause an onset of lymphedema. Skin care recommendations are the same for those at risk for or with existing lymphedema. Washing the skin with a mild soap, applying lotion regularly to avoid cracking of the skin, and using soaps and lotions low in pH and fragrance are important to avoid further dryness and skin irritation.

Occupational therapy practitioners can make additional recommendations on modifications or adaptations to enhance independence as needed. Recommendations for skin care during the radiation process include avoiding wearing underwire bras during breast irradiation, following the radiation oncologist's guidelines for skin care during radiation, never applying lotions or oils to skin in the radiation field before treatment, and avoiding overstretching irradiated tissues if painful. Avoidance of trauma is important and includes wearing protective sleeves that cover the forearms while cooking or using mild insect repellant to avoid inflammation from insect bites during engagement of outdoor activities. General recommendations for those with lymphedema include washing compression garments daily or alternating several garments to avoid excessive moisture or bacterial exposure.

Evidence suggests that those who have greater self-efficacy and self-regulatory abilities to control their lymphedema demonstrate greater adherence to self-management practices (Sherman & Koelmeyer, 2013). Occupational therapy practitioners can work with survivors or their caregivers on integrating self-management strategies into habits and routines that promote the adoption and maintenance of healthy behaviors, potentially affecting self-efficacy and self-regulatory abilities (AOTA, 2015b). Therefore, practitioners should integrate self-management and surveillance

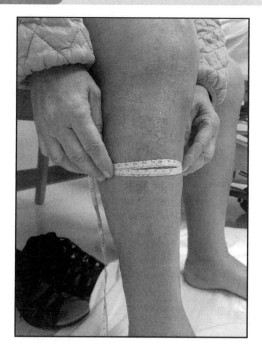

FIGURE 18.6 Client self-measurement for ongoing surveillance.

Source. K. M. Polo. Used with permission.

strategies of lymphedema into intervention practices for promotion of healthy routines within this population.

Healthy habits and routines for those at risk for or with lymphedema include incorporating risk reduction practices to reduce potential onset or exacerbation of lymphedema. Occupational therapy practitioners working with this population should be familiar with lymphedema risk reduction practices, which recommend developing a healthy lifestyle, including following a diet and exercise regimen, getting regular medical checkups, avoiding possible triggers, monitoring for signs of infection or changes in symptoms and circumferential measurements, and developing a healthy skin hygiene regimen (NLN, 2012).

Risk Reduction

The NLN's (2012) position statement on lymphedema risk reduction practices cautions survivors and health care providers on possible triggers to avoid an onset or exacerbation of lymphedema. Avoiding injury or trauma to the affected area includes any situation that might typically cause swelling in a person without lymphedema, such as falls, burns, scratches, punctures, and breaks in the skin. Other things to avoid include injections and blood draws, exposure to extreme cold or prolonged exposure to heat, limb constriction such as wearing tight jewelry or clothing, carrying heavy bags, and blood pressure checks on the at-risk limb (NLN, 2012).

General occupational therapy practitioners can introduce organizing and planning strategies into patients' daily routines to avoid risk of onset; practitioners can suggest planning to rest in cooler areas during exposure to heat during a summer outing or explain how a survivor might pack and carry a bag to accommodate a lighter weight. Table 18.7 lists the NLN's risk reduction practices and

TABLE 18.7.   Risk Reduction Practices

RISK REDUCTION STRATEGY	OCCUPATIONAL THERAPY INTERVENTION
Skin care and hygiene	▪ Client education to develop proper skin hygiene with incorporation of skin checks for dry, cracked skin ▪ Client education to develop a proper daily moisturizing skin care routine (low-pH, unscented lotions are recommended) ▪ Client education to avoid cutting cuticles
Avoid trauma to the affected area	▪ Client education to avoid venipuncture or blood draws in affected limb, if possible ▪ Client education to wear nonconstricting protective gear during high-risk times for trauma; for example, wearing protective gloves or sleeves during gardening or pet care for a client who might be at risk of upper extremity lymphedema
Avoid excessive and prolonged constriction to the affected area	▪ Client education to wear nonconstricting clothing (e.g., not tight sleeves or stockings, tight bra that could lead to excessive pressure from an underwire) ▪ Recommend all clothing be supportive and have smooth compression ▪ Avoid blood pressure checks in the affected limb, if possible
Avoid exposure to excessive heat or cold in the affected limb	▪ Client education about proper sunscreen regimen during hot weather ▪ Client education about wearing proper protection during winter months to avoid frostbite
Avoid stasis in the affected limb	▪ Client education to avoid sitting or standing for a long period for those at risk of lower extremity lymphedema ▪ Recommend intermittent movement breaks, change of position, or elevating the affected limb during activities that might create stasis in the affected lower extremity
Understand pros and cons of prophylactic compression	▪ Client education to review the pros and cons of wearing prophylactic (i.e., risk reduction) compression during air travel

Source. Based on NLN (2012).

highlights how occupational therapy practitioners can integrate these into interventions with clients at risk for lymphedema.

Cancer survivors at risk for or with lymphedema often limit their daily activity for fear of an onset or exacerbation. A systematic review of the literature indicated strong evidence that exercise was found not to cause an onset of lymphedema or make existing lymphedema worse; exercise, in fact, improves mood, QoL, and ROM and facilitates weight loss (Hunter et al., 2017). Therefore, occupational therapy practitioners can feel confident in suggesting

physical activity to clients with lymphedema (Hunter et al., 2017). Practitioners who work with cancer survivors to develop healthy exercise and physical activity regimens should take into consideration the NLN's position statement on exercise (NLN, 2011b).

Indeed, occupational therapy practitioners have the skill set to provide intervention to those with or at risk for lymphedema in various practice settings (see Case Example 18.1). Practitioners can make suggestions for adapting, modifying, or improving engagement in these tasks for either the client or their caregiver.

CASE EXAMPLE 18.1. BERNITA: EARLY DETECTION OF LYMPHEDEMA ONSET

Bernita is a 46-year-old, slightly obese woman who was diagnosed with Stage II breast cancer, requiring a right mastectomy with an axillary lymph node biopsy and radiation. She will undergo reconstructive surgery and has an expander placed for preparation. She works full-time at a local post office as a front desk clerk and would like to return once she has medical clearance. She has been off of work for 10 weeks and is nearing the end of her family medical leave. Bernita was referred to outpatient occupational therapy services by her oncologist because of chest wall tightness and restricted ROM in the right shoulder, leading to an inability to reach items off a high shelf; and issues with sleep participation because of pain; and because she wants to return to work in the near future.

Targeting outcomes
Bernita's history is negative for lymphedema; however, she has known risk factors, including lymph node biopsy, surgery, radiation, and obesity. In addition to addressing her occupational performance deficits from ROM and pain, the occupational therapist chooses to adopt a lymphedema prevention and health and wellness approach by using an early surveillance protocol, including upper-extremity (UE) objective circumferential measurements (see Table 18.8) and asking about self-reported signs and symptoms (see Table 18.9).

After collecting early surveillance objective measures and early signs and symptoms reports, the occupational therapist chooses to focus on a prevention, health, and wellness approach to Bernita's treatment plan. Goals are selected to improve Bernita's ability to reach items off high shelves, find positioning strategies for decreased pain and improved sleep participation, make plans to improve her performance of specified work demands, and integrate a self-management approach for ongoing surveillance of lymphedema onset into her daily routine. Additionally, targeting risk reduction practices through patient education for ongoing surveillance is prioritized.

Intervention
While working with Bernita on self-management approaches for early detection of lymphedema, the occupational therapist creates an education sheet on how she can integrate objective measurements and presents a list of common signs and symptoms of an onset of lymphedema. Bernita also identifies that she will have her husband perform the objective circumferential measurements of her arms on the first day of every month and record them in a journal to monitor volume changes. The therapist and Bernita work toward improving Bernita's abilities to reach items from higher surfaces and identifying positioning strategies for improved sleep participation.

TABLE 18.8. Initial Evaluation Objective Circumferential Measurements for Bernita		
LANDMARK	**RIGHT UPPER EXTREMITY***	**LEFT UPPER EXTREMITY**
Mid-hand	20.2 cm	21.2 cm
Wrist	18.0 cm	18.1 cm
Elbow	29.4 cm	29.8 cm
10 cm distal to the lateral epicondyle	26.9 cm	26.5 cm
10 cm proximal to the lateral epicondyle	36.2 cm	36.1 cm
Upper arm just below the axilla	37.5 cm	38.8 cm

*These measurements indicate that the entire upper extremity, and therefore the entire column, are at risk.

(Continued)

CASE EXAMPLE 18.1. BERNITA: EARLY DETECTION OF LYMPHEDEMA ONSET *(Cont.)*

TABLE 18.9. Reported Signs and Symptoms of Lymphedema at Initial Evaluation of Bernita

QUESTION	RESPONSE
Does your jewelry or clothing feeling uncomfortable or tight?	No
Do you have any feelings or sensations of heaviness, tightness, fullness, or stiffness?	No
Do you have any aching in your arm?	No
Have you observed any swelling or increase in arm girth?	No

One day Bernita comes to the appointment with new complaints of aching and tightness in her right UE. Upon these complaints, the occupational therapist decides to reassess Bernita's objective circumferential measurements (see Table 18.10) and list of signs and symptoms of lymphedema for a potential onset (see Table 18.11).

Analyzing the collected data, the occupational therapist determines that Bernita's right UE's mid-hand circumferential measurement has increased (reassessment 22.5 cm – 20.2 cm baseline = 2.3 cm) more than 2 cm in girth, warranting immediate referral. Additionally, Bernita has reported two new signs of an onset of lymphedema (aching and sensations of heaviness and tightness) in her right UE. The noted increase in girth and newly reported symptoms prompt the practitioner to immediately refer Bernita to her clinical oncologist for written orders for evaluation and treatment from a trained lymphedema therapist.

TABLE 18.10. Reevaluation Objective Circumferential Measurements of Bernita

LANDMARK	BASELINE ASSESSMENT		REASSESSMENT	
	Right upper extremity*	Left upper extremity	Right upper extremity*	Left upper extremity
Mid-hand	20.2 cm	21.2 cm	22.5 cm**	21.4 cm
Wrist	18.0 cm	18.1 cm	18.4 cm	18.2 cm
Elbow	29.4 cm	29.8cm	29.7cm	29.6 cm
10 cm distal to the lateral epicondyle	26.9 cm	26.5 cm	27.1 cm	26.6 cm
10 cm proximal to the lateral epicondyle	36.2 cm	36.1 cm	36.6 cm	36.4 cm
Upper arm just below the axilla	37.5 cm	38.8 cm	37.7 cm	38.7 cm

*These measurements indicate that the entire upper extremity, and therefore the entire column, are at risk.
**Indicates an increase of >2 cm.

TABLE 18.11. Reported Signs and Symptoms of Lymphedema at Reevaluation of Bernita

QUESTION	RESPONSE
Does your jewelry or clothing feeling uncomfortable or tight?	No
Do you have any feelings or sensations of heaviness, tightness, fullness, or stiffness?	**Yes***
Do you have any aching in your arm?	**Yes***
Have you observed any swelling or increase in arm girth?	No

Note. *Denotes positive signs and symptoms of lymphedema.

SUMMARY

The multifactorial nature of lymphedema makes it extremely important that occupational therapy practitioners adopt a preventive and risk reduction approach to self-management of this chronic condition. Although many occupational therapy practitioners do not hold special certification in lymphedema management, they do have the training, knowledge, and skills to incorporate self-management approaches into interventions to improve the health, wellness, and QoL for those survivors with or at risk of lymphedema.

All occupational therapy practitioners should understand how to monitor for early signs and symptoms of lymphedema by adopting prospective surveillance methods, such as assessing objective circumferential measurements and monitoring self-report symptomology, for triage to a trained lymphedema therapist when an onset is suspected. Triage is critical because occupational therapy practitioners often are on the front line of patient care, working with at-risk survivors on occupational performance issues, and timely referral when lymphedema is suspected may reduce the potential for this condition to become irreversible or chronic in nature.

Occupational therapy practitioners can provide interventions based on a self-management approach by educating clients on the risks associated with lymphedema and integrating risk reduction practices and self-surveillance into daily routines to decrease the risk of developing or furthering lymphedema.

REFERENCES

American Occupational Therapy Association. (2014). Occupational therapy practice framework: Domain and process (3rd ed.). *American Journal of Occupational Therapy, 68*(Suppl. 1), S1–S48. http://doi.org/10.5014/ajot.2014.682006

American Occupational Therapy Association. (2015a). *The role of occupational therapy in chronic disease management.* Retrieved from https://www.aota.org/~/media/Corporate/Files/AboutOT/Professionals/WhatIsOT/HW/Facts/FactSheet_ChronicDisease Management.pdf

American Occupational Therapy Association. (2015b). *The role of occupational therapy with health promotion.* Retrieved from https://www.aota.org/~/media/Corporate/Files/AboutOT/Professionals/WhatIsOT/HW/Facts/FactSheet_HealthPromotion. pdf

Armer, J. M., Hulett, J. M., Bernas, M., Ostby, P., Stewart, B. R., & Cormier, J. N. (2013). Best-practice guidelines in assessment, risk reduction, management, and surveillance for post-breast cancer lymphedema. *Current Breast Cancer Reports, 5,* 134–144. https://doi.org/10.1007/s12609-013-0105-0

Armer, J. M., & Stewart, B. R. (2005). A comparison of four diagnostic criteria for lymphedema in a post-breast cancer population. *Lymphatic Research and Biology, 3,* 208–217 https://doi.org/10.1089/lrb.2005.3.208

Asmussen, P., & Strößenreuther, R., (2012). Compression therapy. In M. Földi & E. Földi (Eds.), *Földi's textbook of lymphology* (pp. 499–560). Munich: Elsevier.

Baxter, M. F., Newman, R., Longprè, S. M., & Polo, K. M. (2017). Occupational therapy's role in cancer survivorship as a chronic condition. *American Journal of Occupational Therapy, 71,* 1–7. https://doi.org/10.5014/ajot.2017.713001

Binkley, J. M., Harris, S. R., Levangie, P. K., Pearl, M., Guglielmino, J., Kraus, V., & Rowden, D. (2012). Patient perspectives on breast cancer treatment side effects and the prospective surveillance model for physical rehabilitation for women with breast cancer. *Cancer, 118*(S8), 2207–2216. https://doi.org/10.1002/cncr.27469

Brown, C. J., Chu, C. S., Cheville, A. L., & Schmitz, K. H. (2013). The prevalence of lymphedema symptoms among survivors of long-term cancer with or at risk for lower limb lymphedema. *American Journal of Physical Medicine & Rehabilitation, 92,* 223–231. https://doi.org/10.1097/PHM.0b013e31826edd97

Chance-Hetzler, J., Armer, J., Van Loo, M., Anderson, B., Harris, R., Ewing, R., & Stewart, B. (2015). Prospective lymphedema surveillance in a clinic setting. *Journal of Personalized Medicine, 5,* 311–325. https://doi.org/10.3390/jpm5030311

Cormier, J. N., Askew, R. L., Mungovan, K. S., Xing, Y., Ross, M. I., & Armer, J. M. (2010). Lymphedema beyond breast cancer: A systematic review and meta-analysis of cancer-related secondary lymphedema. *Cancer, 116,* 5138–5149. https://doi.org/10.1002/cncr.25458

Földi, E., & Földi, M., (2012). Lymphostatic diseases. In M. Földi & E. Földi (Eds.), *Földi's textbook of lymphology* (pp. 175–259). Munich: Elsevier.

Fu, M. R., Ridner, S. H., Hu, S. H., Stewart, B. R., Cormier, J. N., & Armer, J. M. (2013). Psychological impact of lymphedema: A systematic review of literature from 2004 to 2011. *Psycho-Oncology, 22,* 1466–1484. https://doi.org/10.1002/pon.3201

Greene, A. (2015). Epidemiology and morbidity of lymphedema. In A. Greene, S. Slavin, & H. Brorson (Eds.), *Lymphedema* (pp. 33–44). Cham, Switzerland: Springer.

Hayes, S. C., Rye, S., Battistutta, D., DiSipio, T., & Newman, B. (2010). Upper-body morbidity following breast cancer treatment is common, may persist longer-term and adversely influences quality of life. *Health and Quality of Life Outcomes, 8,* 92. https://doi.org/10.1186/1477-7525-8-92

Hunter, E. G., Gibson, R. W., Arbesman, M., & D'Amico, M. (2017). Systematic review of occupational therapy and adult cancer rehabilitation: Part 1. Impact of physical activity and symptom management interventions. *American Journal of Occupational Therapy, 71,* 1–11. https://doi.org/10.5014/ajot.2017.023564

International Society of Lymphology. (2016). The diagnosis and treatment of peripheral lymphedema: 2016 consensus document of the International Society of Lymphology. *Lymphology, 49,* 170–184.

Jammallo, L. S., Miller, C. L., Singer, M., Horick, N. K., Skolny, M. N., Specht, M. C., . . . Taghian, A. G. (2013). Impact of body mass index and weight fluctuation on lymphedema risk in patients treated for breast cancer. *Breast Cancer Research and Treatment, 142,* 59–67. https://doi.org/10.1007/s10549-013-2715-7

Karadibak, D., & Yavuzsen, T. (2015). Evaluation of kinesthetic sense and hand function in women with breast cancer-related lymphedema. *Journal of Physical Therapy Science, 27,* 1617–1675. https://doi.org/10.1589/jpts.27.1671

Lasinski, B. B., Thrift, K. M., Squire, D., Austin, M. K., Smith, K. M., Wanchai, A., . . . Armer, J. M. (2012). A systematic review of the evidence for complete decongestive therapy in the treatment of lymphedema from 2004 to 2011. *PM&R, 4,* 580–601. https://doi.org/10.1016/j.pmrj.2012.05.003

Lorig, K. R., & Holman, H. R. (2003). Self-management education: History, definition, outcomes, and mechanism. *Annals of Behavioral Medicine, 26,* 1–7. https://doi.org/10.1207/S15 324796ABM2601_01.

Lymphoedema Framework. (2006). *Best practice for the management of lymphoedema: International consensus.* London: MEP Ltd.

McLaughlin, S. A. (2012). Lymphedema: Separating fact from fiction. *Oncology Journal, 26,* 242–249.

Merchant, S. J., & Chen, S. L. (2015). Prevention and management of lymphedema after breast cancer treatment. *Breast Journal, 21,* 276–284. https://doi.org/10.1111/tbj.12391

National Lymphedema Network. (2010). *Position statement of the National Lymphedema Network: Training of lymphedema therapists.* Retrieved from https://lymphnet.org/position-papers

National Lymphedema Network. (2011a). *Position statement of the National Lymphedema Network: The diagnosis and treatment of lymphedema.* Retrieved from https://lymphnet.org/position-papers

National Lymphedema Network. (2011b). *Position statement of the National Lymphedema Network: Exercise.* Retrieved from https://lymphnet.org/position-papers

National Lymphedema Network. (2011c). *Position statement of the National Lymphedema Network: Screening and measurement for early detection of breast cancer-related lymphedema.* Retrieved from https://lymphnet.org/position-papers

National Lymphedema Network. (2012). *Position statement of the National Lymphedema Network: Lymphedema risk reduction practices.* Retrieved from https://lymphnet.org/position-papers

National Lymphedema Network. (2018). *Infection and other complications.* Retrieved from https://lymphnet.org/position-papers

Paskett, E. D., Naughton, M. J., McCoy, T. P., Case, L. D., & Abbott, J. M. (2007). The epidemiology of arm and hand swelling in premenopausal breast cancer survivors. *Cancer Epidemiology Biomarkers & Prevention, 16,* 775–782. https://doi.org/10.1158/1055-9965.EPI-06-0168

Sherman, K. A., & Koelmeyer, L. (2013). Psychological predictors of adherence to lymphedema risk minimization guidelines among women with breast cancer. *Psycho-Oncology, 22,* 1120–1126. https://doi.org/10.1002/pon.3111

Shigaki, C. L., Madsen, R., Wanchai, A., Stewart, B. R., & Armer, J. M. (2013). Upper extremity lymphedema: Presence and effect on functioning five years after breast cancer treatment. *Rehabilitation Psychology, 58,* 342–349. http://doi.org/10.1037/a0034657

Silver, J. K., Baima, J., & Mayer, R. S. (2013). Impairment-driven cancer rehabilitation: An essential component of quality care and survivorship. *CA: A Cancer Journal for Clinicians, 63,* 295–318. https://doi.org/10.3322/caac.21186

Smoot, B., Wong, J., Cooper, B., Wanek, L, Topp, K., Byl, N., & Dodd, M. (2010). Upper extremity impairments in women with or without lymphedema following breast cancer treatment. *Journal of Cancer Survivorship, 4,* 167–178. https://doi.org/10.1007/s11764-010-0118-x

Tidhar, D., Armer, J. M., Deutscher, D., Shyu, C. R., Azuri, J., & Madsen, R. (2015). Measurement issues in anthropometric measures of limb volume change in persons at risk for and living with lymphedema: A reliability study. *Journal of Personalized Medicine, 5,* 341–353. https://doi.org/10.3390/jpm5040341

Viehoff, P. B., Gielink, P. D. C., Damstra, R. J., Heerkens, Y. F., Van Ravensberg, D. C., & Neumann, M. H. A. (2015). Functioning in lymphedema from the patients' perspective using the *International Classification of Functioning, Disability and Health (ICF)* as a reference. *Informa Healthcare, 54,* 411–421. https://doi.org/10.3109/0284186X.2014.952389

Chemotherapy-Induced Peripheral Neuropathy

19

Shelby Ubrich, MOT, OTR, and Asfia Mohammed, MOT, OTR

LEARNING OBJECTIVES

After completing this chapter, readers should be able to
- Comprehend the etiology and pathology of chemotherapy-induced peripheral neuropathy (CIPN) performance across the lifespan,
- Identify appropriate assessments for determining the negative effect of CIPN on occupational performance during the evaluation process across the lifespan, and
- Apply common occupational therapy interventions to decrease the negative effect of CIPN on occupational performance across the lifespan.

KEY TERMS AND CONCEPTS

- Chemotherapy-induced peripheral neuropathy
- Chemotherapy-related neurotoxicity
- Dysesthesias
- Epidermis–dermis–fascia technique
- Exercise
- Paresthesias
- Peripheral neuropathy
- Sensory reeducation

INTRODUCTION

Chemotherapy-induced peripheral neuropathy (CIPN) is a commonly experienced adverse side effect that can be caused by some chemotherapy treatments. Common chemotherapy agents that may cause CIPN include platinum compounds, taxanes, vinca alkaloids, thalidomide, and bortezomib (Park et al., 2013). *Peripheral neuropathy* is a disease or degenerative state of the peripheral nerves that affects motor, sensory, or autonomic systems, resulting in potential muscle weakness and atrophy, pain, and numbness. CIPN can cause damage to both motor and sensory nerves, although it is more common among sensory nerves ("Peripheral neuropathy," n.d.). Damage to the sensory nerves can lead to symptoms of *paresthesias* (prickly sensation), *dysesthesias* (painful sensation), and numbness of the hands and feet in a "glove–stocking" distribution (Park et al., 2013). These sensory symptoms can affect cancer survivors' functional status and quality of life (QoL) by causing ataxia, pain, and severe numbness.

The common chemotherapy agents previously listed have been shown to affect components of the nervous system, in particular the dorsal root ganglion (DRG). The DRG is not protected by the blood–nerve barrier and thus is more vulnerable to neurotoxic damage (Park et al., 2013). The platinum-derived agents have been shown to cause nerve cell death in the DRG, in turn causing peripheral neuropathy (Park et al., 2013).

One study of 4,179 patients reported that 68.1% of patients presented with CIPN symptoms within the first month of receiving chemotherapy, 60% reported CIPN at 3 months, and 30% reported it at 6 months or later (Seretny et al., 2014). These data suggest that CIPN does have the potential to subside over time for a small percentage of cancer survivors, but multiple studies have suggested that the prevalence of CIPN is underreported. Numerous researchers and clinicians have called for a gold standard assessment to identify the incidence and prevalence of CIPN with more accuracy (Park et al., 2013).

CIPN is also reported among pediatric cancer patients, but its prevalence and impact are not well known (Moore & Groninger, 2013). In a pilot study assessing use of the Pediatric-Modified Total Neuropathy Score (Ped–mTNS), Gilchrist et al. (2009) indicated that 60% of children reported sensory symptoms and 55% reported motor symptoms. Symptoms observed among pediatric patients include lack of energy, pain, drowsiness, nausea, cough, and lack of appetite (Moore & Groninger, 2013). These symptoms can lead to impairments in daily activities, play, leisure, and education. The side effects of CIPN are linked to functional limitations such as difficulty carrying a heavy object, turning and pivoting, picking up a backpack, and lifting things from the floor (i.e., from a squat) or down from overhead. Adults with CIPN report impairments in common occupations, such as cooking, cleaning, driving, sleeping, functional mobility, exercising, and socializing (Speck et al., 2012).

The impact of CIPN on occupational performance and engagement in daily activities is severe and may result in loss of roles and routines when symptoms limit participation. Occupational therapy intervention is essential for modifying and adapting everyday activities to minimize clients' impairment and increase their participation and performance, leading to an increased QoL. This chapter describes CIPN across the lifespan and reviews evidence for prevention and occupational therapy treatment.

CIPN DEFINING FEATURES ACROSS THE LIFESPAN

Chemotherapy-related neurotoxicity is the result of adverse side effects that can present in the central nervous system or peripheral nervous system, severely affecting QoL (Taillibert et al., 2016). Such neurotoxicities can lead to dose limitations and even discontinuation of treatment dependent on the severity of side effects, which in turn affects the efficacy of treatment (Taillibert et al., 2016). The impact on the peripheral nervous system can be manifested in its three divisions: (1) sensory, (2) motor, and (3) autonomic (Gilchrist, 2012). Sensory and motor symptoms are described in Exhibit 19.1. Patients may also experience a loss of proprioception, spatial awareness, and orientation within the body (Moore & Groninger, 2013). The presentation of CIPN has been reported to be very consistent across the lifespan. Both pediatric and adult patients experience similar symptoms; however, pediatric prevalence and treatment have not been widely investigated.

The severity of symptoms depends on the dosage and regimen of administration of the chemotherapies known to cause CIPN. In many cases, when the presence of CIPN is noted, the dosage is decreased or the regimen is altered to prevent increased severity of CIPN symptoms. Neuropathy-related risk factors can also affect the severity of symptoms, such as underlying neuropathy, alcohol usage, folate or Vitamin B12 deficiency, and hereditary sensory–motor neuropathy (Taillibert et al., 2016).

Both sensory and motor symptoms of CIPN have been reported to negatively affect functional performance. Patients with metastatic breast cancer described difficulty with walking, socializing, driving, standing, cooking, climbing stairs, maintaining balance and steadiness, opening containers, holding onto objects, flipping pages of paper, fastening jewelry, exercising, and sleeping (Speck

et al., 2012). Loss of proprioception can lead to impaired safety and increased risk of falls because it decreases awareness of foot placement (Moore & Groninger, 2013). Pediatric patients have reported symptoms of CIPN that affect occupational performance such as fatigue, pain, and muscle weakness (Moore & Groninger, 2013).

Along with sensory and motor impairments, studies have also shown that symptoms of CIPN can adversely affect long-term QoL, psychosocial function, and sleep. Social isolation and psychological distress were also reported as direct impacts of losing engagement in meaningful activities (Hong et al., 2014). Another study also noted that the estimated reductions in QoL (comprising physical well-being, social well-being, emotional well-being, and functional well-being) among patients undergoing cancer treatment who were experiencing CIPN ranged from 15%–20% (Matsuoka et al., 2018).

Among pediatric and adult patient populations, the goal of pain management is to provide a reduction of symptoms. Currently, there are no options that will completely relieve motor or sensory symptoms of CIPN (Moore & Groninger, 2013). Table 19.1 presents some options to manage symptoms of CIPN (Moore & Groninger, 2013).

OCCUPATIONAL THERAPY'S ROLE IN MANAGING CIPN ACROSS THE LIFESPAN

Because of the complex presentation of CIPN, occupational therapy intervention can vary from patient to patient. Studies have reported that occupational therapy intervention is primarily focused on adaptation and remediation through sensory and functional activities (Pergolotti et al., 2016).

Occupational Profile

Occupational therapy intervention for patients experiencing CIPN begins with developing an occupational profile to understand the extent and experience of the impairments (American Occupational Therapy Association [AOTA], 2017). To compile a robust occupational profile, occupational therapy practitioners collect information to identify patients' concerns related to occupations, meaningful activities, aspects of the environment or client factors limiting engagement, and occupational history that has been affected by CIPN (AOTA, 2014, 2017).

EXHIBIT 19.1. CIPN Symptoms	
SENSORY SYMPTOMS	**MOTOR SYMPTOMS**
▪ Loss of intervention in a glove and stocking distribution ▪ Tactile allodynia (pain from stimuli not typically painful [heightened sensitivity]) ▪ Cold allodynia ▪ Hypersensitivity ▪ Loss of both vibration sensitizing and deep tendon reflexes ▪ Pain that is described as burning, tingling, painful numbness, or electric ▪ Decreased proprioception ▪ Impaired spatial awareness and orientation within the body	▪ Decline in muscle strength ▪ Atrophy ▪ Balance deficits ▪ Gait abnormalities ▪ Decreased manual dexterity

Note. CIPN = chemotherapy-induced peripheral neuropathy.

TABLE 19.1. Therapeutic Symptom Management of CIPN

AGENT	POPULATION	MANAGEMENT
Gabapentin	Adult and pediatric	Has been used effectively to treat neuropathic pain
Pyridostigmine	Adult and pediatric	Assists with neuropathy-related bowel immotility
Nortriptyline	Adult (toxic even in low doses for pediatric patients)	Works by blocking the reuptake of serotonin and norepinephrine in the pain-modulating system within the central nervous system
Opioids: morphine, oxycodone, and fentanyl Tramadol (not for pediatrics)	Adult and pediatric	Can help with painful neuropathies to help manage pain until other agents are effective
Acupuncture	Adult and pediatric	▪ Found to improve sensation and gait, resulting in decreased analgesic use ▪ Low risk of adverse events when provided by a trained professional
Transcutaneous nerve stimulation	Adult and pediatric	Improves neuropathy symptoms, including numbness, pain, and allodynia among diabetic neuropathy patients
Physical rehabilitation	Adult and pediatric	▪ Improves functional outcomes by increasing fine motor dexterity, gait and balance stability, and engagement in ADLs and IADLs ▪ Helps pediatric clients continue to work to meet appropriate developmental milestones

Note. ADLs = activities of daily living; CIPN = chemotherapy-induced peripheral neuropathy; IADLs = instrumental activities of daily living.

Analyzing Occupational Performance

After establishing a robust occupational profile, occupational therapy practitioners analyze clients' current occupational performance: They observe clients' performance in meaningful activities, administer assessments to identify and measure the level of impairments and skills, create goals with the client to address desired outcomes, and determine the mode of intervention on the basis of best practice (AOTA, 2014).

Assessments that can be conducted to establish a baseline include functional assessments such as the Functional Independence Measure (Deutsch et al., 1996), Activity Measure for Post-Acute Care (Jette et al., 2014), range of motion (ROM), manual muscle testing, various sensory tests, and the Functional Assessment of Cancer Therapy–, as in Chapter 17– General (FACT–G; Cella et al., 1993). The FACT–G measures a patient's functional, social, physical, and emotional well-being (Cella et al., 1993). Other important assessments that can provide insight into the patient's daily routine include the Role Checklist (Oakley et al., 1986) and the Model of Human Occupation Screening Tool (Parkinson et al., 2001). The established baseline then allows occupational therapy practitioners to fully see the impact of the client's symptoms on their engagement or lack of engagement in ADLs or IADLs.

Intervention

Occupational therapy intervention may include therapeutic use of occupations and activities, preparatory methods and tasks, education and training, advocacy, and group interventions (AOTA, 2014). Occupational therapy sessions may incorporate preparatory activities, such as aerobic exercise, thermal therapy, stretching, and strengthening,

as recommended by Davies (2013). Education and training can include incorporating energy conservation techniques to enhance occupational performance as well as establishing routines to maximize time management and participation. Most important, occupational therapy intervention can include adapting tasks and environments to optimize occupational performance in desired occupations and activities. Patients have reported that functional engagement decreases their CIPN symptoms (Speck et al., 2012).

Occupational therapy practitioners may also find themselves needing to advocate for services that may benefit cancer survivors with CIPN. For example, practitioners may need to initiate a consultation for counseling services if the client is struggling with anxiety or stress that is affecting occupational performance. Anxiety and stress can exacerbate CIPN symptoms and require appropriate intervention (Davies, 2013). Occupational therapy intervention may also focus on empowering clients to obtain resources to enhance occupational participation and increase well-being (AOTA, 2014).

Occupational therapy practitioners establish treatment plans that are directed by the selection and implementation of various approaches to intervention (AOTA, 2014). Approaches to intervention include health promotion, remediation, restoration, maintenance, modification, and prevention. Occupational therapy practitioners use these approaches to select appropriate practice models, frames of reference, or treatment theories to guide intervention (AOTA, 2014).

One example of restorative intervention that has been used to treat CIPN includes stimulation to promote nerve conduction through the use of Kinesio Taping® to increase blood flow and nerve conduction to the extremities (Lee & Mohammed, 2018). Other interventions shown to have positive benefits in preventing secondary musculoskeletal impairments, in turn bringing patients closer to their functional baseline, include active ROM exercises and strengthening or simple active movement (Kim et al., 2015).

Promoting clients' awareness through education about CIPN before chemotherapy is initiated can provide substantial benefits. Because one of the factors used to manage the severity of CIPN is the dosage and administration of the aggravating chemotherapy, it is very important that clients are aware of the signs of CIPN. Recognizing the signs and symptoms of CIPN can drive clients to report any symptoms to their oncologist right away, which may lead to dosage reduction immediately. This limits the prolonged exposure to the problematic chemotherapy agent, decreasing the severity of CIPN among clients treated with the aggravating chemotherapies.

Modification and adaptation of therapeutic occupations and activities have been shown to improve functional outcomes through the increase of functional participation (Speck et al., 2012). Modifications can include building up utensil grips to compensate for decreased grip strength, wearing clothing that is not a noxious stimulus, or sitting down to engage in activities previously performed by standing to increase safety in response to numbness in lower extremities.

Environmental modifications can be made as well. Some environmental modifications include reorganizing cabinets to place important items within reach; removing fall hazards such as throw rugs, clutter, and wires; and adding light to dark areas that the client frequently visits. Community tasks can also be modified. For example, clients can use an electric scooter in a store if they are not able to tolerate walking around during shopping or obtain a handicap parking sticker to limit the distance from the parking lot to the store.

Commonly Used Assessments Specific to Sequelae

Although there is no gold standard assessment tool for CIPN among adults, occupational therapy practitioners can use a limited number of assessments to fully identify clients' impairments to develop client-centered interventions that support functional performance. Some commonly used assessments to measure client factors include

- ROM;
- Manual muscle testing;
- Grip strength;
- Pinch strength;
- Sensation;
- Various assessments of the arm, shoulder, and hand;
- Brief Fatigue Inventory (MD Anderson Cancer Center, 2018); and
- Pittsburgh Sleep Quality Index (Buysse et al., 1989; see Table 19.2).

Several grading systems also are used clinically to classify the severity of CIPN, such as the National Cancer Institute's Common Terminology Criteria for Adverse Events (CTCAE; Brewer et al., 2016) and the Total Neuropathy Score (TNS; Gilchrest et al., 2009). In a review by Cavaletti et al. (2007), the TNS showed more sensitivity to changes in CIPN. The Ped–mTNS is currently noted in the literature for assessing peripheral neuropathy in the pediatric

population (school-age children ages 5–18 years). Alternatively, in the pediatric population, the CTCAE was formerly the most commonly used measure for peripheral neuropathy (Gilchrist et al., 2009). However, the CTCAE is very extensive and broad in its scope and lacks the ability to identify the specific characteristics of CIPN. The Ped–mTNS identifies deficits specifically related to pin sensibility, vibration sensation, muscle strength, and deep tendon reflexes (Gilchrist et al., 2009).

After using appropriate assessments to gather necessary information regarding clients' functional capacity and deficits, occupational therapy practitioners should develop an intervention plan to address clients' needs for management of symptoms as a result of CIPN for improved functional engagement in all occupations and improved QoL. Reassessment of symptoms and occupational performance is completed intermittently, and appropriate revisions to the intervention plan are made throughout treatment.

Client factors such as neuromusculoskeletal and movement-related functions are traditionally measured through routine assessment of ROM, manual muscle testing, grip strength, and pinch strength. The Nine Hole Peg Test (Mathiowetz et al., 1985) provides a more objective measure of finger dexterity that can demonstrate progress or regression over time, which allows for improved prognostication of the outcome of functional performance of tasks (Kim et al., 2015; Wang et al., 2015). Sensory function is measured by presence or absence of pain; clients' ability to recognize light touch or deep touch, sharp or dull sensations, and temperature; stereognosis; and proprioception (Kim et al., 2015).

The Semmes Weinstein Monofilament Test (Weinstein, 1993) can be used to measure a more precise degree of sensory loss and is very sensitive to comparison of sensory loss with the return of sensations. The Moberg Pickup Test (Ng et al., 1999) is even more functionally representative of fine motor dexterity and sensation because it uses small everyday objects to be picked up, held, manipulated, and identified.

More specifically defined functional assessments of patient perception include the Disabilities of the Arm, Shoulder, and Hand (DASH; Hudak et al., 1996) and the Manual Ability Measure (MAM; Chen et al., 2005; Pergolotti et al., 2016). These assessments can be used as precursor and distinguishing tools for intervention focus because they use practical, everyday functional tasks to identify clients' perceived ability to perform such tasks and further reflect with actual performance in treatment sessions. The DASH and MAM present the opportunity for increased awareness, self-initiated problem solving, and identification of possible modifications facilitated by the occupational therapy practitioner (Chen et al., 2005; Hudak et al., 1996; Pergolotti et al., 2016).

Global and specific mental functions are also client factors to be assessed and accounted for through the typical interview process, including the use of specific measures related to fatigue and sleep. The side effects of CIPN clients experience and the extent of such interference can greatly affect their state of fatigue and sleep, which, in turn, affects their functional status in daily occupations. The Brief Fatigue Inventory (MD Anderson Cancer Center, 2018) can be used to assess the severity of fatigue experienced as a result of

TABLE 19.2. CIPN Assessment Tools	
ASSESSMENT	**BRIEF DESCRIPTION**
ROM	Evaluation of active or passive ROM
Manual muscle testing	Evaluation of strength
Jamar dynamometer and pinch gauge (Bechtol, 1954)	▪ Jamar dynamometer measures grip strength ▪ Pinch gauge measures tip, key, and palmar pinch
Nine Hole Peg Test (Mathiowetz et al., 1985; Wang et al., 2015)	▪ Assesses finger dexterity ▪ Involves picking up, holding, and manipulating pegs for placement into and removal from board as fast as possible
Moberg Pickup Test (Ng et al., 1999)	▪ Assesses finger dexterity and sensation ▪ Involves picking up, holding, manipulating, and identifying small objects ▪ Timed, quick, and inexpensive
Sensation	▪ Pain ▪ Light touch versus deep touch ▪ Sharp versus dull ▪ Hot versus cold ▪ Stereognosis ▪ Proprioception
Semmes Weinstein Monofilament Test (Weinstein, 1993)	▪ Set of monofilaments that vary in thickness and diameter and are used to map out sensory loss ▪ The results are useful in comparing sensory loss with the return of sensations
Disabilities of the Arm, Shoulder, and Hand (Hudak et al., 1996)	▪ Questionnaire asks about symptoms and ability to perform certain activities ▪ 30 items
Manual Ability Measure (Chen et al., 2005)	▪ Questionnaire on perceived ease or difficulty that a person may experience when performing unilateral and bilateral ADLs ▪ 20-item and 36-item versions scored on a 4-point scale
Brief Fatigue Inventory (MD Anderson Cancer Center, 2018)	Short scale that quickly assesses severity of fatigue experienced by cancer patients as well as fatigue's impact on patients' ability to function over the previous 24 hours
Pittsburgh Sleep Quality Index (Buysse et al., 1989)	▪ Used to measure adults' quality and patterns of sleep ▪ Differentiates "poor" from "good" sleep quality by measuring 7 areas (subjective quality, latency, duration, habitual efficiency, disturbances, medications, and daytime dysfunction) over the past month

Note. ADLs = activities of daily living; CIPN = chemotherapy-induced peripheral neuropathy; ROM = range of motion.

various treatment symptoms, such as CIPN, and the Pittsburgh Sleep Quality Index (Buysse et al., 1989) measures the quality and patterns of sleep. Therefore, it is important to be familiar with many assessments to fully address clients' current needs for improved management of CIPN and functional status.

Occupational Therapy Interventions Focused on Sequelae

Occupational therapy intervention requires a multifaceted approach when addressing cancer survivors' functional abilities and limitations affected by CIPN. No one intervention approach is best or suitable to meet the needs of every individual living with CIPN. Some commonly used interventions to manage the impact of CIPN include increased awareness of deficits and safety concerns, adaptation and compensatory strategies, neuromuscular electrical stimulation, sensory reeducation, use of compression stockings, exercise, Kinesio Taping, and education about coping

strategies. See Table 19.3 for a brief description of proposed interventions.

Awareness of CIPN

The promotion of increased awareness pertains to insight into clients' current functional status and limitations, with emphasis on safe performance of tasks in various environments. Individuals living with CIPN are at a significantly greater risk of falling and injuring themselves secondary to impaired sensation, proprioception, and muscle strength and control (Gewandter et al., 2013; Holz et al., 2017; Veale, 2016). Thus, it is particularly important to be fully aware of one's surroundings at all times with respect to flat surfaces without and with transitions to uneven terrain, which are more difficult to negotiate with impaired sensation or strength (Holz et al., 2017; MD Anderson Cancer Center, 2017).

Occupational therapy practitioners may need to make modifications to the environment, such removing tripping hazards (e.g., loose rugs, extension cords,

TABLE 19.3.   CIPN Interventions

INTERVENTION	BRIEF DESCRIPTION
Increased awareness	▪ Self-awareness and insight into current functional status and limitations ▪ Awareness of skin integrity ▪ Safe performance in various environments
Adaptation and compensatory strategies	▪ Modifications to environment, tools, or techniques, with emphasis on task analysis
Neuromuscular electrical stimulation	▪ Transcutaneous electrical nerve stimulation units use electrical fields to directly affect the transmission of pain ▪ Evidence is limited for the cancer population
Sensory reeducation	▪ Various textures ▪ Vibration ▪ Tactile input ▪ Proprioception
Compression stockings	▪ Reduce pain ▪ Provide more tactile input
Exercise	▪ Improves functional strength for safe performance of functional mobility and participation in all occupations
Kinesio Taping	▪ Alleviates compression of nerves ▪ Provides pain relief
Coping strategies	▪ Mindfulness ▪ Coping skills ▪ Meditation ▪ Yoga ▪ Diaphragmatic breathing ▪ Sleep hygiene

Note. CIPN = chemotherapy-induced peripheral neuropathy.

unnecessary obstacles) and adding appropriate durable medical equipment (e.g., shower chair, tub transfer bench, bedside commode), rails, or grab bars in areas of concern for loss of balance, such as transitions within the home and bathrooms (Holz et al., 2017; Pergolotti et al., 2016). Additional considerations include daily skin checks for detection of any cuts or injuries that may put clients at increased risk for infection because of impaired sensation. Practicing proper hygiene and wearing loose cotton socks with protective shoes for good support are also important for maintaining skin integrity and safety with balance (MD Anderson Cancer Center, 2017). Heightened sensory experiences, such as severe pain, and significantly decreased sensory experiences, such as numbness, can greatly affect functional independence and safety for individuals living with CIPN. Compression stockings have been shown to decrease the sensation of pain (e.g., pins and needles, burning) as well as improve sensory feedback, allowing for improved functional independence with occupations (Holz et al., 2017).

Modifying techniques and the environment

Task analysis is key to breaking down tasks into smaller parts, making modifications to the techniques clients are using, and altering the environmental components for functional independence. Adaptations and compensatory strategies evolve from increased awareness of functional

deficits and active problem solving to improve functional capacity and, ultimately, performance of occupations. Adaptations or modifications can consist of adaptive equipment from built-up foam tubing, nonslip materials, button hooks, rocker knives, and the use of other adaptive tools to perform functional tasks to maintain independence as well as the use of assistive devices during such tasks for improved balance and overall safety (Kim et al., 2015; Pergolotti et al., 2016; Speck et al., 2012).

The implementation of coping skills along with environmental modifications can further support task analysis. Self-management strategies are effective in reducing the impact of CIPN symptoms during engagement in occupations (Holz et al., 2017; Speck et al., 2012). Some reported self-management strategies include

▪ Focus on movement to reduce symptoms,
▪ Attitude awareness,
▪ Mindfulness,
▪ Meditation,
▪ Yoga,
▪ Diaphragmatic breathing, and
▪ Sleep hygiene.

Establishing and restoring function

Neuromuscular reeducation and sensory reeducation are intervention approaches used for restoration of function. Although there is limited evidence for the cancer population, making this is an area of further opportunity for research, the use of neuromuscular electrical stimulation (e.g., transcutaneous electrical nerve stimulation) can help with chronic pain related to CIPN when it is resistant to conservative treatment. It can be administered by an occupational therapist as well as many other medical professionals (Holz et al., 2017; Kim et al., 2015; Taillibert et al., 2016; Veale, 2016). Sympathetic nerve blocks and sympathetic neurolysis, which is delivered by an injection and spinal cord or peripheral nerve stimulators, are permanent implantable devices administered by a physician. Because they are more invasive interventions, they are less commonly seen (Kim et al., 2015).

Sensory reeducation focuses primarily on desensitization and restoration of sensory function with exposure to various textures, vibration, tactile input, and proprioception. For instance, various textures are introduced at areas of sensory loss and areas of normal sensation to allow the brain to process and compare the tactile input for sensory retraining. As mentioned previously, compression stockings can also help increase tactile input for improved sensory feedback as well as decrease pain (Holz et al., 2017). Increased attention to tasks using vision to provide the brain with necessary feedback is also recommended secondary to impaired sensation.

The literature shows the most promising support for use of exercise, which has been reported to consistently improve symptoms of CIPN and overall functional well-being (Holz et al., 2017; Kim et al., 2015; Speck et al., 2012; Taillibert et al., 2016; Veale, 2016). *Exercise* aimed at improving active ROM, strength, balance, stability, and posture has a restorative focus as it relates to functional participation in occupation (Kim et al., 2015). Exercise should be noted as improving weakness, fatigue, and other neuromuscular deficits as a result of CIPN symptoms rather than as having a direct impact on the symptoms of CIPN (Veale, 2016). Thus, it can be concluded that exercise has an impact on functional independence, QoL, and the reduction of falls (Veale, 2016).

Kinesio Tape has been used to minimize the effects of certain neurologic conditions, such as cerebral palsy (Kinesio University, 2013). The Kinesio Tex Gold Finger Print, in comparison with the Kinesio Tex Classic, was designed to be particularly effective with circulatory, lymphatic, and neurological treatments. This is possible because the fingerprint advancement allows for a more microtargeted fingerprint pattern in the adhesion of the tape.

The *epidermis–dermis–fascia technique* (EDF) is a dermal taping technique that may lead to positive responses in the brain (Kinesio University, 2013). It has been used to counter certain neurologic conditions such as cerebral palsy. The EDF technique for management of CIPN involves thinly cut strips placed superficially with 0%–5% tension anchored on the distal aspect of the limb traveling along the affected area proximally. See Figures 19.1–19.3 for a visual of this EDF technique. The EDF technique is thought to lift the epidermal layers, providing increased blood flow among the epidermis, dermis, and fascia and decreasing the noxious sensation to the affected areas (Lee & Mohammed, 2018). Although no formal studies have been conducted on the use of this

FIGURE 19.1. EDF technique for CIPN on toes.

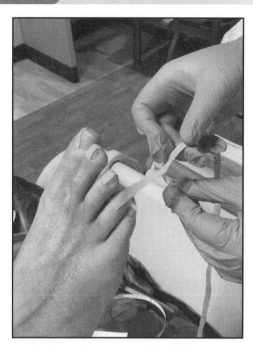

Note. CIPN = chemotherapy-induced peripheral neuropathy; EDF = epidermis–dermis–fascia.
Source. A. Mohammed. Used with permission.

FIGURE 19.2. EDF technique for CIPN: Applying tape over the back of toes.

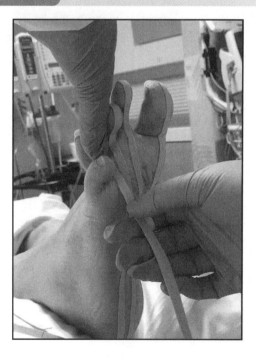

Note. CIPN = chemotherapy-induced peripheral neuropathy; EDF = epidermis–dermis–fascia.
Source. A. Mohammed. Used with permission.

FIGURE 19.3. EDF technique for CIPN on bottom of foot.

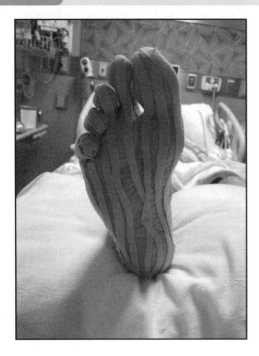

Note. CIPN = chemotherapy-induced peripheral neuropathy; EDF = epidermis–dermis–fascia.
Source. A. Mohammed. Used with permission.

technique for CIPN management, patients have reported that the presence of the tape has allowed them to tolerate functional mobility and grooming while standing (Lee & Mohammed, 2018). Further research on the use of Kinesio Tape with CIPN management is warranted. Case Example 19.1 describes the use of kineseotaping to manage CIPN with one adult patient with leukemia, and Case Example 19.2 describes CIPN management of one pediatric cancer survivor.

SUMMARY

CIPN is a common, recognizable side effect of cancer treatment that requires proper identification of its functional impact on occupational performance and engagement in occupations for clients to achieve independence and fulfillment. Although a gold standard assessment tool is yet to be identified, skilled clinicians can implement a variety of assessments and modalities to improve clients' QoL.

Occupational therapy practitioners have a unique opportunity to comprehensively identify how CIPN affects clients' roles and routines from a holistic approach and recognition of physical, sensory, functional, and psychological components. These client factors are collectively addressed by a compilation of modes of intervention, including modification, restoration, and promotion of awareness. Although the negative side effects of CIPN may improve over time with a multifaceted approach of interventions, the overall goal is symptom management

CASE EXAMPLE 19.1. MRS. MARTIN: LIVING WITH AND MANAGING CIPN

Occupational profile

Mrs. Martin is a 61-year-old woman presenting to occupational therapy services with a cancer diagnosis of myelodysplastic syndrome with a planned haploidentical stem cell transplant (SCT), which is a type of allogeneic transplant using cells from a half-matched donor. She is admitted to the inpatient unit in acute care for her chemotherapy induction 6 days before her scheduled SCT. Mrs. Martin is referred to occupational therapy services for participation in an exercise group during her prolonged hospitalization. Before admission, she was living with her mother and was independent with all ADLs in the home.

Mrs. Martin is a retired schoolteacher and reports her hobbies as playing board games and doing puzzles. Her home is 160 miles from the hospital, and she arrived with her mother in their own car. On discharge, she will need to stay locally for 100 days to ensure continued recovery and good health, with immediate availability to return to the hospital should any complications arise. At discharge, she will be staying at a

hospitality apartment that is one level with no steps to negotiate and with access to a walk-in shower. Mrs. Martin has no durable medical equipment (DME) of her own; however, she does have a wheelchair available to her at the hospitality home for use during her stay.

Analysis of occupational performance

At initial evaluation through informal questioning and interviewing, Mrs. Martin was noted to be independent with all functional mobility and ADLs and reported no complaints with IADLs. The only complaint she reported was some discomfort in her knees with mobility secondary to comorbid arthritis. She presented with no impairments in all areas of client factors and performance skills, so the occupational therapist initially took preventive and maintenance approaches in establishing the intervention plan for Mrs. Martin, given her treatment course and expected prolonged hospitalization.

(Continued)

CASE EXAMPLE 19.1. MRS. MARTIN: LIVING WITH AND MANAGING CIPN *(Cont.)*

Intervention process

The occupational therapist initially provided education to address the importance of consistent out-of-bed activity (6–8 hours per day) and continued participation in habits, roles, and routines in the hospital environment as similarly and consistently as possible to those of her home environment. The therapist also provided initial teaching of an upper-extremity home exercise program that included resistance exercise bands to help Mrs. Martin maintain her current strength and endurance and prevent deconditioning with extended hospitalization.

The occupational therapist provided specific education for performance of resistive exercises only as appropriate with regard to platelet count, with completion of exercises with active range only and no resistance when platelets dropped below 20,000 platelets per microliter, as tolerated, because resistive exercises are contraindicated below this level. Mrs. Martin was to perform the home exercise program independently on a daily basis three times per day, 10 repetitions each time, as tolerated. Group exercise class was also offered, and Mrs. Martin was encouraged to attend three times per week at 1-hour durations for improved strength, endurance, and quality of life with her prolonged medical needs and hospitalization and the accompanying risk for deconditioning.

Occupational therapy interventions focused on sequelae

Mrs. Martin was seen for 1–2 individual treatment sessions per week during her first month of hospitalization because she was not attending the group exercise sessions and was mostly observed performing ADLs and functional mobility with supervision and fair compliance with out-of-bed activity. These individual treatment sessions focused on therapeutic exercise, compensatory strategies, positioning, and DME recommendations (i.e., bedside commode, tub bench, handheld showerhead) to increase Mrs. Martin's safety and independence with ADLs.

At about the 1-month mark, Mrs. Martin presented with decreased out-of-bed tolerance and increased need for assistance, requiring a rolling walker and increased assistance with ADLs secondary to significant complaints of neuropathic pain in her bilateral lower extremities (BLEs) affecting her functional mobility for participation in ADLs. Thus, treatment interventions became more focused on sensory reeducation with exposure to various textures, positioning with elevation of BLEs, and introduction of epidermis-dermis-fascia (EDF) technique with Kinesio Tape for alleviation of debilitating pain from CIPN.

The occupational therapist applied a test strip of Kinesio Tape for 24 hours to clear Mrs. Martin of any skin integrity concerns before proceeding with the Kinesio Tape technique for CIPN. No skin integrity concerns were noted, so the therapist applied Kinesio Tape to Mrs. Martin's BLEs (feet) for improved comfort and pain relief from CIPN, using the EDF technique with no tension. After cleansing and drying both feet, the therapist applied thin strips of fingerprint Kinesio Tape from the anterior position, anchored on the nail beds and traveling along the affected area proximally, and secured at the posterior position of the heel with no tension on the dorsum of each foot.

Mrs. Martin was educated on having Kinesio Tape removed if it was bothersome to any degree, including itching or redness; instruction was also given for slow, controlled removal and use of adhesive remover if needed. Fortunately, Mrs. Martin presented with no complaints before, during, or after taping throughout use of the treatment intervention during hospitalization.

The occupational therapist first trialed the EDF technique with Kinesio Tape on the dorsum aspect of Mrs. Martin's feet, before further trialing it on the ventral aspect of her feet, to identify the effectiveness of the intervention to the most problematic area, given that Mrs. Martin had reported that her pain was most significant at the dorsum aspect compared with the ventral. She was instructed to wear any given application for only 5 days at a time and to ensure proper cleansing and drying of skin (with no use of lotions) before reapplication of Kinesio Tape while performing routine skin checks.

On follow-up, Mrs. Martin reported significant improvement in functional participation in mobility and ADLs in her hospital room, secondary to decreased pain in BLEs with use of Kinesio Tape with the EDF technique. The occupational therapist provided family training during the second and third applications secondary to effectiveness of the intervention to allow for continued implementation and improved functional independence with ADLs and functional mobility during hospitalization in preparation for discharge to home. Despite improvements in pain management and functional performance, recommendations for DME (i.e., bedside commode, shower chair, grab bars, a handheld showerhead) were still warranted in the home setting because of fall safety concerns and fatigue management needs affected by the presence of CIPN.

CASE EXAMPLE 19.2. KELLY: CHILDHOOD WITH CIPN

Kelly is an 11-year-old girl with a history of acute lymphoblastic leukemia who has not achieved remission despite treatment. Her course of treatment was complicated by severe colitis and *Clostridium difficile* infection as well as strokelike symptoms associated with methotrexate toxicity. Kelly's treatment course also included high doses of vincristine. On initial evaluation, she was living with her parents and three older sisters, was completing some homeschooling, and reported enjoying art and video games; however, she reported difficulty engaging in leisure activities.

Kelly presented with gross weakness ("fair minus" or 3 minus/5 at shoulders, and "good minus" or 4 minus/5 distally to upper extremities [UEs]). She had decreased dorsiflexion to her right foot, significant tightness with shortening of her hamstrings, and in long sitting was unable to achieve full extension of her right knee. Kelly had a recent fall at home and was fearful of mobility in the hospital setting with her occupational therapist. She became very aggravated and anxious on initiation of occupational therapy sessions, often working herself up to the point of throwing up in an attempt to avoid mobility.

Initial sensation impairments were difficult to assess in relation to her behaviors because she would not directly communicate or answer the occupational therapist's questions. Impairments noted were based on the functional impairments observed, which included poor functional mobility, fair static and poor dynamic standing balance, impaired postural alignment, fear of mobility, decreased engagement in self-care activities, and impaired ability to reach overhead (which included maintaining standing balance with attempt to brush her hair).

Kelly also displayed significant body image impairments related to treatment interventions. She was resistive to adaptive equipment, including an ankle–foot orthosis (AFO) and assistive device for mobility. She was very self-conscious about engagement in ADL routines near the bathroom mirror because her hair was falling out.

Kelly also displayed further symptoms associated with peripheral neuropathy to bilateral hands, including impaired ability to hold a writing tool, impaired digit opposition, decreased gross grasp, impaired fine motor control, and impaired ability to maintain a hand hold on heavy objects (e.g., a full cup). Again, despite noted impairments, she was resistive to formal assessment.

Despite multiple impairments and a long cancer treatment, Kelly was new to therapy services and remained difficult to engage, although multiple occupational therapists met with her to see whether she would respond differently on the basis of personality and rapport.

In an effort to maximize safety and fall prevention in the setting of poor patient engagement, the focus was initially on fitting and trialing the AFO and on using adaptive devices for functional mobility to allow Kelly to engage in mobility in both home and community settings. This would also increase Kelly's confidence in standing and ease her ability to complete her ADL routine, especially those tasks requiring the use of her UEs overhead and with reach out of her base of support.

An AFO was fitted with the assistance of an orthotist, and a rolling walker was provided. Kelly and her family were educated on effects of high-dose chemotherapy agents, the benefits of assistive devices, and the importance of Kelly's consistent engagement in therapeutic interventions and ADL routines to improve her safety; decrease falls risk; and aid in consistent improvement to strength, balance, and endurance. This required frequent reeducation because Kelly was highly sedentary and often received the occupational therapist in the side-lying position in bed.

Kelly displayed significant improvements in postural alignment, standing balance, functional mobility, and endurance with just the initiation of an AFO. However, outside her therapy sessions, she resisted using her AFO and completely refused to use a rolling walker. In this particular case, family dynamics also played a role in consistency of engagement in interventions because both parents worked full-time and were caring for another child with a chronic illness. Focus shifted to improving proprioceptive input to Kelly's feet (e.g., consistent use of sneakers during mobility both in and outside the home), mirror therapy for visual input to postural alignment and step pattern, and high-level weight-bearing activities (e.g., dancing, Hula-Hoop, pushing activities).

Cotreatments were completed occasionally with physical therapy to maximize consistency and follow-through. Kelly became resistive to this after two sessions as well, reporting, "I don't want to do anything fun, just let me do my exercises and be done." She would no longer engage in leisure activities as part of therapeutic intervention. Focus again shifted to dynamic movements and ability to transition from tailored sitting on the floor to standing to allow engagement in play with her sisters in her home environment. Kelly was again fearful and aggressive in this area, but with consistency from the occupational therapist, she was able to improve from maximum assistance to standing from a seated position to minimal assistance without use of the AFO.

At this stage, Kelly's treatment remains largely outpatient, and because of the previously mentioned family dynamics, consistency in engagement in outpatient therapy has remained minimal. The occupational therapist sees Kelly intermittently during inpatient admissions, and Kelly remains grossly at minimal assist level for a basic self-care routine; however, she continues to display impairments in the areas of gross motor movements (jumping, skipping, running) and fine motor coordination (impaired ability to hold a writing utensil, difficulty cutting food, and impaired digit opposition). She also remains a high falls risk associated with limitations in balance, postural alignment, and endurance associated with compensatory movements related to peripheral neuropathy and right foot drop.

because most clients have some degree of residual side effects that influence their functional performance and QoL over the lifespan.

REFERENCES

American Occupational Therapy Association. (2014). Occupational therapy practice framework: Domain and process (3rd ed.). *American Journal of Occupational Therapy, 68*(Suppl. 1), S1–S48. https://doi.org/10.5014/ajot.2014.682006

American Occupational Therapy Association. (2017). AOTA occupational profile template. *American Journal of Occupational Therapy, 71,* 7112420030. https://doi.org/10.5014/ajot.2017.716S12

Bechtol, C. O. (1954). Grip test: The use of a dynamometer with adjustable handle spacings. *Journal of Bone and Joint Surgery, 36A*(4), 820–824.

Brewer, J. R., Morrison, G., Dolan, M. E., & Fleming, G. F. (2016). Chemotherapy-induced peripheral neuropathy: Current status and progress. *Gynecologic Oncology, 140,* 176–183. https://doi.org/10.1016/j.ygyno.2015.11.011

Buysse, D. J., Reynolds, C. F., Monk, T. H., Berman, S. R., & Kupfer, D. J. (1989). The Pittsburgh Sleep Quality Index (PSQI): A new instrument for psychiatric research and practice. *Psychiatry Research, 28,* 193–213. https://doi.org/10.1016/0165-1781(89)90047-4

Cavaletti, G., Frigeni, B., Lanzani, F., Platti, M., Rota, S., Briani, C., . . . Italian NETox Group. (2007). The Total Neuropathy Score as an assessment tool for grading the course of chemotherapy-induced peripheral neurotoxicity: Comparison with the National Cancer Institute Common Toxicity Scale. *Journal of the Peripheral Nervous System, 12,* 210–215. https://doi.org/10.1111/j.1529-8027.2007.00141.x

Cella, D. F., Tulsky, D. S., Gray, G., Sarafian, B., Linn, E., Bonomi, A., . . . Brannon, J. (1993). The Functional Assessment of Cancer Therapy scale: Development and validation of the general measure. *Journal of Clinical Oncology, 11,* 570–579. https://doi.org/10.1200/JCO.1993.11.3.570

Chen, C., Granger, C., Peimer, C., Moy, O., & Wald, S. (2005). Manual Ability Measure (MAM-16): A preliminary report on a new patient-centered and task-oriented outcome measure of hand function. *Journal of Hand Surgery, 30,* 207–216. https://doi.org/10.1016/j.jhsb.2004.12.005

Davies, P. S. (2013). Chronic pain management in the cancer survivor: Tips for primary care providers. *Nurse Practitioner, 38*(6), 28–38. https://doi.org/10.1097/01.NPR.0000429893.95631.63

Deutsch, A., Braun, S., & Granger, C. V. (1996). The Functional Independence Measure (FIM Instrument) and the Functional Independence Measure for Children (WeeFIM Instrument): Ten years of development. *Clinical Reviews in Physical and Rehabilitation Medicine, 8,* 267–281.

Gewandter, J. S., Fan, L., Magnuson, A., Mustian, K., Peppone, L., Heckler, C., . . . Mohile, S. G. (2013). Falls and functional impairments in cancer survivors with chemotherapy-induced peripheral neuropathy (CIPN): A University of Rochester CCOP study. *Supportive Care in Cancer, 21,* 2059–2066. https://doi.org/10.1007/s00520-013-1766-y

Gilchrist, L. (2012). Chemotherapy-induced peripheral neuropathy in pediatric cancer patients. *Seminars in Pediatric Neurology, 19,* 9–17. https://doi.org/10.1016/j.spen.2012.02.011

Gilchrist, L. S., Tanner, L., & Hooke, M. C. (2009). Measuring chemotherapy-induced peripheral neuropathy in children: Development of the Ped-mTNS and pilot study results. *Rehabilitation Oncology, 27*(3), 7–15.

Holz, S. C., Wininger, Y. D., Cooper, C., & Smith, S. R. (2017). Managing neuropathy after chemotherapy in patients with cancer. *Archives of Physical Medicine and Rehabilitation, 98,* 605–607. https://doi.org/10.1016/j.apmr.2016.08.461

Hong, J. S., Tian, J., & Wu, L. H. (2014). The influence of chemotherapy-induced neurotoxicity on psychological distress and sleep disturbance in cancer patients. *Current Oncology, 21,* 174–180. https://doi.org/10.3747/co.21.1984

Hudak, P., Amadio, P. C., Bombardier, C., & Upper Extremity Collaborative Group. (1996). Development of an upper extremity outcome measure: The DASH (Disabilities of the Arm, Shoulder, and Hand). *American Journal of Industrial Medicine, 29,* 602–608. https://doi.org/10.1002/(SICI)1097-0274(199606)29:6<602::AID-AJIM4>3.0.CO;2-L

Jette, D. U., Stilphen, M., Ranganathan, V. K., Passek, S. D., Frost, F. S., & Jette, A. M. (2014). Validity of the AM-PAC "6-Clicks" inpatient daily activity and basic mobility short forms. *Physical Therapy, 94,* 379–391. https://doi.org/10.2522/ptj.20130199

Kim, J. H., Dougherty, P. M., & Abdi, S. (2015). Basic science and clinical management of painful and non-painful chemotherapy-related neuropathy. *Gynecologic Oncology, 136,* 453–459. https://doi.org/10.1016/j.ygyno.2015.01.524

Kinesio University. (2013). *KT3: Clinical concepts and advanced taping methods.* Albuquerque, NM: Kinesio Taping Association International.

Lee, C., & Mohammed, A. (2018, April). *Therapeutic use of K-tape to minimize neuropathy induced functional deficits in the cancer population.* Poster presented at the American Occupational Therapy Association Annual Conference, Salt Lake City.

Mathiowetz, V., Weber, K., Kashman, N., & Volland, G. (1985). Adult norms for the Nine-Hole Peg Test of finger dexterity. *Occupational Therapy Journal of Research, 5,* 24–28. https://doi.org/10.1177/153944928500500102

Matsuoka, H., Nakamura, K., Matsubara, Y., Ida, N., Saijo, M., Ogawa, C., & Masuyama, H. (2018). The influence of chemotherapy-induced peripheral neuropathy on quality of life of gynecologic cancer survivors. *International Journal of Gynecologic Cancer, 28,* 1394–1402. https://doi.org/10.1097/igc.0000000000001320

MD Anderson Cancer Center. (2017). *Peripheral neuropathy.* Retrieved from https://www.mdanderson.org/patient-education/Endocrine/Peripheral-Neuropathy_docx_pe.pdf

MD Anderson Cancer Center. (2018). *Brief Fatigue Inventory (BFI).* Retrieved from https://www.mdanderson.org/research/departments-labs-institutes/departments-divisions/symptom-research/symptom-assessment-tools/brief-fatigue-inventory.html

Moore, R. J., & Groninger, H. (2013). Chemotherapy-induced peripheral neuropathy in pediatric cancer patients. *Cureus, 5*(6), e124. https://doi.org/10.7759/cureus.124

Ng, C., Ho, D., & Chow, S. (1999). The Moberg Pickup Test: Results of testing with a standard protocol. *Journal of Hand Therapy, 12,* 309–312. https://doi.org/10.1016/s0894-1130(99)80069-6

Oakley, F. M., Kielhofner, G., Barris, R., & Reichler, R. (1986). The Role Checklist: Development and empirical assessment of reliability. *Occupational Therapy Journal of Research, 6,* 158–170. https://doi.org/10.1177/153944928600600303

Park, S. B., Goldstein, D., Krishnan, A. V., Lin, C. L., Friedlander, M. L., Cassidy, J., . . . Kiernan, M. C. (2013). Chemotherapy-induced peripheral neurotoxicity: A critical analysis. *CA: A Cancer Journal for Clinicians, 63,* 419–437. https://doi.org/10.3322/caac.21204

Parkinson, S., Forsyth, K., & Kielhofner, G. (2001). *The Model of Human Occupation Screening Tool (MOHOST).* Chicago: Model of Human Occupation Clearinghouse, University of Illinois at Chicago.

Pergolotti, M., Williams, G. R., Campbell, C., Munoz, L. A., & Muss, H. B. (2016). Occupational therapy for adults with cancer: Why it matters. *Oncologist, 21,* 314–319. https://doi.org/10.1634/theoncologist.2015-0335

Peripheral neuropathy. (n.d.). In *Merriam-Webster Online.* Retrieved from https://www.merriam-webster.com/dictionary/peripheral%20neuropathy

Seretny, M., Currie, G. L., Sena, E. S., Ramnarine, S., Grant, R., MacLeod, M. R., . . . Fallon, M. (2014). Incidence, prevalence, and predictors of chemotherapy-induced peripheral neuropathy: A systematic review and meta-analysis. *Pain, 155,* 2461–2470. https://doi.org/10.1016/j.pain.2014.09.020

Speck, R. M., DeMichele, A., Farrar, J. T., Hennessy, S., Mao, J. J., Stineman, M. G., & Barg, F. K. (2012). Scope of symptoms and self-management strategies for chemotherapy-induced peripheral neuropathy in breast cancer patients. *Support Care Center, 20,* 2433–2439. https://doi.org/10.1007/s00520-011-1365-8

Taillibert, S., Rhun, E. L., & Chamberlain, M. C. (2016). Chemotherapy-related neurotoxicity. *Current Neurology and Neuroscience Reports, 16*(9), 81. https://doi.org/10.1007/s11910-016-0686-x

Veale, P. (2016, August 26). *Rehabilitation management for chemo-induced peripheral neuropathy.* Retrieved from http://www.rehabpub.com/2016/08/rehabilitation-management-chemo-induced-peripheral-neuropathy/

Wang, Y.-C., Bohannon, R. W., Kapellusch, J., Garg, A., & Gershon, R. C. (2015). Dexterity as measured with the 9-Hole Peg Test (9-HPT) across the age span. *Journal of Hand Therapy, 28,* 53–60. https://doi.org/10.1016/j.jht.2014.09.002

Weinstein, S. (1993). Fifty years of somatosensory research. *Journal of Hand Therapy, 6,* 11–22. https://doi.org/10.1016/S0894-1130(12)80176-1

Psychosocial Issues

Kathleen Lyons, ScD, OTR/L

LEARNING OBJECTIVES

After completing this chapter, readers should be able to
- Identify appropriate instruments and referral resources to use in screening for distress, anxiety, and depression in cancer survivors across the lifespan;
- Understand the potential for cancer survivors to experience posttraumatic growth and enhanced well-being after cancer diagnosis across the lifespan;
- Articulate the rationale for using occupational engagement to enhance the mental health of cancer survivors across the lifespan; and
- Foster well-being of cancer survivors via occupational engagement across the lifespan.

KEY TERMS AND CONCEPTS

- Anxiety
- Avoidance behavior
- Cognitive–behavioral therapy
- Depression
- Distress
- Distress Thermometer
- Fear of recurrence
- Occupational engagement
- Posttraumatic growth
- Posttraumatic stress
- Transdiagnostic approach

INTRODUCTION

Treatment advances and rising survival rates have prompted health care practitioners to characterize cancer as a chronic illness (Phillips & Currow, 2010) as opposed to the terminal diagnosis it was once assumed to be. Despite this, few people receive a cancer diagnosis without feeling shocked and aware of their own mortality (Singer, 2018). Responses to this acute awareness of mortality vary among individuals. Some people experience psychosocial challenges of distress, anxiety, or depression. Others report the phenomenon of ***posttraumatic growth,*** which occurs when the cancer experience prompts increased resilience and mental health (Zamora et al., 2017). Additionally, people can experience both psychosocial challenges and growth at points along the cancer experience (Jim & Jacobsen, 2008; Schroevers et al., 2011).

This chapter explores these psychosocial issues from the perspective of occupational therapy. The chapter's central thesis is that occupation is a powerful medium through which to tackle psychosocial challenges and promote psychosocial growth. Keeping our primary focus on promoting and enabling occupational engagement is our profession's unique contribution to cancer rehabilitation.

DEFINING FEATURES OF THE PSYCHOSOCIAL SEQUELAE ASSOCIATED WITH CANCER

Posttraumatic Growth

Posttraumatic growth refers to both a process and an outcome whereby a person experiences improved adaptation, awareness, and psychological functioning after confronting an upsetting event (Tedeschi et al., 1998). Such improvements have been reported by pediatric cancer survivors (Zamora et al., 2017), adult cancer survivors (Mehrabi et al., 2015), and parents of pediatric cancer survivors (Barakat et al., 2006). Survivors of childhood cancers and adult cancer survivors have reported improvements in areas such as resilience and personal strength, spirituality, appreciation of life, social relationships, and recognition of new possibilities for life choices (Tedeschi & Calhoun, 2004; Zamora et al., 2017). Although many studies describe the features of posttraumatic growth, less is known about when and how it develops in survivors (Zamora et al., 2017).

Psychosocial Challenges

Distress

The National Comprehensive Cancer Network (NCCN; 2017) defines **distress** as an unpleasant emotional experience that can hamper the ability to cope with cancer or its treatment. Distress is a normal reaction to a life-threatening illness. The degree of distress a person experiences can range from very mild feelings of sadness or vulnerability to more disabling extremes of panic or emotional crisis. It is important to note that not all distress is intense enough to become disabling. Indeed, some distress can be a catalyst for adaptive coping and growth. However, significant untreated distress can lead to low adherence to cancer treatment or other health-promoting behaviors (NCCN, 2017).

Anxiety

Anxiety is an emotional state that is felt as tension, worry, or irritability and is manifested in physical symptoms like elevated blood pressure or sleep disruptions (Kazdin, 2000). Anxiety can develop into a clinical disorder when the worrisome thoughts become difficult to manage and interfere with daily life and activities for 6 months. In particular, cancer survivors can experience **fear of recurrence** where the preoccupying anxieties center on cancer recurrence. This can include a hypervigilance to physical symptoms, such as pain or swollen lymph nodes, that could signal the cancer's return (Yi & Syrjala, 2017).

Significant anxiety during treatment can also develop into **posttraumatic stress**, leading to intrusive thoughts (Jim & Jacobsen, 2008), hyperarousal, or emotional numbness (Yi & Syrjala, 2017). In general, people with an anxiety disorder tend to avoid situations that provoke anxious symptoms. Although avoidance behavior generally reduces anxiety in the short-term, it eventually fails to reduce anxiety and leads to severely restricted routines and activity patterns when used as a long-term coping strategy (Kazdin, 2000).

Depression

Depression is characterized by persistent anhedonia (i.e., loss of enjoyment in activities), sadness, poor sleep or appetite, low energy, or poor concentration (World Health Organization, 2012). Depression is one of the most disabling conditions a person can experience, and it affects multiple life domains, including work, home management, and family roles (Bruce, 2000). Similar to the description for anxiety, **avoidance behavior** is a large factor in what makes depression so debilitating (Kanter et al., 2010). Avoiding stressful or averse situations can temporarily reduce distress or sadness but ultimately exacerbates depression by severely restricting routines and limiting the opportunities for experiencing positive emotions during activities.

Age Considerations Across the Lifespan

Cancer can occur at any point across the lifespan, and an individual's age and developmental stage are important factors to consider when exploring psychosocial issues (Lebel et al., 2013; NCCN, 2017). When cancer occurs in adolescence, it comes at a time when youth are developing independence and responsibility and are renegotiating relationships with parents (Arnett, 2000). Cancer and its treatment disrupt those developmental tasks, which can be challenging for many people. On the other hand, younger cancer survivors have generally been more likely to report posttraumatic growth (Kolokotroni et al., 2014; Sansom-Daly & Wakefield, 2013). Kolokotroni and colleagues hypothesize that the cancer diagnosis at a younger age can generate both more distress and more opportunities for posttraumatic growth.

Parental report of distress, anxiety, and depression do not perfectly correlate with the self-report of children or adolescents with cancer. In a recent study, parents rated their child's level of distress, anxiety, or depression higher than the child rated their level of distress, and the disagreement between scores was higher when parental distress was high (Abate et al., 2018). Psycho-oncology research also suggests that family functioning is important to consider in pediatric oncology (Erker et al., 2018) because poorer family functioning and support are associated with greater reports of distress in adolescent and young adult cancer survivors (Sansom-Daly & Wakefield, 2013).

In general, adolescents to middle-aged adults with cancer are more likely to report psychosocial challenges than are older adults with cancer (NCCN, 2017). One proposed explanation is the non-normative aspect of cancer in those early life stages (Lebel et al., 2013). By older adulthood, many people have experienced a chronic illness or have seen peers struggle with life-threatening illness. In a sense, cancer is not a completely unexpected event in older adulthood. Alternatively, when cancer occurs in middle adulthood, it comes at a time when most peers are healthy and productivity demands are high in terms of school, work, or family responsibilities. That said, it is important to not make assumptions regarding the level of distress a certain person is experiencing and to screen for psychosocial challenges regardless of age or developmental stage.

Factors Associated With Psychosocial Issues

It is beyond the scope of this chapter to provide current estimates of the prevalence of distress, depression, and anxiety in cancer survivors because prevalence varies according to cancer site, age, race, and time since diagnosis (Traeger et al., 2014). In general, approximately one-third of adult cancer survivors experience a clinically significant psychosocial challenge (Singer, 2018). Phrased another way, the majority of cancer survivors do not experience disabling psychosocial challenges. Even so, occupational therapy practitioners should screen for clinical or subclinical distress that could temporarily or periodically affect occupational engagement.

NCCN's (2017) clinical practice guidelines for distress management refer to several factors that have been associated with increased risk for moderate to severe distress, including

- History of psychiatric disorder, substance abuse, or sexual abuse;
- Cognitive impairment;
- Presence of comorbid conditions;
- Uncontrolled symptoms;

- Communication (e.g., barriers of language or literacy, barriers of a physical nature);
- Living alone;
- Female gender; and
- Having young children.

Unfortunately, many of these factors are not amenable to intervention (e.g., history of psychiatric illness, gender, living situation, family constellation).

Psycho-oncologists have studied coping strategies of cancer survivors to identify malleable attitudes that could affect mental health during and after cancer treatment. That literature has generally found the following:

- People who endorse conditional goal setting (i.e., happiness or social acceptance depends on achieving a certain goal or condition) are at risk for psychosocial challenges (Street, 2003).
- People who use avoidant coping (i.e., avoiding things that trigger negative memories or emotions) report more negative changes in life since their cancer diagnosis (Schroevers et al., 2011).
- People who ruminate (i.e., focus attention on source of distress and possible causes and consequences as opposed to solutions) and catastrophize (i.e., predict a negative outcome and assume it will be unbearable) experience more sadness, depression, or anger (Schroevers et al., 2008).

On the other hand, six coping strategies have been associated with cancer survivors reporting positive changes since diagnosis (Schroevers et al., 2011), which can be seen as an expression of posttraumatic growth:

1. Goal reengagement, such as directing renewed energy toward important and achievable goals (Wrosch et al., 2003);
2. Involvement in pleasant activities (Kanter et al., 2010; Schroevers et al., 2008);
3. Positive reappraisal or positive reframing such as interpreting events and behaviors from an affirmative and optimistic mindset (Rajandram et al., 2011);
4. Active coping, in which one uses their resources to attempt to address a problem (Carroll, 2013);
5. Acceptance (i.e., willingness to admit that a challenging situation is occurring; Elumelu et al., 2015; Scheier & Carver, 2001); and
6. Religious coping (Elumelu et al., 2015; Rajandram et al., 2011).

The coping strategies listed here are not inherently adaptive or maladaptive, but the overuse or exclusive use of them can become problematic. Avoidance and denial both temporarily keep the reality of a situation away until the person can face and deal with it, which may be helpful for a survivor at a given moment in time (Jim & Jacobsen, 2008; Sansom-Daly & Wakefield, 2013; Singer, 2018). The role of cancer occupational therapy practitioners is to accept the reality of the cancer diagnosis and to look for opportunities to strengthen the psychological growth (Singer, 2018). Essentially, the coping strategies that relate to posttraumatic growth can all be mobilized and enacted through occupational engagement. It is the doing, being, and becoming aspects of occupational engagement that help people stay fully engaged in life, despite whatever challenges they may be facing (Wilcock, 1999).

OVERVIEW OF OCCUPATIONAL THERAPY'S ROLE IN MANAGING PSYCHOSOCIAL ISSUES ACROSS THE LIFESPAN

All occupational therapy practitioners, in all areas of cancer rehabilitation practice, have two responsibilities in promoting mental health across the lifespan in light of the psychosocial issues that can arise during cancer diagnosis and treatment:

1. Be alert to and screen for distress, anxiety, and depressive symptoms that warrant a referral to mental health services.
2. Foster occupational engagement that has the potential to enhance mental health.

Screening and Referral to Mental Health Services

Distress, anxiety, and depression can not only reduce quality of life (QoL), but each has the potential to become disabling enough to interfere with cancer treatment and possibly survival (NCCN, 2017). Many oncology practices screen for distress with the goal of avoiding these negative consequences by referring patients who need additional support to the appropriate services. In many ways, distress screening is the most logical gateway to mental health referrals.

The **Distress Thermometer** was developed by NCCN (2017). It asks a person to rate their level of distress on a 0–10 scale. After the person gives a quantitative rating, they are asked to identify the source of distress in the categories of physical, practical, family, emotional, or religious problems. A score of 4 or higher is traditionally used as a prompt to conduct further screening (and evaluation, if warranted) for depression or anxiety. For this reason, the Distress Thermometer is not traditionally seen as a standalone screening instrument, but one that directs subsequent assessment and actions. NCCN has a published algorithm that providers can use to structure further screening and referrals to other disciplines such as social work, psychology or psychiatry, and spiritual counseling (NCCN, 2017).

The Distress Thermometer has been adapted for use in pediatrics (Patel et al., 2011); some practices use the standard Distress Thermometer for parents of children with cancer and use the adapted pediatric version for the patients (Kazak et al., 2012). The Psychosocial Assessment Tool© (PAT) is another screening tool used in pediatric oncology (Kazak et al., 2001). The PAT uses parent reporting to screen for distress in seven domains of family functioning: structure/resources, family problems, social support, stress reactions, family beliefs, child problems, and sibling problems.

Occupational therapy practitioners can play an important role in developing and implementing screening programs for distress, anxiety, and depression. Table 20.1 contains information about screening instruments and factors to consider. Before implementing a screening program, it is important to establish robust referral mechanisms so patients can be referred to evidence-based interventions when warranted.

TABLE 20.1.   Screening for Psychosocial Challenges

INFORMATION TYPE	DISTRESS	ANXIETY	DEPRESSION
Definition	The "unpleasant emotional experience of a psychological (cognitive, behavioral, emotional), social, and/or spiritual nature that may interfere with the ability to cope effectively with cancer, its physical symptoms and its treatment." (NCCN, 2017, p. 7)	Emotional state characterized by feelings of worry, tension, and physical symptoms (Kazdin, 2000)	Mental disorder characterized by persistent sadness, anhedonia, poor sleep or appetite, low energy, or poor concentration (WHO, 2012)
Examples of screening tools for adults	Distress Thermometer (NCCN, 2017)	■ Generalized Anxiety Disorder 7 item screener (GAD–7; Spitzer et al., 2006) ■ Hospital Anxiety and Depression Scale (HADS; Zigmond & Snaith, 1983) ■ Brief Symptom Inventory (Derogatis, 2000)	■ Patient Health Questionnaire (PHQ–9; Kroenke & Spitzer, 2002) ■ Hospital Anxiety and Depression Scale (HADS; Zigmond & Snaith, 1983) ■ Brief Symptom Inventory (Derogatis, 2000)
Examples of screening tools for children and adolescents	■ Brief Symptom Inventory (Derogatis, 2000) ■ Distress Thermometer adapted for pediatrics (Patel et al., 2011) ■ Psychosocial Assessment Tool (Kazak et al., 2001)	Beck Youth Inventory anxiety module (for ages 7–18 years; Beck et al., 2005)	Beck Youth Inventory depression module (for ages 7–18 years; Beck et al., 2005)
Guidelines	■ A score of <4 on the Distress Thermometer (adults) is interpreted as "mild distress" and a score of ≥4 is interpreted as moderate to severe distress. Moderate to severe distress should trigger further screening for anxiety or depression (Yi & Syrjala, 2017). ■ NCCN (2017) guidelines provide an algorithm for screening and referral. NCCN recommends screening for distress at the initial cancer visit and again at regular intervals. ■ There do not seem to be established cutoff scores for the pediatric version of the Distress Thermometer; one study suggested a cutoff of 5 or 6 may yield better specificity without substantial loss of sensitivity as compared to the traditional cutoff of 4 points (Wiener et al., 2017).	On the GAD–7, a score of 5–9 indicates mild anxiety, 10–14 indicates moderate anxiety, and ≥15 indicates severe anxiety (Spitzer et al., 2006).	On the PHQ–9, a cutoff of ≥10 has 88% sensitivity and 88% specificity for detecting actual cases of clinical depression (Kroenke & Spitzer, 2002).
Unique considerations	Distress is a natural reaction to a life-threatening disease, and not all levels of distress are disabling.	Cancer survivors are particularly at risk for anxiety related to fear of cancer recurrence. Anxiety can also extend to posttraumatic stress.	Depression is one of the most disabling mental health disorders.
Role of occupational therapy	■ Facilitate screening and referrals to mental health services; ■ Determine the degree to which distress, anxiety, or depression is affecting occupational engagement; and ■ Help people find ways to effectively and enjoyably complete their daily occupations.		

Note. NCCN = National Comprehensive Cancer Network; WHO = World Health Organization.

Evidence-Based Interventions

Table 20.2 contains a list of interventions that have at least provisional evidence supporting their use to address distress, anxiety, or depression experienced by adult cancer survivors. Some of these interventions (e.g., relaxation techniques, physical activity) can be administered or overseen by an occupational therapy practitioner. Practitioners including these interventions in their practice as a way to foster mental health will need to stay current with the research evidence to ensure that they are conducting these interventions in the manner that has been shown to be effective in studies (e.g., recommending the appropriate "dose" and type of exercise or relaxation strategy).

Resources such as the Cochrane Collaboration can be useful (www.cochranelibrary.com). Cochrane produces systematic reviews so that patients, providers, and researchers have access to high-quality evidence that can inform decision making in health care. A Cochrane Collaboration report indicates there is some evidence to suggest that psychosocial interventions can improve emotional well-being of cancer survivors (Galway et al., 2012). Occupational therapy practitioners can use that and other reviews to identify interventions they would like to incorporate into their practice.

Evidence-based psychosocial interventions are developing for pediatric cancer survivors. In a recent systematic review, 33 studies of psychosocial interventions for pediatric cancer survivors (under age 21 years) or family members were found (Peikert et al., 2018). The interventions ranged from groups to individual face-to-face programs to computer-based interventions. The targeted outcomes were reducing psychological burden, improving social support, and improving physical and psychological well-being. The authors reported that most of the psychosocial interventions show promise in reducing psychosocial burden, but the majority of the studies lacked a comparison condition, and the risk of bias was high. As suggested earlier, occupational therapy practitioners who want to deliver evidence-based psychosocial interventions in pediatrics need to review the intervention components (e.g., dose, content, delivery mechanism) of published studies to determine what can be feasibly implemented in a given setting.

Occupational Engagement

Although the previously described interventions are important tools in the toolkit of strategies to improve mental health, the remainder of the chapter targets a powerful tool that has not received as much explicit attention in cancer rehabilitation: *occupational engagement*. **Occupational engagement** is the act of performing a personally selected and meaningful occupation within a specific setting and context (American Occupational Therapy Association, 2014).

Contemporary clinical psychology is moving toward a transdiagnostic approach to treatment of anxiety and depression (Newby et al., 2015). The **transdiagnostic approach** involves targeting the underlying maladaptive processes that are seen in a broad array of emotional disorders as opposed to creating distinct treatment protocols for each variation of anxiety disorder or depressive disorder (Craske, 2012). As mentioned before, people struggling with depression or anxiety commonly cope by avoiding the

TABLE 20.2. Evidence-Based Interventions to Address Psychosocial Challenges of Cancer Survivors		
INTERVENTION	**USED WITH ADULTS**	**USED WITH CHILDREN AND ADOLESCENTS**
Mindfulness-based therapy (Yi & Syrjala, 2017; Zhang et al., 2015)	X	
CBT (Hunter et al., 2017b; NCCN, 2017; Patel et al., 2009; Poggi et al., 2009; Yi & Syrjala, 2017; Zhang et al., 2017)	X	X
Psychotherapy (NCCN, 2017)	X	
Psychoeducational interventions (Galway et al., 2012; Hunter et al., 2017b; NCCN, 2017)	X	
Peer support (Peikert et al., 2018)		X
Social skills training (Barrera et al., 2018)		X
Family or couples therapy (NCCN, 2017; Peikert et al., 2018)	X	X
Hope therapy (Shekarabi-Ahari et al., 2012)		X
Hypnosis (Yi & Syrjala, 2017)	X	
Self-management training (Yi & Syrjala, 2017)	X	
Medication (NCCN, 2017; Yi & Syrjala, 2017)	X	
Relaxation techniques (Greenlee et al., 2014); stress management training (Hunter et al., 2017b)	X	
Physical activity (NCCN, 2017; Yi & Syrjala, 2017)	X	
Yoga (Greenlee et al., 2014; Hunter et al., 2017a)	X	

Note. Based on reviews or meta-analyses of individual studies. CBT = cognitive–behavioral therapy; NCCN = National Comprehensive Cancer Network.

situations that provoke uncomfortable emotions. Although avoidance can reduce anxiety or negative affect in the short term, it ultimately becomes disabling because it decreases activity levels and reduces the opportunities for pleasurable or productive activities that allow people to enact their values (Kanter et al., 2010). Therefore, a common feature of *cognitive–behavioral therapies* (CBTs) for depression and anxiety focuses on performing productive or pleasurable activities that reflect a person's values, despite the presence of worrisome or negative affect (Hayes, 2004; Hegel & Arean, 2003; Kanter et al., 2010). The idea of performing activities despite the presence of worrisome or negative affect is akin to the occupational therapy goal of promoting occupational engagement despite any challenges presented by physical or mental illness.

Although occupational therapy practitioners are experts in facilitating occupational engagement, most do not have the advanced and specialized training to deliver CBTs. Therefore, occupational therapy cannot replace the mental health services that are warranted for cancer survivors who are experiencing clinically significant levels of anxiety and depression. However, the aim of this chapter is to help occupational therapy practitioners realize that their primary therapeutic modality (i.e., therapeutic occupation) has the potential to influence mental health. Occupational therapy focused on enabling occupation can not only complement mental health services for those patients with clinically significant levels of anxiety and depression but also has the potential to enhance mental health or promote resilience in patients who have subclinical levels of anxiety and depressive symptoms (i.e., levels that fail to rise to the level of diagnosable depressive or anxiety disorder).

Evaluation

After screening for distress, depression, or anxiety, occupational therapy practitioners should make sure they ask about and understand the ways in which distress, depression, and anxiety are affecting occupational engagement as part of the evaluation process. For example, mild anxiety or depression may reduce an individual's enjoyment of previously pleasurable activities such as parenting tasks. Or moderate anxiety may make it hard to concentrate and perform school activities accurately. Moderate to severe depressive symptoms could be more disabling, leading to absenteeism at work. In essence, the evaluation process should include a discussion of the ways in which distress, anxiety, or depressive symptoms are interfering with valued occupations.

As with any occupational therapy service, when using occupational engagement to address psychosocial challenges, practitioners should create an occupational profile and evaluate occupational performance. Several assessments can be used for this purpose. Depending on the setting and the time constraints, practitioners could use a screening tool such as the Model of Human Occupation Screening Tool (Parkinson et al., 2006) to focus the evaluation process. Evaluation instruments for adults include the Canadian Occupational Performance Measure (Law et al., 2019), the Activity Card Sort (Baum & Edwards, 2008; Lyons et al., 2010), the Occupational Circumstances Assessment Interview and Rating Scale (Forsyth et al., 2006), or the Occupational Self-Assessment (Baron et al., 2006). Evaluation instruments for occupational performance in pediatrics include the Short Child Occupational Profile (Bowyer et al., 2008) and the Child Occupational Self Assessment (Kramer et al., 2014).

Whatever assessment is chosen, occupational therapy practitioners must determine the occupations that are necessary for fulfilling valued roles in the patient's life. They must also determine occupations that are pleasurable for each person. Engaging in productive activities that are related to valued roles and pleasurable activities are targets of CBTs because of their antidepressant effects (Kanter et al., 2010). At the end of the occupational therapy evaluation, practitioners should have a clear idea of what activities compose patients' definition of a meaningful life and the ways in which those activities are currently difficult because of psychosocial challenges.

Treatment Approaches

Much of the psycho-oncology literature focuses on techniques for symptom reduction (e.g., helping people create or maintain stress management strategies such as mindful meditation or exercise). Table 20.3 includes examples of approaches to intervention that address psychosocial challenges. As noted earlier, these approaches can be integrated

---

TABLE 20.3.   Approaches to Intervention

APPROACH TO INTERVENTION	EXAMPLES
Create/promote (health promotion)	• Promote healthy habits, including sleep hygiene, proper nutrition, physical activity, yoga, and stress management/relaxation techniques
Establish/restore	• Support participation in evidence-based treatments for depression and anxiety (e.g., CBTs, mindfulness-based therapy, psychotherapy, hope therapy, family or couples therapy, hypnosis, medication) • Social skills training
Modify (compensation/adaptation)	• Problem solving to promote adaptive coping
Prevent (disability prevention)	• Prospective screening for distress and psychosocial challenges along the cancer diagnosis and treatment continuum • Support groups

Note. CBTs = cognitive–behavioral therapies.

into occupational therapy treatment plans in many settings. Table 20.4 contains examples of occupational therapy interventions that can address psychosocial challenges.

The words of Scheier and Carver (2001) should offer guidance to occupational therapy practitioners. They suggest one aim of psycho-oncology is to help people avoid "a kind of functional death in which the person prematurely disengages from the opportunities of life" (p. 27). Understandably and necessarily, most people reduce their activity level during cancer treatment. However, if a person discontinues all of their pleasurable or productive activities, they may increase the risk of distress, anxiety, or depression. Occupational therapy can help cancer survivors enhance their well-being by strategically incorporating at least one pleasurable, comforting, or productive activity into their daily routine. Case Examples 20.1 and 20.2 illustrate how this can be done in a pediatric or adult setting.

Exhibit 20.1 includes a template for an activity-planning structure that can be used with cancer survivors to help them find ways to engage in valued occupations despite challenges created by physical, psychological, environmental, or scheduling barriers (Lyons et al., 2019; Lyons, Newman, Adachi-Mejia et al., 2018). In pilot studies, this structure has been shown to increase activity level for personally chosen activities (Lyons et al., 2019; Lyons, Newman, Kaufman et al., 2018) and increase QoL (Lyons et al., 2015). The activity-planning structure helps people use their limited energy wisely while creating opportunities to experience positive affect and make progress toward long-term goals.

The first step of the activity-planning structure is to identify an activity that has the potential to influence mood (i.e., a pleasurable activity, something comforting or calming) or

TABLE 20.4.   Occupational Therapy Interventions

OCCUPATIONAL THERAPY INTERVENTIONS	EXAMPLES
Occupations and activities	▪ Encouragement of participation in meaningful occupations ▪ Physical activity or exercise or mind–body modalities
Preparatory methods and tasks	▪ Stress management techniques, including progressive muscle relaxation or prayer
Education and training	▪ Psychoeducation for patients, caregivers, and family members regarding adaptive coping and psychosocial sequelae of cancer
Advocacy	▪ Promotion of distress screening across the cancer continuum
Group interventions	▪ Support groups

EXHIBIT 20.1.   Activity Planning Worksheet

MY ACTIVITY PRESCRIPTION FOR THE COMING WEEK

Motivation (Why do this activity?)

Obstacles (What might make this activity hard/impractical/impossible?)

Activity prescription (What activity? How often in the next 7 days?)

Any special considerations of when, where, who, and how?

How did it go?   Lessons learned for next time:

Monday	Tuesday	Wednesday	Thursday	Friday	Saturday	Sunday	Satisfaction (0–10)
Yes No Goal	Yes No Goal	Yes No Goal	Yes No Goal	Yes No Goal	Yes No Goal	Yes No Goal	Effort: Outcome:

an activity that expresses one's values or identity. After an activity is identified, the survivor describes all of the barriers that might make it hard to engage in the activity within the next 7 days (e.g., fatigue, appointments, standards for perfection).

The second step is to create a goal for doing the activity within the next 7 days. In essence, the survivor is creating their own "activity prescription" to follow in the coming week. The short time frame provides enough opportunity to do the activity but it is not so long that a person can keep putting it off. A helpful goal is

- *Behavioral:* Something you do, not the outcome you want;
- *Observable:* Not just that you will feel better; you will know if you met the goal because it is measurable in some way; and
- *Achievable:* Something you feel confident you can do if you put a little effort into it.

The third step is to create a detailed action plan to delineate who will be involved (and how their cooperation will be secured), exactly when the activity will be done, where the activity will occur, and how it will be done. A useful action plan targets all of the barriers that are identified in the first step. A useful action plan also includes a Plan B to address any foreseeable challenges that might arise (e.g., it rains when you planned to take a walk outside, the kids get sick when you had planned to do a social activity outside the home). Plan B allows survivors to determine ways to not let that challenge thwart progress to the goal (e.g., dance to music inside, play a game with the kids that is social).

After the survivor has the action plan, they execute it. The occupational therapy practitioner should follow up in a subsequent session to celebrate and affirm successes or to process struggles. Although a survivor may not fully meet goals initially, they can learn valuable lessons that can help foster effective activity planning. Sometimes they learn that the goal

CASE EXAMPLE 20.1. MARIA: ADDRESSING PSYCHOSOCIAL ISSUES DURING LYMPHEDEMA TREATMENT

Maria is a 45-year-old woman referred to occupational therapy because of lymphedema after a right-side mastectomy for Stage III breast cancer. She finished treatment 3 months ago. Before her surgery, she scored a 5 on the Distress Thermometer (NCCN, 2020) but declined a referral to mental health services. She was treated with medication for a depressive disorder in her early 20s and said she does not want to "go down that path" again. She preferred to talk with her priest who supported her during treatment.

Maria is engaged during occupational therapy and follows instructions because she wants to "get this swelling under control and get back to my life." Lymphedema has affected her body image and makes it hard to perform some leisure activities she enjoys such as baking and salsa dancing. She states she is putting those activities "on hold" until she feels better. She is making good progress with the lymphedema control but reports frustration that this will be something she has to monitor and manage for the foreseeable future. In each session, she reports she is becoming more worried about her arm and that her life will "never return to normal."

Mike, the occupational therapist, decides to readminister the Distress Thermometer so he can assess Maria's level of discomfort with her situation. Her score has increased to a 6, and subsequent screening with the Hospital Anxiety and Depression Scale (Zigmond & Snaith, 1983) suggests that she is struggling with anxiety. Maria agrees with the assessment and agrees to consider a referral to mental health only when Mike explains that medication is not the only treatment available to her and describes some behavioral treatments.

At the same time, Mike asks Maria about her weekly routine and asks if she has other pleasurable activities to look forward to now that she has put her favorite activities of baking and dancing on hold. With regret, she reports she does not really have anything that took

the place of those occupations. Although reluctant to pursue those activities, she agrees it might be helpful to have an enjoyable activity to look forward to. After deliberation, she decides to try coloring in the evenings to "calm her nerves." With Mike's guidance, she uses the activity-planning worksheet to set a goal for coloring and to make a detailed plan of when, where, and how she will accomplish it.

At the following session, Maria reports she had a good experience doing the coloring, and Mike and Maria revisit the worksheet and set a new goal for the coming week. After 2 weeks of this, Mike asks if she has considered trying dancing or baking again. Maria ambivalently reports that her friends have been encouraging her and her husband to join them for a night of salsa dancing. With encouragement, she uses the activity worksheet to plan what she will wear, when she will practice dancing with her husband before they go out, and how she might manage her cancer-related fatigue. Mike and Maria discuss the dance steps that are most difficult and how she can make adjustments with her husband to allow her to safely and comfortably perform them.

The following week, Maria reports that she had a lot of fun dancing with her husband, and it helped them laugh with each other again. Although she was frustrated with how tired she got when dancing and how much she had to think about her outfit and her body, she says she loved seeing her friends again and getting "lost in the music." She says she has decided to accept the referral to mental health. Seeing her friends again made her realize how much she had been holding in, "holding her breath, waiting for the next shoe to drop." Maria says she wants to find other ways to "let her breath out." She continues with her lymphedema treatment but also continues to identify a weekly activity prescription to fuel her recovery and well-being.

CASE EXAMPLE 20.2. CONNOR: ADDRESSING PSYCHOSOCIAL ISSUES DURING STEM CELL TRANSPLANTATION

Connor is a 12-year-old male being treated for acute lymphoblastic leukemia. He was referred to inpatient occupational therapy when admitted for a stem cell transplant (SCT). The program's psychosocial screening program noted high levels of anxiety in both Connor (a score of 7 on the pediatric Distress Thermometer) and his widowed father (a score of 6 on the Distress Thermometer). Consequently, Connor and his father were referred to the social worker on the SCT team.

During the initial occupational therapy evaluation, Connor reports significant frustration over missing extracurricular school events and sadness over a loss of contact with friends who are uncomfortable around him because they know he has to avoid crowds and exposure to infections. He also reports that he struggles with anxiety during the chemotherapy treatments and is fearful of having a bad reaction or feeling nauseous. Additionally, he worries that his older brother resents the disruption to their lives and routines that his illness has caused. He cannot articulate any coping strategies that help him, but he is willing to learn and try any techniques. His favorite occupations are basketball, video games, and board games like chess.

Initial occupational therapy sessions focus on exploring various relaxation techniques that could help Connor during reinfusion of stem cells the following week and in future treatments. In addition to providing detailed information about what to expect, Connor and the occupational therapy assistant explore different digital files he could listen to with his earbuds. After experimenting with progressive muscle relaxation, guided imagery, and music, Connor has an action plan to use music during the treatment and can independently share the plan with the team.

During occupational therapy sessions, Connor also talks about his sadness over missing his friends and feeling like a burden to his brother. He has been told that he will have very little energy in the coming weeks as his immune system rebuilds, so he feels nervous about reaching out to his friends. He is, however, willing to find a fun way to pass time with his brother when he comes to visit. The occupational therapy assistant uses the activity-planning worksheet to help him identify an enjoyable game to play during the visit and a way to invite his brother to join him.

The next day, Connor reports that while he played the game with his brother, he had a really helpful talk with him. His brother was surprised and saddened by Connor's feelings of guilt and the loss of connection he feels with his friends. His brother reassured him that he only wants Connor to get well again. His brother also suggested that they set up a chat group on social media with Connor's friends. His brother offered to post an update each day so Connor's friends would know what was going on with Connor, and they could comment. His brother said he could manage the chat (e.g., post pictures Connor chose and post Connor's replies) until Connor had enough energy to post updates himself. In that way, Connor could communicate through his brother and receive well wishes without having to expend the energy until he was ready.

When Connor is discharged from the hospital, he reports feeling good about being able to use his chosen relaxation techniques when he feels like he needs them. His brother is glad to have an important role in supporting his brother, and Connor's friends send daily messages with pictures and funny stories from school that help Connor feel included and remembered.

---

was too aggressive or there was an additional barrier that they need to account for in future action planning (Lyons, Newman, Kaufman et al., 2018). The role of the occupational therapy practitioner is to use activity analysis skills to help cancer survivors set achievable goals and develop effective action plans that address psychological, physical, and environmental barriers.

SUMMARY

This chapter addresses three main psychosocial issues from the perspective of occupational therapy. First, practitioners need to screen for distress, anxiety, and depression because, if left untreated, these mental disorders can affect not only a person's QoL, but also their treatment adherence and possibly survival (NCCN, 2017). Reviews of psycho-oncology studies demonstrate wide variation in how people respond to cancer and inconsistencies in what predicts better or worse outcomes (Sansom-Daly & Wakefield, 2013). Therefore, screening is important because we cannot assume someone is or is not experiencing psychosocial challenges without exploring it with them.

The second issue involves referring cancer survivors to appropriate psychological or spiritual services. It does not help to screen for psychosocial challenges if a robust treatment service is not available. Many resources are available to practices and providers who are interested in providing evidence-based care; these include the Cochrane Library and the NCCN Guidelines (NCCN, 2017).

Finally, occupational therapy practitioners must work with survivors to ensure that psychosocial challenges interfere as little as possible with occupational engagement. Participation in meaningful occupation is our primary therapeutic modality. Participation in meaningful activity can also have an antidepressant effect that is important to harness.

REFERENCES

Abate, C., Lippé, S., Bertout, L., Drouin, S., Krajinovic, M., Rondeau, É., . . . Sultan, S. (2018). Could we use parent report as a valid proxy of child report on anxiety, depression, and distress? A systematic investigation of father–mother–child triads in children successfully treated for leukemia. *Pediatric Blood & Cancer, 65*(2), e26840. https://doi.org/10.1002/pbc.26840

American Occupational Therapy Association. (2014). Occupational therapy practice framework: Domain and process (3rd ed.). *American Journal of Occupational Therapy, 68*(Suppl. 1), S1–S48. https://doi.org/10.5014/ajot.2014.682006

Arnett, J. J. (2000). A theory of development from the late teens through the twenties. *American Psychologist, 55,* 469–480. https://doi.org/10.1037/0003-066X.55.5.469

Barakat, L. P., Alderfer, M. A., & Kazak, A. E. (2006). Posttraumatic growth in adolescent survivors of cancer and their mothers and fathers. *Journal of Pediatric Psychology, 31,* 413–419. http://doi.org/10.1093/jpepsy/jsj058

Baron, K., Kielhofner, G., Iyenger, A., Goldhammer, V., & Wolenski, J. (2006). *User's manual: Occupational Self-Assessment* (Version 2.2). Chicago: University of Illinois at Chicago.

Barrera, M., Atenafu, E. G., Sung, L., Bartels, U., Schulte, F., Chung, J., . . . McConnell, D. (2018). A randomized control intervention trial to improve social skills and quality of life in pediatric brain tumor survivors. *Psycho-Oncology, 27,* 91–98. https://doi.org/10.1002/pon.4385

Baum, C. M., & Edwards, D. (2008). *Activity Card Sort* (2nd ed.). Bethesda, MD: AOTA Press.

Beck, J. S., Beck, A. T., Jolly, J. B., & Steer, R. A. (2005). *Beck Youth Inventories for Children and Adolescents manual* (2nd ed.). San Antonio: Psych Corps.

Bowyer, P. L., Kramer, J., Ploszaj, A., Ross, M., Schwartz, O., Kielhofner, G., & Kramer, K. (2008). *The Short Child Occupational Profile (SCOPE)* (Version 2.2). Chicago: University of Illinois at Chicago.

Bruce, M. L. (2000). Depression and disability. In G. M. Williamson, D. R. Shaffer, & P. A. Parmelee (Eds.), *Physical illness and depression in older adults* (pp. 11–29). New York: Kluwer Academic/Plenum.

Carroll, L. (2013). Active coping. In M. D. Gellman & J. R. Turner (Eds.), *Encyclopedia of behavioral medicine.* New York: Springer. https://doi.org/10.1007/978-1-4419-1005-9

Craske, M. G. (2012). Transdiagnostic treatment for depression and anxiety. *Depression and Anxiety, 29,* 749–753. https://doi.org/10.1002/da.21992

Derogatis, L. (Ed.). (2000). *Brief Symptom Inventory (BSI): Administration, scoring, and procedure manual.* Minneapolis: NCS Pearson.

Elumelu, T. N., Asuzu, C. C., & Akin-Odanye, E. O. (2015). Impact of active coping, religion and acceptance on quality of life of patients with breast cancer in the department of radiotherapy, UCH, Ibadan. *BMJ Supportive & Palliative Care, 5,* 175–180. https://doi.org/10.1136/bmjspcare-2012-000409

Erker, C., Yan, K., Zhang, L., Bingen, K., Flynn, K. E., & Panepinto, J. (2018). Impact of pediatric cancer on family relationships. *Cancer Medicine, 7,* 1680–1688. https://doi.org/10.1002/cam4.1393

Forsyth, K., Deshpande, H., Kielhofner, G., Henrikkson, C., Haglund, L., Olson, L., . . . Kulkarni, S. (2006). *Occupational Circumstances Assessment Interview and Rating Scale (OCAIRS)* (Version 4.0). Chicago: University of Illinois at Chicago.

Galway, K., Black, A., Cantwell, M., Cardwell, C. R., Mills, M., & Donnelly, M. (2012). Psychosocial interventions to improve quality of life and emotional wellbeing for recently diagnosed cancer patients. *Cochrane Database of Systematic Reviews, 11,* CD007064. https://doi.org/10.1002/14651858.CD007064.pub2

Greenlee, H., Balneaves, L. G., Carlson, L. E., Cohen, M., Deng, G., Hershman, D., . . . Tripathy, D. (2014). Clinical practice guidelines on the use of integrative therapies as supportive care in patients treated for breast cancer. *JNCI Monographs, 2014*(50), 346–358. https://doi.org/10.1093/jncimonographs/lgu041

Hayes, S. C. (2004). Acceptance and commitment therapy, relational frame theory, and the third wave of behavioral and cognitive therapies. *Behavior Therapy, 35,* 639–665. https://doi.org/10.1016/S0005-7894(04)80013-3

Hegel, M. T., & Arean, P. A. (2003). *Problem-solving treatment for primary care: A treatment manual for depression, Project IMPACT.* Hanover, NH: Dartmouth College.

Hunter, E. G., Gibson, R. W., Arbesman, M., & D'Amico, M. (2017a). Systematic review of occupational therapy and adult cancer rehabilitation: Part 1. Impact of physical activity and symptom management interventions. *American Journal of Occupational Therapy, 71,* 7102100030. http://doi.org/10.5014/ajot.2017.023564

Hunter, E. G., Gibson, R. W., Arbesman, M., & D'Amico, M. (2017b). Systematic review of occupational therapy and adult cancer rehabilitation: Part 2. Impact of multidisciplinary rehabilitation and psychosocial, sexuality, and return-to-work interventions. *American Journal of Occupational Therapy, 71,* 7102100040. http://doi.org/10.5014/ajot.2017.023572

Jim, H. S. L., & Jacobsen, P. B. (2008). Posttraumatic stress and posttraumatic growth in cancer survivorship: A review. *Cancer Journal, 14,* 414–419. https://doi.org/10.1097/PPO.0b013e31818d8963

Kanter, J. W., Busch, A. M., & Rusch, L. C. (2010). *Behavioral activation.* New York: Routledge.

Kazak, A. E., Brier, M., Alderfer, M. A., Reilly, A., Parker, S. F., Rogerwick, S., . . . Barakat, L. P. (2012). Screening for psychosocial risk in pediatric cancer. *Pediatric Blood & Cancer, 59,* 822–827. https://doi.org/10.1002/pbc.24166

Kazak, A. E., Prusak, A., McSherry, M., Simms, S., Beele, D., Rourke, M., . . . Lange, B. (2001). The Psychosocial Assessment Tool (PAT)©: Pilot data on a brief screening instrument for identifying high risk families in pediatric oncology. *Families, Systems, & Health, 19,* 303–317. https://doi.org/10.1037/h0089454

Kazdin, A. E. (Ed.). (2000). *Encyclopedia of psychology.* Washington, DC: American Psychological Association.

Kolokotroni, P., Anagnostopoulos, F., & Tsikkinis, A. (2014). Psychosocial factors related to posttraumatic growth in breast cancer survivors: A review. *Women & Health, 54,* 569–592. https://doi.org/10.1080/03630242.2014.899543

Kramer, J., ten Velden, M., Kafkes, A., Basu, S., Federico, J., & Kielhofner, G. (2014). *Child Occupational Self Assessment* (Version 2.2). Chicago: University of Illinois at Chicago.

Kroenke, K., & Spitzer, R. L. (2002). The PHQ-9: A new depression diagnostic and severity measure. *Psychiatric Annals, 32*(9), 509–515. https://doi.org/10.3928/0048-5713-20020901-06

Law, M., Baptiste, S., Carswell, A., McColl, M. A., Polatajko, H., & Pollock, N. (2019). *Canadian Occupational Performance Measure* (5th ed., rev.). Altona, Manitoba: COPM, Inc.

Lebel, S., Beattie, S., Ares, I., & Bielajew, C. (2013). Young and worried: Age and fear of recurrence in breast cancer survivors. *Health Psychology, 32,* 695–705. https://doi.org/10.1037/a0030186

Lyons, K. D., Bruce, M. A., Hull, J. G., Kaufman, P. A., Li, Z., Stearns, D. M., . . . Hegel, M. T. (2019). Health through activity:

Initial evaluation of an in-home intervention for older adults with cancer. *American Journal of Occupational Therapy, 73,* 7305205070. https://doi.org/10.5014/ajot.2019.035022

Lyons, K. D., Hull, J. G., Kaufman, P. A., Li, Z., Seville, J., Ahles, T. A., . . . Hegel, M. T. (2015). Development and initial evaluation of a telephone-delivered, behavioral activation, and problem-solving treatment program to address functional goals of breast cancer survivors. *Journal of Psychosocial Oncology, 33,* 199–218. https://doi.org/10.1080/07347332.2014.1002659

Lyons, K. D., Li, Z., Tosteson, T. D., Meehan, K., & Ahles, T. A. (2010). Consistency and construct validity of the Activity Card Sort (modified) in measuring activity resumption after stem cell transplantation. *American Journal of Occupational Therapy, 64,* 562–569. https://doi.org/10.5014/ajot.2010.09033

Lyons, K. D., Newman, R., Adachi-Mejia, A. M., Whipple, J., & Hegel, M. T. (2018). Content analysis of a participant-directed intervention to optimize activity engagement of older adult cancer survivors. *OTJR: Occupation, Participation and Health, 38,* 38–45. https://doi.org/10.1177/1539449217730356

Lyons, K. D., Newman, R. M., Kaufman, P. A., Bruce, M. L., Stearns, D. M., Lansigan, F., . . . Hegel, M. T. (2018). Goal attainment and goal adjustment of older adults during person-directed cancer rehabilitation. *American Journal of Occupational Therapy, 72,* 7202205110. http://doi.org/10.5014/ajot.2018.023648

Mehrabi, E., Hajian, S., Simbar, M., Houshyari, M., & Zayeri, F. (2015). Post-traumatic growth: A qualitative analysis of experiences regarding positive psychological changes among Iranian women with breast cancer. *Electronic Physician, 7,* 1239–1246. https://doi.org/10.14661/1239

National Comprehensive Cancer Network. (2017). *NCCN clinical practice guidelines in oncology: Distress management.* Retrieved from https://www.nccn.org/professionals/physician_gls/pdf/distress.pdf

National Comprehensive Cancer Network. (2020). *NCCN Distress Thermometer and problem list for patients.* Retrieved from https://www.nccn.org/patients/resources/life_with_cancer/pdf/nccn_distress_thermometer.pdf

Newby, J. M., McKinnon, A., Kuyken, W., Gilbody, S., & Dalgleish, T. (2015). Systematic review and meta-analysis of transdiagnostic psychological treatments for anxiety and depressive disorders in adulthood. *Clinical Psychology Review, 40*(Suppl. C), 91–110. https://doi.org/10.1016/j.cpr.2015.06.002

Parkinson, S., Forsyth, K., & Kielhofner, G. (2006). *A user's manual for Model of Human Occupation Screening Tool (MOHOST)* (Version 2.0). Chicago: University of Illinois at Chicago.

Patel, S. K., Katz, E. R., Richardson, R., Rimmer, M., & Kilian, S. (2009). Cognitive and problem solving training in children with cancer: A pilot project. *Journal of Pediatric Hematology/Oncology, 31,* 670–677. https://doi.org/10.1097/MPH.0b013e3181b25a1d

Patel, S. K., Mullins, W., Turk, A., Dekel, N., Kinjo, C., & Sato, J. K. (2011). Distress screening, rater agreement, and services in pediatric oncology. *Psycho-Oncology, 20,* 1324–1333. https://doi.org/10.1002/pon.1859

Peikert, M. L., Inhestern, L., & Bergelt, C. (2018). Psychosocial interventions for rehabilitation and reintegration into daily life of pediatric cancer survivors and their families: A systematic review. *PLoS One, 13,* e0196151. https://doi.org/10.1371/journal.pone.0196151

Phillips, J. L., & Currow, D. C. (2010). Cancer as a chronic disease. *Collegian, 17*(2), 47–50. https://doi.org/10.1016/j.colegn.2010.04.007

Poggi, G., Liscio, M., Pastore, V., Adduci, A., Galbiati, S., Spreafico, F., . . . Massimino, M. (2009). Psychological intervention in young brain tumor survivors: The efficacy of the cognitive behavioural approach. *Disability and Rehabilitation, 31,* 1066–1073. https://doi.org/10.1080/09638280802509546

Rajandram, R. K., Jenewein, J., McGrath, C., & Zwahlen, R. A. (2011). Coping processes relevant to posttraumatic growth: An evidence-based review. *Supportive Care in Cancer, 19,* 583–589. https://doi.org/10.1007/s00520-011-1105-0

Sansom-Daly, U. M., & Wakefield, C. E. (2013). Distress and adjustment among adolescents and young adults with cancer: An empirical and conceptual review. *Translational Pediatrics, 2*(4), 167–197. http://tp.amegroups.com/article/view/2851

Scheier, M. F., & Carver, C. S. (2001). Adapting to cancer: The importance of hope and purpose. In A. Baum & B. L. Andersen (Eds.), *Psychosocial interventions for cancer* (pp. 15–36). Washington, DC: American Psychological Association. https://doi.org/10.1037/10402-002

Schroevers, M., Kraaij, V., & Garnefski, N. (2008). How do cancer patients manage unattainable personal goals and regulate their emotions? *British Journal of Health Psychology, 13,* 551–562. http://doi.org/10.1348/135910707X241497

Schroevers, M., Kraaij, V., & Garnefski, N. (2011). Cancer patients' experience of positive and negative changes due to the illness: Relationships with psychological well-being, coping, and goal reengagement. *Psycho-Oncology, 20,* 165–172. http://doi.org/10.1002/pon.1718

Shekarabi-Ahari, G., Younesi, J., Borjali, A., & Ansari-Damavandi, S. (2012). The effectiveness of group hope therapy on hope and depression of mothers with children suffering from cancer in Tehran. *Iranian Journal of Cancer Prevention, 5*(4), 183–188. https://www.ncbi.nlm.nih.gov/pmc/PMC4209570/

Singer, S. (2018). Psychosocial impact of cancer. In U. Goerling & A. Mehnert (Eds.), *Psycho-Oncology* (pp. 1–11). New York: Springer. https://doi.org/10.1007/978-3-319-64310-6_1

Spitzer, R. L., Kroenke, K., Williams, J. B. W., & Lowe, B. (2006). A brief measure for assessing generalized anxiety disorder: The GAD-7. *Archives of Internal Medicine, 166,* 1092–1097. https://doi.org/10.1001/archinte.166.10.1092

Street, H. (2003). The psychosocial impact of cancer: Exploring relationships between conditional goal setting and depression. *Psycho-Oncology, 12,* 580–589. http://doi.org/10.1002/pon.677

Tedeschi, R. G., & Calhoun, L. G. (2004). Posttraumatic growth: Conceptual foundations and empirical evidence. *Psychological Inquiry, 15*(1), 1–8. https://doi.org/10.1207/s15327965pli1501_01

Tedeschi, R. G., Park, C. L., & Calhoun, L. G. (1998). Posttraumatic growth: Conceptual issues. In R. C. Tedeschi, C. L. Park, & L. C. Calhoun (Eds.), *Posttraumatic growth: Positive changes in the aftermath of crisis* (pp. 1–22). Mahwah, NJ: Lawrence Erlbaum Associates. https://doi.org/10.4324/9781410603401

Traeger, L., Cannon, S., Keating, N. L., Pirl, W. F., Lathan, C., Martin, M. Y., . . . Park, E. R. (2014). Race by sex differences in depression symptoms and psychosocial service use among non-Hispanic black and white patients with lung cancer. *Journal of Clinical Oncology, 32,* 107–113. https://doi.org/10.1200/JCO.2012.46.6466

Wiener, L., Battles, H., Zadeh, S., Widemann, B. C., & Pao, M. (2017). Validity, specificity, feasibility and acceptability of a brief pediatric Distress Thermometer in outpatient clinics. *Psycho-Oncology, 26,* 461–468. https://doi.org/10.1002/pon.4038

Wilcock, A. A. (1999). Reflections on doing, being, becoming. *Australian Occupational Therapy Journal, 46*(1), 1–11. https://doi.org/10.1046/j.1440-1630.1999.00174.x

World Health Organization. (2012). *Depression fact sheet.* Retrieved from https://www.who.int/news-room/fact-sheets/detail/depression

Wrosch, C., Scheier, M. F., Miller, G. E., Schulz, R., & Carver, C. S. (2003). Adaptive self-regulation of unattainable goals: Goal disengagement, goal reengagement, and subjective well-being. *Personality and Social Psychology Bulletin, 29,* 1494–1508. https://doi.org/10.1177/0146167203256921

Yi, J. C., & Syrjala, K. L. (2017). Anxiety and depression in cancer survivors. *Medical Clinics of North America, 101,* 1099–1113. https://doi.org/10.1016/j.mcna.2017.06.005

Zamora, E. R., Yi, J., Akter, J., Kim, J., Warner, E. L., & Kirchhoff, A. C. (2017). "Having cancer was awful but also something good came out" Post-traumatic growth among adult survivors of pediatric and adolescent cancer. *European Journal of Oncology Nursing, 28*(Suppl. C), 21–27. https://doi.org/10.1016/j.ejon.2017.02.001

Zhang, M.-F., Wen, Y.-S., Liu, W.-Y., Peng, L.-F., Wu, X.-D., & Liu, Q.-W. (2015). Effectiveness of mindfulness-based therapy for reducing anxiety and depression in patients with cancer: A meta-analysis. *Medicine, 94*(45), e0897–e0900. https://doi.org/10.1097/MD.0000000000000897

Zhang, M., Huang, L., Feng, Z., Shao, L., & Chen, L. (2017). Effects of cognitive behavioral therapy on quality of life and stress for breast cancer survivors: A meta-analysis. *Minerva Medica, 108*(1), 84–93. https://doi.org/10.23736/S0026-4806.16.04528-6

Zigmond, A., & Snaith, R. (1983). The Hospital Anxiety and Depression Scale. *Acta Psychiatrica Scandinavica, 67,* 361–370. https://doi.org/10.1111/j.1600-0447.1983.tb09716.x

PART V.

Cancer and Participation in Occupations Across the Lifespan

Activities of Daily Living and Instrumental Activities of Daily Living

Caitlyn Lombardo, MSOT, OTR/L, CLT, and Chrysanne Karnick, MOT, OTR/L, CAPS, CLT

21

LEARNING OBJECTIVES

After completing this chapter, readers should be able to
- Understand how to evaluate a cancer survivor's ADL and IADL dysfunction as it relates to their cancer diagnosis and its treatments;
- Recognize client factors in the cancer population that may contribute to ADL and IADL dysfunction;
- Identify appropriate functional assessments to use with their clients during ADL and IADL performance; and
- Recognize strategies to use ADL and IADL as occupation-based occupational therapy intervention for cancer survivors.

KEY TERMS AND CONCEPTS

- ADLs
- Apraxia
- Cancer-related fatigue
- Care of others
- Care of pets
- Chemotherapy-induced peripheral neuropathy
- Child rearing
- Communication management
- Dressing
- Driving and community mobility
- Feeding
- Financial management
- Functional mobility
- Health management and maintenance
- Home establishment and management
- IADLs
- Internal pouch
- Meal preparation and cleaning
- Neobladder
- Oncology
- Ostomy
- Personal device care
- Religious and spiritual activities and expression
- Safety and emergency maintenance
- Sexual activity
- Shopping
- Swallowing and eating
- Toileting and toilet hygiene
- Urinary diversion

INTRODUCTION

This chapter helps occupational therapy practitioners understand how a cancer diagnosis and its treatments may affect cancer survivors' participation in ADLs and IADLs. Occupational therapy practitioners working in cancer rehabilitation may apply the knowledge they gain in this chapter to assessment of how cancer can lead to ADL and IADL dysfunction and the client factors and performance patterns commonly affected in this population. Knowledge of how cancer and its treatments affect ADLs and IADLs will facilitate occupational therapy practitioners' clinical reasoning during both evaluation and treatment of their clients.

Participation in ADLs and IADLs is beneficial for the overall health of cancer survivors and in promoting and maintaining participation in meaningful activities. Therefore, occupational therapy practitioners should support their clients' participation in ADLs and IADLs to help limit or reverse cancer-related disability (Pergolotti et al., 2015). The ultimate objective of this chapter is to ensure that occupational therapy practitioners know how to evaluate and treat ADL and IADL dysfunction when working in cancer rehabilitation.

ADLs AND IADLs AS OCCUPATION ACROSS THE LIFESPAN

Occupational therapy practitioners may encounter oncology survivors across the cancer care continuum and in varied practice settings, including early intervention, school-based services, acute care hospitals, inpatient rehabilitation centers, subacute rehabilitation, nursing homes, home care, and outpatient settings. *Oncology* is a medical specialty focusing on the diagnosis and treatment of cancer (National Cancer Institute, n.d.). Clients across the lifespan may deal with various cancer diagnoses and difficulties with ADLs and IADLs. *ADLs* are defined as "activities oriented toward taking care of one's own body" and *IADLs* are defined as "activities to support daily life within the home and community that often require more complex interactions than those used in ADLs" (American Occupational

Therapy Association [AOTA], 2014, p. S19). See Table 21.1 for examples of ADLs and IADLs as occupations and Table 21.2 for definitions of occupations.

Feeding

Impairments in the ability to feed oneself are commonly associated with *chemotherapy-induced peripheral neuropathy* (CIPN; see Chapter 19, "Chemotherapy-Induced Peripheral Neuropathy," for more specific information on CIPN), a commonly experienced adverse side effect that can be caused by some chemotherapy treatments. CIPN may lead to weakness and deficits in dexterity throughout the upper extremity (UE), which can limit a person's ability to set up their food, including opening containers and holding utensils while bringing food to their mouth (Tofthagen et al., 2013).

TABLE 21.1. ADLs and IADLs as Occupation

ADL/IADL	TASK ANALYSIS	COMMON ONCOLOGICAL AREAS TO ADDRESS
Feeding	▪ Opening containers ▪ Holding utensils ▪ Bringing food to the mouth	▪ CIPN ▪ Gustatory changes ▪ Postural changes ▪ Tumor location
Toileting	▪ Obtaining and using toileting supplies ▪ Managing clothing ▪ Maintaining toileting position ▪ Transferring to and from toileting position ▪ Cleaning body ▪ Caring for menstrual and continence needs	▪ Surgical anatomical changes ▪ External appliances
Dressing	▪ Obtaining articles of clothing ▪ Threading limbs into clothing ▪ Pulling clothing over upper body or hips ▪ Fastening buttons and clasps	▪ Surgical precautions ▪ Left neglect ▪ Peripheral neuropathy
Functional mobility	▪ Bed mobility ▪ Transfering to standing ▪ Ambulation ▪ Community mobility	▪ Fatigue ▪ Sensation loss ▪ Balance ▪ Pulmonary reserve ▪ Difficulty sequencing tasks
Personal device care	▪ Manipulating items ▪ Ensuring safety	▪ Hand strength and dexterity ▪ Apraxia and sequencing difficulties
Sexual activity	▪ Positioning ▪ Sexual desire	▪ Body image changes ▪ CRF
Care of others	▪ Maintaining independence to provide care to others	▪ Cancer treatment–related cognitive impairment ▪ CRF
Care of pets	▪ Providing care and supervision to support the needs of a pet	▪ Cancer treatment–related cognitive impairment ▪ CRF
Child rearing	▪ Providing care and supervision to support the developmental needs of a child	▪ Cancer treatment–related cognitive impairment ▪ CRF
Communication management	▪ Speaking ▪ Writing ▪ Typing ▪ Gestures	▪ Surgical changes ▪ Respiratory status ▪ Cancer treatment–related cognitive impairment ▪ Dexterity
Driving	▪ Hand–eye coordination ▪ Posture ▪ Safety awareness	▪ Ocular impairments ▪ Safety awareness insight
Financial management	▪ Attention ▪ Executive function	▪ Cancer treatment–related cognitive impairment
Health management	▪ Physical fitness ▪ Nutrition ▪ Decreased health risk behaviors ▪ Medication routines	▪ Cancer treatment–related cognitive impairment ▪ Fine motor coordination ▪ CRF

(Continued)

TABLE 21.1.   ADLs and IADLs as Occupation *(Cont.)*

ADL/IADL	TASK ANALYSIS	COMMON ONCOLOGICAL AREAS TO ADDRESS
Home maintenance	• Obtaining, maintaining, and repairing personal and household possessions	• Cancer treatment–related cognitive impairment • Environmental isolation restrictions
Meal preparation and clean-up	• Planning, preparing, and serving well-balanced, nutritious meals • Cleaning up food and utensils after meals	• Cancer treatment–related cognitive impairment • Fine motor coordination • CRF • Gustatory reception changes
Safety emergency and maintenance	• Knowing and performing preventive procedures to maintain a safe environment • Recognizing sudden, unexpected hazardous situations • Initiating emergency action to reduce the threat to health and safety	• Cancer treatment–related cognitive impairment • CRF
Shopping	• Acknowledging energy levels • Safety education	• CRF • Pulmonary reserve

Note. ADL = activity of daily living; CIPN = chemotherapy-induced peripheral neuropathy; CRF = cancer-related fatigue; IADL = instrumental activities of daily living.

TABLE 21.2.   Definitions of Occupations

CATEGORY	DESCRIPTION
Feeding	Setting up, arranging, and bringing food [or fluid] from the plate or cup to the mouth; sometimes called *self-feeding*
Swallowing and eating	Keeping and manipulating food or fluid in the mouth and swallowing it; *swallowing* is moving food from the mouth to the stomach
Functional mobility	Moving from one position or place to another (during performance of everyday activities) . . . includes functional ambulation and transportation of objects
Toileting and toilet hygiene	Obtaining and using toileting supplies, managing clothing, maintaining toileting position, transferring to and from toileting position, cleaning body, and caring for menstrual and continence needs (including catheter, colostomy, and suppository management), as well as completing intentional control of bowel movements and urination and, if necessary, using equipment or agents for bladder control (Uniform Data System for Medical Rehabilitation, 1996, pp. III-20, III-24)
Dressing	Selecting clothing and accessories appropriate to time of day, weather, and occasion; obtaining clothing from storage area; dressing and undressing in a sequential fashion; fastening and adjusting clothing and shoes; and applying and removing personal devices, prosthetic devices, or splints
Personal device care	Using, cleaning, and maintaining personal care items, such as hearing aids, contact lenses, glasses, orthotics, prosthetics, adaptive equipment, glucometers, and contraceptive and sexual devices
Sexual activity	Engaging in activities that result in sexual satisfaction and/or meet relational or reproductive needs
Care of others	Arranging, supervising, or providing care for others
Care of pets	Arranging, supervising, or providing care for pets and service animals
Child rearing	Providing care and supervision to support the developmental needs of a child
Communication management	Sending, receiving, and interpreting information using a variety of systems and equipment, including writing tools, telephones, keyboards, audiovisual recorders, computers or tablets, communication boards, call lights, emergency systems, Braille writers, telecommunication devices for deaf people, augmentative communication systems, and personal digital assistants
Driving and community mobility	Planning and moving around the community and using public or private transportation such as driving, walking, biking, or accessing and riding in buses, taxi cabs, or other transportation systems
Financial management	Using fiscal resources, including alternate methods of financial transaction and planning and using finances with long-term and short-term goals

(Continued)

TABLE 21.2.   Definitions of Occupations *(Cont.)*

POPULATION	POTENTIAL ACTIVITIES
Health management and maintenance	Developing, managing, and maintaining routines for health and wellness promotion, such as physical fitness, nutrition, decreased health risk behaviors and medication routines
Home establishment and management	Obtaining and maintaining personal and household possessions and environment (e.g., home, yard, garden, appliances, vehicles), including maintaining and repairing personal possessions (e.g., clothing, household items) and knowing how to seek help or whom to contact
Meal preparation and cleaning	Planning, preparing, and serving well-balanced, nutritious meals and cleaning up food and utensils after meals
Religious and spiritual activities and expression	Participating in religion, "an organized system of beliefs, practices, rituals, and symbols designed to facilitate closeness to the sacred or transcendent" (Moreira-Almeida & Koenig, 2006, p. 844), and engaging in activities that allow a sense of connectedness to something larger than oneself or that are especially meaningful, such as taking time out to play with a child, engaging in activities in nature, and helping others in need (Spencer et al., 1997)
Safety and emergency maintenance	Knowing and performing preventive procedures to maintain a safe environment; recognizing sudden, unexpected hazardous situations; and initiating emergency action to reduce the threat to health and safety; examples include ensuring safety when entering and exiting the home, identifying emergency contact numbers, and replacing items such as batteries in smoke alarms and light bulbs
Shopping	Preparing shopping lists (grocery and other); selecting, purchasing, and transporting items; selecting method of payment; and completing money transactions; included are Internet shopping and related use of electronic devices such as computers, cell phones, and tablets

Source. Excerpted from "The Occupational Therapy Practice Framework: Domain and Process (3rd ed.)," by the American Occupational Therapy Association, 2014, *American Journal of Occupational Therapy, 68,* pp. S19–S20. Copyright © 2014 by the American Occupational Therapy Association. Used with permission.

Occupational therapy practitioners should provide cancer survivors with therapeutic exercises for the neuropathy and with adaptive equipment, such as built-up handles, to increase ease and independence with feeding. Many pediatric survivors may have issues with feeding related to physically holding a bottle or utensils as a result of weakness or neuropathy, sensory issues related to food avoidance, or a decrease in their developmental reflexes (e.g., rooting reflex).

Swallowing and Eating

Swallowing and eating are early developmental skills that are essential for children to achieve. Cancer treatment that includes medications and surgical interventions can put pediatric survivors, especially developing infants, at risk for developmental delay of these skills. These survivors may have difficulty with aspects of swallowing and eating. Occupational therapy practitioners should collaborate with speech–language pathologists to educate survivors and their caregivers on eating and swallowing strategies to increase safety and independence.

Functional Mobility

Many occupations involve an aspect of *functional mobility,* which ranges from small positional changes to larger motions involving transporting oneself or items to complete a task. Cancer and its treatments can have significant negative effects on functional mobility. For example, when a person is diagnosed with lung cancer, engagement in functional mobility is at risk for decline because of decreased respiratory capacity and the effects of surgical and other cancer treatments. Adults with lung cancer commonly experience a decline in their ability to perform ADLs, "specifically, bathing, dressing, getting in and out of a chair, and using the toilet, after their diagnosis" (Pergolotti et al., 2014, p. 603).

When a survivor has a reduced lung capacity after lung surgery, movements such as getting in and out of bed, getting on and off a toilet, and walking to and from the bathroom can be challenging. If occupational therapy practitioners are working with a survivor who has had recent lung surgery, it is crucial to ensure safe transfer training and incorporate energy conservation techniques (ECTs). It may be beneficial to introduce the use of an adaptive device, such as a rollator to use when gathering items and moving them around the home, to maximize safety and allow rest when necessary.

Toileting and Toilet Hygiene

The ability to independently perform toileting and toilet hygiene can be affected by many factors, and many cancer survivors experience deficits in these occupations. For example, survivors with bladder cancer may have urinary diversion during the surgical removal of the tumor. *Urinary diversion* is a surgical procedure that reroutes the normal flow of urine out of the body when urine flow is blocked. There are several options for this surgery, depending on tumor involvement and surgeon and patient preference. Survivors may have an ostomy with a bag, a neobladder, or an internal pouch after surgery (Hedgepeth et al., 2010). An *ostomy* is an artificial opening surgically made in the abdomen to allow for the removal of waste materials. A *neobladder* is a continent urinary reservoir made from a segment of bowel or stomach, with implantation of ureters and urethra, that is used to replace the bladder after cystectomy. An *internal pouch* is an artificial bladder created to hold urine after bladder removal.

Each of these options requires survivors to learn new skills related to toileting, new toileting positions, and strategies to manage new equipment. After surgery for bladder cancer, occupational therapy practitioners should assess fine motor control, provide therapeutic exercise as appropriate, and educate survivors on new toileting schedules and body positioning. The new appliance may affect the client's body image, and therefore occupational therapy practitioners should provide psychosocial support as needed (Hedgepeth et al., 2010).

Dressing

When cancer survivors have a primary cancer, such as osteosarcoma, or a metastatic cancer to the bone at the pelvis or femur, they often have the tumor removed, followed by a total hip replacement (Grimer et al., 2005; Kabukcuoglu et al., 1999). Occupational therapy practitioners should provide education on maintaining total hip precautions during transfers, dressing, bed mobility, IADLs, and any other occupation survivors find meaningful.

Some cancers, such as osteosarcoma affecting the knee area, can result in amputation. Approximately 50% of cancer survivors with osteosarcoma of the knee undergo amputation (Luetke et al., 2014). Donning and doffing prosthetic devices becomes an ADL that must be addressed, as well as selecting appropriate clothing and accessories to wear with the prosthetic during occupational therapy treatment.

Personal Device Care

Cancer survivors who require hearing aids or glasses must be able to manipulate the device appropriately to ensure it is in working order. When working with a survivor who is experiencing CIPN, occupational therapy practitioners must be sure to address any deficits regarding fine motor coordination and dexterity. Survivors may be at risk for developing deficits in hand strength and coordination after chemotherapy treatments that affect their ability to maintain and use personal care devices such as hearing aids and glasses. If survivors are unable to check the battery on a hearing aid or ensure that the screws on their glasses are tight, they may not be able to use these devices.

Not using, or being able to use, devices may put survivors at risk for dangerous situations if they cannot hear or see appropriately. If they are unable to see or hear properly, survivors could also be at risk for not engaging in activities they might enjoy, such as going out to a restaurant with friends if they are not able to read from a menu or listen to a specials list from the server. According to Sau et al. (2015), using personal devices "also helps [survivors] to occupy their time by doing those activities [on a] regular basis and help[s] to integrate with social life" (p. 430). Occupational therapy practitioners should address any deficits with a range of interventions, including participation in functional tasks and interventions to increase range of motion (ROM), strength, and coordination.

Personal Hygiene and Grooming

Cancer survivors may experience various challenges to personal hygiene and grooming, depending on the type of cancer they have and its treatments. For example, when the client is a survivor diagnosed with a brain tumor, it is important to understand the location of the lesion and the potential effects on daily life. One deficit that can cause potential safety hazards is *apraxia,* the inability to execute a voluntary motor movement despite being able to demonstrate normal muscle function, which can lead to difficulty with the use of tools or the familiar objects used to perform daily occupations. "Apraxic behavior in tool use is primarily attributed to the impaired or lost access to the tool-related knowledge, concepts of use, and problem solving" (Bieńkiewicz, 2014, p. 353).

For example, a survivor who had a *craniotomy,* a surgical opening in the skull to remove a tumor, may have difficulty identifying and using tools properly, such as a toothbrush or toothpaste for oral hygiene. When provided with tools to complete the toothbrushing task, the survivor may not be able to sequence removing the toothpaste cap, applying the toothpaste to the brush, and bringing the brush to their mouth. They may skip steps or attempt to use the toothbrush incorrectly, like a comb or another object.

Occupational therapy practitioners should make a goal and work with the patient on safe and correct setup, sequencing, and completion of the task to increase overall independence. This may require breaking down each aspect of the task, modifying setup location, or involving caregivers as needed to ensure safety is maintained.

Sexual Activity

Sexual activity is an important occupation that may be greatly affected by cancer diagnosis and treatment. Cancer survivors may have to respond to and manage treatment side effects and changes in body image. Pergolotti et al. (2016) noted that large numbers of older adults are surviving cancer but report having fair or poor health during and after cancer treatment. They may experience poorer perceived health due to *cancer-related fatigue* (CRF; see Chapter 15, "Cancer-Related Fatigue," for more information). CRF differs from "typical" fatigue that is caused by lack of sleep or tiredness in several ways. First, fatigue among cancer survivors is more persistent, more devastating, and longer lasting. Second, it is physical, mental, and emotional. Third, it is not relieved by adequate sleep or rest (Charalambous et al., 2016).

Sexual activity positively affects a person's quality of life (QoL) when their need for sexual satisfaction is being met. Occupational therapists can use assessments of fatigue, such as the Cancer Fatigue Scale (Schwartz, 1998) or the Brief Fatigue Inventory (Mendoza et al., 1999), to assess the effect of CRF on a client's daily life (Charalambous et al., 2016). Occupational therapy practitioners can then introduce energy conservation strategies and positioning to increase comfort. Practitioners should aim to increase QoL and satisfaction for survivors experiencing a decrease in sexual activity secondary to CRF.

Care of Others

Many cancer survivors are responsible not only for their own self-care on a daily basis but also for the care of others such as a child, a parent, a partner, or others. Cancer and its treatment can greatly affect the ability of survivors to perform caregiving occupations.

For example, a survivor with rectal cancer may be faced with recovery after an *abdominoperineal resection* (APR). This is a standard surgical procedure used to remove rectal cancer that lies close to the anus. After an APR procedure, the anus is removed with the cancer, and the cut end of the large bowel is attached to the abdominal wall to form a colostomy. During the recovery process, a common precaution is that patients are not allowed to sit at the edge of a bed or in a chair for approximately 6 weeks. Occupational therapy practitioners must ensure that survivors are able to complete all basic ADLs without sitting. This presents an obvious challenge for survivors who have caregiving responsibilities. Occupational therapy practitioners should assess all caregiving responsibilities such as preparing a meal for an elder parent or washing and drying baby clothes for a new grandchild.

Care of Pets

Care of pets is a common and often overlooked occupation in occupational therapy intervention planning. When meeting a cancer survivor who has a pet, occupational therapy practitioners should address any deficits that a client may be facing with this occupation. People often consider their pets to be family members. Survivors who undergo cancer treatments such as surgery, chemotherapy, or radiation may need modifications to successfully perform their role of caregiver to their pets.

For example, after abdominal surgeries, there is a risk for pain, especially when bending, and there are often restrictions on how much a survivor can lift. Modifications that could be made to feed a pet include raising the height of a food bowl or taking small portions of food from a large bag instead of lifting and pouring into a bowl.

Child Rearing

A diagnosis of cancer not only alters a cancer survivor's life, but it may also alter their children's lives. Helping a child to achieve all developmental milestones promotes improved QoL. In turn, the reaction of children to their parent's cancer experience may affect the parent. As Gazendam-Donofrio et al. (2008) noted, "it is possible that the children's emotional and behavioral functioning, which may be affected by their parent's cancer, affects how the parents function" (p. 134).

Occupational therapy practitioners may encounter the effects of cancer in multiple and sometimes unanticipated settings. For example, an occupational therapy practitioner in a school system may be notified that a child they are working with has a parent who has been diagnosed with colorectal cancer, and the practitioner may be called on to assist the parent and child. The practitioner may consider including both the parents and the child in occupational therapy assessment and intervention if appropriate.

Communication Management

When a cancer survivor is faced with life-altering situations such as a loss of communication, occupational therapy practitioners can play a major role in assisting the survivor to modify approaches to communication. For example, survivors with cancer affecting their respiratory status and requiring mechanical ventilation are at high risk for not being able to communicate their needs. These survivors may need to be involved in making critical medical decisions to determine the next course of action, and having the ability to communicate their wishes is paramount.

Encountering such situations is becoming more common. Ten Hoorn et al. (2016) noted that "current practice in the intensive care unit is to use less sedation in mechanically ventilated patients, which increases the number of patients potentially able to communicate while mechanically ventilated and awake" (p. 333). Occupational therapy practitioners can determine an appropriate method to facilitate communication with staff and family members. After assessment, practitioners can determine whether a patient can use low-tech levels of communication, such as eye gaze, gestures, pointing toward pictures on a communication board, or writing with pen and paper, or high-tech levels of communication such as a computer tablet to type (Ten Hoorn et al., 2016). The practitioner can then assist the survivor to achieve appropriate positioning to be able to communicate their needs and wishes.

Driving and Community Mobility

Many cancer survivors experience challenges to safe driving and community mobility during the active phase of their treatment and after cessation. Cancers can affect body structures and systems, and both cancer and its treatment can affect vision, coordination, cognition, and other aspects of function that are necessary to safely drive or to use public transportation.

For example, consider clients who have been diagnosed with a form of hematological disorder and who may be able to receive an allogenic hematopoietic stem cell transplant (SCT) to increase their chance of survival. Some may experience a common set of complications known as *graft-versus-host disease (GVHD)*, a condition that can occur after SCT in which the donor immune cells attack the recipient's tisues that "is a major cause of morbidity that compromises patients' quality of life" (Saboo et al., 2015, p. 1670).

Ocular GVHD generally manifests as dry eye disease, with symptoms of ocular discomfort, pain, redness, grittiness, and blurred vision. Any of these symptoms could put a person at risk when returning to driving or any form of community mobility. Occupational therapy practitioners are able to assist clients with off-the-road and on-the-road assessment, evaluation, and interventions to ensure the safety of their clients during this occupation or make a referral to an appropriate practitioner for these services.

Financial Management

Many cancer survivors experience chemotherapy-induced cognitive dysfunction as a result of chemotherapy treatments (see Chapter 17, "Cancer-Related Cognitive Impairment," for more information). With improving survival rates, increasing numbers of people are experiencing adverse side effects of treatment.

Survivors treated with chemotherapy may experience an increased difficulty in multitasking and processing, which are essential skills for managing one's finances, because of deficits in memory, executive functioning, and processing (Selamat et al., 2014). It may be difficult for clients to balance a checkbook, set up automatic payments for recurring monthly expenses, or plan for retirement secondary to deficits in concentration, attention, and memory. Occupational therapy practitioners can intervene with clients to increase performance in these occupations, with a focus on maintaining independence with financial management.

Health Management and Maintenance

Cancer survivors are often encouraged by their oncologist to improve their physical health and wellness before cancer treatment (see Chapter 10, "Prehabilitation," for more information; Kushi et al., 2006). Occupational therapy practitioners can help clients develop appropriate plans for health and wellness promotion, including physical fitness, nutrition, decreased health risk behaviors, and medication routines that account for the client's disease status (in particular any disease in the bones or spine) and lab values (including hemoglobin and platelets; AOTA, 2014). Medication routines can be affected by cognitive changes or fine motor control deficits related to cancer and cancer treatment. Occupational therapy practitioners should help survivors address the factors that are the most meaningful to them and to safely improve participation in health and wellness promotion.

Home Establishment and Management

Home establishment and management is a complex IADL that encompasses obtaining, maintaining, and repairing personal and household possessions as well as the environment (AOTA, 2014). Many cancer survivors experience a disruption in their ability to successfully perform home establishment and management. For example, after a bone marrow transplant, many survivors are told by their oncologist not to engage in yardwork or gardening because of the increased risk for infection during these tasks (Partridge-Hinckley et al., 2009). After chemotherapy and bone marrow transplant, survivors may also have mild cognitive impairment, which affects their ability to know how or from whom to seek help to complete these tasks while they are not allowed to (Kelly et al., 2017). Occupational therapy practitioners should provide education on why these precautions are important and address any impairments in executive function and judgment that affect their client's independence with home establishment and management.

Meal Preparation and Clean-Up

Participating in meal preparation and cleaning is multifaceted and can be affected by cancer and cancer treatment in many ways. As mentioned before, cognitive deficits or CRF can greatly affect function and participation in these tasks. Cancer survivors who have undergone surgery may benefit from education regarding energy conservation for meal preparation, such as ordering meals or groceries online, preparing larger amounts of food at once, and using

a rollator to move plates and utensils from the table to sink to clean.

Religious and Spiritual Activities and Expression

Participation in religion and engagement are often important to cancer survivors. These activities may also improve emotional well-being and decrease psychological distress (Gall et al., 2000).

Physical changes from cancer can affect a person's ability to participate in religious or spiritual activities. For example, a client with a lower-extremity amputation may find it difficult to repeatedly sit and stand during a Christian mass, or a Muslim client with an amputation may not be able to prostrate during *sujud*. Cancer survivors often avoid crowded locations because of their decreased immune system, and these precautions as well as frequent hospitalizations or treatments can affect clients' participation in their preferred method of religious or spiritual activities. They may not be able to attend their preferred place for religious worship, and the occupational therapy practitioner can help the client identify additional ways to continue their spiritual activities and expressions during their treatment. For example, an immunocompromised client may not be able to attend services in person but can access virtual services.

Safety and Emergency Maintenance

Performing each aspect of safety and emergency maintenance requires intact cognitive function, especially in the areas of executive function, memory, and attention. Player et al. (2014) found that up to 70% of women who have completed chemotherapy for breast cancer report signs of mild cognitive impairment, or "chemo brain." The areas most often affected are executive function, memory, and attention. The women in this study reported the greatest difficulty managing all the aspects of their household, which includes safety and emergency maintenance. Occupational therapy practitioners need to identify these sometimes subtle changes in cognition during and after chemotherapy treatment, help the clients identify these changes, and create comprehensive treatment plans to address deficits and ensure safety in these sometimes complex emergency situations.

Shopping

Shopping in the community may require increased energy, depending on the method of mobility and availability of assistance from others. This may prove extremely challenging for some cancer survivors. For example, survivors with lung cancer may require supplemental oxygen after surgery or because of their disease.

When addressing the occupation of shopping, occupational therapy practitioners can be instrumental in increasing clients' independence and ease during the activity by focusing on education, including education on issues such as oxygen tank and line management, ways to incorporate breathing into functional activities, how to incorporate exercise into activity, and any specific areas within the realm of shopping that the client is having difficulty with (Maekura et al., 2015).

FACTORS THAT MAY CONTRIBUTE TO OCCUPATIONAL IMPAIRMENT IN ADLs AND IADLs

Client Factors

Cancer and its treatments can have negative effects on multiple client factors and, in turn, affect occupational performance. There are five main client factors: (1) values, (2) beliefs, (3) spirituality, (4) body functions, and (5) body structures (see Table 21.3).

Performance Skills

When analyzing an activity and examining performance skills, occupational therapy practitioners should examine the client's demonstrated abilities. To complete an ADL, survivors must combine various performance skills. There are three main types of performance skills: (1) motor, (2) process, and (3) social interaction (see Table 21.4).

Performance Patterns

Identifying what habits, routines, roles, and rituals are most important to cancer survivors undergoing cancer diagnosis and treatment is crucial. Survivors often experience a change in their occupational performance patterns. Daily performance may change from going to work and caring for others or pets to creating new routines, such as identifying what clothes are the best to wear while getting chemotherapy, arriving at a center for chemotherapy, picking what lunch to eat during chemotherapy treatment, and identifying how to spend the time while receiving chemotherapy. After chemotherapy, the survivor's routines may require taking care of their household while they still feel healthy, having all items they need when they are nauseous, or finding family or friends to stay with them while they recover from treatment. Such dramatic changes in performance patterns affect occupational performance.

Occupational therapy practitioners should identify how to maximize clients' independence through education on energy conservation, pacing, and structuring days around chemotherapy treatment to maximize performance in meaningful tasks. Cancer survivors may benefit from cooking large batches of meals or deep cleaning before chemotherapy to decrease the need for cooking and cleaning after treatment, when they may feel weak or nauseous. Occupational therapy practitioners can help identify performance patterns that are most important to survivors and create an intervention plan structured around these meaningful tasks.

Adolescent and young adult survivors may see their habits, routines, and roles changed dramatically. For example, a survivor in college may reside on a campus and live with their friends and roommates with relative autonomy. After diagnosis and treatment, the survivor may have to return home to their parents' house and give up this newfound autonomy. Occupational therapy practitioners should work

TABLE 21.3. Client Factors

CLIENT FACTORS	EXAMPLE	TREATMENT IDEA
Values	Spending time with family members	Participate in preparing a family meal for a holiday celebration
Beliefs	Hard work pays off	Include therapeutic exercise during sessions to focus on core strengthening to increase the client's independence with household maintenance work
Spirituality	Finding purpose in life	Incorporate mindfulness into a session to help the client focus on finding their purpose in life
Body functions and body structures	Specific mental functions that affect a client's attention	Increase the client's ability to concentrate on reading medication labels to correctly manage medications

TABLE 21.4. Performance Skills

PERFORMANCE SKILL	EXAMPLE OF DEFICIT	TREATMENT IDEAS
Motor skills	Loss of grip or grip strength due to CIPN	Address oral care, with focus on grip of toothpaste, brush, cup, and toothpaste cap
Process skills	Navigation	Help client learn to move the wheelchair safely and without bumping into obstacles in their bathroom so they can complete toileting as independently as possible
Social interaction skills	Cannot appropriately regulate their interactions with the bank teller	Address distractibility and impulsivity during social interactions in controlled environments, progressing to uncontrolled environments

Note. CIPN = chemotherapy-induced peripheral neuropathy.

with survivors to identify ways they can create new routines, habits, and roles or adapt their performance patterns to increase their participation in meaningful activities and regain some of their lost autonomy.

Context and Environment

Occupational therapy practitioners should consider the contexts and social and physical environments in which specific occupations occur (AOTA, 2014). The physical environments in which cancer survivors operate can dramatically change during cancer treatment. For example, a survivor going through a bone marrow transplant may be restricted to their private hospital room for several weeks. Often these survivors are required to stay in their hospital room at all times or are only allowed to leave their room in context of mobility in a controlled environment because of their compromised immune system (Biagioli et al., 2017). Some survivors are negatively affected by prolonged isolation.

For example, a survivor who works outdoors and enjoys outdoor leisure tasks may find it difficult to adjust to several weeks indoors, where they cannot work on typical projects. Another survivor who works from home and enjoys more sedentary leisure tasks, such as doing puzzles or reading books, may easily adapt to a new physical environment during hospitalization. The social environment also changes with prolonged hospitalization.

The expectations of and relationships with friends and family may be significantly affected by a potentially life-threatening diagnosis. Family and friends may change their approach to social interactions. Occupational therapy practitioners may observe family members providing assistance for all ADLs and IADLs even though the survivor could easily complete the occupations independently. For example, a parent may feed their teenage son even though he can independently feed himself and would feed himself in a different environment.

When treating a client, occupational therapy practitioners need to consider all aspects of context—cultural, personal, temporal, and virtual (AOTA, 2014). Practitioners need to be aware of the cultural context of their client. For example, they should have an awareness of the cultural norms around end-of-life care and dying. In some languages and cultures, the word *hospice* cannot be translated, and a client or their family members may not be familiar with the word and have difficulty understanding the concept of hospice care.

Personal and temporal context can play a role in how survivors approach their treatment. One survivor may want to participate in any treatment or trial that could extend life, despite the side effects, whereas another survivor with a different personal or temporal context may focus on QoL over extending life through further treatment.

The virtual context is becoming increasingly relevant to occupational therapy clients and intervention. Online support groups and social media can provide support and connectivity for survivors going through treatment. Ensuring that clients can access technology and appropriately use their devices can be an important part of occupational therapy treatment. Addressing any fine motor, cognitive, or visual deficits to allow for participation in the virtual context can allow survivors to participate in socialization and their daily occupations.

OCCUPATIONAL THERAPY EVALUATION OF ADLs AND IADLs

Occupational Profile

The occupational profile is the first step in the occupational therapy evaluation process. It gives occupational therapy practitioners an understanding of the client's occupational history and experiences, patterns of daily living, interests, values, and needs (AOTA, 2014). To gain an understanding of the client's occupational profile, practitioners need to understand why the client needs occupational therapy services and how their performance of occupations has been affected.

The questions occupational therapy practitioners ask cancer survivors may be similar to the questions they would ask other clients. Information about home setup, social support, values, habits, needs, participation in ADLs and IADLs, barriers, concerns, and strengths should be identified. Some additional questions and discussion for cancer survivors may include the following:

- *"Where are you in your cancer treatment, and what treatment will be next?"* Understanding the survivor's course of treatment will help the practitioner develop appropriate intervention plans and determine the frequency and location of treatment. A survivor getting outpatient radiation therapy or chemotherapy may not be able to be referred to an inpatient rehabilitation hospital, and planning will need to be focused on home or outpatient therapy. A survivor with frequent visits to the oncologist for blood work or transfusions might benefit from an occupational therapy schedule based around those appointments.
- *"How do you feel after treatment?"* A survivor who has undergone chemotherapy before may have a good understanding of how they will feel each day after treatment. Occupational therapy practitioners should incorporate this information into treatment when discussing energy conservation or participation in occupations as well as when planning timing of therapy sessions.
- *"Do you have any neuropathy, and when did it begin? How does it affect your function?"* CIPN is a common side effect and often affects a client's participation in fine motor tasks. Intervention should address CIPN with a focus on both remediation and compensation.
- *"Have you had an increase in fatigue? Has it affected your participation in meaningful tasks?"* Education on CRF and ECTs can improve a client's participation in occupations.

Different cancer diagnoses and treatments will elicit additional questions from the occupational therapy practitioner on the basis of the client's medical history. For example, for a survivor with ovarian or breast cancer who has had surgery with lymph node removal, the occupational therapy practitioner would question and assess for signs and symptoms of lymphedema. For a survivor with a progressive cancer, such as a glioblastoma, the practitioner must have a thorough understanding of the progression of symptoms when creating intervention plans and goals.

For a survivor with cancer, patterns of daily living may have dramatically changed after diagnosis. An understanding of the client's interests, values, and needs will focus occupational therapy intervention sessions on what is most meaningful to the client. Occupational therapy practitioners should consider additional questions related to cancer and its treatment for this population to create a comprehensive occupational profile.

Analysis of Occupational Performance

Once an occupational therapy practitioner has developed an occupational profile, the next step in the process is to analyze occupational performance. There are many parts to this process that are linked together. It is important to always keep a holistic view of the occupational profile, functional impairments, and how they relate to everyday ADL and IADL tasks, as well as to be realistic about goal setting. Practitioners must choose appropriate assessments to use during an evaluation as well as choose appropriate tasks for survivors to participate in (see Table 21.5 for commonly used ADL and IADL assessments). It is essential to collaborate with the survivor when goal setting as well as to keep goals functional and measurable. Case Examples 21.1–21.5 reflect realistic settings that occupational therapy practitioners might encounter during their career with oncology survivors.

TABLE 21.5.   Commonly Used Assessments for ADLs and IADLs

ASSESSMENT	AUTHORS	AGES	PURPOSE	AREAS ADDRESSED
Activity Measure for Post Acute Care	Jette et al. (2008)	Adults	Used across diagnoses, conditions, and settings where post-acute care is provided	▪ Basic mobility ▪ ADLs ▪ Applied cognitive
Katz Index of Independence in Activities of Daily Living	Katz et al. (1963)	Geriatric	Assesses functional status, in particular the client's ability to perform ADLs independently	▪ Bathing ▪ Dressing ▪ Toileting ▪ Transferring ▪ Continence ▪ Feeding
Modified Barthel Index	Mahoney & Barthel (1965)	Adults and geriatric population	Shows the degree of independence of a patient without assistance	▪ Bowel and bladder control ▪ Grooming ▪ Toileting ▪ Feeding ▪ Transfers ▪ Walking ▪ Dressing ▪ Climbing stairs ▪ Bathing
Performance Assessment of Self Care Skills, Version 4.0	Rogers & Holm (2014)	Adults	Observation-based performance rating of ADL in clinic or home	▪ 3 ADLs ▪ 5 functional mobility tasks ▪ 18 IADLs
Executive Function Performance Test	Baum et al. (2008)	30–90-year-olds	Top-down assessment identifying executive function skills needed to perform common daily occupations for independent living	▪ Initiation ▪ Organization ▪ Sequencing ▪ Judgment ▪ Understanding of task completion
Contextual Memory Test	Toglia (1993)	18 years and older	Assesses awareness of memory capacity, recall of line-drawn items, and strategy use	Memory strategies to complete tasks
Catherine Bergego Scale	Chen et al. (2012)	Adults with stroke	Identify unilateral behavioral neglect	Severity of unilateral behavioral neglect
Arnadottir OT-ADL Neurobehavioral Evaluation (now the A-ONE)	Arnadottir (1990)	16 years and older	Identify neurobehavioral deficits, how they affect functional performance of ADLs, and relation to cortical lesions	▪ Dressing ▪ Grooming ▪ Transfers ▪ Mobility ▪ Feeding ▪ Communication
Multiple Errands Test	Shallice & Burgess (1991)	Adolescents to adults	Assess executive function and problem solving in relatively open-ended situations	Executive function, initiation and problem solving needed during ADLs

Note. ADLs = activities of daily living; IADLs = instrumental activities of daily living.

CASE EXAMPLE 21.1. MR. JONES IN ACUTE CARE

Mr. Jones is a 58-year-old man who has been diagnosed and living with lung cancer for the past 3 years. He is a husband, father of two, and works for the U.S. Postal Service. During the 2 weeks before his admission to the hospital, he noticed some shortness of breath while working his usual route delivering mail. He found himself taking more breaks during the day than normal.

Mr. Jones woke his wife one evening with complaints of severe shortness of breath, so she took him to the emergency room. He was admitted to the hospital, and during the next 12 hours he continued to decompensate, to the point where he was admitted to the intensive care unit (ICU) and placed on a ventilator secondary to respiratory insufficiency and hypotension. The next morning the team in the ICU placed an order for an occupational therapy evaluation. The occupational therapist reviewed Mr. Jones's chart and coordinated with the nurse and respiratory therapist taking care of him to see him for his occupational therapy evaluation.

The occupational therapist identified significant edema to Mr. Jones's upper and lower extremities. Because he was on a ventilator and unable to talk, the occupational therapist began to identify the most effective form of communication for Mr. Jones. He could respond by opening his eyes to his name and attempt to wave to the therapist; however, this was difficult because of his upper extremity (UE) edema. He was awake, alert, and able to follow all instructions during the initial interactions.

The occupational therapist provided Mr. Jones with a built-up pen and paper stabilized on a clipboard so he could attempt to write to communicate; however, his grip was poor. The occupational therapist then positioned a computer tablet on the bedside table for Mr. Jones to type his answers regarding his social history about where he lives, his family, his job requirements, and his hobbies.

At that moment, Mr. Jones communicated to her that his biggest complaint was the discomfort from the ventilator tubing in his mouth and the constant pooling of oral secretions. The occupational therapist introduced a suction tool that he could grip, with assistance, to bring to his mouth and complete modified oral hygiene. Mr. Jones relaxed and coordinated his breathing with the ventilator.

The occupational therapist provided education on UE exercises and positioning that would help to reduce edema and improve Mr. Jones's ability to move his own arms, grip a pen, and hold a tissue to wipe his mouth to increase his comfort while on the ventilator. In later sessions, the occupational therapist focused on

- UE range of motion and strengthening exercises,
- Increasing sitting tolerance at the edge of the bed,
- Transfer training to a chair and toilet,
- Increasing standing tolerance at a sink for grooming,
- Performing standing bathing tasks or modifying with shower chair to conserve energy,
- Dressing with adaptive equipment if necessary, and
- Improving communication strategies while on the ventilator.

CASE EXAMPLE 21.2. MRS. SINGH AT INPATIENT REHABILITATION

Mrs. Singh is a 67-year-old woman diagnosed with acute myeloid leukemia. She had several rounds of chemotherapy and reached complete remission. She was then admitted for an allogeneic stem cell transplant. During her transplant, she was isolated in a private hospital room for 4 weeks because of her impaired immune system.

Mrs. Singh was later found to have graft-versus-host disease (GVHD). Her GVHD was treated with medication after a prolonged stay in the hospital. Mrs. Singh was admitted to a rehabilitation facility for further inpatient rehabilitation services.

During the evaluation, Mrs. Singh presented with decreased independence with her ADLs, IADLs, and transfers. After a prolonged hospitalization, Mrs. Singh has decreased strength throughout her upper and lower extremities. Scarring on her skin from the GVHD limits range of motion (ROM) in her digits, elbows, and shoulders, which affects her function.

Mrs. Singh enjoys cooking for her family, going to her local temple, and playing cards with her friends. She has been using a wheelchair for mobility because of weakness and decreased ROM.

Intervention with Mrs. Singh focuses on

- Manual therapy to address scarring and improve skin mobility;
- Active and passive ROM throughout the upper extremities (UEs) within her tolerance;
- "Wall writing" to improve digit, elbow, and shoulder ROM;
- Exercise putty to improve hand strength;
- UE exercises to improve strength;
- Performing ADL tasks first sitting and then standing to improve endurance;
- Performing cooking tasks sitting and then standing to improve independence with IADLs;
- Folding laundry in standing to improve UE ROM, strength, and balance with UE unsupported;
- Playing familiar card games to improve fine motor control while reaching outside of the midline to retrieve cards every round; and
- Transfer training to toilet, shower, bed, car, couch, and chairs with and without armrests at various heights.

Mrs. Singh enjoys participation both in therapeutic exercises and in ADL, leisure, and IADL tasks. On discharge from the rehabilitation hospital, she can dress and bathe herself, perform cooking and cleaning tasks, and engage in leisure tasks with her friends. She can perform community mobility and transfer to chairs without armrests that are present at her temple.

CASE EXAMPLE 21.3. ELLA IN OUTPATIENT OCCUPATIONAL THERAPY

Ella is a 14-year-old girl who has acute lymphocytic leukemia and has undergone all treatment of a bone marrow transplant. She is in 8th grade and enjoys playing the violin in her school orchestra. She is beginning to transition back into school full-time. She has many medical appointments during the week and is looking forward to working with the occupational therapist to improve the weakness and neuropathy that she experiences in both of her upper extremities (UEs).

Ella's occupational therapy evaluation is scheduled at 4:00 p.m. following her day at school. Her main complaints when she meets with the occupational therapist are that her books feel heavy when she has to carry them from class to class and that her fingers feel tired during music class. She has full range of motion throughout her UEs; however, her manual muscle test reveals slightly decreased strength, and she scores 4 out of 5 throughout. Her sensation is slightly diminished distally in both hands. The following are examples of interventions the occupational therapist could implement with Ella:

- UE strengthening
- Fine motor coordination exercises with exercise putty
- Core strengthening exercises
- Exploring different backpacks for school.

CASE EXAMPLE 21.4. MRS. CHEN IN HOME CARE

Mrs. Chen is a 52-year-old woman diagnosed with breast cancer. She has had lumpectomy, chemotherapy, and radiation. Since completing treatment, she has increased fatigue and weakness, which affect her ability to participate in her daily occupations. At her doctor's appointment, Mrs. Chen reports having difficulty caring for herself, having all meals delivered, and spending most of her time in bed because of fatigue and weakness. Her doctor refers her for occupational therapy services in the home.

Mrs. Chen works as a kindergarten teacher but is on medical leave during treatment. She enjoys reading, gardening, and creating unique lesson plans for her students. During the evaluation, the occupational therapist finds that Mrs. Chen requires contact guard assistance for transfers. She has fair static and dynamic standing balance and requires frequent rest breaks because of fatigue. Mrs. Chen reports impaired mood as a result of difficulty participating in her normal routine.

Occupational therapy intervention focuses on
- Education on cancer-related fatigue (CRF) and ways to decrease fatigue;
- Education on energy conservation techniques (ECTs);
- Participation in gardening tasks in standing and kneeling, with a focus on incorporating ECTs and rest breaks to increase the amount of time she is able to participate in gardening before having to take rest breaks;
- Participation in lesson planning and creating new arts and craft projects for her students; and
- While standing, incorporation of learned techniques to create a large folding thank you card for her students and colleagues who sent her get well messages

Mrs. Chen was able to incorporate what she learned about CRF and ECTs to improve her endurance and participation in ADLs, IADLs, and leisure tasks. Working on lesson planning for work and gardening helped her return to a more typical routine, and creating a thank you card for her students and colleagues improved her mood.

CASE EXAMPLE 21.5. NOHA IN EARLY INTERVENTION

Noha is a 9-month-old girl who was diagnosed at age 6 months with a neuroblastoma. Her tumor was in her abdomen, and she stopped eating around age 6 months. She was in the hospital for several months and, during that time, was given food by bottle or spoon despite attempting to resist all feeding. She became aversive to feeding because of this negative association of being forced food when resisting. She showed no signs of aspiration, and her oral–motor skills were intact. Food aversion was related to sensory issues only.

On meeting Noha and her family, the occupational therapist determines what activities and milestones Noha has met and what deficits need to be addressed. Noha's father's biggest concern during the evaluation is that Noha is not eating anything by mouth and has become aversive to the sight of the bottle and spoon. Noha eats dissolvable cookies exclusively. The occupational therapist puts emphasis on the family's feeding interactions with Noha outside of occupational therapy sessions to improve carryover of techniques learned during intervention sessions.

During the sessions, the occupational therapist focuses on the following areas related to feeding:
- The therapist uses play with a bottle and spoon without the intention of feeding to decrease Ella's aversion to the sight of the items.

(Continued)

CASE EXAMPLE 21.5. NOHA IN EARLY INTERVENTION *(Cont.)*

- The therapist addresses Ella's tactile awareness of food through play. She uses various types of food with different textures in different containers, including cups, trays, and plates.
- The therapist conducts structured sessions with decreased environmental stimulation. All occupational therapy sessions are performed with play at beginning of session, and then, once she is comfortable with the occupational therapist, Noha is transitioned to her high chair during the session for improved carryover of feeding tasks with family.
- Family members are given recommendations for types of food to have on hand for the following sessions to progress to new textures and types of foods.

- Family members are given activities to perform outside of occupational therapy sessions, using what was positive during the session to carry over during the day (e.g., feeding with a type of food that was successful).
- Types of food and food textures are changed regularly so Noha does not get into a food jag where she then refuses that type of food and eliminates one more item from her diet.

The occupational therapist sees Noha for 4 weeks, 4 times per week, with carryover by parents. At the end of the 4 weeks Noha is able to eat and drink from a bottle and can use a spoon with assistance to feed herself at the appropriate developmental level.

OCCUPATIONAL THERAPY INTERVENTIONS FOR ADLs AND IADLs

Pilegaard et al. (2017) noted that "research shows that most people with advanced cancer have difficulties performing and participating in everyday activities" (p. 745). Occupational therapy practitioners are trained to analyze any daily task and help clients work toward achieving the task as independently as possible. When working with the cancer population, it is extremely important to remember that the cancer survivor's personal interests and goals will drive the sessions. No matter where a survivor is along the continuum of cancer care, it is important to help them be as independent in their ADLs and IADLs as possible to maintain their QoL.

SUMMARY

Cancer and its treatments can significantly affect the ability of cancer survivors to perform ADLs and IADLs in their typical contexts and environments. Comprehensive evaluation of ADLs and IADLs is a critical component of occupational therapy intervention with cancer survivors. Evaluation must include analysis of how cancer and its treatments affect the cancer survivor's participation in ADLs and IADLs, including client factors and performance patterns. Identifying the survivor's goals and priorities through development of the occupational profile guides selection of appropriate assessments for occupational therapy intervention.

After treatment, cancer survivors may present with treatment-related deficits, such as fatigue, CIPN, or chemotherapy-induced cognitive impairment. These deficits may present additional challenges to ADL and IADL performance, providing an opportunity for the occupational therapy practitioner to improve the survivor's occupational performance, participation, and QoL.

REFERENCES

American Occupational Therapy Association. (2014). Occupational therapy practice framework: Domain and process (3rd ed.). *American Journal of Occupational Therapy, 68*(Suppl. 1), S1–S48. https://doi.org/10.5014/ajot.2014.682006

Arnadottir, G. (1990). *The brain and behavior: Assessing cortical dysfunction through activities of daily living.* Philadelphia: Mosby.

Baum, C. M., Connor, L. T., Morrison, T., Hahn, M., Dromerick, A. W., & Edwards, D. F. (2008). Reliability, validity, and clinical utility of the Executive Function Performance Test: A measure of executive function in a sample of people with stroke. *American Journal of Occupational Therapy, 62,* 446–455. https://doi.org/10.5014/ajot.62.4.446

Biagioli, V., Piredda, M., Alvaro, R., & de Marinis, M. G. (2017). The experiences of protective isolation in patients undergoing bone marrow or haematopoietic stem cell transplantation: Systematic review and metasynthesis. *European Journal of Cancer Care, 26,* e12461. https://doi.org/10.1111/ecc.12461

Bieńkiewicz, M. M. N., Brandi, M.-L., Goldenberg, G., Hughes, C. M. L., & Hermsdörfer, J. (2014). The tool in the brain: Apraxia in ADL. Behavioral and neurological correlates of apraxia in daily living. *Frontiers in Psychology, 5,* 353. https://doi.org/10.3389/fpsyg.2014.00353

Charalambous, A., Kaite, C., Constantinou, M., & Kouta, C. (2016). Translation and validation of the Cancer-Related Fatigue Scale in Greek in a sample of patients with advanced prostate cancer. *BMJ Open, 6,* e011798. https://doi.org/10.1136/bmjopen-2016-011798

Chen, P., Hreha, K., Fortis, P., Goedert, K. M., & Barrett, A. M. (2012). Functional assessment of spatial neglect: A review of the Catherine Bergego Scale and an introduction of the Kessler foundation neglect assessment process. *Topics in Stroke Rehabilitation, 19,* 423–435. https://doi.org/10.1310/tsr1905-423

Gall, T. L., Miguez de Renart, R. M., & Boonstra, B. (2000). Religious resources in long-term adjustment to breast cancer. *Journal of Psychosocial Oncology, 18,* 21–37. https://doi.org/10.1300/J077v18n02_02

Gazendam-Donofrio, S. M., Hoekstra, H. J., van der Graaf, W. T. A., Pras, E., Visser, A., Huizinga, G. A., & Hoekstra-Weebers,

J. E. H. M. (2008). Quality of life of parents with children living at home: When one parent has cancer. *Supportive Care in Cancer, 16,* 133–141. https://doi.org/10.1007/s00520-007-0299-7

Grimer, R. J., Bielack, S., Flege, S., Cannon, S. R., Foleras, G., Andreeff, I., . . . Gosheger, G. (2005). Periosteal osteosarcoma: A European review of outcome. *European Journal of Cancer, 41,* 2806–2811. https://doi.org/10.1016/j.ejca.2005.04.052

Hedgepeth, R. C., Gilbert, S. M., He, C., Lee, C. T., & Wood, D. P., Jr. (2010). Body image and bladder cancer specific quality of life in patients with ileal conduit and neobladder urinary diversions. *Urology, 76,* 671–675. https://doi.org/10.1016/j.urology.2010.01.087

Jette, A., Haley, S. M., Coster, W., & Ni, P. (2008). *Boston University Activity Measure for Post Acute Care™ (AM–PAC).* Boston: Boston University Health and Disability Research Institute.

Kabukcuoglu, Y., Grimer, R. J., Tillman, R. M., & Carter, S. R. (1999). Endoprosthetic replacement for primary malignant tumors of the proximal femur. *Clinical Orthopaedics and Related Research, 358,* 8–14.

Katz, S., Ford, A. B., Moskowitz, R. W., Jackson, B. A., & Jaffe, M. W. (1963). The Index of ADL: A standardized measure of biological and psychosocial function. *JAMA, 185,* 914–919. https://doi.org/10.1001/jama.1963.03060120024016

Kelly, D. L., Buchbinder, D., Duarte, R. F., Auletta, J. J., Bhatt, N., Byrne, M., . . . Shah, A. J. (2017). Neurocognitive dysfunction in hematopoietic cell transplant recipients: Expert review from the Late Effects and Quality of Life Working Committee of the CIBMTR and Complications and Quality of Life Working Party of the EBMT. *Biology of Blood and Marrow Transplantation, 24,* 228–241. https://doi.org/10.1016/j.bbmt.2017.09.004

Kushi, L. H., Byers, T., Doyle, C., Bandera, E. V., McCullough, M., McTiernan, A., . . . Thun, M. J. (2006). American Cancer Society guidelines on nutrition and physical activity for cancer prevention: Reducing the risk of cancer with healthy food choices and physical activity. *CA: A Cancer Journal for Clinicians, 56,* 254–281, quiz 313–314. https://doi.org/10.3322/caac.20140

Luetke, A., Meyers, P. A., Lewis, I., & Juergens, H. (2014). Osteosarcoma treatment—where do we stand? A state of the art review. *Cancer Treatment Reviews, 40,* 523–532. https://doi.org/10.1016/j.ctrv.2013.11.006

Maekura, R., Hiraga, T., Miki, K., Kitada, S., Miki, M., Yoshimura, K., . . . Mori, M. (2015). Personalized pulmonary rehabilitation and occupational therapy based on cardiopulmonary exercise testing for patients with advanced chronic obstructive pulmonary disease. *International Journal of Chronic Obstructive Pulmonary Disease, 10,* 1787–1800. https://doi.org/10.2147/COPD.S86455

Mahoney, F. I., & Barthel, D. W. (1965). Functional evaluation: The Barthel Index. *Maryland State Medical Journal, 14,* 61–65.

Mendoza, T. R., Wang, X. S., Cleeland, C. S., Morrissey, M., Johnson, B. A., Wendt, J. K., & Huber, S. L. (1999). The rapid assessment of fatigue severity in cancer patients: Use of the Brief Fatigue Inventory. *Cancer, 85,* 1186–1196. https://doi.org/10.1002/(sici)1097-0142(19990301)85:5<1186::aid-cncr24>3.0.co;2-n

Moreira-Almeida, A., & Koenig, H. G. (2006). Retaining the meaning of the words religiousness and spirituality: A commentary on the WHOQOL SRPB group's "A Cross-Cultural Study of Spirituality, Religion, and Personal Beliefs as Components of Quality of Life" (62: 6, 2005, 1486–1497). *Social Science and Medicine, 63,* 843–845. https://doi.org/10.1016/j.socscimed.2006.03.001

National Cancer Institute. (n.d.). Oncology. *NCI dictionary of cancer terms.* Retrieved from https://www.cancer.gov/publications/dictionaries/cancer-terms/def/oncology

Partridge-Hinckley, K., Liddell, G. M., Almyroudis, N. G., & Segal, B. H. (2009). Infection control measures to prevent invasive mould diseases in hematopoietic stem cell transplant recipients. *Mycopathologia, 168,* 329–337. https://doi.org/10.1007/s11046-009-9247-z

Pergolotti, M., Cutchin, M. P., Weinberger, M., & Meyer, A.-M. (2014). Occupational therapy use by older adults with cancer. *American Journal of Occupational Therapy, 68,* 597–607. https://doi.org/10.5014/ajot.2014.011791

Pergolotti, M., Deal, A. M., Lavery, J., Reeve, B. B., & Muss, H. B. (2015). The prevalence of potentially modifiable functional deficits and the subsequent use of occupational and physical therapy by older adults with cancer. *Journal of Geriatric Oncology, 6,* 194–201. https://doi.org/10.1016/j.jgo.2015.01.004

Pergolotti, M., Williams, G. R., Campbell, C., Munoz, L. A., & Muss, H. B. (2016). Occupational therapy for adults with cancer: Why it matters. *Oncologist, 21,* 314–319. https://doi.org/10.1634/theoncologist.2015-0335

Pilegaard, M. S., Ia Cour, K., Gregersen Oestergaard, L., Johnsen, A. T., Lindahl-Jacobsen, L., & Brandt, A. (2017). The "Cancer Home-Life Intervention": A randomised-controlled trial evaluating the efficacy of an occupational therapy–based intervention in people with advanced cancer. *Palliative Medicine, 32,* 744–756. https://doi.org/10.1177/0269216317747199

Player, L., Mackenzie, L., Willis, K., & Loh, S. Y. (2014). Women's experiences of cognitive changes or "chemobrain" following treatment for breast cancer: A role for occupational therapy. *Australian Occupational Therapy Journal, 61,* 230–240. https://doi.org/10.1111/1440-1630.12113

Rogers, J. C., & Holm M. B. (2014). *Performance Assessment of Self-Care Skills (Version 4.0).* Retrieved from https://www.ono.ac.il/wp-content/uploads/PASS-Home-Test-Manual.pdf

Saboo, U. S., Amparo, F., Abud, T. B., Schaumberg, D. A., & Dana, R. (2015). Vision-related quality of life in patients with ocular graft-versus-host disease. *Ophthalmology, 122,* 1669–1674. https://doi.org/10.1016/j.ophtha.2015.04.011

Sau, K., Amin, K. P., Sharma, A., & Fakorede, S. O. (2015). Participation in activities of daily living can reduce loneliness in older adults. *Indian Journal of Psychiatry, 57,* 430–431. https://doi.org/10.4103/0019-5545.171857

Schwartz, A. L. (1998). The Schwartz Cancer Fatigue Scale: Testing reliability and validity. *Oncology Nursing Forum, 25,* 711–717.

Selamat, M. H., Loh, S. Y., Mackenzie, L., & Vardy, J. (2014). Chemobrain experienced by breast cancer survivors: A meta-ethnography study investigating research and care implications. *PLoS One, 9,* e108002. https://doi.org/10.1371/journal.pone.0108002

Shallice, T., & Burgess, P. W. (1991). Deficits in strategy application following frontal lobe damage in man. *Brain, 114,* 727–741. https://doi.org/10.1093/brain/114.2.727

Spencer, J., Davidson, H., & White, V. (1997). Help clients develop hopes for the future. *American Journal of Occupational Therapy, 51,* 191–198. https://doi.org/10.5014/ajot.51.3.191

Ten Hoorn, S., Elbers, P. W., Girbes, A. R., & Tuinman, P. R. (2016). Communicating with conscious and mechanically ventilated critically ill patients: A systematic review. *Critical Care, 20,* 333. https://doi.org/10.1186/s13054-016-1483-2

Tofthagen, C., Visovsky, C. M., & Hopgood, R. (2013). Chemotherapy-induced peripheral neuropathy: An algorithm to guide nursing management. *Clinical Journal of Oncology Nursing, 17,* 138–144. https://doi.org/10.1188/13.CJON.138-144

Toglia, J. P. (1993). *Contextual Memory Test.* San Antonio, TX: NCS Pearson.

Uniform Data System for Medical Rehabilitation. (1996). *Guide for the Uniform Data Set for Medical Rehabilitation (including the FIM instrument).* Buffalo, NY: Author.

Sleep and Rest

Megan Bailey, OTD, OTR/L, and Robin Newman, OTD, OT, OTR, CLT, FAOTA

22

LEARNING OBJECTIVES

After completing this chapter, readers should be able to
- Explain the scope of sleep-related problems for cancer survivors across the lifespan,
- Analyze the client factors and environmental factors that may contribute to sleep disturbances for cancer survivors across the lifespan,
- Provide examples of the impact that sleep-related challenges may have on the health and occupational performance of cancer survivors across the lifespan,
- Apply knowledge of sleep assessments to a case study scenario, and
- Evaluate sleep-related intervention approaches for case study scenarios.

KEY TERMS AND CONCEPTS

- Cancer-related fatigue
- Chronic insomnia
- Circadian rhythm sleep–wake disorders
- Cognitive–behavioral therapy
- Cosleeping
- Hypersomnias
- Insomnias
- Parasomnias
- Perpetuating factors
- Precipitating factors
- Predisposing factors
- Rest
- Sleep
- Sleep efficiency
- Sleep hygiene
- Sleep-movement disorders
- Sleep-related breathing disorders

INTRODUCTION

Sleep and rest are occupations that are central to people's lives and affect their health and wellness as well as their ability to perform other valued occupations. This is true across cultures and throughout the lifespan. According to the *Occupational Therapy Practice Framework: Domain and Process* (*OTPF*; 3rd ed.; American Occupational Therapy Association [AOTA], 2014), the occupation of *sleep* can be defined as

> taking care of personal needs for sleep, such as ceasing activities to ensure onset of sleep, napping, and dreaming; sustaining a sleep state without disruption; and performing nighttime care of toileting needs and hydration; also includes negotiating the needs and requirements of and interacting with others within the social environment such as children or partners, including providing nighttime caregiving such as breastfeeding and monitoring the comfort and safety of others who are sleeping. (p. S20)

Similarly, *rest* can be defined as

> engaging in quiet and effortless actions that interrupt physical and mental activity, resulting in a relaxed state; included are identifying the need to relax; reducing involvement in taxing physical, mental, or social activities; and engaging in relaxation or other endeavors that restore energy and calm and renew interest in engagement. (AOTA, 2014, p. S20)

For cancer survivors, sleep patterns may be disrupted by both the cancer and its treatment. People with cancer experience myriad sleep problems, including difficulty falling asleep, problems maintaining sleep, poor *sleep efficiency* (i.e., the ratio of time asleep to time in bed), early awakening, and excessive daytime sleepiness (Roscoe et al., 2007).

The scope of the problem is significant, with 30%–50% of individuals with cancer reporting a form of impaired sleep quality compared with 15% of the general population (OncoLink, 2018). Among individuals with advanced cancer, this number may be much greater; one study reported that 72% of patients surveyed experienced sleep disturbances (Fiorentino & Ancoli-Israel, 2007). Research suggests that pediatric cancer patients and survivors may experience even higher rates of sleep disturbances, with estimates as high as 87% (Zupanec et al., 2010).

Although sleep problems are widespread, they remain both underdiagnosed and undertreated (Zhou, Partridge, & Recklitis, 2017). Left untreated, problems with sleep often continue into survivorship and may evolve into chronic conditions (Mustian et al., 2013). Prolonged sleep problems, such as *chronic insomnia* (i.e., insomnia that occurs at least 3 nights per week and lasts for more than 3 weeks), are associated with many negative physical and psychosocial health outcomes among a population already at higher risk for health issues (Zhou, Partridge, & Recklitis, 2017).

This chapter provides an overview of the sleep-related challenges faced by cancer survivors as well as evidence-based assessments and interventions to address these challenges.

SLEEP AND REST AS OCCUPATION

AOTA (2017) described the importance of sleep as an occupation:

> Restful and adequate sleep provides the foundation for optimal occupational performance, participation, and engagement in daily life, a concept that is historically consistent with the development of occupational therapy. The effect of sleep on function and participation is incorporated into the repertoire of occupational therapy practitioners and addressed across the lifespan. (para. 1)

Sleep influences physical and psychological health, and inadequate sleep may further affect illness and recovery (Collins et al., 2017).

Chronic sleep problems also have the potential to greatly affect quality of life. Within the scope of occupational therapy practice, problems with sleep may affect participation in ADLs, IADLs, play, work, leisure, and social participation. Therefore, occupational therapy practitioners are well suited to address the occupation of sleep and rest to support the highest level of participation in meaningful daily activities.

DEFINING SLEEP DISORDERS

There are six major categories of sleep disorders (National Sleep Foundation, n.d.; OncoLink, 2018):
1. *Insomnias:* Sleep disorders characterized by difficulty falling asleep or staying asleep
2. *Hypersomnias:* A group of sleep disorders characterized by excessive daytime sleepiness that may even occur after one receives adequate sleep
3. *Sleep-related breathing disorders:* A group of sleep disorders characterized by abnormal respiration during sleep
4. *Circadian rhythm sleep–wake disorders:* A group of sleep disorders characterized by insomnia or excessive sleepiness caused by desynchronization between internal sleep–wake rhythms and the light–darkness cycle
5. *Parasomnias:* A group of sleep disorders that involve unwanted events or experiences that occur while one is falling asleep, sleeping, or waking up
6. *Sleep-movement disorders:* A group of sleep disorders characterized by movement before or during sleep.

Cancer survivors may experience a range of symptoms that may or may not qualify as a specific sleep disorder. The most common form of sleep disorder in this population is insomnia (OncoLink, 2018). According to the *International Classification of Sleep Disorders,* one must meet the following criteria to qualify for a diagnosis of insomnia (American Academy of Sleep Medicine, 2014):

TABLE 22.1.   Negative Health Outcomes Associated With Sleep Disturbance

HEALTH CATEGORY	ASSOCIATION OUTCOMES
Physical health	▪ Increased risk of cardiovascular disease ▪ Increased risk of obesity ▪ Increased risk of diabetes ▪ Increased risk of mortality ▪ Increased vasomotor and endocrine symptoms
Psychological and emotional health	▪ Increased fatigue ▪ Increased anxiety ▪ Cognitive challenges ▪ Increased risk of depressive disorders ▪ Social skills deficits ▪ Emotional regulation deficits

- Difficulty sleeping, characterized by either (or both) 30 minutes or more to fall asleep or more than 30 minutes of nighttime awakenings
- A ratio of total sleep time to time spent in bed of less than 85%
- Sleep disturbance occurring at least 3 nights per week
- Sleep disturbance that causes significant impairment in daytime functioning or marked distress.

Even if the individual does not meet the criteria for an official diagnosis, sleep problems can still be debilitating and have a far-reaching impact on daily functioning. Many cancer survivors experiencing problems with sleep also experience fatigue. Although there is a strong correlation between the experiences and symptoms of cancer-related fatigue and sleep disturbances, they are distinct constructs (Roscoe et al., 2007). The American Cancer Society (2018) describes *cancer-related fatigue* as "not the tired feeling people remember having before they had cancer . . . . People describe it as feeling weak, listless, drained, or 'washed out'" (para. 1–2).

Evidence suggests that poor sleep is associated with myriad physical and psychological health problems, as detailed in Table 22.1 (Fernandez-Mendoza & Vgontzas, 2013; Harvard Medical School, Division of Sleep Medicine, 2007).

CONTRIBUTING FACTORS AND MECHANISMS OF SLEEP AND REST DISTURBANCES

Sleep disturbances can begin before cancer treatment, can continue during treatment, and may persist for years after the completion of treatment (Zhou et al., 2018). As a result, it is important to appreciate the risk factors that can contribute to sleep and rest disturbances across the cancer continuum and across the lifespan. They include the cancer itself, cancer treatment, biological processes, environmental factors, psychosocial disturbances, and comorbid medical disorders (Ancoli-Israel, 2009; Daniel et al., 2016).

Savard and Morin (2001) described factors affecting sleep disturbances in cancer survivors using the three P Model of Insomnia developed by Spielman (1986):

predisposing, precipitating, and perpetuating factors. *Predisposing factors* are factors that increase the cancer survivor's general vulnerability to develop sleep disturbance. *Precipitating factors* trigger the onset of sleep disturbances in cancer survivors. *Perpetuating factors* are factors that contribute to the maintenance of sleep disturbance over time in cancer survivors (Savard & Morin, 2001). To better understand the etiology of clients' sleep disturbances, it is important for occupational therapists to consider which of these factors warrant further assessment as part of a comprehensive occupational therapy evaluation. See Table 22.2 for an overview of the key contributing factors to sleep challenges for individuals with cancer.

Contextual factors are also critical contributing factors to sleep challenges. Exhibit 22.1 provides guiding questions that occupational therapy practitioners can use to facilitate a conversation regarding the context of the client's sleep problems.

Although risk factors are experienced across the lifespan, certain bedtime challenges may be unique to children and their caregivers. Of particular concern is the use of *cosleeping,* which is the practice of sleeping in the same bed or room with one's child ("Co-sleeping," n.d.). Although it is natural that parents or caregivers want to comfort a child with cancer, the use of cosleeping as a strategy to support sleep may lead to long-term sleep disturbances for both the child and the caregiver (Daniel et al., 2016). This is consistent with research examining sleep among healthy children that indicates that cosleeping is often associated with poorer child sleep outcomes (Simard et al., 2008). Cosleeping may result from the caregivers' attempt to alleviate sleep disturbances associated with their child's illness. Many parents indicate that although they intended cosleeping to be a short-term measure, their child became reliant on it. In some instances, cosleeping was associated with night waking, thereby disrupting sleep for both the caregiver and the child (Williams & McCarthy, 2014).

SLEEP DISTURBANCES' EFFECT ON OCCUPATIONAL PERFORMANCE

Sleep disturbances may have a pervasive impact on individuals' ability to perform valued occupations across the lifespan. For children, sleep disturbances can affect ADLs; family functioning; and social functioning, including play and school functioning (Daniel et al., 2016). For adolescents and young adults, sleep disturbances have been associated with challenges with physical coordination, emotional regulation, social skills, and cognitive function (Olson, 2014), which can particularly affect IADLs, formal education participation, work, leisure, and social participation.

Loh et al. (2017) found that older adults with cancer who experienced sleep deficits were more likely to report challenges performing the following daily activities:
- Shopping
- Cooking
- Managing medications
- Using the phone
- Doing housework
- Managing finances
- Driving and using public transportation.

In addition, of the study participants who reported having sleep challenges, 68% reported requiring assistance with at least one IADL, and 76% reported limitations in physical activity.

EVALUATING SLEEP AND REST

Sleep disorders are often overlooked by both survivors and medical providers and are consistently underdiagnosed in the cancer setting (Savard & Morin, 2001; Zhou et al., 2018). Sleep problems are often viewed as a "normal" response to a recent cancer diagnosis and temporary in nature (Dahlya et al., 2013; Zhou, Partridge, Syrjala, et al., 2017). In a study of the 25 National Cancer Institute (NCI)–designated comprehensive cancer centers and National Cancer Care Network (NCCN) members' survivorship programs, Zhou, Partridge, Syrjala, et al. (2017) found that more than 56% of survivorship programs were screening fewer than 25% of survivors for sleep problems. No program was providing more than 50% of survivors with optimal insomnia-related care (Zhou, Partridge, Syrjala, et al., 2017).

Without routine screening and diagnosis, however, survivors do not have the opportunity to receive evidence-based interventions for their sleep problems, which results in ongoing occupational performance problems that can persist through treatment and well into survivorship. Despite NCCN and NCI recommendations for survivors to discuss sleep problems with their providers, there is a clear gap in communication about sleep-related issues during medical encounters (NCCN, 2015; NCI, 2013; Zhou et al., 2017). Occupational therapy practitioners can serve an important role in addressing this gap by routinely asking survivors about their sleep, their perceptions of sleep problems, and how sleep problems affect their occupational performance (Ancoli-Israel, 2009; Zhou et al., 2017).

In addition, sleep can be evaluated and further understood as a part of a cluster of symptoms, including fatigue, depression, anxiety, and pain (Palesh et al., 2010). As a result, occupational therapy practitioners should evaluate these symptoms to understand their potential impact on the occupation of sleep (refer to Chapters 15, 16, and 20 on fatigue, pain, and psychosocial issues, respectively, for additional details). Last, occupational therapy practitioners can calculate sleep efficiency—the number of minutes of sleep divided by the number of minutes in bed multiplied by 100 (Berger et al., 2005)—to determine whether cancer survivors are meeting acceptable age-related norms for sleep (Linder & Christian, 2013). For children, a good night's sleep is calculated at 90% sleep efficiency, whereas 95% sleep efficiency is considered a good night's sleep for adults.

Providing timely screening of sleep challenges for individuals with cancer is essential to proactively address clients' concerns. A comprehensive assessment of a client's sleep challenges should include an evaluation of key factors highlighted in Table 22.2. These factors include predisposing, precipitation, and perpetuating factors that include the client's diagnosis and treatment, side effects, and behaviors, as well as psychosocial and environmental factors. Table 22.3 provides an overview of common assessments of sleep.

Table 22.2.   Factors Impacting Sleep Disruptions in Cancer Survivors

TYPE OF FACTOR	EXAMPLES OF FACTOR
Predisposing factors	▪ Personal or family history of insomnia ▪ Psychiatric Disorders such as anxiety disorder or depression ▪ Higher BMI ▪ Poorer functional status ▪ Aging ▪ Hyper-arousability
Precipitating factors	Cancer and cancer treatment ▪ Hospitalization ▪ Surgery ▪ Chemotherapy ▪ Radiation ▪ Hormonal therapy ▪ Medications ▪ Bone marrow transplant ▪ Tumors that increase steroid production Side effects and late effects ▪ Delirium ▪ Menopausal symptoms ▪ Pain ▪ Fatigue ▪ Nausea and vomiting ▪ Altered circadian rhythm ▪ Pruritis ▪ Body temperature changes ▪ Shortness of breath ▪ Functional loss Environment ▪ Changes in sleep environment (e.g., being in the hospital instead of home) ▪ Increased noise levels and lighting in institutional settings, such as hospitals or inpatient rehabilitation settings ▪ Changes in sleep routines, including the ability to nap during the day or receiving medical procedures in the evening Psychosocial ▪ Worry about survival ▪ Depression ▪ Anxiety ▪ Emotional burden ▪ Family stress and coping Comorbid medical disorders ▪ Other primary sleep disorders ▪ Headaches
Perpetuating factors	▪ Irregular sleep–wake schedule ▪ Engaging in sleep interfering activities in the bedroom ▪ Spending excessive amounts of time in bed ▪ Daytime napping ▪ Faulty attitudes and beliefs about sleep ▪ Eating or drinking alcohol before bed ▪ Tobacco use ▪ Caffeine use ▪ Limited physical activity ▪ Cosleeping

Note. BMI = body mass index.
Sources. Ancoli-Israel, 2009, 2015; Daniel et al., 2016; Fiorentino & Ancoli-Israel, 2007; Hinds et al., 2007; O'Donnell, 2004; Savard & Morin, 2001; Spielman, 1986.

EXHIBIT 22.1.	Context and Environment: Questions to Guide Client Evaluation

Physical
- Does the home environment support rest or sleep?
  - For example, does excessive noise or light affect the individual's ability to fall asleep or stay asleep?
- Does the hospital environment support rest or sleep?
  - For example, are patients being woken up during the night for medical care? Are there differences between the physical environments of the home and hospital that create sleep challenges?

Social
- What are the expectations of the people with whom the survivor has contact or relationships regarding rest and sleep?
  - For example, does the family understand and help to fulfill the sleep needs of the children?
- How do the sleep habits of a roommate in an inpatient facility affect the client's ability to sleep?

Cultural
- What value is placed on sleep and rest in the family unit?
- How does the individual's community view sleep routines?
  - For example, does a teenager's peer group encourage staying up late?
- Does a child's family value consistency in bedtime routine?

Personal
- What is the survivor's socioeconomic status, and how might this support or inhibit access to restful periods, rest time, and sleep?
- How does the client's identity influence their beliefs and values regarding sleep?
- Does the client engage in use of caffeine, alcohol, or nicotine? If so, how do these behaviors affect the client's sleep patterns?
- Is the client taking any medications that may affect sleep?

Temporal
- How does the client's ability to sleep vary at different times of day?
- Does the client set a regular bedtime at a consistent time of day?

Virtual
- Does the client use technology right before going to bed or in the bedroom?
- Where does the client keep their phone in the bedroom?
- Does the client's use of technology support or inhibit their ability to fall asleep?
  - For example, does the client listen to music or use a white noise machine to support their ability to fall asleep?

Note. BMI = body mass index; *OTPF = Occupational Therapy Practice Framework: Domain and Process* (AOTA, 2014).

INTERVENTION STRATEGIES

A range of medical providers have a role to play in implementing interventions for individuals with cancer to address their sleep concerns. Table 22.4 outlines the primary types of interventions occupational therapists use, as part of an interprofessional collaboration, to address sleep-related challenges, as classified by the *OTPF* (AOTA, 2014; Carlson & Garland, 2005; Denlinger et al., 2018; Mustian et al., 2013; Zhou, Partridge, & Recklitis, 2017; Zhou, Partridge, Syrjala, et al., 2017).

Occupational therapy practitioners play a particularly crucial role in addressing maladaptive habits and routines that may negatively affect sleep quality. Such interventions are often referred to as *sleep hygiene* and involve optimizing environmental and personal factors to improve occupational performance in the area of sleep, which falls directly within the occupational therapy scope of practice. Denlinger et al. (2018) recommended the following as part of a comprehensive sleep hygiene intervention:

- Participate in regular physical activity in the morning, afternoon, or both. Avoid moderate to strenuous physical activity within 3 hours of bedtime.
- Increase exposure to bright light during the day.
- Reduce exposure to bright light (e.g., computer, phone screen, light sources close to the eye) within a few hours before bedtime and during the night.
- Avoid heavy meals and limit fluid intake within 3 hours of bedtime.
- Avoid alcohol and nicotine use too close to bedtime.
- Limit caffeine consumption and avoid caffeine consumption at least 4 hours before bedtime.
- Enhance the sleep environment (e.g., dark, quiet room; comfortable temperature).
- Set aside a "worry time" before bedtime, which includes a time to review the day and plan for the next day.
- Avoid looking at the clock when awake during the night.
- Maintain a regular bedtime and wake time every day.
- If necessary, limit to one short nap per day in the afternoon (no longer than 30 minutes).
- Turn off electronics and light-emitting sources at bedtime.

See Case Example 22.1 to learn more about the evaluation, intervention planning, and treatment process for an individual with cancer experiencing sleep challenges.

COGNITIVE–BEHAVIORAL THERAPY PILOT FOR CANCER SURVIVORS

Cognitive–behavioral therapy (CBT; i.e., a psychotherapy treatment focused on changing patterns of thinking and behavior) is typically considered the gold standard treatment for insomnia. Although extensive research has not yet been done on the use of CBT to improve sleep for

TABLE 22.3.   Brief Description of Sleep Assessments

ASSESSMENT	DESCRIPTION
Self-report measures	
Sleep log (National Sleep Foundation, n.d.)	A record of the client's sleep habits, including bedtime and hours slept per night as well as the impact of sleep on daily routines and activities. Sleep logs are usually kept for 1–2 weeks.
Insomnia Severity Index (Morin, 1993)	A 7-question self-report evaluation that uses a 5-point Likert scale to identify the nature and severity of insomnia.
Pittsburgh Sleep Quality Index (Buysse et al., 1989)	A self-report measure to assess quality and patterns of sleep, according to the following 7 components: subjective sleep quality, sleep latency, sleep duration, habitual sleep efficiency, sleep disturbances, use of sleeping medications, and daytime dysfunction over the past month.
Epworth Sleepiness Scale (Johns, 1991)	An 8-question self-report measure that uses a 4-point Likert scale to evaluate the client's level of daytime sleepiness.
Children's Sleep Habits Questionnaire (Owens et al., 2000)	A 45-item parent-report sleep questionnaire for school-age children. In addition to giving an overall score, the report measures the following 8 subscales: Bedtime Resistance, Sleep Onset Delay, Sleep Duration, Sleep Anxiety, Night Wakings, Parasomnias, Sleep Disordered Breathing, and Daytime Sleepiness. The questionnaire has also been adapted for use with infants.
PROMIS Sleep Disturbance Short Form (Yu et al., 2011)	An 8-question self-report form created by the American Psychological Association to evaluate problems with sleep that affect sleep quality. Available in adult and child forms.
Interview (American Occupational Therapy Association, 2017)	Suggested questions: ▪ How long have you experienced difficulty sleeping? ▪ Describe your activities during the hour before you go to bed. ▪ How long does it take you to fall asleep? ▪ How many times do you typically wake up during the night? ▪ How long does it take you to fall back to sleep? ▪ How many hours do you typically sleep each night? ▪ Why do you feel you have difficulty sleeping? ▪ Do you take naps during the day? If so, for how long? ▪ Do you feel sleepy during the day? If so, what is the impact of your sleepiness on your ability to perform important activities such as work, caregiving, and going to school? ▪ What is the impact of your important daily activities such as work, school, or caregiving, on your ability to sleep? ▪ Do you exercise? How often?
Objective measures	
Polysomnography (PSG)	PSG is often considered the gold standard for measuring sleep disturbances. PSG takes overnight sleep measurements of brain waves, eye movement, and muscle tension. This test is not administered by an occupational therapist but rather by a polysomnographic technologist.

cancer survivors, preliminary studies are showing positive results.

For example, Zhou, Partridge, and Recklitis (2017) conducted a study of 38 adults cancer survivors who reported insomnia symptoms for an average of 2.4 years. Fewer than 1 in 3 survivors had reported insomnia symptoms to their cancer providers within the past year. Survivors were then enrolled in a 3-session CBT program delivered over a 1-month period. Significant group improvements were reported for measures of sleep efficiency, sleep quality, and insomnia symptoms. The study's results suggest that CBT may be a promising intervention for treating insomnia in cancer survivors.

See Case Example 22.2 for an example of the assessment and intervention process for a pediatric client with cancer experiencing sleep challenges in a hospital setting.

SUMMARY

Sleep is a critically important occupation that affects both individuals' health and their ability to participate in other valued occupations; as such, problems related to sleep can have a far-reaching effects on many areas of life, including IADLs, social participation, work, and leisure activities. In addition, sleep challenges often co-occur with other cancer-related symptoms, such as pain, psychosocial distress, and cancer-related fatigue, which can further compound the effects of sleep on occupational performance. Individuals with cancer disproportionately experience sleep-related challenges that affect individuals across the lifespan, including children and adolescents as well as individuals with different types of cancer.

Occupational therapy practitioners are well positioned to address the sleep challenges of individuals with cancer

TABLE 22.4. Primary Interventions to Address Sleep-Related Challenges

OTPF APPROACH TO INTERVENTION	INTERVENTION TYPE	EXAMPLES
Restore	Cognitive–behavioral	▪ Sleep restrictions ▪ Sleep-related self-talk patterns ▪ Stimulus control
Modify	Environmental	▪ Sleep hygiene interventions (for more details, see Denlinger et al., 2018)
Restore	Lifestyle	▪ Established sleep routines ▪ Caregiver education ▪ Exercise programs ▪ Smoking cessation education ▪ Limited caffeine and alcohol intake ▪ Nutritional education
Restore	Mindfulness-based stress reduction	▪ Relaxation techniques ▪ Mindfulness exercises ▪ Breathing exercises
Restore	Addressing contributing factors	▪ Pain reduction interventions ▪ Fatigue management interventions ▪ Mental health interventions

Note. OTPF = Occupational Therapy Practice Framework: Domain and Process (AOTA, 2014).

CASE EXAMPLE 22.1. ELIZABETH: SLEEP DISTURBANCES AFTER BREAST CANCER TREATMENT

Elizabeth is a 46-year-old woman referred to occupational therapy because of upper extremity (UE) dysfunction following a left-side mastectomy for Stage II triple negative breast cancer. She finished treatment 1 month ago, including chemotherapy and radiation. She is currently on a leave of absence from her job as an elementary schoolteacher in a nearby town but is planning on returning to work in 6 weeks.

Elizabeth has a supportive family, including her husband and two young daughters, and a network of extended family, friends, and coworkers who assisted with child care during treatment. Before her cancer treatment, Elizabeth took great joy in cooking for her family, exercising, taking care of her home, and actively participating in her children' activities.

The occupational therapist performed an evaluation using the following assessments:

▪ Goniometry
▪ Visual Analogue Scale (McCormack et al., 1988)
▪ Pittsburgh Sleep Quality Index (PSQI; Buysse et al., 1989)
▪ Canadian Occupational Performance Measure (COPM; Law et al., 2019).

Assessment results and occupational analysis

Range of motion assessment revealed limitations in left shoulder flexion, shoulder abduction, and external rotation. Elizabeth reported pain with these shoulder movements and told the occupational therapist that she "can't find a comfortable sleep position" as a result of the pain in her arm. The Visual Analogue Scale revealed a rating of 3/10 pain at rest and 7/10 pain with activity. Elizabeth reported that the pain she felt in her UE had been keeping her awake at night. The PSQI score confirmed that Elizabeth was experiencing poor sleep.

The COPM revealed occupational performance challenges in the areas of sleep, rest, driving, and participating in activities with her children (see Exhibit 22.2). Elizabeth explained that her performance on the identified occupations was affected by daytime sleepiness, pain, and worry about the future. She reported that she was not sleeping well and could not rest because she was trying to catch up on everything she needed to do before she returned to work in 6 weeks. She said that she had been relying on coffee to "keep [her] awake." She was particularly upset about missing her daughter's soccer games because of her daytime sleepiness.

Elizabeth reported that she was relieved to let someone know her sleep was disrupted. She did not want to complain about it because she was so thankful to be alive and hoped her sleep would just get better with time. Her goal for occupational therapy was to be able to return to her usual activities, especially sleep, without pain.

To score the PSQI, the occupational therapist calculated Elizabeth's sleep efficiency on the basis of the information provided. On the PSQI, Elizabeth reported that she typically slept approximately 5 hours per night (300 minutes) and shared that she spent

(Continued)

CASE EXAMPLE 22.1. ELIZABETH: SLEEP DISTURBANCES AFTER BREAST CANCER TREATMENT (Cont.)

approximately 8 hours in bed (480 minutes). Sleep efficiency is calculated as the number of minutes of sleep divided by the number of minutes in bed multiplied by 100. Elizabeth's sleep efficiency was 62.5%. The occupational therapist shared that a good night's sleep for adults is calculated at 95% and was optimistic that occupational therapy intervention would support better sleep for Elizabeth. The global PSQI score ranges from 0–21, with lower scores suggesting better sleep. Elizabeth's score was 17, suggesting a significant sleep problem.

The occupational therapist then administered the COPM to gain a better understanding of the occupational performance challenges Elizabeth was experiencing because of her breast cancer. The therapist asked Elizabeth to rate on a scale of 1–10 the importance of the occupational performance challenges she selected and then to rate her performance and satisfaction on a scale of 1–10, with higher numbers signifying greater performance and satisfaction. Exhibit 22.3 details the results of Elizabeth's COPM and self-ratings of her occupational performance challenges.

Intervention

The occupational therapist, in collaboration with Elizabeth, set a 6-week plan to support optimal UE function and occupational performance, with a focus on rest and sleep. The plan also included consulting with a psychologist to support adjustment to survivorship. During weekly occupational therapy sessions, Elizabeth incorporated a variety of strategies into her daily routine to support optimal sleep and rest. The occupational therapist recommended the following sleep hygiene strategies to support sleep, which Elizabeth found helpful (Denlinger et al., 2018):

- Enhancing Elizabeth's sleep environment by adjusting her bedroom temperature to keep it cooler, drawing the shades to keep the room dark, and using a body pillow to minimize pain;
- Setting aside worry time before bed, including a dedicated time when Elizabeth can review the day and plan for the next day;
- Engaging in regular physical activity in the morning or afternoon, while her children are in school;
- Limiting use of electronics before bed; and
- Limiting caffeine before bedtime.

The occupational therapist also incorporated strategies to manage pain, fatigue, and emotional distress, including:

- Seat belt pillow to minimize pain across the mastectomy site;
- Energy conservation strategies such as pacing activities, prioritizing, and planning ahead (Packer et al., 1995); and
- Relaxation techniques.

Outcome of intervention

After 6 weeks of intervention, Elizabeth demonstrated significant improvements in UE function, pain management, and sleep. She actively incorporated the sleep hygiene strategies into her daily and nightly routine and was able to sleep through the night with 85% sleep efficiency. She reported that she had enough energy and alertness to attend one of her daughter's soccer games per week. Elizabeth said that she would continue to incorporate the sleep hygiene and pain management strategies into her daily routine as she returned to work. She reported that she would continue to meet with the psychologist weekly for continued support as she transitioned back to work.

EXHIBIT 22.2.	Elizabeth's Canadian Occupational Performance Measure		
OCCUPATIONAL PERFORMANCE CHALLENGE	**IMPORTANCE**	**PERFORMANCE**	**SATISFACTION**
Sleeping	10	3	1
Rest	10	1	1
Driving	10	5	2
Activities with children	10	3	1

in both inpatient and outpatient settings. Despite NCI (2013) guidelines, individuals with cancer do not consistently receive screenings for sleep challenges; therefore, occupational therapists can both provide screenings and advocate for improved interprofessional collaboration to ensure that clients receive regular, timely screenings. Occupational therapists may then choose to conduct more formal sleep assessments and interventions that address clients' health and psychosocial risk factors and the environment.

CASE EXAMPLE 22.2. ALEXIS: PEDIATRIC CLIENT EXPERIENCING SLEEP CHALLENGES

Alexis is an 8-year-old girl who loves art and horseback riding. She lives with her older brother and parents in the suburbs of Boston. Alexis is currently undergoing treatment for acute lymphoblastic leukemia at a children's hospital. She was hospitalized 3 weeks ago for prolonged neutropenia and fevers as a side effect of chemotherapy. Her parents visit her daily and appreciate being involved in her care.

Since hospitalization, Alexis has spent most of her days in bed because of fevers, lack of energy, and nausea. As a result, she has experienced deconditioning from the prolonged hospitalization and is having trouble performing ADLs such as dressing, bathing, and eating. Her physician has referred her to occupational therapy to increase her independence in ADL performance.

During her initial occupational therapy evaluation, Alexis explains that one of the reasons she is so tired during the day and unable to perform her ADLs independently is that she is having difficulty sleeping through the night. She says that she is awakened multiple times over the course of the night when the nurses check on her and turn on the light. Alexis's nurse confirms that Alexis must have her vital signs checked every 4 hours overnight. Once Alexis is woken up, she is distracted by the sound of pumps beeping with her IV medications and finds it difficult to fall back asleep. She says she hates being in the hospital and misses her bedroom back at home. In addition, Alexis's parents fill out the Children's Sleep Habits Questionnaire (Owens et al., 2000) and explain that Alexis regularly sleeps in a cool, dark room with her stuffed animal, Peaches.

The occupational therapist could use many possible intervention approaches. The therapist could consider modifying the environment and implementing sleep hygiene measures, as recommended by Denlinger et al. (2018), such as establishing regular bedtime and wake time routines and minimizing light and noise in the room. This intervention would require an interdisciplinary collaboration between the occupational therapist and nursing staff to determine how the team could improve Alexis's sleep hygiene while adhering to the necessary medical safety guidelines. For example, the therapist might work with the nursing and medical staff to find a regular time every day that could be designated as Alexis's rest time, during which she would not receive any services. In fact, many of the other children on the unit could benefit from having a similar designated rest time, and this could become a unitwide practice.

As another approach to intervention, the occupational therapist could address Alexis's preferences for her bedroom at home and take steps to recreate her home sleep environment as much as possible in the hospital setting. For example, Alexis's parents should bring her stuffed animal, Peaches, to the hospital to make the environment more familiar and comfortable.

REFERENCES

American Academy of Sleep Medicine. (2014). *International classification of sleep disorders* (3rd ed.). Darien, IL: Author.

American Cancer Society. (2018). *What is cancer-related fatigue?* Retrieved from https://www.cancer.org/treatment/treatments-and-side-effects/physical-side-effects/fatigue/what-is-cancer-related-fatigue.html

American Occupational Therapy Association. (2014). Occupational therapy practice framework: Domain and process (3rd ed.). *American Journal of Occupational Therapy, 68*(Suppl. 1), S1–S48. https://doi.org/10.5014/ajot.2014.682006

American Occupational Therapy Association. (2017). *Occupational therapy's role in sleep.* Retrieved from https://www.aota.org/About-Occupational-Therapy/Professionals/HW/sleep.aspx

Ancoli-Israel, S. (2009). Recognition and treatment of sleep disturbances in cancer. *Journal of Clinical Oncology, 27,* 5864–5866. https://doi.org/10.1200/JCO.2009.24.5993

Ancoli-Israel, S. (2015). Sleep disturbances in cancer: A review. *Sleep Medicine Research, 6,* 45–49. https://doi.org/10.17241/smr.2015.6.2.45

Berger, A. M., Parker, K. P., Young-McCaughan, S., Mallory, G. A., Barsevick, A. M., Beck, S. L., & Hall, M. (2005). Sleep/wake disturbances in people with cancer and their caregivers: State of the science. *Oncology Nursing Forum, 32,* e98–e126. https://doi.org/10.1188/05.ONF.E98-E126

Buysse, D., Reynolds, C., Monk, T., Berman, S., & Kupfer, D. (1989). The Pittsburgh Sleep Quality Index: A new instrument for psychiatric practice and research. *Psychiatry Research, 28,* 193–213. https://doi.org/10.1016/0165-1781(89)90047-4

Carlson, L., & Garland, S. (2005). Impact of Mindfulness-Based Stress Reduction (MBSR) on sleep, mood, stress and fatigue symptoms in cancer outpatients. *International Journal of Behavioral Medicine, 12,* 278–285. https://doi.org/10.1207/s15327558ijbm1204_9

Collins, K. P., Geller, D. A., Antoni, M., Donnell, D. M., Tsung, A., March, J. W., . . . Steel, J. L. (2017). Sleep duration is associated with survival in advanced cancer patients. *Sleep Medicine, 32,* 208–212. https://doi.org/10.1016/j.sleep.2016.06.041

Co-sleeping. (n.d.). In *Merriam-Webster Online.* Retrieved from https://www.merriam-webster.com/dictionary/co-sleeping

Dahlya, S., Ahluwalia, M. S., & Walia, H. K. (2013). Sleep disturbances in cancer patients: Underrecognized and undertreated. *Cleveland Clinic Journal of Medicine, 80,* 722–732. https://doi.org/10.3949/ccjm.80a.12170

Daniel, L. C., Schwartz, L. A., Mindell, J. A., Tucker, C. A., & Bakarat, L. P. (2016). Initial validation of the Sleep Disturbances in Pediatric Cancer Model. *Journal of Pediatric Psychology, 41,* 588–599. https://doi.org/10.1093/jpepsy/jsw008

Denlinger, C. S., Sanft, T., Baker, K. S., Broderick, G., Demark-Wahnefried, W., Friedman, D. L., . . . Freedman-Cass, D. A. (2018). Survivorship, Version 2.2018, NCCN clinical practice guidelines in oncology. *Journal of the National Comprehensive Cancer Network, 16*(10). https://doi.org/10.6004/jnccn.2018.0078

Fernandez-Mendoza, J., & Vgontzas, A. (2013). Insomnia and its impact on physical and mental health. *Current Psychiatry Reports, 15,* 418. https://doi.org/10.1007/s11920-013-0418-8

Fiorentino, L., & Ancoli-Israel, S. (2007). Sleep dysfunction in patients with cancer. *Current Treatment Options in Neurology, 9,* 337–346. https://doi.org/10.1007/BF02938540

Harvard Medical School, Division of Sleep Medicine. (2007). *Sleep and disease risk.* Retrieved from http://healthysleep.med.harvard.edu/healthy/matters/consequences/sleep-and-disease-risk

Hinds, P. S., Hockenberry, M., Rai, S. H., Zhang, L., Razzouk, B. I., McCarthy, K., . . . Rodriguez-Galindo, C. (2007). Nocturnal awakenings, sleep environment interruptions, and fatigue in hospitalized children with cancer. *Oncology Nursing Forum, 34,* 393–402. https://doi.org/10.1188/07.ONF.393-402

Johns, M. (1991). A new method for measuring daytime sleepiness: The Epworth Sleepiness Scale. *Sleep, 14,* 50–55. https://doi.org/10.1093/sleep/14.6.540

Law, M., Baptiste, S., Carswell, A., McColl, M., Polatajko, H., & Pollock, N. (2019). *Canadian Occupational Performance Measure* (5th ed., rev.). Altona, Man, Canada: COPM, Inc.

Linder, L. A., & Christian, B. J. (2013). Nighttime sleep characteristics in hospitalized school-aged children with cancer. *Journal for Specialists in Pediatric Nursing, 18,* 13–24. https://doi.org/10.1111/jspn.12005

Loh, K. P., Pandya, C., Kadambi, S., Flannery, M., Reizine, N., Magnuson, A., . . . Mohile, S. G. (2017). Associations of sleep disturbance with physical function and cognition in older adults with cancer. *Support Care Cancer, 25,* 3161–3169. https://doi.org/10.1007/s00520-017-3724-6

McCormack, H. M., Horne, D. J., & Sheather, S. (1988). Clinical applications of Visual Analogue Scales: A critical review. *Psychological Medicine, 18*(4), 1007–1019. https://doi.org/10.1017/s0033291700009934

Morin, C. M. (1993). *Insomnia, psychological assessment and management.* New York: Guilford Press.

Mustian, K., Sprod, L., Janelsins, M., Peppone, L., Palesh, O., Chandwani, K., . . . Morrow, G. (2013). Multicenter, randomized controlled trial of yoga for sleep quality among cancer survivors. *Journal of Clinical Oncology, 31,* 3233–3243. https://doi.org/10.1200/JCO.2012.43.7707

National Cancer Institute. (2013). *Follow-up care after cancer treatment.* Retrieved from http://www.cancer.gov/cancertopics/factsheet/Therapy/followup

National Comprehensive Cancer Network. (2015). *NCCN clinical practice guidelines in oncology: Survivorship.* Retrieved from https://www.nccn.org/professionals/physician_gls/default.aspx

National Sleep Foundation. (n.d.). *Sleep diary.* Retrieved from https://sleepfoundation.org/sites/default/files/SLEEPDiaryv6.pdf?utm_source=feedburner&utm_medium=feed&utm_campaign=Feed%3A%20nsfalert%20%28Newsletter%20-%20NSF%20Alert%29

O'Donnell, J. F. (2004). Insomnia in cancer patients. *Clinical Cornerstone, 6,* S6–S14. https://doi.org/10.1016/S1098-3597(05)80002-X

Olson, K. (2014). Sleep-related disturbances among adolescents with cancer: A systematic review. *Sleep Medicine, 15,* 496–501. https://doi.org/10.1016/j.sleep.2014.01.006

OncoLink. (2018, July 16). Sleep problems (insomnia) in the cancer patient. *OncoLink.* Retrieved from https://www.oncolink.org/support/side-effects/insomnia/sleep-problems-insomnia-in-the-cancer-patient

Owens, J., Spirito, A., & McGuinn, M. (2000). The Children's Sleep Habits Questionnaire (CSHQ): Psychometric properties of a survey instrument for school-aged children. *Sleep, 23,* 1043–1051.

Packer, T. L., Brink, N., & Sauriol, A. (1995). *Managing fatigue: A six-week course for energy conservation.* Tucson, AZ: Therapy Skill Builders.

Palesh, O. G., Roscoe, J. A., Mustian, K. M., Roth, T., Savard, J., Ancoli-Israel, S., . . . Morrow, G. R. (2010). Prevalence, demographics, and psychological associations of sleep disruption in patients with cancer: University of Rochester Cancer Center–Community Clinical Oncology Program. *Journal of Clinical Oncology, 28,* 292–298. https://doi.org/10.1200/JCO.2009.22.5011

Roscoe, J., Kaufman, M., Matteson-Rusby, S., Palesh, O., Ryan, J., Kohli, S., . . . Morrow, G. (2007). Cancer-related fatigue and sleep disorders. *Oncologist, 12*(Suppl. 1), 35–42. https://doi.org/10.1634/theoncologist.12-S1-35

Savard, J., & Morin, C. M. (2001). Insomnia in the context of cancer: A review of a neglected problem. *Journal of Clinical Oncology, 19,* 895–908. https://doi.org/10.1200/JCO.2001.19.3.895

Simard, V., Nielsen, T. A., Tremblay, R. E., Boivin, M., & Montplaisir, J. Y. (2008). Longitudinal study of preschool sleep disturbance: The predictive role of maladaptive parental behaviours, early sleep problems, and child/mother psychological factors. *Archives of Pediatrics and Adolescent Medicine, 162,* 360–367. https://doi.org/10.1001/archpedi.162.4.360

Spielman, A. J. (1986). Assessment of insomnia. *Clinical Psychology Review, 6,* 11–25. https://doi.org/10.1016/0272-7358(86)90015-2

Williams, L. K., & McCarthy, M. C. (2014). Parent perceptions of managing child behavioral side-effects of cancer treatment: A qualitative study. *Child: Care, Health and Development, 41,* 611–619. https://doi.org/10.1111/cch.12188

Yu, L., Buysse, D. J., Germain, A., Moul, D. E., Stover, A., Dodds, N. E., Johnston, K. L., & Pilkonis, P. A. (2011). Development of short forms from the PROMIS sleep disturbance and Sleep-Related Impairment item banks. *Behavioral Sleep Medicine, 10*(1), 6–24. https://doi.org/10.1080/15402002.2012.636266.

Zhou, E. S., Clark, K., Recklitis, C. J., Obenchain, R., & Loscalzo, M. (2018). Sleepless from the get go: Sleep problems prior to initiating cancer treatment. *International Journal of Behavioral Medicine, 25,* 502–516. https://doi.org/10.1007/s12529-018-9715-2

Zhou, E., Partridge, A., & Recklitis, C. (2017). A pilot trial of brief group cognitive–behavioral treatment for insomnia in an adult cancer survivorship program. *Psycho-Oncology, 26,* 843–848. https://doi.org/10.1002/pon.4096

Zhou, E., Partridge A., Syrjala, K., Michaud, A., & Recklitis, C. (2017). Evaluation and treatment of insomnia in adult cancer survivorship programs. *Journal of Cancer Survivorship, 11,* 74–79. https://doi.org/10.1007/s11764-016-0564-1

Zupanec, S., Jones, H., & Stremler, R. (2010). Sleep habits and fatigue of children receiving maintenance chemotherapy for ALL and their parents. *Journal of Pediatric Oncology Nursing, 27,* 217–228. https://doi.org/10.1177/1043454209358890

Play and Leisure

23

Christine Connelly, MSOT, OTR/L, and Brianne Morris, MOT, OTR/L

LEARNING OBJECTIVES

After completing this chapter, readers should be able to
- Understand typical development of play and leisure interests across the lifespan and recognize the importance of play and leisure as an occupation for cancer survivors;
- Comprehend how cancer-related dysfunction in client factors, performance skills and patterns, and capacity for interacting with environments compromises development and participation in play and leisure;
- Assess impairment in play and leisure skills and behaviors, and identify the underlying cancer-related deficits in client factors, performance skills and patterns, and capacity for interacting with environments;
- Identify and describe occupational therapy interventions to address the psychosocial effects of cancer care and treatment, develop the component skills of play and leisure, and promote play and leisure behaviors; and
- Explain the importance of family and caregiver education to create opportunities and environments that foster optimal play skills and leisure interest development for cancer survivors.

KEY TERMS AND CONCEPTS

- Developmental play
- Distraction play
- Flow
- Free play
- Immunocompromised
- Intrinsic motivation
- Isolation
- Leisure
- Medical play
- Occupation
- Play
- Play-based assessment
- Play theory
- Play therapy
- Preparation play
- Prolonged hospitalization

INTRODUCTION

Exploration and participation in play and leisure activities allow for improved self-concept and the ability to partake in daily activities that promote social, personal, and physical development (Darcy et al., 2014). Because of complications that result from a cancer diagnosis, treatment side effects, and shifts in environments, cancer survivors experience changes in physical, cognitive, and emotional development that affect their participation in daily activities, socialization, and play and leisure experiences. For child, adolescent, and adult cancer survivors, a disruption in daily activities, work, play, and leisure has a significant impact on emotional and physical quality of life (QoL; Hwang et al., 2015). Because play and leisure participation is essential to overall health, well-being, and adjustment, occupational therapy is necessary to identify and treat underlying deficits caused by cancer and cancer treatments.

To understand how cancer affects individuals' performance in play and leisure activities, it is important to be aware of some common themes of cancer-related impairment:

- Diagnosis during critical points of childhood development impedes the initial development of specific body functions and skills, hindering play and leisure.
- Cancer survivors often experience a significant decline or disruption in play and leisure activity exploration, pursuit, and participation as a result of isolation, treatment schedules, and loss of interest and motivation.
- Limited exposure to and appropriate participation in play causes delays in cognition, language, and social skills (Stagnitti & Lewis, 2015; Turhan et al., 2018; Westby, 2000).
- Delayed or maladaptive behaviors, play, and social skills develop as a result of reduced expectations, altered environmental conditions, and a lack of social boundaries.
- The most common treatment side effects that affect play and leisure include reduced energy, drive, and motivation; pain; impaired strength; and neurocognitive dysfunction or the presence of precautions (e.g., low laboratory values, reduced weight-bearing ability, peripheral neuropathy; Marusak et al., 2017; Mohammadi et al., 2017; Zheng et al., 2018).

- Disruptions of established leisure participation have significant effects on overall well-being, sense of self, and stress relief.

Occupational therapy practitioners are equipped to use play and leisure to both assess and intervene with the client factors, performance skills and patterns, and contexts and environments affected by cancer to establish, restore, or modify optimal performance throughout treatment into survivorship (American Occupational Therapy Association [AOTA], 2008; Baxter et al., 2017). This chapter explores how cancer affects play and leisure development, exploration, and participation across the lifespan. Additionally, it assists in identifying play and leisure deficits among cancer survivors and in developing occupational therapy interventions while integrating family and caregivers into the client's goals of care.

PLAY AND LEISURE AS OCCUPATION

For children and youths, *occupations* are activities that enable them to learn and develop life skills (e.g., school-related activities), foster creativity and enjoyment (e.g., play and leisure), and thrive as both a means and an end (e.g., self-care, relationships with others; AOTA, 2015). *Play* is a subjective experience that is intrinsically motivated, freely chosen, and pleasurable for the play participant and that is exploratory, fun, and safe in nature (Hughes, 2010; Piaget, 1962). It is a dynamic process that is essential to children's growth, development, and learning from infancy into adulthood (Brown & Vaughan, 2010). Play and leisure are fundamental domains of childhood as well as principal occupations across the lifespan (Henry, 2008). Active engagement in play and leisure pursuits allows children to make sense of the world around them and develop physical coordination, emotional maturity, social skills, and self-confidence to explore new experiences and environments.

Clients diagnosed with cancer at any point in the lifespan undergo treatment that may consist of surgery, chemotherapy, radiation, immunotherapy, and hormonal therapy, singularly or in combination. These treatments can cause significant physical and psychosocial difficulties and negative effects, which affect the client's ability or motivation to participate in meaningful play and leisure activities (Hwang et al., 2015; see Chapter 2, "Cancer Treatment Approaches Across the Lifespan," for more information on treatment of cancer). Research demonstrates that the lack of exposure to play and leisure opportunities deprives children of optimal learning and development (AOTA, 2008).

The foundational play components and developmental process lay a framework for success in physical, cognitive, and social–emotional development. *Play theory* categorizes play by the activity in which one is engaged (e.g., sensorimotor, social, parallel, symbolic, cooperative), which changes over time with different interactions, abilities, and social norms (Lynch & Moore, 2016). By considering the different stages and types of play, occupational therapy practitioners can take the components of play and examine changes in client factors and performance skills and patterns and explore how experiences and environment affect play performance and participation. Table 23.1 presents

TABLE 23.1.   Stages of Play

STAGE	AGE	DESCRIPTION	PURPOSE AND BENEFITS
Solitary play	Begins at birth, occurs lifelong	Child is engrossed in independent play, even with others around	- Building from "unoccupied play" within the first 3 months of life - Discovering how body moves and position in space provides basis for future exploration and play development - Understanding personal play space and toys - Building ability to entertain oneself - Developing attention and concentration
Onlooker or spectator play	2 years	Child observes and notices others but does not engage with them	- Learning how to play - Can benefit from being allowed to watch others and not being pushed in until ready
Parallel play	2–3 years	Children play side by side using their own materials, watching and listening but not yet interacting	- Learning ownership and valuable social skills to transition to social play
Associative play	3–4 years	Beginning of group play; children participate in the same play, although independently	- Learning to interact with peers to practice language and social skills, help resolve conflicts, and develop friendships
Cooperative play	4+ years/later preschool to middle childhood	Children play together to accomplish a joint goal, supporting self and others; involves various play roles and scenarios	- Encouraging "grown-up" play themes - Learning to accept and create roles - Building negotiation and leadership skills - Developing problem-solving skills

Note. Created with modifications from Parten (1932).

TABLE 23.2. Types of Play as It Relates to Occupation

PLAY OCCUPATION	DEVELOPMENT PURPOSE	KEY COMPONENTS AND SKILL DEVELOPMENT	RELEVANCE TO CANCER POPULATION
Birth to 2 years			
Sensorimotor or exploratory play	▪ Called "practice play" by Piaget (1962) ▪ Evolves into functional play	▪ Motivation to play ▪ Exploration of sensations and movements ▪ Sensory development ▪ Visual development (gaze, hand to mouth, eye–hand) ▪ Spatial relations ▪ Awareness of surroundings	Educating caregivers on context setup and providing opportunities to explore safely; variations of play materials Examples: • Tummy time • Crawling • Teething toys • Squeeze toys • Play mats • Mirrors
Social play	▪ Promotes attachment, bonding, relating to others ▪ Progresses from solitary to onlooker to parallel play	▪ Visual development ▪ Attachment ▪ Relating to others ▪ Attunement ▪ Caregiver–child bonding ▪ Emotional sharing ▪ Soothing in stressful situations	Educating parents on developmentally appropriate activities Examples: ▪ Play with parents ▪ Peekaboo
Functional or object play	▪ Helps children explore different materials and understand function of objects ▪ Provides setup for pretend play	▪ Visual attention ▪ Eye–hand coordination ▪ Fine motor skills: grasping–releasing, reaching, transferring objects, manipulating ▪ Container play ▪ Cause and effect ▪ Motor action sequences ▪ Problem solving	Providing appropriate and safe play materials and modeling use Examples: ▪ Blocks ▪ Stacking rings ▪ Nesting cups ▪ Container play ▪ Push–pull toys
Physical play or gross motor play	▪ Promotes coordination, balance, proprioception, and motor control	▪ Movement transitions from stationary to mobile; is object and action driven ▪ Gross motor skills: crawling, standing, climbing, throwing, kicking; transitions ▪ Negotiation of environment and spatial relations ▪ Pushing and pulling objects ▪ Riding ▪ Dancing	Promoting staying active and ways to set up context to explore Providing modifications for fatigue, pain, coordination difficulties Examples: ▪ Ball skills ▪ Swinging ▪ Climbing
Symbolic or pretend play	▪ Begins around 2 years of age ▪ Facilitates understanding roles, promotes creativity, promotes regulation	▪ Use unrealistic and realistic props to act out basic actions ▪ Understand roles ▪ Practice skills of living ▪ Imitation ▪ Creativity ▪ Imagination ▪ Emotional regulation ▪ Self-referencing ▪ Play-based referencing	Promoting opportunities to engage in novel play and foster creativity to expand play repertoire Examples: ▪ Drinking from a cup ▪ Feeding a doll with a spoon or bottle
Early childhood: Ages 2–5 years			
Dramatic or fantasy play	▪ Helps children begin to understand and experience different roles and functioning within community (e.g., family, character, functional) ▪ Frees children from established patterns	▪ Use imagination ▪ Take turns ▪ Cooperate ▪ Share ▪ Develop language ▪ Allows for forms of abstraction—time, place, amount, words, ideas	Serving as diversionary play to allow for transformation of "normal" or role play stressful situations Examples: ▪ Dressing up ▪ Playing doctor to ease medical procedures

(Continued)

TABLE 23.2. Types of Play as It Relates to Occupation *(Cont.)*

PLAY OCCUPATION	DEVELOPMENT PURPOSE	KEY COMPONENTS AND SKILL DEVELOPMENT	RELEVANCE TO ONCOLOGY POPULATION
Constructive play	▪ Teaches manipulation, building, problem-solving skills ▪ Manipulation of objects progresses to manipulation of words, concepts, and ideas	▪ Manipulating objects ▪ Stacking ▪ Building ▪ Constructing ▪ Imagination and creativity ▪ Experimentation ▪ Problem solving	Fostering opportunities to handle different materials and improve fine motor coordination and strength Examples: ▪ Building tower or sandcastle ▪ Legos ▪ Puzzles ▪ Couch pillow fort
Physical or rough-and-tumble play	▪ Transitions from exploratory play	▪ Helps with social awareness, fairness, and altruism ▪ Symbolic play and games evolve into organized games or sports	Educating caregivers on opportunities for safe physical play Examples: ▪ Playing on a playground ▪ Running ▪ Jumping
		Middle childhood: Ages 6–10 years	
Games with rules	▪ Primary form of physical and social play	▪ Rule following ▪ Turn taking ▪ Winning or losing ▪ Social contracts	Promoting opportunities for both winning and losing Examples: ▪ Board games ▪ Computer games ▪ Tag variations ▪ Basketball
Crafts and hobbies	▪ Developed form of constructive play	▪ Creativity ▪ Organize and solve problems ▪ Further development of gross and fine motor skills	Educating on exploring and hobbies, maximizing independence Examples: ▪ Collections ▪ Bike riding ▪ Roller skating ▪ Building sets ▪ Wood working ▪ Jewelry making
Organized sports	▪ Functioning as a team	▪ Cooperation ▪ Teamwork ▪ Rules ▪ Roles ▪ Formal peer groups	Promoting opportunities winning and losing, following rules, socializing with similar aged peers and being part of a group Examples: ▪ Sports team ▪ Dance group ▪ Scouting
Social play	▪ Interactions to allow for participation in adult world	▪ Reciprocity ▪ Sharing ▪ Cooperation ▪ Friendship and belonging ▪ Moral reasoning ▪ Values	Creating opportunities to engage with friends in person when possible or virtually Examples: ▪ Computer or video games with friends
		Later childhood into adolescence	
Hobbies and recreation	▪ Promotes leisure exploration and participation	▪ Self-awareness and sense of identity ▪ Sense of enjoyment and accomplishment ▪ Thought processes become formal operations	Strengthening skills to return to preferred hobbies or recreation activities or explore new activities Examples: ▪ Reading ▪ Collections ▪ Crafting ▪ Photography ▪ Running

(Continued)

TABLE 23.2.   Types of Play as It Relates to Occupation *(Cont.)*

PLAY OCCUPATION	DEVELOPMENT PURPOSE	KEY COMPONENTS AND SKILL DEVELOPMENT	RELEVANCE TO ONCOLOGY POPULATION
Organized sports	• Aids in further skill development and competitiveness	• Cooperation and competitiveness • Stress relief • Health benefits	Strengthening skills to return to preferred sports or making modifications (e.g., fabricate custom chest plate to protect Mediport) when cleared to return Examples: ▪ Lacrosse ▪ Baseball
Social play	▪ Continues further development ▪ Transitions to spending time together rather than playing together ▪ Experiences may become more celebratory or ritual in nature	▪ Self-awareness ▪ Socialization ▪ More intimate communication ▪ Variety of social experiences	Maintaining friendships during treatment Examples: ▪ Hang out with friends ▪ Go to the movies ▪ Listen to music ▪ Go to dances and parties

Note. Created with modifications from Brown and Vaughan (2010), Case-Smith (2015), Hughes (2010), and Westby (2000).

the stages of play development, and Table 23.2 presents the types of play as they relate to occupational performance.

Play

From birth through childhood, children move through the stages of play outlined in Table 23.2 in a relatively ordered sequence. During this time, children experience and learn vital information about themselves and others, including how their body moves, properties of play materials, cause and effect, ownership, attention, the roles they and others hold, sharing, turn taking, and higher level social interaction skills such as negotiation and leadership (Case-Smith, 2015; Parten, 1932; Westby, 2000).

Children diagnosed with cancer within the first 2 years of life may lack development of exploratory and social play skills as a result of disruptions in their ability to actively engage in exploratory play and social interactions with siblings, parents, and peers. Research shows that early experiences can affect children's development in both a cumulative and a possibly delayed manner, so early intervention is essential (Marusak et al., 2017).

Adolescents and adults diagnosed with cancer may experience changes in strength, endurance, and opportunities to participate in games with peers or organized sports, which limits engagement in preferred activities and causes further muscle weakness and mental health side effects (e.g., anxiety, depression). Play serves as an avenue through which overall skill development occurs and positively affects anxiety, coping skills, and overall adjustment, which are essential in the cancer population (Ullan et al., 2014).

Evidence demonstrates that play, especially *free play,* or unstructured, voluntary and individually initiated play, promotes brain development and neural connections, which facilitate creativity, memory, problem solving, decision making, conflict resolution, social–emotional growth, leadership skill development, and higher academic performance (Gray, 2013; Pellis et al., 2010). The developmental stages and types of play promote learning and social interaction, create understanding of different environments and

rules of engagement, and allow children to practice skills they will need in the future (Brown & Vaughan, 2010; Parten, 1932)

Leisure

Play provides the groundwork for leisure interest exploration and participation. *Leisure* pursuits are similar to play in that the experience is intrinsically motivated, fun, and chosen to occur during one's free time. Leisure is a subjective experience characterized by time, activity, and experience for engagement in individually meaningful activities. When engaged in leisure activities, individuals can experience feelings of freedom, reward, pleasure, relaxation, and decreased awareness of the passage of time (Keats et al., 1999; Sellar & Stanley, 2010). Research demonstrates that participation in leisure activities can improve self-esteem, self-awareness, sense of identity, life satisfaction, overall health and wellness, and occupational balance (Sellar & Stanley, 2010). Shared leisure activities provide opportunities for independence in structuring one's time and developing peer relationships (Kleiber et al., 2002).

There is a positive correlation between health and leisure participation, whereby individuals experience improved self-perception, stress reduction, and overall physical function (Hutchinson et al., 2003). Having an excess of leisure or nonobligatory time without meaningful engagement can lead to boredom and depression, which many cancer survivors experience because of shifts in time, routines, and productivity (e.g., school, work). When survivors are engaged in meaningful play and leisure activities with the "just-right challenge," they can experience *flow,* a mental state of being fully immersed in the task at hand, and may experience decreased awareness of the passage of time (Sellar & Stanley, 2010).

Evidence shows that people need a balance of individual skill and task difficulty to avoid anxiety, frustration, or fear of failure on the one hand, and boredom, routine, and loss of interest on the other. It is essential to maintain, promote, modify, and explore play and leisure participation across the cancer care continuum to support physical and psychosocial health as well as reduce the risk of recurrence or secondary cancers (Daunhauer & Cermak, 2008; McCullough et al., 2016).

Play and Leisure During Illness

The onset of illness causes a profound change of a reality that was once comfortable and predictable as clients experience fewer interactions with friends and family and decreased engagement in everyday rituals. Hospitalization is a stressful, threatening experience with significant emotional effects that cause stress; anxiety; maladaptive behaviors; withdrawal; regression in development; and disruptions in sleep, self-care, and play routines (Bohg et al., 1986).

Many children undergoing treatment exhibit limited playfulness and decreased repertoire of play activities, resourcefulness, mature reciprocal play, sharing, and willingness to lose in cooperative game play (Kielhofner et al., 1983; Tanta & Knox, 2015). Older children, adolescents, and adults may experience a loss of motivation or skills needed to engage in once-meaningful play and leisure activities. Occupational therapy intervention in hospital environments can decrease anxiety and stress, providing a sense of control and leading to improvements in emotional and physical well-being, adjustment, and coping with illness and hospitalization (Haiat et al., 2003).

Supporting and promoting play and leisure in the naturally occurring contexts of home, hospital, and the community is essential throughout treatment and into survivorship.

Occupational therapy practitioners need to thoroughly evaluate foundational components and individual factors of play and leisure across the lifespan to promote successful occupational performance. Through assessment and intervention, occupational therapy practitioners can cultivate success using restoration, modification, and preventive capacities to foster occupational performance in play and leisure.

FACTORS THAT MAY CONTRIBUTE TO OCCUPATIONAL IMPAIRMENT IN PLAY AND LEISURE

Client Factors

Several body functions are necessary for successful play and leisure performance. People rely on sensory, mental, neuromusculoskeletal, cardiopulmonary, and various other organ systems to develop, explore, and participate in play and leisure tasks. A cancer diagnosis and its respective treatments can cause secondary impairments in these body functions, affecting clients in all stages of the cancer continuum (Darcy et al., 2015; Hwang et al., 2015; Phillips et al., 2015). Identifying and treating the client factors affected by cancer that influence play development and leisure engagement is critical for the cancer survivor's overall development and QoL.

Table 23.3 provides a comprehensive summary of the key client factors and performance skills affected by cancer diagnosis and treatment that influence play and leisure

TABLE 23.3. Effect of Cancer on Client Factors and Performance Skills in Context of Play and Leisure Development and Participation

BODY FUNCTIONS AND STRUCTURES	CANCER DIAGNOSIS AND TREATMENT EFFECTS	DYSFUNCTION IN PLAY- AND LEISURE-RELATED PERFORMANCE SKILLS
Sensory		
Pain	- Cancer-related pain - Procedural and postsurgical pain - Treatment-induced bone pain - Neuropathic pain	- Avoidance of extremity or whole-body movements - Poor activity tolerance preventing play and leisure participation - Increased attraction to sedentary activities (e.g., television, video games)
Touch	- CIPN - Numbness - Heightened tactile sensitivity	- Impaired balance preventing safe engagement in gross motor play and leisure activities (e.g., negotiating playgrounds, sports) - Decreased tolerance for manipulation of hard-edged toys or game pieces (e.g., connecting and separating Legos) - Poor tactile discrimination affecting ability shuffle, deal, or hold playing cards - Limited sensory feedback provided by various textures during play (e.g., play dough, finger paint)
Mental		
Energy and drive	- Cancer-induced fatigue and decreased levels of energy - Reduced appetite secondary to nausea - Reprioritization of needs and wants and changes in motivation	- Decreased internal motivation and interest in play or leisure activities - Limited initiation of and engagement in preferred play activities - Diminished exploration of novel play or leisure activities

(Continued)

TABLE 23.3. **Effect of Cancer on Client Factors and Performance Skills in Context of Play and Leisure Development and Participation** *(Cont.)*

BODY FUNCTIONS AND STRUCTURES	CANCER DIAGNOSIS AND TREATMENT EFFECTS	DYSFUNCTION IN PLAY- AND LEISURE-RELATED PERFORMANCE SKILLS
Emotional regulation	▪ Steroid-induced emotional lability, moodiness ▪ Heightened anxiety and stress causing decreased frustration tolerance and coping skills ▪ Impaired impulse control from instant gratification ▪ Fear of medical personnel, unknown procedures, and prognosis affecting trust and ability to transition	▪ Unable to cope with losing or failing at preferred play or leisure tasks ▪ Difficulty participating in competitive games ▪ Avoidance of novel activities and games secondary to fear of failing ▪ Difficulty transitioning to novel people, separating from parents, establishing rapport ▪ Immature social skills and poor turn taking ▪ Decreased cooperative, collaborative, and reciprocal play skills
Cognition and executive functioning	▪ Medication-related neurotoxicity ▪ Chemotherapy-induced cognitive processing delays ▪ Neurocognitive changes from brain tumor location, resection, or radiation ▪ Limited exposure to learning environments	▪ Decreased understanding of toy or tool use impeding initiation of play ▪ Impaired problem-solving, sequencing, and organizing skills to engage in multistep activities or follow directions for hobbies or game and sports play (e.g., cooking, board and card games, Lego® models) ▪ Decreased experience and creative thought for pretend and imaginary play themes ▪ Impaired judgment and safety awareness limiting independent transportation to activities and social outings
Attention and memory	▪ Increased distractibility from overstimulated hospital environment ▪ Reduced short-term memory from neurotoxic effects of chemotherapy, medications, or location of cancer	▪ Difficulty retaining game-play rules ▪ Inability to engage in play or game activity to completion ▪ Impaired concentration (e.g., difficulty with book reading)
Neuromusculoskeletal		
Bone and joint mobility and stability	▪ Diminished bone integrity and stability from disease or metastases with subsequent weight-bearing restrictions ▪ Steroid-induced avascular necrosis ▪ GVHD-induced muscle contractures ▪ Diminished shoulder ROM secondary to inactivity ▪ Upper extremity guarding and shoulder tightness at CVC site ▪ Decreased dorsiflexion strength with ankle–foot ROM restrictions	▪ Dependence on adaptive device to maintain weight bearing, inhibiting play positions and overall activity engagement ▪ Impaired overhead reach for gross motor play and exercise (e.g., ball throw and catch, yoga, dance) ▪ Inefficient grasp patterns impeding drawing, writing, coloring, and painting skills ▪ Impaired bending and floor-to-stand transfer skills limiting floor-based play or exercise activities
Muscle power, strength, and endurance	▪ Steroid-induced myopathy with proximal weakness ▪ Generalized weakness and deconditioning from inactivity ▪ Brain cancer causing neurological compromise and hemiparesis	▪ Insufficient muscle strength to transition between play positions, engage in gross motor activities, and carry or lift play and leisure objects (e.g., climbing on playground) ▪ Lack of bilateral coordination to engage in bimanual play and leisure activities (e.g., jump rope, doll dressing, musical instruments) ▪ Poor postural endurance and difficulty maintaining upright seated positioning for engagement in tabletop activities
Voluntary movement	▪ Neurological deficits, including ataxia ▪ Impaired gross and fine motor coordination ▪ Neurotoxic medication–induced tremors	▪ Difficulty engaging in activities requiring coordination and timing (e.g., sports, dance) ▪ Impaired distal control preventing participation in fine motor–based activities (e.g., beading, knitting, assembling models)

(Continued)

TABLE 23.3.   Effect of Cancer on Client Factors and Performance Skills in Context of Play and Leisure Development and Participation *(Cont.)*

BODY FUNCTIONS AND STRUCTURES	CANCER DIAGNOSIS AND TREATMENT EFFECTS	DYSFUNCTION IN PLAY- AND LEISURE-RELATED PERFORMANCE SKILLS
Organ structures and systems		
Cardiovascular	▪ Steroid-induced hypertension ▪ Tachycardia ▪ Postoperative hypotension, dizziness ▪ Chemotherapy-related cardiomyopathy	▪ Restricted from engaging in cardiovascular activities (e.g., running, sports) ▪ Limited to seated or sedentary play and leisure activities
Respiratory	▪ Dyspnea and shortness of breath from infection-induced PNA or pneumonitis ▪ Reduced lung capacity secondary to resections, infectious agents, fluid overload, pneumothorax ▪ Pulmonary compromise requiring supplemental oxygen delivery ▪ Surgical incision (postthoracotomy) causing shoulder ROM limitations	▪ Limited exercise and activity tolerance for movement-based play and cardiovascular exercise ▪ Impaired overhead reach and increased guarded posture preventing engagement in throwing, catching, climbing
Hematological	▪ Reduced lab values (HgB, Plts, WBC) resulting in decreased energy and tachycardia, risk of bleeding and infection ▪ Blood clots, DVT ▪ CVC, central line, or Mediport insertion for lab draws and treatment infusions	▪ Difficulty with high-energy exercise and activity secondary to fatigue from low blood counts ▪ Unable to engage in high-impact or contact activities (e.g., rough-and-tumble play, basketball, skiing) ▪ Restricted to engaging in resistive and repetitive exercise routines (e.g., weight training, Pilates reformer)
Immunological	▪ Diminished immune system requires isolation from peers and family ▪ PPE worn by family or self ▪ Increased acquired infection	▪ Decreased engagement in play with siblings and peers ▪ Limited learning, practice, and repetition of play experiences ▪ Confined to solitary play or play with adults and health care professionals instead of shared and cooperative play with peers ▪ Surrounded by people wearing masks; unable to see facial expressions to link with pretend play experiences
Digestive	▪ Feeding tubes ▪ Nausea and vomiting resulting in prolonged bedrest ▪ Malnourishment and weight loss	▪ Compromised bonding experience with caregiver during feeding preventing development of early reciprocal communication skills ▪ Decreased tolerance of tummy time secondary to feeding tube placement ▪ Avoidance of out-of-bed positioning or mobility to prevent nausea limiting opportunities for participation ▪ Reduced energy reserves and stamina needed to sustain play or leisure activity until completion
Skin	▪ Scleroderma from GVHD ▪ Subcutaneous CVC insertion for lab draws and infusions ▪ Peripheral or central line with connection to IV pole	▪ Poor self-image secondary to observable skin changes resulting in social isolation ▪ Skin and joint tightness limiting ROM and ability to move arms and legs freely during play ▪ Restricted from playing contact sports with Mediport insertion ▪ Fear of pain with frequent accessing of Mediport adding to client anxiety and tendency to "shut down" and disengage socially ▪ Limited movement options secondary to restrictions with IV pole attachment (e.g., no running, no rough-and-tumble play)

Note. CIPN = chemotherapy-induced peripheral neuropathy; CVC = central venous catheter; DVT = deep vein thrombosis; GVHD = graft-versus-host disease; HgB = hemoglobin; Plts = platelets; PNA = pulmonary nodular amyloidosis; PPE = personal protective equipment; ROM = range of motion; WBC = white blood cell count.
Sources. Adapted from American Occupational Therapy Association (2014), Marusak et al. (2017), Ness et al. (2009), Phillips et al. (2015), and Pruitt & Nagarajan (2009).

development and participation. Body functions such as energy and drive, pain, and cognition, along with the immunological and digestive body systems, are highlighted as client factors particularly unique to cancer that significantly interfere with play and leisure participation (AOTA, 2014).

Energy and drive

Cancer's effect on clients' energy levels and drive greatly influences engagement in play and leisure. Pain, heightened fatigue levels, and reduced appetite as a result of cancer and its treatment contribute to reduced energy levels. Because the clients' drive, or need to fulfill a desire or want, is directly influenced by energy, clients experiencing lowered energy reserves have less motivation for activity engagement. Actions or behaviors motivated by internal reasons, or **intrinsic motivation,** is a key element that factors into one's ability to actively participate in, experience, and continue play, so cancer survivors are at great risk for losing the drive to play (Knox & Mailloux, 1997). Without the initial drive and internal motivation to engage in play or leisure activities, the benefits of these occupations will not be reinforced, thereby making cancer survivors even less inclined to engage in such activities.

Pain

Phillips et al. (2015) stated that approximately 12% of childhood cancer survivors ages 20–49 years reported having pain as a result of cancer diagnosis and treatment. However, a higher percentage of survivors reported pain while in active treatment of cancer (Baxter et al., 2017). Pain can occur as a result of the cancer disease process, diagnostic medical procedures, and treatment (Chauhan et al., 2010). Pain incurred by medical procedures for diagnostic or treatment purposes is the more commonly reported type of pain experience among pediatric clients with cancer (Scarponi & Pession, 2016).

Pain's emotional and psychological impact on clients of any age interferes with their ability to sustain attention on a task, their ability to engage socially, and their overall motivation for play and leisure activities. However, the act of engaging in preferred play and leisure activities can be an effective intervention to distract a client from the pain experience (Ullán et al., 2014). With successful efforts to alleviate pain through cancer treatment, analgesics, or even play therapy (described in the "Evidence-Based Interventions" section of this chapter), an increase in activity level, play, and socialization can be achieved for clients with cancer (Chauhan et al., 2010; Scarponi & Pession, 2016). For more information, see Chapter 16, "Cancer-Related Pain."

Neurocognitive impairment

Phillips et al. (2015) reported that 35% of childhood cancer survivors have some presentation of neurocognitive impairment. (For more information, see Chapter 17, "Cancer-Related Cognitive Impairment.") Turhan et al. (2018) found that pediatric clients who received chemotherapy, radiation therapy, or both for leukemia treatment presented with late neurological and cognitive effects, including reduced IQ and academic skills compared with siblings. Contributing components of impaired neurocognitive impairment included difficulties with attention, memory, executive functioning, and coping (Turhan et al., 2018).

For example, survivors who have trouble with executive functioning skills experience challenges following multistep directions to participate in board games or step-by-step building or craft activities. Lack of sustained attention also inhibits their capacity to stay on a play task or learn new skills needed for novel leisure activities. Play ideas and patterns are underdeveloped, because pediatric survivors are unable to attend, ideate, organize, or sequence

imaginative play themes (Fink et al., 2012). Because play is the foundation for language, comprehension, and pragmatic skill development, any reduction or compromise in play experiences will subsequently compound the cognitive deficits of cancer survivors (Stagnitti & Lewis, 2015).

Digestive and immunological systems

Every organ system is susceptible to the destructive effects of cancer. The digestive and immunological systems particularly become part of the cancer sequelae that significantly interrupt clients' ability to enjoy or participate in play or leisure activities. The digestive system becomes significantly compromised as a result of chemotherapy treatment. Frequent bouts of nausea and vomiting put survivors in such an uncomfortable state that they often attempt to seek comfort by lying still, closing their eyes, staying in bed, and avoiding engagement in any activities.

Digestion difficulties also affect feeding and mealtime routines. In extreme cases, survivors rely on feeding tubes and nutritional IV fluids to receive nourishment. For infants particularly, this passive means of feeding removes bonding experiences between parent and child. The infant misses opportunities for unoccupied sensorimotor and exploratory play, which is an essential precursor to more developed play types. A gastronomy tube or percutaneous endoscopic gastronomy causes sensitivity to the abdominal area, which may cause discomfort while clients are prone and prevent infants from engaging in tummy-time play, reducing the musculoskeletal benefits gained from this position. Older children do not experience the oral sensory and tactile benefits of eating, which prevents them from developing a foundation to feel confident exploring various textures during play.

Cancer survivors may also be **immunocompromised,** or have an impaired immune system with a greater risk for infection because of chemotherapy treatment, steroids, and other medications. As a result of being highly susceptible to infection, survivors are typically restricted in terms of the types of environments they can be in and the number and age of people they surround themselves with, and they often have to wear masks and gloves in public spaces. Exposure to and interactions with a variety of people provide the opportunity to develop language and social skills, adapt to unpredictability, and form a sense of self. Survivors with reduced exposure to people resort to more solitary play activities, which reduces opportunities for cooperative play and the development of social skills. The cancer population most susceptible to a disruption in play behaviors and leisure engagement as a result of their prolonged immunocompromised state is clients requiring a stem cell transplant (SCT; see Chapter 2, "Cancer Treatment Approaches Across the Lifespan," for more on SCT).

During a prolonged inpatient hospital admission for SCT, cancer survivors are confined to the hospital room secondary to being at significant risk for infection. The small space of a hospital room does not afford the ability to move and explore as survivors would in their own home, school, or playground. In addition to limited environmental and socialization options for exploration, survivors have to avoid exposure to any old or used objects and toys that cannot be properly disinfected. This prevents children from bringing their favorite toy or stuffed animal into the hospital for comfort or play. Koukourikos et al. (2015) confirmed that a stuffed animal can help soothe pediatric clients during medical tests and treatments and reduce behavior regressions. Plush or stuffed toys are also effective in distracting pediatric clients experiencing postoperative pain (Ullán et al., 2014).

Familiar play objects and the act of play in a hospital setting can help pediatric cancer survivors feel a sense of control and normalize an environment that might otherwise feel scary (Darcy et al., 2015). This is especially important for clients with terminal illness (Koukourikos et al., 2015). Being immunocompromised with a *prolonged hospitalization,* an acute hospital admission lasting greater than 1–2 weeks, also directly affects the client's environment and context of play and leisure, which is discussed later in this chapter.

Performance Skills

The collective client factors affected by cancer ultimately inhibit development of the performance skills needed for successful play and leisure participation. The impact can be observed in different degrees of severity compromising motor, processing, and social interaction skills. For example, the physical manifestations that result from a cancer diagnosis and treatment side effects can range from subtle numbness and tingling in the fingertips (i.e., chemotherapy-induced peripheral neuropathy [CIPN]) to complete paresis of the arms and legs, as seen in leptomeningeal disease. (See Chapter 19, "Chemotherapy-Induced Peripheral Neuropathy," for more on CIPN).

The severity of motor skills affected by cancer diagnosis and treatment will correlate to the degree of impact it has on a client's physical performance. A similar range of severity applies to cognitive processing and social skills. Survivors may report occasional short-term memory difficulties, or they can have profound cognitive deficits resembling those of a client after stroke or traumatic brain injury. The social interaction skills affected can also vary widely; some clients demonstrate no social deficits at all, whereas others lose their expressive language skills entirely or exhibit emotional outbursts in response to simple demands.

In terms of the types of play children engage in (see Table 23.2), children need all performance skill areas to succeed in play's variations. Applying activity analysis, occupational therapy practitioners can predict that any motor skill deficit will encumber play and leisure that rely heavily on physical manipulation or movement (e.g., sensorimotor and exploratory play, play involving gross motor skills, functional and object play, constructive play, rough-and-tumble play, crafts and hobbies, sports). However, a processing difficulty affecting the capacity to attend, initiate or terminate, sequence, and organize or problem solve will hinder the client's ability to engage in pretend, dramatic, imaginary, constructive, and symbolic play as well as in games with rules and reading. Slowed cognitive processing combined with impaired judgment will also impede the ability to drive safely, reducing independent access to favored leisure outings. Finally, any type of activity that is not solitary in nature and requires expressive and receptive language, turn taking, impulse control, and emotional regulation (e.g., social play, associative play, cooperative play, organized sports) will be greatly affected by challenges in the skill area of social interaction.

The cancer diagnosis and severity of treatment side effects may dictate the types of play and leisure activities cancer survivors gravitate toward or reveal the play type that survivors are deficient in on the basis of the strength or weakness of performance skills. For example, pediatric survivors with relapsed leukemia requiring prolonged strict *isolation*, or the elimination of clients' exposure to people and environments to prevent acquiring infection, often demonstrate difficulty with processing and social interaction skills secondary to a lack of exposure to same-age peers and to learning and play environments. As a result, survivors gravitate toward solitary or parallel play activities that require limited interaction (e.g., functional or object play, constructive play, craft activities).

Survivors may often rely on repetitive play patterns with a decreased repertoire of imaginative themes. In extreme cases, perseverative or compulsive behaviors can sometimes replace play in this population (e.g., snipping repetitively with scissors, excessively sorting and categorizing game cards, lining up trains). Survivors can also demonstrate immature social interaction and negotiation skills or even a complete disregard for a playmate's presence.

While in isolation, cancer survivors also resort to using technology in substitution for active play and leisure, which further promotes sedentary behavior. Survivors who solely rely on technology for play and leisure are prone to impaired performance skills, including motor development, creativity, impulse control and waiting skills, respect, and turn taking. They demonstrate increases in overall anxiety, a reliance on being entertained, and decreased attention span (Arbesman et al., 2013; Sosa, 2016). In general, both pediatric and adult survivors undergoing cancer treatment spend a significant amount of time playing games and watching videos on tablets and smartphones as a distraction technique while just waiting for appointments or going through an unpleasant medical procedure. For developing survivors, this "screen time" further limits development of physical and mental skills as compared with free play, physical play, or exploratory play. With the rise in technology and screen time and decrease in active free play, play skills lack the necessary elements for motor, processing, and social skill development.

Performance Patterns

Cancer-related symptoms, treatment protocols, and side effects all contribute to a disruption in the roles and everyday routines of cancer survivors (Darcy et al., 2015). As a direct effect of the environmental changes they experience for treatment needs, hospitalizations, and infection control, the roles and routines inherent to the environments clients miss are affected. The roles of playmate, teammate, or club member are put on hold as survivors are removed from the leisure activities that support these identities. Play, school, and leisure involvement are reprioritized. Medical treatment needs override school attendance in the acute stages of diagnosis, and conserving energy for school, rather than engaging in outdoor play, takes a higher priority for cancer survivors (Tsimicalis et al., 2017). These shifts in priorities and changes in life roles ultimately affect survivors' self-concept and result in decreased reports of QoL (Hwang et al., 2015; Manav & Ocakci, 2016).

Cancer survivors' typical, everyday routines are disrupted because of intensive treatment schedules, hospitalizations, symptom presentation, and overall activity intolerance. Survivors are restricted from participation in some of their favored active leisure activities as a result of safety precautions from the diagnosis or treatment effects. The need for this routine change influences the physical and social expectations placed on survivors by the family, caregivers, medical personnel, and sometimes themselves. Decreased importance is placed on active play and leisure engagement as survivors and caregivers support more sleep and sedentary tasks in an effort to "help" rest from treatments.

To provide comfort during a challenging time, caregivers do more for their family member with cancer, despite what the person is still capable of. This "passive parenting" fosters a sense of learned helplessness that creates an unbalanced dynamic between the survivor and caregiver, leading to decreased activity participation and ultimately a decline in function and independence levels (Brand et al., 2017). To keep cancer survivors happy, caregivers often suspend boundary and limit setting, and survivors no longer have a sense of consequence. Without consequence, survivors may develop maladaptive coping behaviors such as difficulty taking direction from caretakers or hospital personnel. Brand et al. (2017) encourages caregivers to promote and enforce rules to provide a sense of order and security for their children. Survivors are also often given material rewards after difficult medical procedures or gifted with an abundance of toys, games, and activities to ease the burden of their diagnosis. However, these items depreciate in value because survivors feel no intrinsic reward, and the play and leisure accessories eventually lose their appeal. Therefore, it is important to differentiate between rewarding and gifting, and to pair each act with appropriate behaviors or events so that clients continue to value the toys and games provided and recognize their self-worth in the process.

Without school or work schedules to abide by, cancer survivors have little daily structure and no events to encourage early rise times or consistent bedtimes. This affects sleep and wake cycles and patterns, which results in poor sleep hygiene, exacerbates fatigue, and creates a further decrease in motivation for active play or leisure engagement during the day. Survivors often perform ADLs and play and leisure activities within the confines of the home or at the hospital bedside, which further reduces movement opportunities throughout the day.

The change in roles and routines of clients with cancer reduces expectations, limits internal gratification and satisfaction, and decreases structure and behavior patterns. This compromises clients' drive and motivation to engage in play and leisure activities they once deemed pleasurable. Occupational therapy practitioners can play an integral part in helping cancer survivors reestablish routines and redefine their roles. Managing both direct and indirect side effects of cancer is essential to helping reintegrate typical patterns, routines, and environments (Tsimicalis et al., 2017).

Context and Environment

An environment that allows for spontaneous exploration, object and person availability, opportunity for choice, and

internal control promotes a healthy development of play skills among children (Knox & Mailloux, 1997). Interference with any of these components will result in immature or underdeveloped play skills, which can ultimately inhibit leisure interest formation.

Darcy et al. (2015) identified the environment of children with cancer as instrumental in influencing everyday life functioning and experiences, including play, recreation, and leisure. Valuable time socializing with peers, siblings, and colleagues is lost with frequent or extended absences from school or work as a result of symptoms, side effects, the need to relocate for specialized treatments, or prolonged hospitalization (da Silva & Cabral, 2015; Tsimicalis et al., 2017). As a result, opportunities for play skill development and leisure activity engagement diminish substantially. Both acute and prolonged hospitalizations can affect play and leisure development in multiple ways.

- *Time in bed.* Cancer survivors hospitalized for treatment are prone to decreased engagement in physical activity and a tendency to engage in ADLs, television watching, and sedentary play activities all in bed (Götte et al., 2014). Götte et al. (2014) found that more than 50% of survivors hospitalized for leukemia or bone cancer treatment remained in bed longer than 23 hours per day. Continuous bedrest reduces the drive and motivation for play and leisure participation, further limiting experiences and opportunities the occupation provides. As a result, the need for play and leisure intensifies, because it serves as both an emotional outlet and a platform for movement and cognitive processing.
- *Hospital control.* A hospital environment dictates the space, resources, and people available to experience play and leisure opportunities. The hospital also restricts access to favored toys, peers, and siblings and provides little space and opportunity for spontaneous exploration and movement (Götte et al., 2014). As a result, engagement in typical play patterns and behaviors is hampered.
- *Isolation precautions.* A hospital playroom or recreation room can offer novel play experiences and leisure opportunities, which can be very useful for motivating clients with cancer. However, not all cancer survivors have the ability to use a playroom or recreation room because of isolation precautions. Also, these rooms typically consist of toys, games, crafts, and electronics that require decreased physical activity and promote sedentary play (da Silva & Cabral, 2015).
- *Medical equipment.* In the hospital setting, it is common for play to involve medical equipment, such as syringes and gloves because this is what is readily available and familiar to pediatric cancer survivors. Engaging in play with hospital supplies can have profound psychosocial benefits in addition to providing opportunities for symbolic and pretend play (Scarponi & Pession, 2016).
- *Lack of peers.* Adults become pediatric cancer survivors' primary playmates in the hospital, which eliminates the experience of unpredictable play that typically occurs with same-age peers. In an attempt to comfort children with cancer, health care professionals, caregivers, and other adults typically avoid engaging in any play themes

or competitive activities that may result in conflict or stress during play. As a result, children do not have the opportunity to develop coping or conflict resolution skills as they would when playing with a same-age peer.

Beyond hospitalization, cancer survivors likely need modifications and adaptations to the school or home environment to successfully engage in play and leisure activities, which can lead to isolation or social exclusion if clients have difficulty reintegrating with peers (Darcy et al., 2014). Health care providers, teachers, and caregivers must promote an environment of inclusion and assistance to bridge the gap between a client and their peer or sibling. Occupational therapy practitioners are skilled at assessing and adapting the environment, modeling age-appropriate play behaviors, and making recommendations to optimize play and leisure opportunities in any circumstance.

OCCUPATIONAL THERAPY EVALUATION OF PLAY AND LEISURE

Evaluating cancer survivors is multifaceted; many unique implications and precautions affect various domains of development and the ability to participate in meaningful occupations. Within this population, the relatively predictable trajectory of development and participation is influenced by various challenges and stresses along with an element of trauma (Koukourikos et al., 2015; Li et al., 2016; Silva et al., 2017). Therefore, it is paramount to establish trust and rapport with both the survivor and caregivers, keeping questions client centered and highlighting elements of play and leisure in treatment discussion. Creating a positive relationship cultivates cooperation and decreases anxiety about the evaluation and treatment process, allowing for better representation of skills (Dudgeon et al., 2015).

Cancer survivors may experience significant changes in mood, self-esteem, self-concept, and socialization, becoming less independent and more reliant on caregivers. Building rapport through active listening and interest in the client's priorities, values, and goals allows for better understanding of leisure capacity (Keats et al., 1999; Sellar & Stanley, 2010). To best assess play and leisure exploration and participation, evaluation should consist of a detailed occupational history and a thorough assessment of client factors, performance skills and patterns, and clinical observations.

Occupational Profile

The occupational profile of the cancer survivor within play and leisure assessment consists of understanding the occupation itself, the environment, patterns, and routines. Having a comprehensive understanding of diagnosis, treatment, and related dysfunction allows occupational therapy practitioners to ask leading questions for appreciation of the individual's profile. Practitioners can ask the following guiding questions related to play and leisure assessment:

- What play and leisure activities are meaningful to you [your child]?

- What are your favorite play and leisure activities?
- Describe what you like about this play or leisure activity.
- How often are you able to engage in this play or leisure activity?
- When do you play or participate in this activity (e.g., time of day, duration, cycle of treatment)?
- Where do you play or engage in leisure (e.g., in bed, at home, in the hospital playroom)?
- What changes or patterns have you noticed with different cycles or aspects of treatment?
- Describe the type of play (e.g., how do you play: parallel, symbolic, games with rules).
- Describe the nature of play (e.g., playful, repetitive, novel, expanded routines).
- Describe the quality of play (e.g., physical, sedentary, manipulative).
- How have diagnosis, treatment, and symptoms affected play and leisure participation?
- Describe any changes in cognition, processing, memory, attention, sensory perception, strength, range of motion (ROM), endurance, coordination, balance, mood and affect, behavior, energy, motivation, and drive.
- What are your goals to improve your play or leisure performance or participation?

Analysis of Occupational Performance

Examination of the client's medical history and understanding of the current and projected cancer treatment, possible side effects, and prognosis are essential to evaluation and creation of the occupational therapy plan of care. Knowledge of treatment side effects helps occupational therapy practitioners to fully assess client factors and performance skills, guides the questions asked, and focuses evaluation as it relates to occupation. For example, one may experience changes in cognition (i.e., attention and memory) from cranial radiation or chemotherapy, peripheral neuropathy from vincristine, or myopathy and behavioral changes from high-dose steroids. These changes can affect attention to task, the ability to expand on learned experiences and problem solve, and the ability to manipulate necessary toys or tools for independence in preferred play or leisure activities.

Occupational therapy practitioners also need to consider the various cancer-specific precautions, including low laboratory values, Mediport access, bone metastases, spinal precautions, and neuropathy. Having a comprehensive understanding of cancer-related dysfunction (use Table 23.3 as a reference) and obtaining the occupational profile facilitate assessment of specific client factors, performance skills, and performance patterns that affect participation. For example, a survivor may experience ROM deficits because of muscle weakness, pain, contractures, or port sensitivity, which can be assessed with goniometer measurements or functional observations of reaching, bending, grasp, and tool manipulation. Another survivor who has undergone prolonged hospitalization may present with fear of movement and new people, preference for sedentary play, and limited exploration or repertoire of play skills and routines. Table 23.4 features common deficits that affect play and leisure within the oncology population, with examples of assessment approaches.

Table 23.4 Occupational Therapy Assessment of Cancer-Related Deficits on Play and Leisure Skills

CANCER-RELATED SYMPTOMS AND DEFICITS	ASSESSMENT TOOL OPTIONS	FUNCTIONAL ASSESSMENT AND CLINICAL OBSERVATIONS
Neurocognitive toxicity	▪ MOCA (Nasreddine et al., 2005) ▪ DAYC–2 (Voress & Maddox, 2013) ▪ HELP (Furuno et al., 1994) ▪ Bayley–III (Bayley, 2005) ▪ BDI–2 (Newborg, 2005)	▪ Cause–effect pop toys ▪ Memory games ▪ Card games ▪ Reading sample ▪ Puzzles, shape sorters ▪ Board games ▪ Copying ▪ Word search ▪ Clinical observations of sequencing, initiation, attention, and memory
Sensory impairments and processing changes	▪ SPM (Miller-Kuhaneck et al., 2007) ▪ Sensory Profile (Dunn, 1999)	▪ Tolerance for tactile, vestibular, and proprioceptive activities ▪ Clinical observations of arousal and activity levels, impulse control
Pain	▪ Rating scale (1–10) ▪ Wong-Baker FACES Pain Rating Scale (Wong-Baker, 2015)	▪ Observation of pain through various positions while engaging in play
Limited ROM	▪ Goniometer ▪ Functional movement patterns	▪ Functional reaching for toys ▪ Throwing and catching ▪ Transitions, bending, squatting ▪ Grasp patterns on blocks
Decreased strength and muscle endurance	▪ MMT ▪ Dynamometer ▪ Pinch meter ▪ PDMS–2 (Folio & Fewell, 2000) ▪ BOT–2 (Bruininks & Bruininks, 2005) ▪ Bayley–III ▪ BDI–2 ▪ HELP	▪ Grip and pinch patterns to operate toys ▪ Fine motor force production (e.g., small pop beads, tongs, scissors, play dough) ▪ Stacking blocks for gradation ▪ Shape sorter, puzzle ▪ Writing or coloring sample ▪ Cutting ▪ Quality and sustainability of movement patterns
Proximal weakness and instability	▪ MMT ▪ Antigravity responses (supine flexion, prone extension)	▪ Ability to open and close accordion tubs or large pop beads ▪ Floor-to-stand transitions ▪ Tolerance for prone, quadruped
Decreased sensation and peripheral neuropathy	▪ Semmes–Weinstein monofilaments ▪ Temperature ▪ Dull versus sharp ▪ Proprioception ▪ Digit opposition with and without vision ▪ PDMS–2	▪ Opening toys and containers ▪ Manipulating small pop beads, pennies for piggy bank ▪ In-hand manipulation ▪ Tolerance for tactile media ▪ Behavioral signs (e.g., pulling at hands or feet, avoiding using hands)
Decreased energy, drive, motivation	▪ COPM (Law et al., 2019) ▪ PedsQL (Varni, 1998) ▪ Visual Fatigue Scale (Lee et al., 1991) ▪ Borg Rating of Perceived Exertion Scale (Borg, 1998) ▪ Play and leisure assessments and inventories in Table 23.5	▪ Clinical observation of endurance while engaged in age-appropriate play and leisure activities ▪ Upright sitting and standing posture and tolerance
Impaired socialization	▪ Faces Anxiety Scale	▪ Board games for turn taking, sharing, interacting ▪ Generating novel play theme ▪ Ideating obstacle course ▪ Quality of symbolic play (e.g., given a doll) ▪ Solitary play preferences ▪ Parallel versus cooperative play ▪ Difficulty with transitions to, between, and from activities and environments

Note. Bayley–III = Bayley Scales of Infant and Toddler Development; BDI–2 = Battelle Developmental Inventory Screening Test; BOT–2 = Bruininks–Oseretsky Test of Motor Proficiency; COPM = Canadian Occupational Performance Measure; DAYC-2 = Developmental Assessment of Young Children; HELP = Hawaii Early Learning Profile; MMT = manual muscle testing; MOCA = Montreal Cognitive Assessment; PDMS–2 = Peabody Developmental Motor Scales; PedsQL = Pediatric Quality of Life Inventory; ROM = range of motion; SPM = Sensory Processing Measure.

Table 23.5   Commonly Used Play and Leisure Assessments

ASSESSMENT	BRIEF DESCRIPTION	REFERENCE
Revised Knox Preschool Play Scale	■ Observational assessment describing play competency among children from birth–6 years of age within 4 dimensions (space management, material management, pretense and symbolic, and participation) ■ Formerly the PPS (Bledsoe & Sherpherd, 1982)	Knox (2008)
ToP	■ Observational assessment including 24 items scored on a 4-point scale to assess individuals' degree of playfulness through intrinsic motivation, internal control, ability to suspend reality, and framing ■ TOES: Supplemental assessment consult with player's motivation for play; to be administered with ToP	Skard & Bundy (2008)
Play History	■ Semistructured interview with caregiver to assess past and present play experiences (sensorimotor, symbolic and simple constructive, dramatic, complex constructive, games, recreational)	Behnke & Fetkovich (1984), Takata (1969)
Pediatric Interest Profiles	■ Three age-appropriate profiles of play and leisure interests for individuals ages 6–21 years that evaluate activities, feelings about activity, perceived skill level, and with whom the individual plays ● Kid Play Profile (ages 6–9) ● Preteen Play Profile (ages 9–12) ● Adolescent Leisure Interest Profile (ages 12–21)	Henry (2000)
Play Scale	■ Assessment outlining pre-symbolic and symbolic play development, focusing on cognitive, social, and language skills ■ Ages 9–60 months (5 years)	Westby (2000)
CAPE	■ Standard prompt cards and response options allow specification of participation in terms of behavioral measurements ■ Looks at the child, action, context, and time	King et al. (2004)
Transdisciplinary Play-Based Assessment	■ Assesses developmental skills, cognition, social–emotional, language, physical, and motor development through naturalistic play	Linder (1993)
COPM	■ Provides framework of retrieving subjective rating of leisure activity difficulties to establish needs and goals ■ Measures satisfaction and performance	Law et al. (2019)
PedsQL	■ Modular instrument to measure HRQoL among children and adolescents ages 2–18 years ■ Includes self-report and parent proxy-report scales consisting of 23 items: Total Health Scale Score, Physical Health Summary Score, and Psychosocial Health Summary Score	Varni (1998)
ACS	■ Designed to use picture cards of adults performing specific activities (leisure, sociocultural, and instrumental activities)	Baum & Edwards (2008)
PACS	■ Interview-style assessment tool composed of pictures to determine child's level of occupational performance and engagement ■ Ages 5–14 years ■ Preschool Activity Card Sort for ages 3–6 years (Berg & LaVesser, 2006)	Berg & LaVesser (2006), Mandich et al. (2004)
Interest Checklist	■ Checklist of 80 items, clustered into 5 categories ■ Used to identify meaningful occupations	Matsutsuyu (1969)
Role Checklist	■ Inventory to identify different roles (e.g., student, hobbies) with temporal and value assessment	Dickerson (1999)
Leisure Satisfaction Scale	■ Measures the degree to which clients feel their general "needs" are being satisfied through leisure (subscales of psychological, educational, social, relaxation, physiological, and aesthetic leisure)	Ragheb & Beard (1991)
OPHI	■ Measures past and current occupational functioning through life history narrative with a rating scale	Kielhofner & Henry (1988)

Note. ACS = Activity Card Sort; CAPE = Children's Assessment for Participation and Enjoyment; COPM = Canadian Occupational Performance Measure; HRQoL = health-related quality of life; PACS = Pediatric Activity Card Sort; PedsQL = Pediatric Quality of Life Inventory; PPS = Preschool Play Scale; ToP = Test of Playfulness; TOES = Test of Environmental Supportiveness.

Commonly Used Assessments for Play and Leisure

Research demonstrates that hospitalized children often exhibit delays in development and social interaction, stress with separation, increased anxiety, decreased endurance and movement, decreased resourcefulness, limited repertoire of activities, and decreased playfulness (Kielhofner et al., 1983; Tanta & Knox, 2015). In addition to assessing the five domains of typical development (i.e., physical, social–emotional, cognitive, communication, adaptive or self-help) and how they relate to play and leisure, it is valuable to use play and leisure based-assessments (see Chapter 4, "Special Considerations for Children With Cancer," for specific implications and assessment of cancer-specific changes).

Because *play* refers to one's state of mind, observations of the client's mood, affect, enjoyment, engagement, and exploration provide a better understanding of playfulness (Henry, 2008; Schaaf, 1990; Tanta & Knox, 2015). Throughout clinical observations of play, it is important to note toy selection, environment exploration, interest in operations, patterns and changes in behaviors, attention, elements of cause-and-effect and imaginative play, referencing, abstraction, preferences for movement or sedentary activities, acceptance of novel or unfamiliar activities, and adaptability to activity and environment (Schaaf, 1990; Westby, 2000).

To assess types and frequency of leisure participation, methods such as time journals or pie charts of one's time are valuable to provide a comprehensive report of temporal aspects of involvement (e.g., what days, what time of day, how much time, how often, what the routine is; Sellar & Stanley, 2010). Because play and leisure are complex occupations, a combination of clinical observations can be used in conjunction with **play-based assessments** and leisure-based assessments, which are outlined in Table 23.5 as a reference.

The Knox Preschool Play Scale (Knox, 2008), Test of Playfulness (Skard & Bundy, 2008), and Play History (Behnke & Fetkovich, 1984; Takata, 1969) are play-based clinical measures created by occupational therapists to identify play-related difficulties and develop play-based interventions as they relate to occupational performance (Henry, 2008; Tanta & Knox, 2015). The Pediatric Quality of Life (Varni, 1998) and Canadian Occupational Performance Measure (Law et al., 2019) are valuable assessment tools for clients with prolonged or frequent hospitalizations to measure satisfaction and performance in meaningful occupations over time with intervention. Table 23.5 references commonly used assessments in play and leisure.

OCCUPATIONAL THERAPY INTERVENTIONS FOR PLAY AND LEISURE

Approaches to Improving Play and Leisure

Occupational therapy practitioners rely on using meaningful, client-driven activities to treat impaired or underdeveloped client factors and performance skills to improve occupations. Meaningful activities in the pediatric, adolescent, and adult populations are often tied to the occupation of play and leisure. Engagement in play and leisure is a fundamental source of pleasure for individuals. "Play is inseparable from the child" (da Silva & Cabral, 2015, p. 341) and should be used by medical professionals and caregivers to maintain QoL and development and also as an intervention to address deficits in the occupation.

Many theoretical ideas of play and how to use it as an intervention tool exist. Play and leisure activities can be used in three capacities:
1. *Intervention* to reduce the adverse psychosocial effects of illness, treatment, and hospitalization;
2. *Modality* to improve developmental skills, client factors, or performance skills; and
3. *Medium* to facilitate play skill behaviors, playfulness, and leisure interests (Chen & Chippendale, 2018; Couch et al., 1998; Li et al., 2016; Parham, 2008; Tanta & Knox, 2015).

As a result of the detrimental, multisystem effects of a cancer diagnosis and treatment, cancer survivors can greatly benefit from all three frameworks of play- and leisure-based interventions to address deficits in this occupation across the cancer continuum.

Occupational therapy practitioners can provide play and leisure as an intervention in any clinical setting, including acute care, inpatient rehabilitation, early intervention, home, school, outpatient clinic, or private practice. Education provided to medical personnel, family and caregivers, teachers, and others involved in a client's care is a critical component of intervention and successful outcomes. Exhibit 23.1 provides examples of play- and leisure-based interventions to address cancer-related symptoms and deficits. All three frameworks of play and leisure as interventions are represented.

Evidence-Based Interventions

Play and leisure as a psychosocial intervention for cancer management

The literature on play with medically involved clients supports it as an intervention to address the adverse psychosocial effects of a diagnosis, hospitalization, and medical treatment. Both play and leisure are occupations that can be used as effective interventions to help cancer survivors normalize a hospital admission, learn about medical procedures and treatments, and reduce anxiety and stress related to pain and the overall hospitalization experience (Koukourikos et al., 2015; Li et al., 2016; Scarponi & Pession, 2016; Ullán et al., 2014). The psychosocial effect of these events can have a profound impact on cancer survivors' energy, drive, and motivation as they lose a sense of control and independence.

It is important to always make survivors active participants in their care, providing education in an effort to help them retain some control (Darcy et al., 2014). Empowering survivors with knowledge and choice gives them back autonomy in a setting that typically dictates most of their experiences. In an acute care hospital setting, occupational therapy practitioners can work closely with child life therapists, who often are the first clinicians to help address

EXHIBIT 23.1. Play and Leisure Interventions for Cancer-Related Symptoms and Deficits

OCCUPATIONAL THERAPY INTERVENTIONS	CANCER-RELATED SYMPTOMS AND DEFICITS ADDRESSED
Psychosocial Interventions for Cancer Management	
Relaxation strategies • Mindfulness and guided meditation • Yoga	• Pain • Anxiety • Nausea and vomiting • Decreased energy, drive, motivation
Energy conservation • Pacing, prioritizing, organization, body mechanic education • Play and leisure schedule with rest breaks and down time • Appropriately sized furniture	• Fatigue • Decreased energy, drive, motivation
Role-playing • Familiar dolls, action figures, puppets to act out unfavorable activities or transitions	• Pain • Anxiety
Play and Leisure Skill Development	
Manipulative and constructive play • Legos, play dough, peg boards, beads, arts and crafts	• Limited ROM and fine motor coordination • Decreased sensation or peripheral neuropathy
Manual therapy • PROM, myofascial release, stretching, Simon Says	• Limited ROM • Pain • Decreased sensation or peripheral neuropathy
Cognition-based activity • Cause–effect toys, matching memory games, direction-based board or card games, constructive play	• Neurocognitive toxicity
Therapeutic exercise and strengthening activities • Multi-surface play (floor, bench, table), play in varied body positions, sport skills (kicking, throwing), yoga, rough-and-tumble play	• Proximal weakness and instability • Decreased strength and muscle endurance • Impaired cardiopulmonary function
Sensory-rich play • Sand, water, toys, slides, swings, finger paint, rice bin hide and seek, stereognosis games Sensory integration • Obstacle courses, sensory diet • Toy, activity and environment adaptation to provide optimal sensory input	• Sensory impairments and processing changes • Decreased sensation or peripheral neuropathy
Play Skill Behavior and Leisure Interest Development	
Environment setup • Provide access to age-appropriate toys, games and activities, dress-up props, easily opened and visually engaging containers • Protective flooring • Appropriately sized furniture	• Decreased energy, drive, motivation • Neurocognitive toxicity • Sensory impairments and processing changes • Decreased strength and muscle endurance
Interest exploration and inventory • Exposure to novel toys and activities with opportunity for learning	• Decreased energy, drive, motivation
Facilitation of pretend, imaginary, and dramatic play • Fantasy play themes • Role-playing • Obstructive play Model themes and behaviors for parents and caregiver • Tea party, rescue missions, superhero stories, puppets, dress-up	• Impaired socialization • Neurocognitive toxicity

Note. PROM = passive range of motion; ROM = range of motion.

the psychosocial fallout of medical treatment and hospital admission.

Li et al. (2016) described four types of hospital-based play interventions used with pediatric survivors:

1. ***Preparation play:*** Use of dolls, medical equipment, and instruments to teach and prepare clients for medical procedures to increase understanding and sense of control

2. ***Medical play:*** Play with real or toy medical equipment to familiarize clients to hospital routines and procedures and allow for expression of feelings and concerns

3. **_Distraction play:_** Use of games, toys, music, bubbles, and so on, in an effort to distract clients' attention away from medical procedures and reduce anxiety
4. **_Developmental play:_** Age-appropriate play activities to promote psychosocial development and prevent regression during hospitalization

These types of play aim to give pediatric survivors a sense of control, provide a medium to express feelings surrounding their disease and hospitalization, decrease anxiety provoked by medical procedures, and facilitate psychosocial development gained from play activities. Scarponi and Pession (2016) also documented group **_play therapy_**, including role playing, imaginary medical games, play with medical supplies, and drawing, as an effective nonpharmacological approach to treating cancer-related pain among pediatric cancer survivors.

Play can also be used to reduce anxiety among older hospitalized children, ages 7–11 years, as documented by reduced cortisol levels (Potasz et al., 2013). Play therapy used for pain management allows pediatric survivors to reduce their anxiety surrounding medical procedures while also providing opportunities to exercise important play skills. Play can be used to allow children to explore and express feelings, to role-play unfamiliar experiences to prepare for an unpleasant medical procedure and reduce anxiety, or as a primary occupation that establishes behavior patterns needed for future roles (Schaaf & Burke, 1997). Role-playing can promote storytelling and exploration of feelings, provide a connection between imagination and reality, and offer a sense of control and hope for a patient coping with a cancer diagnosis (Scarponi & Pession, 2016).

Occupational therapy practitioners working with cancer survivors can use play and leisure interventions to prepare their clients for uncomfortable therapy interventions and distract them from treatments that may cause pain (e.g., initial postoperative mobility, passive ROM to tightened joints, neuropathic sensation with tactile play). Mohammadi et al. (2017) examined play-based occupational therapy as an intervention for two pediatric cancer survivors with leukemia while they received chemotherapy. Play-based therapy used play both as a means (i.e., a modality for skill development) and as an end to increase playful activity engagement to assist with coping. Using pain, fatigue, and anxiety scales as pre- and posttest measures for each occupational therapy session, researchers showed play-based therapy to be effective in improving each of these cancer-related symptoms and chemotherapy side effects. Play used in this capacity can include both unstructured and structured play with reality or fantasy components (e.g., building blocks, puppets, board games).

A systematic review reported the benefits of yoga as an exercise activity to decrease the symptom-related psychosocial distress experienced by cancer survivors (Harder et al., 2012). Chen and Chippendale (2018) also supported using leisure activities as an end to promote a sense of control, increase self-esteem, enhance coping skills, and improve QoL.

Using play and leisure interventions to first address the adverse psychosocial effects of cancer care allows occupational therapy practitioners to establish a trusting relationship with survivors before working on skill development and play and leisure behaviors. Practitioners can rely on therapeutic use of self to provide cancer survivors with the means to develop supportive relationships and coping skills to reconnect to social, play, and leisure opportunities (Hwang et al., 2015). Play and leisure interventions can also address the psychosocial effect of a cancer diagnosis across the full continuum of care. Clients on palliative treatment facing end of life can still greatly benefit from play and leisure interventions if they find a sense of purpose in these meaningful activities. Energy conservation concepts, such as pacing and prioritization, along with activity modification suggestions, can allow survivors undergoing palliative care the opportunity to maximize participation in the activities that still bring them a sense of normalcy and pleasure.

Play and leisure as a modality to develop client factors and performance skills

Occupational therapy practitioners have historically been shown to rely on using play and leisure interventions primarily as a means to address client factors and performance skill development (e.g., sensory, cognitive, motor) rather than play behavior skills or playfulness (Couch et al., 1998; Kuhaneck et al., 2013). Play and leisure interventions used as a modality for skill development typically involve more structured play and therapist-directed activities as the practitioner aims to facilitate development of a specific skill set (e.g., fine motor, visual perception, memory). Because cancer survivors present with multisystem deficits, practitioners can use play and leisure activities effectively to treat these foundational skills needed for improved function and occupational performance. After assessing a survivor and identifying the underlying client factors and performance skills affected by cancer, practitioners can use activity analysis to select toys, games, equipment, and hobbies to develop the specific skill sets that have been affected by cancer.

As a result of prolonged hospitalization with inactivity and bed rest, children and adolescents demonstrate decreased physical development and deconditioning, which places them at further risk for decreased strength, endurance, and coordination in both gross and fine motor activities (Götte et al., 2014). Incorporating exercise as a rehabilitation intervention to address the physical manifestations of cancer is supported in the literature (Silver & Gilchrist, 2011). Promoting a healthy lifestyle and engagement in physical exercises and preferred leisure activities is essential, particularly among the adolescent and adult populations. Götte et al. (2014) promoted regular participation in exercise while cancer survivors are undergoing intensive treatment to combat the effects of hospitalization. Engagement in physical and movement-based play and leisure activities in therapy can improve cancer treatment–related deficits in muscle strength, transfer skills, cardiovascular functioning, endurance, and overall conditioning (Vercher et al., 2016).

Occupational therapy practitioners can address underlying musculoskeletal changes by using the environment and specific toys, games, and activities to maximize movement, strength, stamina, and fine and gross motor coordination in the context of play and leisure. Götte et al. (2014) further supported educating cancer survivors on alternative activity options and sport recommendations that they can successfully engage in. Sports-based activities that incorporate a survivor's interests and abilities are best determined by a qualified health care practitioner (Götte et al., 2014).

Equipment adaptations or bracing considerations may arise for those who want to return to sports safely. For example, occupational therapy practitioners can apply principles of splinting to fabricate a custom chest plate to protect a subcutaneous central line for a client still in active cancer treatment. With medical clearance, a survivor can successfully re-engage in more contact-based sports with this protective plate. As for other client populations, occupational therapy practitioners are equipped to select and modify appropriate play and leisure intervention and treatment activities that are meaningful to the cancer survivor that will address physical, mental, and sensory skill deficits.

Play to facilitate play behavior skills, playfulness, and leisure interest development

Understanding the progression of play skill behaviors and types of play is important for occupational therapy practitioners to successfully cultivate an environment for play and leisure exploration and development. Engaging in play allows survivors to strengthen the skills they need to be successful in play. For cancer survivors limited by the constraints of infection control precautions, environmental adaptations and activity modifications are essential to creating optimal opportunities for play. Having a foldable floor mat and child-sized furniture available in a hospital room can transform the sterile environment into a private playroom.

Recommendations for specific toy or activity options to support different types of play are also important to facilitate appropriate play behaviors and leisure exploration. In addition, the organization and number of toys and activities available affect the quality of play. Having fewer toys promotes longer focus, sustained engagement, quality exploration, and creativity (Dauch et al., 2018). Alternatively, having diverse play materials or a variety of toys may also be beneficial because children with prolonged hospitalizations may be exposed to the same toys for a longer period. Finding a balance between the number and novelty of toys and activities is important.

Occupational therapy practitioner–led play groups provide opportunities for sharing, turn taking, and negotiation, which help foster imagination, flexible thinking, and social skill development (Fabrizi et al., 2016). Cancer survivors have limited social opportunities and access to same-age peers as a result of their compromised immune system and frequent hospitalizations (see Chapter 26, "Social Participation," for more information). Therefore, it is the job of occupational therapy practitioners to act as a survivor's playmate or peer to simulate a developmentally and socially appropriate play and leisure experience.

Initiating fantasy play themes, asking open-ended questions, and creating obstacles or obstructions during play are all strategies to invite the survivor to be an active participant in a cooperative play scenario. Occupational therapy

practitioners can help initiate exploration by giving leisure activity checklists or interest inventories to older survivors who resort to watching television and playing video games as primary leisure activities. Engaging survivors in competitive board games or sport-based activities and facilitating losing experiences is also important in helping to foster healthy coping skills to deal with situations that don't go their way.

Family and Caregiver Education

Educating family members and care providers of cancer survivors is a critical component of successful play and leisure skill development. Play skill behaviors and playfulness are learned, mirrored, and reinforced by family and caregivers (Kolehmainen et al., 2015; Rubin et al., 2014). Parents and caregivers can be educated on how to effectively facilitate active play and leisure participation beyond the therapy session for survivors who experience difficulties in this occupation (Rubin et al., 2014). Occupational therapy practitioners can also act as models to teach caregivers how to interact with the survivor with cancer to maximize play and leisure skill development. Fostering the child–caregiver relationship through play can combat the effects of social and environmental deprivation and result in adaptive play skills and behaviors (Daunhauer & Cermak, 2008).

The following are examples of how occupational therapy practitioners can educate caregivers on how to use play and leisure as an intervention to address psychosocial limitations, client factor and performance skill deficits, and impaired play behaviors and leisure interests:

- Educate caregivers on specific diagnosis- and treatment-related precautions to ensure safe play and leisure practices.
- Encourage role-playing with favored dolls or action figures to act out unfavorable medical or therapy treatments to prepare the client.
- Model safe handling techniques and positioning techniques during play and leisure engagement.
- Provide resources for selecting developmentally and age-appropriate toys and activities to create a just-right challenge.
- Model playful responses to a survivor's play behaviors and instruct family and caregivers to mirror similar responses.
- Emphasize that playfulness can be incorporated and carried out during any occupation throughout the day (Fabrizi et al., 2016).
- Create a play schedule and designate times of day dedicated to play and leisure engagement between caregivers and client.
- Reinforce the importance of providing choices during play to foster feelings of autonomy and empowerment.
- Balance structured and unstructured play and supervised and unsupervised play.
- Encourage caregivers to provide clients with intrinsic rewards (e.g., positive praise) for engaging in play and leisure successfully.
- Facilitate interactions between clients and their siblings, cousins, and peers for sharing, turn taking, and winning and losing opportunities.

CASE EXAMPLE 23.1. SARAH: PLAY AND LEISURE

Sarah is an 8-year-old female who was initially diagnosed at age 5 with pre-B cell acute lymphoblastic leukemia that was treated with chemotherapy. Seven months following completion of treatment, she was discovered to have relapsed disease in her bone marrow and cerebrospinal fluid. Over the next 4 months, Sarah started a new chemotherapy regimen, including intrathecal chemotherapy for central nervous system disease, without evidence of remission, resulting in recommendation for stem cell transplant (SCT). She is now admitted to the hospital for SCT in a private room following strict protective isolation precautions. Occupational therapy services are referred to address functional performance concerns and prevent deconditioning as a result of her extended hospital admission.

The occupational therapist conducts Sarah's initial evaluation in her hospital room with her mother present, consisting of clinical observations, child and parent report, and client-centered assessment tools to obtain baseline data and create an occupational profile. Sarah is in the third grade and lives at home with her mother, father, and two siblings. She has had inconsistent school participation because of frequent hospitalizations and keeps in touch with one close friend. Prior to admission, she actively played with her siblings and cousins at home, but her mother notes she has difficulty making friends and getting along with similar-age peers. Sarah has a dog, which she helps care for at home, and reports that she likes arts and crafts, dancing, and watching TV.

Upon occupational therapy evaluation, Sarah presents with age-appropriate cognition and visual–perceptual motor skills and is within functional limits for all range of motion. However, she demonstrates decreased overall strength, endurance, and motivation, which affects her ability to actively participate in age-appropriate play, ADLs, and school-based tasks. Her mother notes limited participation in self-care routines and decreased sleep hygiene since admission. Sarah is cautious to move and reports discomfort at her Mediport site, which is an implantable subcutaneous catheter for venous access located at the chest wall. The occupational therapist uses the Wong Baker FACES Pain Scale and FACES Anxiety Scale (Wong-Baker FACES Foundation, 2015), in which she noted 3/10 pain at port site and "minimal worry/distress," respectively. She complains of fatigue during the evaluation but performs all functional transfers with close supervision and increased time.

Sarah requires encouragement for continued participation during the evaluation, although the occupational therapist establishes trust and works to build rapport with both Sarah and her mother. At the end of the evaluation, she fills out the Pediatric Quality of Life (Varni, 1998) Self-Report to assess perceived physical and psychosocial health challenges, scoring 35% for overall health-related quality of life. Sarah also completes a modified pediatric interest checklist to identify motivating play activities, which include dance, ball play, painting, and beading. Privately, her mother highlights concern for significant changes in overall mood, motivation, and playfulness since her admission. Through clinical observations, parent report and self-report measures, the following play and work behaviors are identified to address during occupational therapy treatment:

- Gravitates towards solitary play routines and repetitive play themes
- Enjoys arts and crafts and dance, although limited engagement
- Requires encouragement to play in once preferred activities rather than watch TV
- Demonstrates behavioral overreactions to losing or "not getting her way"
- Makes frequent requests for help or assistance.

The occupational therapist recommends Sarah receive occupational therapy twice per week throughout her inpatient stay to improve play and leisure participation and performance in addition to improving strength, endurance, coordination, ADLs, and school-related tasks. Table 23.6 outlines the problem list, interventions, and caregiver education to address Sarah's play behaviors,

TABLE 23.6. Sample Play and Leisure Interventions and Caregiver Education for Sarah

FACTORS AFFECTING PLAY/LEISURE PRIOR TO AND DURING ADMISSION	OCCUPATIONAL THERAPY INTERVENTIONS	CAREGIVER EDUCATION	OUTCOMES
Decreased drive/ motivation	- Stickers provided to document completed therapy sessions - Client interests catalogued and incorporated during play - Novel games introduced to interest in play - Use of arts and crafts activities as reward for participation in cooperative play	- Limit frequent material rewards and immediate gratification - Provide positive verbal praise for participation in play - Acknowledge all attempts to try new things	- Self-initiation of play outside of therapy times - Increased exploration of new play and game options - Decreased TV watching and more time out of bed

(Continued)

CASE EXAMPLE 23.1. SARAH: PLAY AND LEISURE *(Cont.)*

TABLE 23.6.　Sample Play and Leisure Interventions and Caregiver Education for Sarah *(Cont.)*

FACTORS AFFECTING PLAY/LEISURE PRIOR TO AND DURING ADMISSION	OCCUPATIONAL THERAPY INTERVENTIONS	CAREGIVER EDUCATION	OUTCOMES
Decreased energy and activity tolerance	■ Timers set for rest breaks during play activities ■ Endurance-building activities performed and graded as needed (e.g., balloon volleyball, soccer) ■ Play in prone, quadruped, or kneeling as tolerated on floor mat ■ Engagement in virtual dance-based video game	■ Establish daily routine to perform ADLs, play, and school-based activities out of bed ■ Incorporate energy conservation strategies into routines ■ Carryover use of timers during play outside of therapy sessions ■ Engage in movement-based play activities with client	■ Increased activity tolerance with fewer/shorter rest breaks needed ■ Improved self-report of Physical Health Summary on Peds QL (Varni, 1998); 11% increase on total Peds QL score ■ Decreased complaints of fatigue during therapy
Prolonged hospitalization	■ Recommendation for environmental setup to encourage out of bed activities (e.g., child-sized chair/desk, floor mat, recliner chair) ■ Post daily schedule incorporating time for ADLs, play/leisure, school-based activities, meals and rest/TV time	■ Use of floor mat to increase play area and movement opportunities ■ Rotate toys/games to maintain novelty but encourage mastery ■ Establish bedtime routine to promote sleep hygiene to maximize arousal during daytime hours	■ Consistent engagement in daily morning ADL care in bathroom ■ Participates in play activity 1x–2x daily in various room locations (floor mat, desk, etc.)
Isolation from peers and siblings	■ Role play to model same-age peer behavior during play ■ Facilitate turn taking during game play ■ Create obstacles during play requiring problem solving ■ Provide competitive outcomes including losing with scripting to aide coping	■ Role play as same-age peer or playmate to simulate appropriate play interactions ■ Provide obstructive play opportunities for client to problem solve and resolve conflict ■ Encourage communication with siblings, cousins, and friends through phone, tablet, or hospital visits, as permitted	■ Gravitation toward cooperative play activities ■ Improved coping with losing a game ■ Increased ease with turn taking and sharing ■ Reports of improved cooperation with sibling during visits
Anxiety from pain and frequent medical procedures	■ Monitor with the Wong Baker FACES Pain Scale and FACES Anxiety Scale (Wong-Baker FACES Foundation, 2015) during sessions ■ Mindfulness teaching and visualizations to prepare for engagement in specific play tasks ■ Use medical syringes during painting activities ■ Child life involvement for medical play in preparation for procedures	■ Provide calming music and reduce stimulation in room in preparation for medical procedures ■ Alert Sarah of planned activities or procedures in advance to answer questions in preparation ■ Lead Sarah through guided imagery during anxiety-provoking procedures	■ Improved self-report of Psychosocial Health Summary on Peds QL; 11% increase on total Peds QL score ■ Improved positive affect throughout occupational therapy sessions ■ Self-initiation of breathing and relaxation strategies to negotiate unfavorable procedures
Learned helplessness	■ Sticker charts provided to document success with ADL and play activities ■ Consistent prompting and education to "try first, ask second" ■ Provide "just right challenge" to facilitate success during therapy activities	■ Provide delayed assistance when asked for help to encourage Sarah to attempt task first ■ Provide positive verbal praise for attempts made to problem solve with independence ■ Scaffold ADL and play and leisure activities to promote success	■ Increased independence with ADLs ■ Increased attempts to "try first" versus asking for assistance ■ Positive affect demonstrated with success

Note. ADLs = activities of daily living; Peds QL = Pediatric Quality of Life Inventory.

CASE EXAMPLE 23.1. SARAH: PLAY AND LEISURE *(Cont.)*

along with her outcomes throughout a 2-month inpatient admission.

Sarah's mood and participation in therapy fluctuate throughout her hospital admission, and at times she is even resistant to occupational therapy intervention, reporting frustration with her prolonged hospitalization and need for isolation. Gradually, she is more receptive during therapy sessions, increases time spent out of bed, demonstrates fewer maladaptive behaviors, and engages in once preferred play activities such as dancing outside of therapy sessions. Her mother demonstrates carryover of environmental recommendations, role playing as a playmate, providing positive praise as a reward, and

balancing the quantity and type of toys/games presented. After 8 weeks, Sarah is cleared for discharge home and receives the following recommendations:

- Comprehensive home program to continue addressing Sarah's play behaviors, endurance and motivation through established routines (play, ADLs, sleep), environmental adaptations, and play opportunities with siblings and cousins to improve physical and psychosocial health.
- Outpatient occupational therapy evaluation to address strength, endurance, and gross and fine motor coordination for greater independence in ADLs and play and leisure tasks.

- Recommend environmental adaptations to make play and leisure opportunities more accessible.

Occupational therapy practitioners who incorporate play behaviors and a sense of playfulness into a treatment session can simultaneously address psychosocial limitations and impaired client factors or performance skills. Using the full potential of play and leisure activities as occupational therapy interventions can effectively improve the occupation of play and leisure. Modeling play and leisure behaviors for caregivers and providing toy, activity, and environment recommendations will allow cancer survivors to successfully engage in play and leisure throughout the course of their treatment and beyond into survivorship.

SUMMARY

Play and leisure are meaningful, fundamental occupations that promote QoL for people of all ages. The unique multisystem effects of cancer have a compounded effect on client factors, performance skills and patterns, and the capacity for interacting with environments. This disrupts the development and exploration of play and leisure skills and interests, psychosocial functioning, and occupational participation. Engaging in play and leisure allows clients to strengthen physical, cognitive, and social–emotional skills they need to be successful in various occupations, while decreasing global psychosocial stressors of the cancer experience. Therefore, play and leisure are used as both a means and an end to treat cancer-specific deficits through skill and interest development, play behaviors, and activity participation.

The assessment of play and leisure in the oncology population requires the ability to identify cancer-related dysfunction through a detailed occupational profile, use of evaluation tools, and clinical observations during functional performance. Occupational therapy practitioners use a holistic client-centered approach to promote, restore, and modify play and leisure skill development and behaviors in effort to reduce the social–emotional effects of anxiety, stress, and loss of autonomy. Through use of play- and leisure-based interventions and thorough survivor and caregiver education and training, survivors can experience

success in meaningful occupations, improve QoL, and build the carryover skills they need throughout the cancer care continuum.

REFERENCES

American Occupational Therapy Association. (2008). AOTA's societal statement on play. *American Journal of Occupational Therapy, 62,* 707–708. https://doi.org/10.5014/ajot.62.6.707

American Occupational Therapy Association. (2014). Occupational therapy practice framework: Domain and process (3rd ed.). *American Journal of Occupational Therapy, 68*(Suppl. 1), S1–S48. https://doi.org/10.5014/ajot.2014.682006

American Occupational Therapy Association. (2015). *Factsheet: Role of occupational therapy with children and youth.* Retrieved from https://www.aota.org/~/media/Corporate/Files/AboutOT/Professionals/WhatIsOT/CY/Fact-Sheets/Children%20and%20Youth%20fact%20sheet.pdf

Arbesman, M., Bazyk, S., & Nochajski, S. M. (2013). Systematic review of occupational therapy and mental health promotion, prevention, and intervention for children and youth. *American Journal of Occupational Therapy, 67,* e120–e130. https://doi.org/10.5014/ajot.2013.008359

Baum, C. M., & Edwards, D. F. (2008). *The Activity Card Sort* (2nd ed.). Bethesda, MD: AOTA Press.

Baxter, M. F., Newman, R., Longpré, S. M., & Polo, K. M. (2017). Occupational therapy's role in cancer survivorship as a chronic condition. *American Journal of Occupational Therapy, 71,* 7103090010. https://doi.org/10.5014/ajot.2017.713001

Bayley, N. (2005). *Bayley Scales of Infant Development* (3rd ed.). San Antonio: Harcourt Assessment.

Behnke, C. J., & Fetkovich, M. M. (1984). Examining the reliability and validity of the Play History. *American Journal of Occupational Therapy, 38,* 94–100. https://doi.org/10.5014/ajot.38.2.94

Berg, C., & LaVesser, P. (2006). The Preschool Activity Card Sort. *OTJR: Occupation, Participation and Health, 26,* 143–151. https://doi.org/10.1177/153944920602600404

Bledsoe, N. P., & Sherpherd, J. T. (1982). A study of the reliability and validity of a preschool play scale. *American Journal of Occupational Therapy, 36,* 783–788. https://doi.org/10.5014/ajot.36.12.783

Bohg, R., Fernie, D. E., & Klein, E. L. (1986). Unstructured play in hospital settings: An internal locus of control rationale.

Children's Health Care, 15, 101–107. https://doi.org/10.1207/s15326888chc1502_8

Borg, G. (1998). *Borg's Perceived Exertion and Pain Scales.* Champaign, IL: Human Kinetics.

Brand, S., Wolfe, J., & Samsel, C. (2017). The impact of cancer and its treatment on the growth and development of the pediatric patient. *Current Pediatric Reviews, 13*(1), 24–33. https://doi.org/10.2174/1573396313666161116094916

Brown, S., & Vaughan, C. (2010). *Play: How it shapes the brain, opens the imagination and invigorates the soul.* New York: Avery.

Bruininks, R. H., & Bruininks, B. D. (2005). *BOT2: Bruininks–Oseretsky Test of Motor Proficiency—second edition: Manual.* San Antonio: Pearson Assessment.

Case-Smith, J. (2015). Development of childhood occupations. In J. Case-Smith & J. C. O'Brien (Eds.), *Occupational therapy for children and adolescents* (7th ed., pp. 64–101). St. Louis: Elsevier Mosby.

Chauhan, A., Weiss, J., & Warrier, R. (2010). Effective management of pain in pediatric hematology and oncology. *Asian Pacific Journal of Cancer Prevention, 11,* 577–579.

Chen, S. W., & Chippendale, T. (2018). Leisure as an end, not just a means, in occupational therapy intervention. *American Journal of Occupational Therapy, 72,* 7204347010. https://doi.org/10.5014/ajot.2018.028316

Couch, K. J., Deitz, J. C., & Kanny, E. M. (1998). The role of play in pediatric occupational therapy. *American Journal of Occupational Therapy, 52,* 111–117. https://doi.org/10.5014/ajot.52.2.111

Darcy, L., Björk, M., Enskär, K., & Knutsson, S. (2014). The process of striving for an ordinary, everyday life, in young children living with cancer, at six months and one year post diagnosis. *European Journal of Oncology Nursing, 18,* 605–612. https://doi.org/10.1016/j.ejon.2014.06.006

Darcy, L., Enskär, K., Granlund, M., Simeonsson, R. J., Peterson, C., & Björk, M. (2015). Health and functioning in the everyday lives of young children with cancer: Documenting with the International Classification of Functioning, Disability and Health—Children and Youth (ICF–CY). *Child: Care, Health and Development, 41,* 475–482. https://doi.org/10.1111/cch.12191

da Silva, L. F., & Cabral, I. E. (2015). *O resgate do prazer de brincar da criança com câncer no espaço hospitalar* [Rescuing the pleasure of playing for the child with cancer in a hospital setting]. *Revista Brasileira Enfermagem, 68,* 337–342. https://doi.org/10.1590/0034-7167.2015680303i

Dauch, C., Imwalle, M., Ocasio, B., & Metz, A. E. (2018). The influence of the number of toys in the environment on toddlers' play. *Infant Behavior and Development, 50,* 78–87. https://doi.org/10.1016/j.infbeh.2017.11.005

Daunhauer, L. A., & Cermak, S. (2008). Play occupations and the experience of deprivation. In L. D. Parham & L. S. Fazio (Eds.), *Play in occupational therapy for children* (2nd ed., pp. 251–261). St. Louis: Mosby.

Dickerson, A. (1999). *The Role Checklist.* Thorofare, NJ: SLACK.

Dudgeon, B. J., Crooks, J., & Chapelle, E. (2015). Hospital and pediatric rehabilitation services. In J. Case-Smith & J. C. O'Brien (Eds.), *Occupational therapy for children and adolescents* (7th ed., pp. 704–726). St. Louis: Elsevier Mosby.

Dunn, W. (1999). *Sensory Profile.* San Antonio, TX: Psychological Corporation.

Fabrizi, S. E., Ito, M. A., & Winston, K. (2016). Effect of occupational therapy–led playgroups in early intervention on child playfulness and caregiver responsiveness: A repeated-measures design. *American Journal of Occupational Therapy, 70,* 700220020. https://doi.org/10.5014/ajot.2016.017012

Fink, N., Stagnitti, K., & Galvin, J. (2012). Pretend play of children with acquired brain injury: An exploratory study. *Developmental Neurorehabilitation, 15,* 336–342. https://doi.org/10.3109/17518423.2012.655798

Folio, R., & Fewell, R. (2000). *Peabody Developmental Motor Scales* (2nd ed.). San Antonio, TX: Pearson Assessments.

Furuno, S., O'Reilly, K. A., Hosaka, C. M., Inatsuka, T. T., & Zeisolt-Falbey, B. (1994). *Hawaii Early Learning Profile.* Palo Alto, CA: Vort.

Götte, M., Kesting, S., Winter, C., Rosenbaum, D., & Boos, J. (2014). Comparison of self-reported physical activity in children and adolescents before and during cancer treatment. *Pediatric Blood & Cancer, 61,* 1023–1028. https://doi.org/10.1002/pbc.24898

Gray, P. (2013). *Free to learn: Why unleashing the instinct to play will make our children happier, more self-reliant, and better students for life.* New York: Basic Books.

Haiat, H., Bar-Mor, G., & Shochat, M. (2003). The world of the child: A world of play even in the hospital. *Journal of Pediatric Nursing, 18,* 209–214. https://doi.org/10.1053/jpdn.2003.28

Harder, H., Parlour, L., & Jenkins, V. (2012). Randomised controlled trials of yoga interventions for women with breast cancer: A systematic literature review. *Supportive Care in Cancer, 20,* 3055–3064. https://doi.org/10.1007/s00520-012-1611-8

Henry, A. (2000). *Pediatric Interest Profile: Surveys of Play for Children and Adolescents, Kid Play Profile, Preteen Play Profile, Adolescent Leisure Interest Profile.* San Antonio, TX: Therapy Skill Builders.

Henry, A. (2008). Assessment of Play and Leisure in Children and Adolescents. In L. D. Parham & L. S. Fazio (Eds.), *Play in occupational therapy for children* (2nd ed., pp. 95–191). St. Louis: Mosby.

Hughes, F. (2010). *Children, play, and development* (4th ed.). Los Angeles: Sage.

Hutchinson, S., Loy, D., & Kleiber, D. (2003). Leisure as a coping resource: Variations in coping with traumatic illness and injury. *Leisure Sciences, 25,* 143–161. https://doi.org/10.1080/01490400306566

Hwang, E. J., Lokietz, N. C., Lozano, R. L., & Parke, M. A. (2015). Functional deficits and quality of life among cancer survivors: Implications for occupational therapy in cancer survivorship care. *American Journal of Occupational Therapy, 69,* 6906290010. https://doi.org/10.5014/ajot.2015.015974

Keats, M. R., Courneya, K. S., Danielsen, S., & Whitsett, S. F. (1999). Leisure-time physical activity and psychosocial well-being in adolescents after cancer diagnosis. *Journal of Pediatric Oncology Nursing, 16,* 180–188. https://doi.org/10.1177/104345429901600402

Kielhofner, G., Barris, R., Bauer, D., Shoestock, B., & Walker, L. (1983). A comparison of play behavior in nonhospitalized and hospitalized children. *American Journal of Occupational Therapy, 37,* 305–312. https://doi.org/10.5014/ajot.37.5.305

Kielhofner, G., & Henry, A. D. (1988). Development and investigation of the Occupational Performance History Interview. *American Journal of Occupational Therapy, 42,* 489–498. https://doi.org/10.5014/ajot.42.8.489

King, G., Law, M., King, S., Hurley, P., Hanna, S., Kertoy, M., & Young, N. (2004). *Children's Assessment of Participation and Enjoyment (CAPE) and Preferences for Activities of Children (PAC)*. San Antonio, TX: Harcourt Assessment.

Kleiber, D., Hutchinson, S., & Williams, R. (2002). Leisure as a resource in transcending negative life events: Self-protection, self-restoration, and personal transformation. *Leisure Sciences, 24,* 219–235. https://doi.org/10.1080/01490400252900167

Knox, S. (2008). Development and current use of the Revised Knox Preschool Play Scale. In L. D. Parham & L. Fazio (Eds.), *Play in occupational therapy for children* (2nd ed., pp. 55–70). St. Louis: Mosby.

Knox, S., & Mailloux, Z. (1997). Play as treatment and treatment through play. In B. E. Chandler (Ed.), *The essence of play: A child's occupation* (pp. 175–204). Bethesda, MD: American Occupational Therapy Association.

Kolehmainen, N., Ramsay, C., McKee, L., Missiuna, C., Owen, C., & Francis, J. (2015). Participation in physical play and leisure in children with motor impairments: Mixed-methods study to generate evidence for developing an intervention. *Physical Therapy, 95,* 1374–1386. https://doi.org/10.2522/ptj.20140404

Koukourikos, K., Tzeha, L., Pantelidou, P., & Tsaloglidou, A. (2015). The importance of play during hospitalization of children. *Materia Socio-Medica, 27,* 438–441. https://doi.org/10.5455/msm.2015.27.438-441

Kuhaneck, H. M. T., Coombs, K. J., & Pannone, A. K. (2013). A survey of pediatric occupational therapists' use of play. *Journal of Occupational Therapy, Schools, and Early Intervention, 6,* 213–227. https://doi.org/10.1080/19411243.2013.850940

Law, M. C., Baptiste, S., Carswell, A., McColl, M. A., Polatajko, H. J., & Pollock, N. (2019). *Canadian Occupational Performance Measure* (5th ed., rev.). Altona, Man., Canada: COPM, Inc.

Lee, K., Hicks, G., & Nino-Murcia, G. (1991). Validity and reliability of a scale to assess fatigue. *Psychiatry Research, 36,* 291–298. https://doi.org/10.1016/0165-1781(91)90027-M.

Li, W. H. C., Chung, J. O. K., Ho, K. Y., & Kwok, B. M. C. (2016). Play interventions to reduce anxiety and negative emotions in hospitalized children. *BMC Pediatrics, 16,* 36. https://doi.org/10.1186/s12887-016-0570-5

Linder, T. W. (1993). *Transdisciplinary Play-Based Assessment: A functional approach to working with young children* (rev. ed.). Baltimore: Brookes.

Lynch, H., & Moore, A. (2016). Play as an occupation in occupational therapy. *British Journal of Occupational Therapy, 79,* 519–520. https://doi.org/10.1177/0308022616664540

Manav, G., & Ocakci, A. F. (2016). Play model for "evaluation of self-concept of children with cancer." *Iranian Journal of Nursing and Midwifery Research, 21,* 124–130. https://doi.org/10.4103/1735-9066.178227

Mandich, A. D., Polatajko, H. J., Miller, L. T., & Baum, C. (2004). *Paediatric Activity Card Sort (PACS)*. Ottawa, ON: CAOT Publications.

Marusak, H. A., Iadipaolo, A. S., Harper, F. W., Elrahal, F., Taub, J. W., Goldberg, E., & Rabinak, C. A. (2017). Neurodevelopmental consequences of pediatric cancer and its treatment: Applying an early adversity framework to understanding cognitive, behavioral, and emotional outcomes. *Neuropsychology Review, 28,* 123–175. https://doi.org/10.1007/s11065-017-9365-1

Matsutsuyu, J. S. (1969). The Interest Check List. *American Journal of Occupational Therapy, 23,* 323–328.

McCullough, L. E., McClain, K. M., & Gammon, M. D. (2016). The promise of leisure-time physical activity to reduce risk of cancer development. *JAMA Internal Medicine, 176,* 826–827. https://doi.org/10.1001/jamainternmed.2016.1521

Miller-Kuhaneck, H., Henry, D. A., & Glennon, T. J. (2007). *Sensory Processing Measure (SPM)*. Los Angeles: Western Psychological Services.

Mohammadi, A., Mehraban, A. H., & Damavandi, S. A. (2017). Effect of play-based occupational therapy on symptoms of hospitalized children with cancer: A single-subject study. *Asia-Pacific Journal of Oncology Nursing, 4,* 168–172. https://doi.org/10.4103/apjon.apjon_13_17

Nasreddine, Z. S., Phillips, N. A., Bédirian, V., Charbonneau, S., Whitehead, V., Collin, I., . . . Chertkow, H. (2005). The Montreal Cognitive Assessment, MoCA: A brief screening tool for mild cognitive impairment. *Journal of the American Geriatrics Society, 53,* 695–699. https://doi.org/10.1111/j.1532-5415.2005.53221.x

Ness, K. K., Hudson, M. M., Ginsberg, J. P., Nagarajan, R., Kaste, S. C., Marina, N., . . . Gurney, J. G. (2009). Physical performance limitations in the Childhood Cancer Survivor Study cohort. *Journal of Clinical Oncology, 27,* 2382–2389. https://doi.org/10.1200/JCO.2008.21.1482

Newborg, J. (2005). *Battelle Developmental Inventory* (2nd ed.). Itasca, IL: Riverside Publishing.

Parham, L. D. (2008). Play and occupational therapy. In L. D. Parham & L. S. Fazio (Eds.), *Play in occupational therapy for children* (2nd ed., pp. 3–39). St. Louis: Mosby.

Parten, M. (1932). Social participation among preschool children. *Journal of Abnormal and Social Psychology, 27,* 243–269. https://doi.org/10.1037/h0074524

Pellis, S. M., Pellis, V. C., & Bell, H. C. (2010). The function of play in the development of the social brain. *American Journal of Play, 2,* 278–296.

Phillips, S. M., Padgett, L. S., Leisenring, W. M., Stratton, K. K., Bishop, K., Krull, K. R., . . . Mariotto, A. B. (2015). Survivors of childhood cancer in the United States: Prevalence and burden of morbidity. *Cancer Epidemiology, Biomarkers & Prevention, 24,* 653–663. https://doi.org/10.1158/1055-9965.EPI-14-1418

Piaget, J. (1962). *Play, dreams and imitation in childhood*. New York: Routledge.

Potasz, C., De Varela, M. J., De Carvalho, L. C., Do Prado, L. F., & Do Prado, G. F. (2013). Effect of play activities on hospitalized children's stress: A randomized clinical trial. *Scandinavian Journal of Occupational Therapy, 20,* 71–79. https://doi.org/10.3109/11038128.2012.729087

Pruitt, D. W., & Nagarajan, R. (2009). Rehabilitation of the pediatric cancer patient. In M. D. Stubblefield & M. W. O'Dell (Eds.), *Cancer rehabilitation: Principles and practice* (pp. 855–867). New York: Demos Medical.

Ragheb, M. G., & Beard, J. G. (1991). *Leisure Satisfaction Measure*. Enumclaw, WA: Idyll Arbor.

Rubin, D. A., Wilson, K. S., Wiersma, L. D., Weiss, J. W., & Rose, D. J. (2014). Rationale and design of Active Play @ Home: A parent-led physical activity program for children with and without disability. *BMC Pediatrics, 14,* 41. https://doi.org/10.1186/1471-2431-14-41

Scarponi, D., & Pession, A. (2016). Play therapy to control pain and suffering in pediatric oncology. *Frontiers in Pediatrics, 4,* 132. https://doi.org/10.3389/fped.2016.00132

Schaaf, R. C. (1990). Play behavior and occupational therapy. *American Journal of Occupational Therapy, 44,* 68–75. https://doi.org/10.5014/ajot.44.1.68

Schaaf, R. C., & Burke, J. P. (1997). What happens when we play? A neurodevelopmental explanation. In B. E. Chandler (Ed.), *The essence of play: A child's occupation* (pp. 79–105). Bethesda, MD: American Occupational Therapy Association.

Sellar, B., & Stanley, M. (2010). Leisure. In M. Curtin, M. Molineux, & J. Supyk-Mellson (Eds.), *Occupational therapy and physical dysfunction: Enabling occupation* (6th ed., pp. 358–369). London: Churchill Livingstone/Elsevier.

Silva, S. G. T. D., Santos, M. A., Floriano, C. M. F., Damião, E. B. C., Campos, F. V., & Rossato, L. M. (2017). Influence of therapeutic play on the anxiety of hospitalized school-age children: Clinical trial. *Revista Brasileira de Enfermagem, 70,* 1244–1249. https://doi.org/10.1590/0034-7167-2016-0353

Silver, J. K., & Gilchrist, L. S. (2011). Cancer rehabilitation with a focus on evidence-based outpatient physical and occupational therapy interventions. *American Journal of Physical Medicine & Rehabilitation, 90*(Suppl. 1), S5–S15. https://doi.org/10.1097/PHM.0b013e31820be4ae

Skard, G., & Bundy, A. (2008). The Test of Playfulness. In L. D. Parham & L. S. Fazio (Eds.), *Play in occupational therapy for children* (2nd ed., pp. 71–93). St. Louis: Mosby.

Sosa, A. V. (2016). Association of the type of toy used during play with the quantity and quality of parent–infant communication. *JAMA Pediatrics, 170,* 132–137. https://doi.org/10.1001/jamapediatrics.2015.3753

Stagnitti, K., & Lewis, F. M. (2015). Quality of pre-school children's pretend play and subsequent development of semantic organization and narrative re-telling skills. *International Journal of Speech–Language Pathology, 17,* 148–158. https://doi.org/10.3109/17549507.2014.941934

Takata, N. (1969). The play history. *American Journal of Occupational Therapy, 23,* 314–318.

Tanta, K. J., & Knox, S. H. (2015). Play. In J. Case-Smith & J. C. O'Brien (Eds.), *Occupational therapy for children and adolescents* (7th ed., pp. 483–497). St. Louis: Elsevier.

Tsimicalis, A., Genest, L., Stevens, B., Ungar, W. J., & Barr, R. (2017). The impact of a childhood cancer diagnosis on the children and siblings' school attendance, performance, and activities: A qualitative descriptive study. *Journal of Pediatric Oncology Nursing, 35,* 118–131. https://doi.org/10.1177/1043454217741875

Turhan, A. B., Tülin Fidan, S., Yarar, C., Nazlı Sakallı, E., Özdemir, Z. C., & Bör, Ö. (2018). Neurocognitive consequences of childhood leukemia and its treatment. *Indian Journal of Hematology & Blood Transfusion, 34,* 62–69. https://doi.org/10.1007/s12288-017-0846-4

Ullán, A. M., Belver, M. H., Fernández, E., Lorente, F., Badía, M., & Fernández, B. (2014). The effect of a program to promote play to reduce children's post-surgical pain: With plush toys, it hurts less. *Pain Management Nursing, 15,* 273–282. https://doi.org/10.1016/j.pmn.2012.10.004

Varni, J. W. (1998). *The copQL (Pediatric Quality of Life Inventory).* Lyon, France: Mapi Research Trust.

Vercher, P., Hung, Y. J., & Ko, M. (2016). The effectiveness of incorporating a play-based intervention to improve functional mobility for a child with relapsed acute lymphoblastic leukaemia: A case report. *Physiotherapy Research International, 21,* 264–270. https://doi.org/10.1002/pri.1663

Voress, J. K., & Maddox, T. (2013). *Developmental Assessment of Young Children* (2nd ed.). Torrance, CA: Western Psychological Services.

Westby, C. E. (2000). A scale for assessing development of children's play. In K. Gitlin-Weiner, A. Sandgund, & C. Schaefer (Eds.), *Play diagnosis and assessment* (pp. 15–57). New York: Wiley.

Wong-Baker FACES Foundation. (2015). *Wong-Baker FACES® Pain Rating Scale.* Retrieved from http://www.WongBakerFACES.org

Zheng, D. J., Lu, X., Schore, R. J., Balsamo, L., Devidas, M., Winick, N. J., . . . Kadan-Lottick, N. S. (2018). Longitudinal analysis of quality-of-life outcomes in children during treatment for acute lymphoblastic leukemia: A report from the Children's Oncology Group AALL0932 trial. *Cancer, 124,* 571–579. https://doi.org/10.1002/cncr.31085

Education

Laura Stimler, OTD, OTR/L, BCP, C/NDT, and Joshua Skuller, PhD, OTR/L, BCP, ATP

LEARNING OBJECTIVES

After completing this chapter, readers should be able to
- Explain the significance of education as an occupation across the lifespan and distinguish the unique role of occupational therapy to improve education participation for individuals diagnosed with cancer;
- Predict barriers to participation in education for cancer survivors across the lifespan;
- Summarize major legislation, including the Individuals with Disabilities Education Act (IDEA) and Section 504 of the Rehabilitation Act, highlighting their importance to maximizing education participation for cancer survivors;
- Give examples of evidence-based occupational therapy assessment tools and interventions to promote successful and meaningful engagement related to education exploration and participation in cancer rehabilitation; and
- Relate education participation to overall health and its role in promoting active participation in the occupational therapy process during cancer rehabilitation.

KEY TERMS AND CONCEPTS

- Cancer-related cognitive impairment
- Education
- Formal educational participation
- Individuals with Disabilities Education Act
- Informal personal educational needs or interest exploration
- Informal personal education participation
- Section 504 of the Rehabilitation Act

INTRODUCTION

Cancer survivors are documented to have decreased participation in education (Donnan et al., 2015; Pini et al., 2012; Sodergren et al., 2017). This chapter emphasizes the significant impact that education participation has on the overall health of individuals diagnosed with cancer and its vital role in improving active participation in the rehabilitation process. This chapter also explores barriers to participation in education related to client factors, performance skills, contexts, and environments, as outlined in the *Occupational Therapy Practice Framework: Domain and Process* (3rd ed.; *OTPF*; American Occupational Therapy Association [AOTA], 2014). A review of standardized and nonstandardized tools used to measure education participation and exploration is provided, as is a case example illustrating the occupational therapy process in an education setting for an individual diagnosed with cancer. Readers will gain an understanding of the unique role of occupational therapy in cancer rehabilitation as well as legislation in place to support cancer survivors in education settings along the continuum of care.

EDUCATION AS OCCUPATION

AOTA (2014) defines the occupation of *education* as "activities needed for learning and participating in the educational environment" (p. S20). Further, AOTA delineates three specific categories of education in the *OTPF*:
1. *Formal education participation* (i.e., engagement in academic coursework and nonacademic, extracurricular, and vocational events),
2. *Informal personal educational needs or interest exploration* (i.e., obtaining topic-related information outside the scope of a formal education setting), and
3. *Informal personal education participation* (i.e., engagement in training, programs or informal classes that provide instruction on an area of interest).

Table 24.1 provides a representation of the occupation of education, as illustrated in the *OTPF*.

Experiences that foster education participation and exploration are established early in childhood. Socialization, sensory exploration, and cognitive engagement during infancy and through the preschool years are paramount to lay the foundation for future academic

TABLE 24.1.   Occupation of Education, as Described in the *OTPF*

CATEGORY	DESCRIPTION (PER *OTPF*)
Formal educational participation	Participating in academic (e.g., math, reading, degree coursework), nonacademic (e.g., recess, lunchroom, hallway), extracurricular (e.g., sports, band, cheerleading, dances), and vocational (prevocational and vocational) educational activities
Informal personal educational needs or interests exploration (beyond formal education)	Identifying topics and methods for obtaining topic-related information or skills
Informal personal education participation	Participating in informal classes, programs, and activities that provide instruction or training in identified areas of interest

Source. American Occupational Therapy Association, 2014, "Occupational Therapy Practice Framework: Domain and Process (3rd ed.)," *American Journal of Occupational Therapy, 68*(Suppl. 1), p. S20. Copyright © 2014 by the American Occupational Therapy Association. Used with permission.

performance (Frolek Clark & Schlabach, 2013; Harman et al., 2017; Institute of Medicine [IOM] & National Research Council [NRC], 2012). In infants and young children, environmental influences, including routine daily activities (i.e., attending daycare, interacting with friends and family), can help prepare children for education participation and academic performance (IOM & NRC, 2012). During the preschool years, children are expected to perform in a variety of settings and environments, incorporating formal education participation into classrooms, playgrounds, lunchrooms, and playgroups (Willard et al., 2017).

As the trajectory of education continues through elementary and middle school, high school, and college or university levels, environmental and classroom activity demands grow. Students are expected to independently participate in academic and nonacademic activities and extracurricular and vocational activities. Outside of formal school environments, teen and adult learners may show interest in identifying topic-related information through informal personal education exploration such as searching the Internet or visiting the library. Informal personal education participation may involve active engagement in classes related to a specific area of interest (e.g., photography lessons; AOTA, 2014).

Older adults also seek continuing education opportunities to fulfill the desire to maximize learning and stay up to date. In a prospective study, researchers explored motivating factors for 306 adults ages 50 years and older to participate in continuing education. Reasons included increasing knowledge, enriching personal development, gaining more social interaction, using free time profitably, and learning more for the sake of helping others (Cachioni et al., 2014). When working with older adults, occupational therapy practitioners may elect to categorize the occupation of education as a leisure activity as defined by the *OTPF* (AOTA, 2014) because of the voluntary nature and unique motivating factors for continued education among this age group.

During the First International Conference on Health Promotion, the World Health Organization (WHO) identified education as one of the fundamental prerequisites to health during the landmark presentation of the Ottawa Charter for Health Promotion (WHO, 1986). Participation in various occupations, including education, leads to satisfaction of needs, including food, shelter, and income,

as well as achievement of future self-sufficiency and sustainable resources, thus directly affecting health (Wilcock & Hocking, 2015). Cancer and its treatment present significant barriers to education participation throughout the lifespan, while negatively affecting the overall health of survivors (Harman et al., 2017; Strauser et al., 2015; Willard et al., 2017).

FACTORS THAT MAY CONTRIBUTE TO OCCUPATIONAL DYSFUNCTION

Client Factors

Values, beliefs, and spirituality

Cancer can have different effects on values, beliefs, and spirituality for survivors across the lifespan. Participation in desired practices and routines may be interrupted during the active treatment phase for cancer and well into long-term survivorship. As a result, cancer and its treatment may motivate some to achieve and value accomplishments more highly but discourage others by interrupting or preventing educational accomplishment. In an interpretive phenomenological analysis study conducted by Fleischer and Howell (2017), the experiences of eight breast cancer survivors were analyzed using semistructured interviews and a modified version of the Activity Card Sort (ACSm). One participant reported feeling a change regarding the value she placed on advancing her education after treatment. More specifically, this participant reported feeling motivated to complete a degree after her treatment (Fleischer & Howell, 2017).

In a systematic review by Pini et al. (2012), multiple studies highlighted teenage participants' emphasis on peer relationships and the direct impact they have on education engagement. Teenagers also reported valuing the ability to successfully complete regular school curriculums and improving opportunities to educate school staff on the student's condition to improve awareness and understanding. Additionally, school absences are frequently reported in the literature; these result in decreased participation in extracurricular activities (Pini et al., 2012; Sodergren et al., 2017; Strauser et al., 2015). As a result, informal education and extracurricular activities related to religious affiliations (e.g., Bible study, Hebrew school) may be put on hold, thus creating a barrier to active participation in meaningful spiritual activities.

Body functions

Mental functions. The period of growth that occurs immediately after birth through the first few years of life is critical to laying the foundation for overall brain development and establishing a positive trajectory of learning potential and performance (Frolek Clark & Schlabach, 2013; Harman et al., 2017; IOM & NRC, 2012). Active participation in social, emotional, sensory, and motor exploration is imperative for cognitive and communication development during the early childhood years. Multiple studies have recognized close correlations between early cognitive development and success in formal education settings (Froleck Clark & Schlabach, 2013; IOM & NRC, 2012; Myers et al., 2015). A cancer diagnosis during these early years poses a significant risk of interrupting typical development. Pathophysiologic features may be altered because of the cancer disease process and aggressive treatments, including chemotherapy and radiation. Negative long-term neurocognitive effects are well documented. Mental functions and cognitive skills, including attention, information processing, executive functioning, visuospatial skills, verbal memory, visual memory, and academic achievement, are commonly reported as below average in childhood cancer survivors, resulting in barriers to academic attainment and performance later in life (Compas et al., 2017; Donnan et al., 2015).

Cancer-related cognitive impairment (CRCI) is believed to possibly result from proinflammatory cytokines, oxidative stress, mitochondrial damage, and genetic factors (Hutchinson et al., 2017). CRCI has been identified in both pediatric and adult populations and may lead to lower academic attainment, decreased school attendance, and depressive symptoms related to poorer academic achievement (Hutchinson et al., 2017). See Chapter 17, "Cancer-Related Cognitive Impairment," for more information.

Energy and drive, muscle functions. During the teenage years, individuals are expected to participate in developmentally appropriate social and school-related activities that naturally foster work skill attainment. Cancer treatment and long-term effects may disrupt the natural progression of school participation during this critical phase of development (Strauser et al., 2015). Fatigue, weakness, decreased motivation, and time-consuming medical treatments frequently prevent school attendance, participation in extracurricular activities, and selection of postsecondary goals, causing individuals to fall behind their peers (Berg et al., 2009; Pini et al., 2012; Sodergren et al., 2017). Musculoskeletal impairments, including amputation, osteoporosis, joint replacement, osteonecrosis, and decreased strength, have been associated with limitations in school participation among childhood cancer survivors (Ness et al., 2009).

Sensory functions

Visual impairments (i.e., double vision) have been correlated with receiving central nervous system (CNS) radiation treatment in individuals diagnosed with CNS tumors (Bashore & Breyer, 2017). Vision is imperative for full participation in education, including mobility, communication, and learning (Kaldenberg, 2017).

Hearing loss is commonly reported in cancer survivors, specifically those who have received high doses of cisplatin and carboplatin (Gurney et al., 2007). In a study exploring the correlation between hearing loss and parent-reported academic and psychosocial difficulties, Gurney et al. (2007) found survivors of neuroblastoma with hearing loss to be at risk for reading, math, and attention difficulties as well as learning disabilities.

Children diagnosed with cancer of the eye (i.e., retinoblastoma) have been documented to present with developmental delays. In a pilot study exploring a prospective screening protocol, more than 72% of children diagnosed with retinoblastoma were referred to occupational therapy for impairments related to sensory processing, vision, motor skills, speech, and feeding (Sparrow et al., 2016).

Direct correlations between pain, fatigue, decreased coordination, and neurosensory and vestibular function have been made to performance limitations (e.g., attendance at work or school) among survivors of pediatric cancer (Gilchrist & Tanner, 2013; Ness et al., 2009). Sensory symptoms, including decreased light touch sensation, vibration sensation, deep tendon reflexes, and balance problems, have been reported in children diagnosed with chemotherapy-induced peripheral neuropathy (CIPN; Gilchrist & Tanner, 2013). In a study performed by Gilchrist and Tanner (2013), children receiving treatment for cancer received scores significantly worse than the control group on the pediatric-modified Total Neuropathy Score (ped–mTNS; Gilchrist & Tanner, 2013) sensory components as well as balance and manual dexterity.

Cardiovascular, hematological, immunological, and respiratory system functions

One of the largest retrospective cohort studies on pediatric cancer survivors, the Childhood Cancer Survivor Study (CCSS), included multi-institution longitudinal follow-up of more than 14,000 individuals who had survived at least 5 years from the time of diagnosis (i.e., diagnosed before the age of 25 years; Robinson et al., 2009). Dietz et al. (2016) explored the relationship between adverse pulmonary outcomes and functional activities reported in the CCSS. Results indicated that survivors are at increased risk for developing pulmonary conditions, including chronic cough, oxygen need, lung fibrosis, and recurrent pneumonia, when compared to siblings. Additionally, survivors were more likely to report functional activity limitations and may experience self-consciousness, social isolation, hoarseness, and musculoskeletal pain as a result of respiratory complications (Dietz et al., 2016).

Additional analyses have been performed using data from the CCSS; those analyses identified direct relationships between physical performance limitations (i.e., school attendance) and organ system impairments, including musculoskeletal, neurosensory, neurological, endocrine, and cardiopulmonary dysfunction (Ness et al., 2009).

Performance Skills

Motor skills (grips, manipulates, coordinates)

Strong evidence supports the fact that vincristine causes CIPN, resulting in slowed fine motor speed, decreased dexterity, decreased wrist range of motion (ROM), and decreased hand muscle strength. (For more information, please see Chapter 19, "Chemotherapy-Induced Peripheral Neuropathy.") Multiple small studies have reported delayed fine motor skills and performance limitations in children who have received vincristine during induction and delayed intensification phases of treatment up to 2 years after treatment (De Luca et al., 2013; Gilchrist & Tanner, 2013; Sabarre et al., 2014).

During a prospective case series design study, Sabarre et al. (2014) explored the correlation between performance limitations in children diagnosed with acute lymphoblastic leukemia who received maintenance chemotherapy, specifically vincristine. Although results did not reach a statistically significant value, almost 50% of the children on treatment received below-average scores on the manual dexterity section of the Movement Assessment Battery for Children–2 (Sabarre et al., 2014). Children receiving vincristine are at risk for limited fine motor skills that may potentially cause decreased manipulation of writing and eating utensils, snipping with scissors, handwriting, use of mature pinching and grasping patterns, and so on. In turn, these limitations can create barriers to satisfactory participation in educational engagement. Occupational therapy practitioners play a critical role in monitoring individuals being treated with vincristine for changes in motor performance during all phases of treatment and into survivorship.

Process skills (initiates or terminates, continues, sequences, organizes)

Neurocognitive impairments are well documented in pediatric cancer survivors. Limitations in executive function, concentration, memory, task completion, processing speed, initiation, inhibition, planning and organization skills, and attention are frequently identified as barriers to education participation and performance (Donnan et al., 2015; Edelmann et al., 2016). Please see Chapter 17 for more information.

Social interaction (approaches or starts, regulates, questions, replies, expresses emotion, transitions)

Children and adolescents who are undergoing cancer treatment may have issues with their overall ability and interest to interact with others in the educational setting. Absences, dramatic physical changes as a result of weight gain or loss, hair loss, and amputations have been reported to cause decreased confidence and negative body image, leading to decreased peer-relationship development

---

EXHIBIT 24.1.	Cancer-Related Risk Factors for Developing Educational Problems

- Diagnosis of cancer at a very young age
- Numerous or prolonged school absences
- History of learning problems before being diagnosed with cancer
- Cancer treatment that results in reduced energy levels, decreased hearing or vision
- Cancer treatment that results in physical disabilities
- Treatment to the central nervous system
- Brain tumors
- Tumors involving the eye or ear
- Acute lymphoblastic leukemia
- Non-Hodgkin's lymphoma
- Treatment including methotrexate given in high doses intravenously or injected into the spinal fluid (intrathecal or intraommaya)
- Cytarabine, if given in high doses intravenously
- Surgery on the brain
- Radiation to the brain (cranial), ear or infratemporal region (midfacial area behind the cheekbones), total body irradiation
- Cisplatin or carboplatin (may affect hearing)

Source. Adapted from "Educational Issues Following Treatment for Childhood Cancer Health Link," in *Health Link: Healthy Living After Treatment for Childhood Cancer. Educational Issues, Version 4.0,* by Children's Oncology Group, 2013. Used with permission.

(Bashore & Breyer, 2017). Pini et al. (2012) conducted a systematic review on the relationship between a cancer diagnosis and educational engagement and school experiences of teenagers. Incidences of bullying or teasing targeted at disease-related physical changes were reported throughout the literature. As a result, participation in school-related activities was affected because of the hesitation of individuals receiving treatment to approach or transition into a new peer group or situation. Exhibit 24.1 shows cancer-related risk factors for developing educational problems.

Assessing client factors in education

Occupational therapy practitioners use a wide variety of assessment tools when working with the oncology population. Both structured and semistructured interviews or inventories may be helpful to collect information or insight into meaningful values, beliefs, and practices related to education as an occupation. Examples of these include the Canadian Occupational Performance Measure (Law et al., 2019); Occupational Performance History Interview (Kielhofner et al., 2004); Pediatric Activity Card Sort (Mandich et al., 2004), Child Occupational Self Assessment, Version 2.2 (Kramer et al., 2014); and the Short Child Occupational Profile, Version 2.2 (Bowyer et al., 2008).

Additional assessments can be used in education settings to address client factors, including goniometry for ROM, manual muscle testing for strength, monofilaments for sensation, and various pain scales for perceived pain. Although these latter tools may be helpful to provide objective information related to the individual's status, they are not used as frequently as approaches that allow for a more global understanding of school participation.

Performance Patterns

Routines and roles specifically related to the education setting may be altered during and after cancer treatment. Pediatric cancer survivors have reported the need to repeat an entire year of school, leading to fear of not returning to previous peer groups and possibly having to create new friendships (Pini et al., 2012). Frequent changes in schedules and physical appearances and increased number of transitions may lead to decreased confidence. Therefore, students often choose to avoid previous routines and roles involving social activities (Bashore & Breyer, 2017; Pini et al., 2012).

Context and Environment

Different types of access to education needs should be considered to promote full education participation. Factors such as where the child is on the cancer care continuum, how they are feeling, and the need for protective isolation may dictate the location of education services provided. If the child is not medically cleared to participate in a school-based setting, a hospital-based, home, or virtual environment may be appropriate. Figure 24.1 provides an illustration of a home school environment. Medical appointments, hospitalization, illness, protective isolation, anxiety, and disease-related symptoms are causes of frequent school absences, which may result in a part-time school schedule (Donnan et al., 2015; Pini et al., 2012; Upton & Eiser, 2006).

INDIVIDUALS WITH DISABILITIES EDUCATION ACT (IDEA) AND SECTION 504 OF THE REHABILITATION ACT

On occasion, a child with a cancer diagnosis who is returning to school will require the support of special education services. The category of *other health impaired* may be most appropriate because it refers to "having limited strength, vitality, or alertness that can impact participation in the educational environment and adversely affects educational performance" (U.S. Department of Education [ED], 2020). Many times, a child with a cancer diagnosis will return to school and will not need the support of special education as dictated by the ***Individuals with Disabilities Education Act*** (IDEA, 2004; P. L. 108-446) but will require some supports to be in place. In this type of situation, the child's family and school personnel should use ***Section 504 of the Rehabilitation Act of 1973*** (as amended; P. L. 93-112) and Title II of the Americans with Disabilities Act (ADA; P. L. 101-336; 2018). Both of these acts are in effect to ensure nondiscrimination of children with disabilities in their school setting and can apply to preschool, grade school, and secondary school (ADA, 2018; Cahill & Bazyk, 2020; Davies, 2012; ED, 2018).

The ADA and Section 504 often use a definition of *disability* that could be considered broader than that of IDEA and therefore offers accommodations to help the child access their learning environment (Cahill & Bazyk, 2020). Figure 24.2 provides an examples of a typical classroom environment. An evaluation and written plan are required

FIGURE 24.1 Families may elect to educate their child in the home environment because it allows for a flexible approach for children who are frequently immune-suppressed or ill. Networking is commonly used to promote socialization and sharing of resources for families of home schooled children (Swisher, 2017).

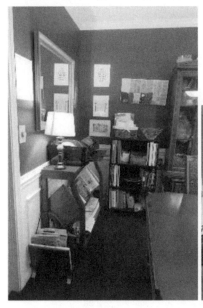
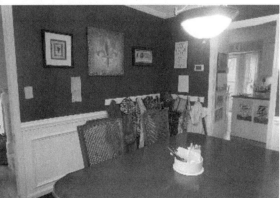

Source. L. Stimler. Used with permission.

FIGURE 24.2	Parents may choose private or public education classroom environments for their school-age child, depending on the child's needs and funding sources (Swisher, 2017).

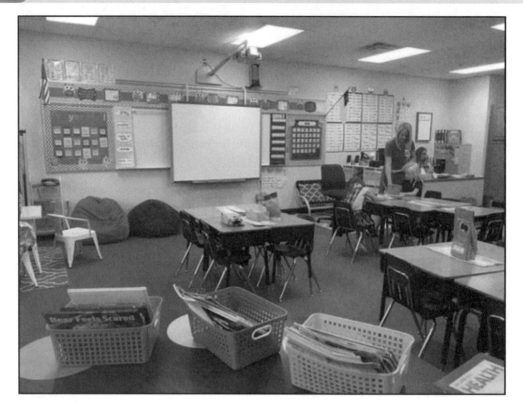

Source. S. Story. Used with permission.

under Section 504 (Davies, 2012). School districts do not receive funding for Section 504 and ADA Title II; however, because both of these are federal laws, school districts that do not comply with these regulations can lose federal funding (Cahill & Bazyk, 2020). Parents should check with their local school district about Section 504 policies. For a comparison of IDEA and Section 504, see Table 24.2.

The definition of *disability* under Section 504 and ADA includes any student with "a physical or mental impairment that substantially limits one or more major life

TABLE 24.2. Comparison Between IDEA and Section 504

	INDIVIDUALS WITH DISABILITIES EDUCATION ACT	**SECTION 504**
Type of law	Education law	Civil rights law
Who is in charge	Special education director	Section 504 coordinator
General purpose of the law	Each child with a disability is guaranteed a free and appropriate education; includes preschool, elementary, and secondary schools	Protects the rights of individuals with disabilities in programs and activities that receive federal assistance from the Department of Education
Name of tool used to implement the law	Individualized education plan	Accommodations (504 Plan)
Types of disabilities	13 disabilities, including other health impairment, which may qualify cancer survivors	All eligible disabilities, including cancer; disability must substantially limit 1 or more major life activities
Safeguards	Parent participation, consent, and notification needed	Notice to parent required
Evaluation of eligibility	An evaluation needed	An evaluation needed

Source. Reprinted from *Living With Cancer: Advocating for Your Child's Educational Needs* by the Leukemia & Lymphoma Society, 2013, p. 9. Copyright © 2013 by the Leukemia & Lymphoma Society. Used with permission.

activities, who has a record of having such an impairment, or is regarding as having such an impairment" (34 C.F.R. 104.3[j][2][i]). Cancer treatment is a lengthy process with many side effects in both the acute and the maintenance phases (Harman et al., 2017). Therefore, children with cancer can benefit from the skilled expertise of an occupational therapy practitioner when returning to school to help determine accommodations to promote school participation. Such examples of accommodations can include but are not limited to keeping a water bottle at the child's desk to help with thirst as a result of treatment, short rest breaks during the school day, frequent trips to the restroom because of increased fluid intake, head coverings in school because of hair loss, and leaving class a few minutes early to navigate the hallways to the next class before the busy class change in the upper grades (Leukemia & Lymphoma Society, 2013). (See Table 24.3 for cognitive accommodation recommendations and Table 24.4 for physical accommodation recommendations.) These accommodations are a part of a written plan discussing how the child will be supported in their education. For the child who demonstrates more significant impairments associated with their cancer

TABLE 24.3. Types of Cognitive Accommodations

COGNITIVE ACCOMMODATION	RATIONALE
The student will be given extra time for classwork, homework, quizzes, and tests.	During and after chemotherapy or radiation treatment, the student may process information and respond more slowly. Students who experience neuropathy in their hands often have difficulty taking notes for long periods.
The student will have a homebound teacher (a licensed teacher provided by the public school) who comes to the child's home to help with assignments.	The student may miss school often because of hospital stays and feeling poorly. The student may need extra help with assignments because of cognitive late effects. A homebound teacher will collect the missed work from school and help the child complete missed assignments.
The student will be assigned a moderate workload that emphasizes quality versus quantity.	A moderate workload allows the student to show that they have mastered the concepts without feeling overwhelmed. After a full school day, the student may be too tired to spend a lot of time on homework.
The student will be permitted an extended school year (during winter, spring, or summer breaks) to allow more time to complete assignments and to stay at their peer grade level.	As a result of learning difficulties arising from cancer treatment, students may need extra time during school breaks to complete schoolwork.

Source. Reprinted from *Living With Cancer: Advocating for Your Child's Educational Needs* by the Leukemia & Lymphoma Society, 2013, p. 13. Copyright © 2013 by the Leukemia & Lymphoma Society. Used with permission.

TABLE 24.4. Types of Physical Accommodations

PHYSICAL ACCOMMODATION	RATIONALE
The student will be given two sets of books, one for use at home and one for use at school.	The student may miss school often because of hospital stays and feeling poorly. Having an extra set of books at home makes it easier for the student to keep up with assignments, especially when absences are unexpected. Also, children experiencing fatigue need lighter backpacks.
The student will be allowed to carry a water or juice bottle throughout the school day.	Students on chemotherapy or other medicines may need to drink extra fluids to prevent dehydration and dry mouth.
The student will be given bathroom, guidance, and clinic passes.	A laminated pass to use when needed allows the student to leave the classroom without drawing attention from the other students.
The student will not be required to participate in physical education activities that involve contact sports, strenuous exercises, and distance running.	Many students return to school with port-a-cath or other central lines in place. They also may be extremely tired from treatment or be at risk for internal bleeding if they suffer from a low platelet count. Strenuous physical activity can tire the student, causing problems with concentration and school performance. For those students with neuropathy in the feet and legs, an exemption from physical activity may be necessary, especially when it requires a lot of running or walking the track.
The student will not be required to participate in the Presidential Youth Fitness Program.	This testing can take too much energy from the child who is physically fragile.
The student will be allowed to wear a hat or scarf throughout the school day.	A student with hair loss may feel uncomfortable. Because most schools have a "no hat" rule, an accommodation should be made.

(Continued)

TABLE 24.4.   Types of Physical Accommodations *(Cont.)*

PHYSICAL ACCOMMODATION	RATIONALE
The student will be allowed to leave class 5 minutes early to get to the next class.	The student may have classes at opposite ends or on different levels of the school building. Hallways can be crowded. The student may need extra time to get to the next class or may need to avoid the inevitable physical contact in a busy school hallway. For those students with neuropathy in the feet and legs, an elevator pass may be needed, if available.
The student will be allowed to have a midmorning and afternoon snack, if needed.	Treatment (especially with steroids) can cause weight loss and increased hunger. A child experiencing weight loss needs snacks to add calories and nutrients to their diet.
The student will be given a shortened school day or rest period, if needed. Intermittent homebound instruction should be offered to make up classes missed because of the child's inability to attend for a full day.	*Intermittent homebound instruction* is the term used when the child can attend school on some days, but gets instructed at home intermittently on the days when they are in clinic, hospitalized, or just not feeling well. Fatigue is most common, but a rest period and/or shortened school day may make it possible for the student to attend school.
The student will be given a locker close to their classes or two lockers (if the classes are spread out or on different floors).	To allow the student to avoid carrying heavy books and notebooks throughout the day, a locker close to their classes can make it possible to change books between classes.
The student will be given a parking space close to the school entrance.	For the student who drives to school, a parking space close to the school entrance will make it easier for them to walk to class without getting tired.
The student will be provided a computer for note taking and assignments.	When handwriting is a challenge, the student can use a computer or other technology to avoid fine motor fatigue and to make assignments easier to read.
The student will be provided a desk suitable for their body size and frame.	A child's body weight on steroids can fluctuate. The child may feel uncomfortable in the initial desk assigned to them and be too embarrassed to say anything.

Source. Reprinted from *Living With Cancer: Advocating for Your Child's Educational Needs* by the Leukemia & Lymphoma Society, 2013, pp. 10–12. Copyright © 2013 by the Leukemia & Lymphoma Society. Used with permission.

diagnosis, the special education team may decide that an evaluation is warranted to determine if the child will benefit from specially designed instruction as dictated through IDEA (see Table 24.2).

For children who are not of school age (younger than age 3 years), a cancer diagnosis could qualify the child for early intervention services through Part C of IDEA. Parents and specialists should check with their state's early intervention program to determine policies and procedures for these services (Myers et al., 2015). Refer to Figure 24.3 for an example of a typical daycare environment for children under 3 years of age.

The transition to a college or vocational school setting is significant because each adult student is responsible for ensuring that their needs are met. Colleges and vocational schools are not required to identify students with disabilities. Students must request accommodations from the appropriate personnel or department, including the student disability services office or 504/ADA coordinator, early if they anticipate having needs. The type of school (i.e., public vs. private university) and funding source will determine on a case-by-case basis whether the school is required to create a 504 plan. Exhibit 24.2 lists reasonable accommodations and auxiliary aids for adult students (Kentucky Protection and Advocacy, 2014). Occupational therapy practitioners have the knowledge base to collaborate with the 504/ADA coordinator or student disability services office to incorporate the use of universal design, accessible curricular materials, and ergonomic needs (Swinth, 2014). Figure 24.4 provides an example of a typical college classroom environment.

OCCUPATIONAL THERAPY EVALUATION OF EDUCATION

Occupational Profile

The occupational profile should illustrate meaningful experiences and priorities for the client. Occupational therapy practitioners can use the following questions related to the occupation of education to create the occupational profile, which is the first step in the evaluation process:

- What do you enjoy about school?
- What is easy for you related to your education or school performance?
- What things are difficult for you?
- What would you like to see changed?
- What has changed since your started chemotherapy?
- What do you find difficult that used to be easy?
- What is preventing you from enjoying learning opportunities?

Upon completion of the occupational profile, occupational therapy practitioners should aim to develop an individualized and client-centered intervention plan. Case Example 24.1 illustrates the occupational therapy process in a school-based setting.

FIGURE 24.3

For babies and toddlers, creating a familiar environment and following a natural routine is important. Children this age have a heightened awareness of changes in their environment and thrive off of routine and familiarity (Wiener & Sourkes, 2014). Immunosuppression may limit opportunities for young children to interact in natural environments, including daycare centers, playgroups, and playgrounds.

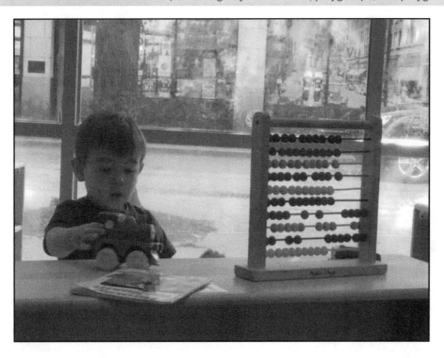

Source. A. Goeing. Used with permission.

Analysis of Occupational Performance

Occupational therapy practitioners in the school-based setting are called to identify barriers to academic and nonacademic performance across multiple school environments and contexts (Frolek Clark et al., 2019). The use of assessments that highlight a broad spectrum of participation considerations are encouraged. The School Function Assessment (Coster et al., 1998) is an occupation-based assessment tool frequently used by occupational therapy practitioners in academic settings (Cahill & Bazyk, 2020). See Table 24.5 for a list of standardized and nonstandardized tools commonly used in school-based settings.

Maintaining family life balance as a parent while advocating for a child diagnosed with cancer presents unique challenges. Identifying appropriate boundaries, discipline, and structure can be difficult, especially when seeing a child experience painful treatments and side effects. Promoting normalcy and natural routines similar to those used before a child was diagnosed is encouraged (Lafond & Leach, 2014). Exhibit 24.3 provides a unique parent perspective on prioritization of school routines for a child diagnosed with cancer.

OCCUPATIONAL THERAPY INTERVENTIONS FOR EDUCATION

Approaches to Improving Education

Occupational therapy practitioners are called to identify barriers to participation, specifically in the area of

EXHIBIT 24.2. Types of Accommodations or Auxiliary Aids for Adult Students

General accommodations

- Assistive technology
- Note takers
- Electronic readers
- Specialized gym equipment
- Reaching device for library use
- Raised-line drawing kits
- Assistive listening devices
- Braille calculators, printers, or writers
- Priority registration
- Relocation of classes
- Accessible parking and/or housing
- Sign language interpreters

Examples of changes in testing

- Electronic responses
- Extended testing time
- Testing over several sessions
- Small group setting
- Private room
- Preferential seating

Source. Reprinted from *504: A College/Vocational School Student's Guide*, by Kentucky Protection and Advocacy, 2014, p. 6. Copyright © 2014 by Kentucky Protection and Advocacy. Used with permission.

FIGURE 24.4 Occupational therapy practitioners may collaborate with the 504/ADA coordinator or student disability services office at the college or university level to incorporate the use of universal design, accessible curricular materials for students, and environmental supports (Swinth, 2014).

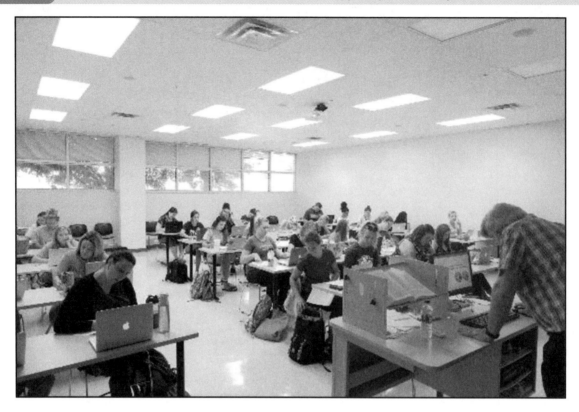

Source. Photograph by Joshua Skuller. Used with permission.

CASE EXAMPLE 24.1. MOISHE: PARTICIPATING IN SCHOOL

Moishe was diagnosed with high-risk acute lymphoblastic leukemia (ALL) at age 8 years after his mother noticed frequent bruising, fatigue, and pallor over the course of a couple of weeks. After a series of blood tests, including a bone marrow aspirate and biopsy, the medical team confirmed the diagnosis of ALL.

His treatment included receiving intense doses of vincristine, L-asparaginase, and methotrexate during the induction phase, and one dose per week during consolidation. Total body irradiation (TBI) was administered during the days before his allogeneic stem cell transplant. Moishe had an elevated risk for rejection of the transplant as a result of having an unrelated, 8/10 human leukocyte antigen–matched donor (Diver, 2015), which resulted in chronic graft-versus-host disease (cGVHD). Complications related to his cGVHD included significant range of motion (ROM) limitations to both upper extremities and diarrhea. Additionally, chemotherapy-induced peripheral neuropathy (CIPN) caused distal weakness, sensory loss, and poor coordination bilaterally, limiting Moishe's fine motor skills throughout his treatment. As

a result of these complications, he required a prolonged hospital stay of 4 months.

During his maintenance phase of chemotherapy, Moishe was medically cleared to return to school. His teacher immediately recognized that he had difficulty with handwriting tasks, keeping up with his peers during physical activities, and poor frustration tolerance when presented with minimal challenges. Because of an overall concern by his teacher and family with academic performance, Moishe was referred to the special education team, including occupational therapy, for a multifaceted evaluation to determine whether he would benefit from special education services.

Evaluation
Occupational profile
Information related to the occupational profile was collected using the Canadian Occupational Performance Measure (COPM; Law et al., 2019) with the help of Moishe's mother. Before his cancer diagnosis, Moishe was active in extracurricular activities including soccer, chess club, and Hebrew school; however, he preferred

(Continued)

CASE EXAMPLE 24.1. MOISHE: PARTICIPATING IN SCHOOL *(Cont.)*

to avoid these activities because of his motor difficulties and fatigue.

His family lived in a two-story home with both parents and three sisters. Upon returning home from his prolonged hospital admission, Moishe reported decreased satisfaction with his performance in the areas of ADLs, play and leisure, school, and social participation.

Analysis of occupational performance

The school-based individual education plan (IEP) evaluation team determined Moishe to be eligible for special education services under the category of "other health impaired" as directed by IDEA (2004). The occupational therapist chose to evaluate Moishe with the following assessment tools: Bruininks–Oseretsky Test of Motor Proficiency (BOT–2; Bruininks & Bruininks, 2006); Evaluation Tool for Children's Handwriting (ETCH) Manuscript (Amundson, 2004); Sensory Profile–2 (SP2) Caregiver Questionnaire and School Companion (Dunn, 2014); and the Child Occupational Self Assessment (COSA), Version 2.2 (Kramer et al., 2014). In addition to these assessments, the occupational therapist also engaged Moishe in conversation about his preferred activities before and after his ALL diagnosis.

Moishe scored below the norm in the Fine Motor Precision, Fine Motor Integration, Manual Dexterity, and Bilateral Coordination subtests on the BOT–2, which is in line with the complications that he experienced as a result of the CIPN and GVHD. The scores on the BOT–2 were also in agreement with scores on the ETCH. Moishe demonstrated 46% legibility for capital letters and 35% legibility for lowercase letters. Much of the illegibility was the result of letters touching each other or reversals, suggesting issues with visual motor skills. He also demonstrated difficulty with in-hand manipulation skills as evidenced by difficulty with complex rotation, translation, and shift. The ETCH also revealed that Moishe wrote 20 letters per minute when timed, which would translate to a first-grade skill (Amundson, 2004). Moishe demonstrated a significant score on the SP2 for the Avoider quadrant with an overall score of 72, placing his responses *much more* than that of his typically developing peers. Further, the SP2 School Companion demonstrated that he was responding much more than his typically developing peers in the areas of visual, touch, and movement.

The occupational therapist administered the COSA, Version 2.2 to get Moishe's perspective on his school performance. Initially Moishe did not want to participate when he saw the checklist, so the occupational therapist quickly downgraded the assessment to the card sort format, and Moishe was more agreeable to participating. Moishe reported that his biggest school-related issues were with completing his work on time, finishing what he is doing without getting too tired, completing tasks with his hands, thinking of ways he can do things, persevering when tasks become difficult, and completing his homework. He reported that he knew all of those should be important to him, but he really thought that getting his work done without getting too tired was the most important. This led Moishe to talk about all of the activities that he liked to do before diagnosis and how he was frustrated that he could not do as much now because he either got too tired or didn't feel well.

Intervention

Intervention plan

Based on the information presented during the assessment process, the occupational therapist developed a treatment plan that initially involved seeing Moishe for 30 minutes weekly for the first 2 months of IEP implementation, along with teacher education, and then reducing that time to twice-monthly occupational therapy sessions for 30 minutes with ongoing teacher education as needed. Occupational therapy–related strategies that were placed on the IEP included sensory processing strategies, fine motor development strategies, visual–motor strategies, and teacher education. The bulk of Moishe's special education services were provided through a collaborative approach in the general classroom to keep him with his peers. IEP goals were developed to address handwriting, completion of work, and frustration tolerance.

Intervention implementation

As part of the teacher training and collaboration, the occupational therapist discussed the possibility of breaking Moishe's tasks down into more manageable chunks. He was having issues with fatigue because of maintenance chemotherapy, and his frustration tolerance was rather low, especially when unable to keep up with his peers. Ideas for breaking the task down were fewer spelling words and doing half of the math problems to show understanding of the concept. Moishe was also given the opportunity to use a keyboard to type his work, which helped with fatigue and handwriting issues.

The occupational therapist noted Moishe's sensory needs, and they worked together to identify a quieter place in the classroom that he could use to complete his work if he was feeling overwhelmed. Moishe said he enjoyed using a study carrel to block all of the extra activity in the room so he could focus on his work. They also discussed using deep pressure strategies, such as wall pushups, chair pulldowns, and arm squeezes, to provide deep pressure so he would be more primed for his work and more accepting of the occasional bumps that happened in the classroom.

The occupational therapist also instructed Moishe and his teachers on the Zones of Regulation® (Kuypers, 2018) program to help them identify when he might be overstimulated in the classroom and would need to take a short break to regroup. During his initial evaluation, Moishe stated that Batman was his favorite superhero. The occupational therapist created a power card (Hilton, 2015) using Batman as the subject to outline the steps Moishe could take when he began to feel upset. *Power cards* are visual

(Continued)

CASE EXAMPLE 24.1. MOISHE: PARTICIPATING IN SCHOOL *(Cont.)*

cues using a child's favorite superhero. The power card was placed on Moishe's desk as to remind him of the steps he could take throughout the day to help reduce frustration.

To improve his fine motor and visual–motor skills, the occupational therapist worked with Moishe at his desk during his morning literacy time when he did the most writing. They worked on hand strengthening and manipulation activities such as pulling small items out of therapy putty using both hands, writing and coloring with smaller tools, and completing worksheets to promote distal control of his pencil. The therapist also began instruction with Handwriting Without Tears® (Olsen, 2018) as a kinesthetic way to relearn writing his letters and to remove some of the visual clutter that can be overwhelming when completing classroom worksheets.

Outcomes

With adaptations to his schoolwork, Moishe was able to complete tasks promptly, which increased his overall confidence as a student. He also enjoyed working on a computer for some of his writing tasks, and his special education teacher created an online document for his journal writing. His transition to school was often difficult in the morning, so Moishe would do his "hand warmups" in the study carrel, which was a calm time for him to organize himself emotionally and prepare to do a Handwriting Without Tears task.

The overall cleaner design (i.e., less visual clutter) of the Handwriting Without Tears program gave Moishe the opportunity to remediate his handwriting skills without extraneous clutter on a worksheet. He was able to use the simplified designs in the workbook to focus on his letters, and within 2 months the occupational therapist was able to document that Moishe was no longer having issues with spacing between letters, and his reversals were also reduced when compared to initial evaluation.

Lastly, Moishe's began to demonstrate stronger self-advocacy skills, something that was not on his IEP. He began to recognize times during the day when he felt more fatigued or frustrated, and he would let his teacher know so they could formulate plans for completion of his tasks.

Intervention Review

At the end of the school year, the occupational therapist re-administered the COSA, Version 2.2, and the COPM. This time Moishe was more interested in completing the checklist form of the COSA than the card sort. He reported that he was still having some difficulty with classroom-related tasks, but they were becoming more important to him, and he was redeveloping his role as a student. His COPM interview also identified that he was becoming more satisfied with his performance as a student. The therapist modified Moishe's treatment plan to reflect these findings and continued to support Moishe's participation in the general classroom and to support the classroom teacher and special education teacher with accommodations by request.

TABLE 24.5.   A Representation of Commonly Used Assessments for Education

TITLE	POPULATION	DESCRIPTION
School Function Assessment (Coster et al., 1998)	▪ Age: Kindergarten–6th grade ▪ Appropriate for children with a range of conditions	Questionnaire used to assess functional performance during nonacademic activities that support academic participation in school settings (i.e., hygiene, handwriting, play, social participation, material management in elementary school setting).
Bruininks-Oserestky Test of Motor Proficiency, 2nd Edition (Bruininks & Bruininks, 2006)	▪ Age: 4–21 years ▪ Appropriate for individuals with developmental disabilities (must be able to follow directions)	Performance-based assessment for motor skills including 8 subtests: Fine Motor Precision, Fine Motor Integration, Manual Dexterity, Bilateral Coordination, Balance, Running Speed and Agility, Upper-Limb Coordination, and Strength. Results may be used to guide academic appointment choices.
Peabody Developmental Motor Scales, 2nd Edition (Folio & Fewell, 2000)	▪ Age: Birth–6 years ▪ Appropriate for individuals with motor, speech–language, and hearing disorders	Performance-based assessment including 6 subtests: Reflexes, Sustained Control, Locomotion, Object Manipulation, Grasping, Visual–Motor Integration. Results highlight strengths and deficits related to motor ability.
Short Child Occupational Profile, Version 2.2 (Bowyer et al., 2008)	▪ Age: 6 months–21 years ▪ Appropriate for a wide range of conditions in natural settings (i.e., home, school, education)	Formal and informal observation, interviews, and other assessments used to collect data related to 6 sections using the Model of Human Occupation concepts (volition, habituation, communication/interaction skills, process skills, motor skills, and the impact of physical and social environments).

(Continued)

TABLE 24.5. A Representation of Commonly Used Assessments for Education *(Cont.)*

TITLE	POPULATION	DESCRIPTION
Sensory Profile 2 (Dunn, 2014)	- Age: Birth–14 years - Appropriate to evaluate sensory processing in individuals in home, clinic, daycare, and school settings	Observation-based and self-report questionnaires used to identify sensory processing patterns that either support or create barriers to daily functioning. Scores correlate with 1 of 4 categories including Seeking/Seeker, Avoiding/Avoider, Sensitivity/Sensor, and Registration/Bystander.
Sensory Profile (Adult/Adolescent; Brown & Dunn, 2002)	- Age: 11–65 years - Appropriate for adolescents and adults to identify personal responses to sensory experiences and strategies to promote function	60-item questionnaire covering taste/smell, movement, visual, touch, activity level, and auditory experiences.
Sensory Processing Measure (SPM; Parham et al., 2007)	- Age: 5–12 years - Appropriate to evaluate behaviors related to sensory processing, praxis, and social participation in children across multiple settings	Observer-rated behavior scale that provides an overview of sensory functioning in multiple environments including the home, main classroom, and school environments.
Sensory Processing Measure–Preschool (Ecker & Parham, 2010)	- Age: 2–5 years - Appropriate to evaluate behaviors related to sensory processing, praxis, and social participation in children across multiple settings	Observer-rated behavior scale that provides an overview of sensory functioning in home and school or daycare environments.
Sensory Integration and Praxis Test (Ayres, 1989)	- Age: 4–8 years - Appropriate for children with sensory integrative and learning deficits	Standardized performance tests (17 subtests) are administered by trained or certified professional. Areas assessed include sensory processing, visual–spatial perception, coordination, and praxis. Scores can be used to identify the sensory integrative component of learning difficulties.
Test of Visual Perceptual Skills, 3rd Edition (TVPS-3; Martin, 2006)	- Age: 4–18.11 years - Appropriate to evaluate perceptual abilities without requiring motor abilities.	Consists of 7 subscales: visual discrimination, visual memory, spatial relationships, form constancy, sequential memory, figure-ground, and visual closure.
Test of Visual–Motor Skills, 3rd Edition, (TVMS–3; Martin, 2010)	- Age: 3–90+ years - Appropriate to assess visual perceptual, motor planning, or execution deficits	Test booklet includes a series of geometric designs of progressive difficulty. Can be used to differentiate visual–motor impairment from perceptual impairment when administered with the TVPS–3.
Developmental Test of Visual Perception, 3rd Edition (Hammill et al., 2013)	- Age: 4–12 years - Appropriate to use to identify visual perceptual skills, visual motor integration, degree of impairment, need for treatment, and progress toward goals	A flipbook that consists of 5 subtests including eye–hand coordination, copying, figure-ground, visual closure, and form constancy.
Canadian Occupational Performance Measure, 5th Edition (Law et al., 2019)	- Age: Various (as young as 7 years) - Appropriate for variety of conditions across developmental stages	Semi-structured interview used to gather information on self-perception of occupational performance and satisfaction in the areas of self-care, productivity, and leisure.
Hawaii Early Learning Profile (Furuno et al., 1994)	- Age: birth–3 years who are developmentally delayed - Appropriate to assess and screen general development in infants and toddlers with disabilities	Nonstandardized scale of items consisting of 685 developmental skills that highlight 6 areas: cognitive, language, gross motor, fine motor, social-emotional, and self-help.
Evaluation Tool of Children's Handwriting (Manuscript: ETCH–M, Cursive: ETCH–C; Amundson, 1995)	- Age: ETCH–M: Grades 1–3 ETCH–C: Grades 3–6 - Appropriate for children in education or clinic settings	Timed performance test that looks at speed and legibility of handwriting during writing activities similar to those required for school participation.

Source. Adapted from *Asher's Occupational Therapy Assessment Tools: An Annotated Index* (4th Ed.), edited by I. E. Asher, 2014, Bethesda, MD: AOTA Press. Used with permission.

EXHIBIT 24.3. Parent Perspective on Education Participation

Participation in school and the educational experience is primary to all children from a developmental and psychosocial perspective. This is especially true with children and adolescents with cancer because so many aspects of their everyday lived experiences are disrupted. Encouraging these children to continue participation at the highest level possible during active treatment and through survivorship is essential. However, it may be difficult for these children to prioritize education during the very taxing active treatment phase.

If an occupational therapist is involved from initial diagnosis and continues through all phases of treatment, then they are ideally positioned to assess for problems that may affect the child's participation in education. This can include issues such as hearing loss, peripheral neuropathies, cognitive deficits, fatigue, and more. The psychosocial impacts can be equally and, in some ways, even more influential on the child's level of engagement. If a child falls behind or becomes overburdened by makeup work, then feelings of frustration, anger, sadness, or anxiety can become associated with school. They can also begin to feel isolated because peer interaction can be limited by illness, isolation precautions, or treatment time. Occupational therapists have the unique opportunity to address both the physical and psychosocial issues that occur. By simultaneously recognizing the emergence and interplay of both of these aspects, an occupational therapist can make a difference in the child's physical ability to participate and boost their motivation to continue engagement during more difficult phases of treatment.

An occupational therapist's ability to recognize the physical and psychosocial deficits that affect education puts them in a position to further support the child through recommendations and referrals to psychology and social work at an early stage. Psychology can assist with emotional and psychosocial issues and complete neuropsychological testing when the occupational therapist detects cognitive deficits. Social work can educate children and parents on programs at the federal, state, and local levels that provide support and allow for service delivery within the schools and, in some cases, facilitate implementation. These additional services can be initiated earlier if occupational therapy is involved from initial diagnosis because they would be the service to recognize when the expertise of these other disciplines can help.

The role that the parents play in their child's education during and after treatment should be carefully considered. The emotional and psychosocial components involved in this population and their families are paramount and not always appropriately addressed. Every parent has to extend some level of discipline or encouragement to their child concerning educational expectations and homework. It can be a trying experience even when dealing with a healthy, typically developing child. The conflicting feelings and heartbreak felt when having to tell your child that they must sit and do homework after a day of treatment or medical tests can be overwhelming.

There is a constant balance that parents must maintain between keeping their child educationally on track and allowing them to engage in activities of their choice. It is often a balance that parents are left to manage on their own, leaving them with feelings of uncertainty as to whether they are getting it right. While it is hard for the child or adolescent to prioritize education because of their physical and emotional state, it can be equally difficult for parents to make it a priority when they are having thoughts that their child may not survive.

Different obstacles to participation develop during transitions and into survivorship. Parents often become versed in complicated medical terminology, treatments, and complications during the initial and active stages of treatment. When transitioning to survivor status, there are new challenges caused by the intensive treatment. These issues are usually addressed in the school, depending on the educational impact. At this time, parents move to new lessons in school coverage of therapy service and individualized education programs. Some of these lessons are hard learned and involve fighting for a child's right to services based on their needs. These rights and services vary significantly between states and school districts, so it is a continual learning process.

—*Dawn Linhardt, OTR/L, CLT, OTDS*, and mother of a pediatric cancer survivor. Used with permission.

---

education, early in the continuum of care. Occupational therapy practitioners are encouraged to identify needs and monitor transitions in late effects clinics and provide self-management strategies and environmental modification recommendations to improve participation (Berg et al., 2009). A literature review by Hay et al. (2015) identified barriers to meeting the needs of students after cancer treatment; these included lack of connectedness between educational and health systems, inadequacies in current legislation, and differences in classification systems. School-based occupational therapy practitioners are ideally positioned to collaborate with teachers, nurses, other school personnel, and families to develop an appropriate individualized education plan or 504 plan, if necessary, with specific strategies using assistive technology, accommodation recommendations, and environmental adaptation (Flegle & Edelbrock, 2019; Hay et al., 2015).

Current evidence supports occupational therapy approaches, including creation of peer support groups, establishment or restoration of performance skills negatively affected by cancer treatment, early intervention to prevent decline, and maintenance or modification to enhance education participation for cancer survivors (Berg et al., 2009;

Hay et al., 2015; Hwang et al., 2015; Willard et al., 2017). See Table 24.6 for additional activities to promote occupational participation in education across the life course.

SUMMARY

Client factors and performance limitations negatively affected by cancer and its treatment are well documented; however, gaps exist along the trajectory of cancer care and rehabilitation, limiting the potential for individuals to receive necessary services into survivorship. This is particularly true during the transition from receiving care in a medical environment to participating in an academic setting because of the lack of connection between these providers. Many side effects of cancer and its treatment are long term and cause barriers to education participation, thus lessening the overall well-being and independence of survivors. There is potential for the significant rise in cancer survivors to have a negative economic impact on the public (Baxter et al., 2017). Occupational therapy practitioners are called to identify needs early along the cancer care continuum and advocate for individuals in the education setting to receive the supportive services they need after a cancer diagnosis.

TABLE 24.6. Education: Activities to Promote Occupational Participation in Education Across the Lifespan

POPULATION	POTENTIAL ACTIVITIES
Children	▪ Promotion of activities that target handwriting, visual motor, visual perceptual, and strengthening activities. ▪ Close monitoring in children with history of chemotherapy-induced peripheral neuropathy to identify motor difficulties (De Luca et al., 2013). ▪ Collaboration with all members of the education and medical staff, including nurses, teachers, nutritionist, physical therapist, speech therapist, etc. (Hay et al., 2015). ▪ Use of hospital-based preschool services and increased parent education regarding the importance of emphasizing academic skills during treatment (e.g., access to academically focused technology, increased emphasis on reading, engagement in age-appropriate toys that focus on preacademic skills; Willard et al., 2017). ▪ Group-based intervention to target social-emotional and executive functioning skills (Willard et al., 2017). ▪ Designation of a school-hospital liaison (Moore et al., 2009; Upton & Eiser, 2006). ▪ Neurocognitive testing in survivors upon entering long-term follow-up (Edelmann et al., 2016). ▪ Identification of potential education needs upon evaluation in late effects or long-term follow-up clinic (Berg et al., 2009). ▪ Provide educational peer workshops including a forum for healthy classmates to ask questions and potentially prevent bullying (Hay et al., 2015; Moore et al., 2009).
Adolescents	▪ Self-management techniques to emphasize sense of empowerment and adaptability to late effects of cancer and treatment, thus maximizing autonomy during daily activities (Barlow et al., 2002; Stinson et al., 2012) ▪ Modification of activity demands related to team activities, school clubs, and sports to avoid exclusion (Berg et al., 2009). ▪ Work in consultation with teachers, physical education teacher, extracurricular faculty, and coaches to maximize participation in the school environment (Berg et al., 2009). ▪ Use of a designated coordinator to facilitate transitions back to the school setting, with increased education for teachers and staff (Pini et al., 2012). ▪ Use of mindfulness techniques to manage stress at school (Malboeuf-Hurtubise et al., 2016). ▪ Creation and usage of digital storytelling for adolescents to communicate with peers and family about experience of cancer and treatment in a nonthreatening manner (Wilson et al., 2016).
Adults	▪ Use a multidisciplinary approach to closely monitor during the transition from an academic or pediatric clinic setting to adult roles (Berg et al., 2009). ▪ Promote increased physical activity levels to decrease fatigue (Dalzell et al., 2017). ▪ Provide education on strategies to improve sleep quality, reduce anxiety and depression, and conserve energy to maximize endurance for education settings. ▪ Use of Skype or other technology when too tired to attend formal education setting or school. ▪ Exercise to reduce cancer-related fatigue and improve quality of sleep (Hunter et al., 2017). ▪ Education, problem-solving, and cognitive–behavioral therapy for management of cancer-related fatigue (Hunter et al., 2017). ▪ Cognitive strategies, assistive technology, and activity adaptation (Hwang et al., 2015).

REFERENCES

American Occupational Therapy Association. (2014). Occupational therapy practice framework: Domain and process (3rd ed.). *American Journal of Occupational Therapy, 68*(Suppl. 1), S1–S48. https://doi.org/10.5014/ajot.2014.682006

Americans with Disabilities Act. (2018). *Information and technical assistance on the Americans with Disabilities Act.* Retrieved from https://www.ada.gov/ada_title_II.htm

Amundson, S. J. (1995). *ETCH test kit: Evaluation tool of children's handwriting.* Homer, AL: OT Kids.

Amundson, S. J. (2004). *Evaluation tool for children's handwriting.* Homer, AK: O.T. Kids, Inc.

Asher, I. E. (2014). *Asher's occupational therapy assessment tools: An annotated index* (4th ed.). Bethesda, MD: AOTA Press.

Ayres, A. J. (1989). *Sensory integration and praxis tests.* Torrance, CA: Western Psychological Services.

Barlow, J., Wright, C., Sheasby, J., Turner, A., & Hainsworth, J. (2002). Self-management approaches for people with chronic conditions: A review. *Patient Education and Counseling, 48*(2), 177–187. https://doi.org/10.1016/S0738-3991(02)00032-0

Bashore, L., & Breyer, E. (2017). Educational and career goal attainments in young adult childhood cancer survivors. *Journal of Specialized Nursing, 22*(2), e12180. https://doi.org/10.1111/jspn.12180

Baxter, M. F., Newman, R., Longpré, S. M., & Polo, K. M. (2017). Occupational therapy's role in cancer survivorship as a chronic condition. *American Journal of Occupational Therapy, 71,* 7103090010. https://doi.org/10.5014/ajot.2017.713001

Berg, C., Neufeld, P., Harvey, J., Downes, A., & Hayashi, R. (2009). Late effects of childhood cancer, participation, and quality of life in adolescents. *Occupational Therapy Journal of Research: Occupation, Participation and Health, 29*(3), 116–124. https://doi.org/10.3928/15394492-20090611-04

Bowyer, P., Kramer, J., Ploszacj, A., Ross, M. Schwartz, O. Kielhofner, G., & Kramer, K. (2008). *Short Child Occupational Profile (SCOPE), Version 2.2.* Chicago: Model of Human Occupation Clearinghouse.

Brown, C., & Dunn, W. (2002). *Adolescent/Adult Sensory Profile.* San Antonio, TX: NCS Pearson.

Bruininks, R. H., & Bruininks, B. D. (2006). *Bruininks–Oseretsky test of motor proficiency* (2nd ed.). San Antonio, TX: NCS Pearson.

Cachioni, M., Ordonez, T. N., da Silva, T. B. L., Batistoni, S. S. T., Yassuda, M. S., Melo, R. C., . . . Lopes, A. (2014). Motivational factors and predictors for attending a continuing education program for older adults. *Educational Gerontology, 40,* 584–596. https://doi.org/10.1080/03601277.2013.802188

Cahill, S., & Bazyk, S. (2020). School-based occupational therapy. In J. Clifford O'Brien & H. Kuhaneck (Eds.), *Case-Smith's occupational therapy for children and adolescents* (8th ed., pp. 627–658). St. Louis: Elsevier Mosby.

Children's Oncology Group. (2013). Educational issues following treatment for childhood cancer. *Health Link: Healthy living after treatment for childhood cancer. Educational Issues, Version 4.0,* 1–4. Retrieved from https://nevaehskcc.org/downloads/educational_issues_Eng.pdf

Compas, B. E., Jaser, S. S., Reeslund, K., Patel, N., & Yarboi, J. (2017). Neurocognitive deficits in children with chronic health conditions. *American Psychologist, 72,* 326–338. https://doi.org/10.1037/amp0000042

Coster, W., Deeney, T., Haltiwanger, J., & Haley, S. M. (1998). *School Function Assessment.* San Antonio, TX: Pearson Education.

Dalzell, M. A., Smirnow, N., Sateren, W., Sintharaphone, A., Ibrahim, M., Mastroianni, L., & O'Brien, S. (2017). Rehabilitation and exercise oncology program: Translating research into a model of care. *Current Oncology, 24*(3), e191–e198. https://doi.org/10.3747/co.24.3498

Davies, P. L. (2012). Pediatric occupational therapy in the United States: Understanding laws, policies, and regulations for practice. In S. J. Lane & A. C. Bundy (Eds.), *Kids can be kids: A childhood occupations approach* (pp. 203–219). Philadelphia: F. A. Davis.

De Luca, C. R., McCarthy, M., Galvin, J., Green, J. L., Murphy, A., Knight, S., & Williams, J. (2013). Gross and fine motor skills in children treated for acute lymphoblastic leukemia. *Developmental Neurorehabilitation, 16*(3), 180–187. https://doi.org/10.3109/17518423.2013.771221

Dietz, A., Chen, Y., Yasui, Y., Ness, K., Hagood, J., Chow, E., . . . Mulrooney, D. A. (2016). Risk and impact of pulmonary complications in survivors of childhood cancer: A report from the Childhood Cancer Survivor Study. *Cancer, 122,* 3687–3696. https://doi.org/10.1002/cncr.30200

Diver, J. (2015). Hematologic and oncologic disorders, bone marrow transplant and graft-versus-host disease. In K. Reuter-Rice & B. Bolick (Eds.), *Pediatric acute care: A guide for interprofessional practice* (pp. 621–628). Burlington, MA: Jones & Bartlett.

Donnan, B. B., Webster, T., Wakefield, C. E., Dalla-Pozza, L., Alvaro, F., Lavoipierre, J., & Marshall, G. M. (2015). What about school? Educational challenges for children and adolescents with cancer. *Australian Educational and Developmental Psychologist, 32*(1), 23–40. https://doi.org/10.1017/edp.2015.9

Dunn, W. (2014). *Sensory Profile 2.* San Antonio, TX: NCS Pearson.

Ecker, C., & Parham, L. D. (2010). *SPM-P kit.* Torrance, CA: Western Psychological Services.

Edelmann, M. N., Daryani, V. M., Bishop, M. W., Liu, W., Brinkman, T. M., Stewart, C. F., . . . Krull, K. R. (2016). Neurocognitive and patient-reported outcomes in adult survivors of childhood osteosarcoma. *JAMA Oncology, 2*(2), 201–208. https://doi.org/10.1001/jamaoncol.2015.4398

Flegle, J. H., & Edelbrock, C. M. (2019). Best practices in supporting students with other health impairments. In G. Frolek Clark, J. E. Rioux, & B. E. Chandler (Eds.), *Best practices for occupational therapy in schools* (2nd ed., pp. 289–295). Bethesda, MD: AOTA Press.

Fleischer, A., & Howell, D. (2017). The experience of breast cancer survivors' participation in important activities during and after treatments. *British Journal of Occupational Therapy, 80*(8), 470–478. https://doi.org/10.1177/0308022617700652

Folio, M. R., & Fewell, R. R. (2000). *Peabody Developmental Motor Scales* (2nd ed.). Austin, TX: Pro-Ed.

Frolek Clark, G., Rioux, J. E., & Chandler, B. E. (Eds.). (2019). *Best practices for occupational therapy in schools* (2nd ed.). Bethesda, MD: AOTA Press.

Frolek Clark, G. J., & Schlabach, T. L. (2013). Systematic review of occupational therapy interventions to improve cognitive development in children ages birth–5 years. *American Journal of Occupational Therapy, 67,* 425–430. https://doi.org/10.5014/ajot.2013.006163

Furuno, S., O'Reilly, K. A., Hosaka, C. M., Inatsuka, T. T., Allman, T. A., & Zeisloft, B. (1994). *Hawaii Early Learning Profile.* Menlo Park, CA: VORT.

Gilchrist, L. S., & Tanner, L. (2013). The pediatric-modified total neuropathy score: A reliable and valid measure of chemotherapy-induced peripheral neuropathy in children with non-CNS cancers. *Support Cancer Care, 21*(3), 847–856. https://doi.org/10.1007/s00520-012-1591-8

Gurney, J. G., Tersak, J. M., Ness, K. K., Landier, W., Matthay, K. K., & Schmidt, M. L. (2007). Hearing loss, quality of life, and academic problems in long-term neuroblastoma survivors: A report from the children's oncology group. *Pediatrics, 120,* e1229–e1236. https://doi.org/10.1542/peds.2007-0178

Hammill, D. D., Pearson, N. A., & Voress, J. K. (2013). *Developmental Test of Visual Perception* (3rd ed.). Austin, TX: Pro-Ed.

Harman, J. L., Wise, J., & Willard, V. W. (2017). Early intervention for infants and toddlers: Applications for pediatric oncology. *Pediatric Blood & Cancer, 65,* e26921. https://doi.org/10.1002/pbc.26921

Hay, G. H., Nabors, M. L., Sullivan, A., & Zygmund, A. (2015). Students with pediatric cancer: A prescription for school success. *Physical Disabilities: Education and Related Services, 34*(2), 1–13. https://doi.org/10.14434/pders.v34i2.19643

Hilton, C. L. (2015). Interventions to promote social participation for children with mental health and behavioral disorders. In J. Case-Smith & J. Clifford O'Brien (Eds.), *Occupational therapy for children and adolescents* (7th ed., pp. 321–345). St. Louis: Elsevier.

Hunter, E. G., Gibson, R. W., Arbesman, M., & D'Amico, M. (2017). Systematic review of occupational therapy and adult cancer rehabilitation: Part 1: Impact of physical activity and symptom management interventions. *American Journal of Occupational Therapy, 71,* 7102100030p1. https://doi.org/10.5014/ajot.2017.023564

Hutchinson, A. D., Pfeiffer, P. M., & Wilson, C. (2017). Cancer-related cognitive impairment in children. *Supportive and Palliative Care, 11*(1), 70–75. https://doi.org/10.1097/SPC.0000000000000258

Hwang, E. J., Lokietz, N. C., Lozano, R. L., & Parke, M. A. (2015). Functional deficits and quality of life among cancer survivors: Implications for occupational therapy in cancer survivorship care. *American Journal of Occupational Therapy, 69,* 6906290010. https://doi.org/10.5014/ajot.2015.015974

Individuals With Disabilities Education Act of 1990, Pub. L. 101–476, renamed the Individuals With Disabilities Education Improvement Act, codified at 20 U.S.C. §§ 1400–1482.

Institute of Medicine & National Research Council. (2012). *From neurons to neighborhoods: An update: Workshop summary.* Washington, DC: The National Academies Press.

Kaldenberg, J. (2017). Visual perceptual dysfunction and low-vision rehabilitation. In A. Wagenfeld, J. Kaldenberg, & D. Honaker (Eds.), *Foundations of pediatric practice for the occupational therapy assistant* (2nd ed., pp. 249–262). Thorofare, NJ: SLACK.

Kentucky Protection and Advocacy. (2014). *504: A college/vocational school student's guide.* Retrieved from http://nebula.wsimg.com/c888fe932e54bc73dd6961be6125c060?AccessKey-Id=65CDDAA309ED09126F01&disposition=0&alloworigin=1

Kielhofner, G., Mallinson, T., Crawford, C., Nowak, M., Rigby, M., Henry, A., & Walens, D. (2004). *Occupational Performance History Interview-II (OPHI-II), Version 2.1.* Chicago: Model of Human Occupation Clearinghouse.

Kramer, J., ten Velden, M., Kafkes, A., Basu, S., Federico, J., & Kielhofner, G. (2014). *Child Occupational Self Assessment, Version 2.2.* Chicago: University of Illinois at Chicago.

Kuypers, L. (2018). *The Zones of Regulation®.* Minneapolis: Kuypers Consulting. Retrieved from http://www.zonesofregulation.com

Lafond, D. A., & Leach, D. D. (2014). The parent's role. In R.I. Hoffman & S. E. Smith (Eds.), *A parent's guide to enhancing quality of life in children with cancer* (pp. 13–26). Beltsville, MD: American Childhood Cancer Organization.

Law, M., Baptiste, S., Carswell, A., McColl, M. A., Polatajko, H., & Pollock, N. (2019). *Canadian Occupational Performance Measure* (5th ed., rev.). Altona, Man., Canada: COPM, Inc.

Leukemia & Lymphoma Society. (2013). *Learning and living with cancer: Advocating for your child's educational needs.* Rye Brook, NY: Author.

Malboeuf-Hurtubise, C., Achille, M., Muise, L., Beauregard-Lacroix, R., Vadnais, M., & Lacourse, E. (2016). A mindfulness-based meditation pilot study: Lessons learned on acceptability and feasibility in adolescents with cancer. *Journal of Child and Family Studies, 25,* 1168–1177. https://doi.org/10.1007/s10826-015-0299-z

Mandich, A., Polatajko, H. J., Miller, L., & Baum, C. (2004). *Pediatric Activity Card Sort.* Ottawa: Canadian Association of Occupational Therapists.

Martin, N. A. (2006). *Test of Visual-Perceptual Skills* (3rd ed.). Novato, CA: Academic Therapy Publications.

Martin, N. A. (2010). *Test of Visual-Motor Skills-3.* Novato, CA: Academic Therapy Publications.

Moore, J. B., Kaffenberger, C., Goldberg, P., Oh, K. M., & Hudspeth, R. (2009). School reentry for children with cancer: Perceptions of nurses, school personnel, and parents. *Journal of Pediatric Oncology Nursing, 26*(2), 86–99. https://doi.org/10.1177/1043454208328765

Myers, C. T., Case-Smith, J., & Cason, J. (2015). Early intervention. In J. Case-Smith & J. Clifford O'Brien (Eds.), *Occupational therapy for children and adolescents* (7th ed., pp. 636–663). St. Louis: Elsevier Mosby.

Ness, K. K., Hudson, M. M., Ginsberg, J. P., Nagarajan, R., Kaste, S. C., Marina, N., . . . Gurney, J. G. (2009). Physical performance limitations in the Childhood Cancer Survivor Study cohort. *Journal of Clinical Oncology, 27,* 2382–2389. https://doi.org/10.1200/JCO.2008.21.1482

Olsen, J. Z. (2018). *Letters and Numbers for Me Teacher's Guide.* Cabin John, Maryland: Learning Without Tears.

Parham, L. D., & Ecker, C. (2007). *SPM comprehensive kit.* Torrance, CA: Western Psychological Services.

Parham, L. D., Ecker, C., Miller Kuhaneck, H., Henry, D. A. & Glennon, T. J. (2007). *Sensory Processing Measure (SPM): Manual.* Torrance, CA: Western Psychological Services.

Pini, S., Hugh-Jones, S., & Gardner, P. H. (2012). What effect does a cancer diagnosis have on the educational engagement and school life of teenagers? A systematic review. *Psycho-Oncology, 21*(7), 685–694. https://doi.org/10.1002/pon.2082

Robinson, L. L., Armstrong, G. T., Boice, J, D., Chow, E. J., Davies, S. M., Donaldson, S. S., . . . Zeltzer, L. K. (2009). The Childhood Cancer Survivor Study: A National Cancer Institute-supported resource for outcome and intervention research. *Journal of Clinical Oncology, 27*(14), 2308–2318. https://doi.org/10.1200/JCO.2009.22.3339

Sabarre, C. L., Rassekh, S. R., & Zwicker, J. G. (2014). Vincristine and fine motor function of children with acute lymphoblastic leukemia. *Canadian Journal of Occupational Therapy, 81,* 256–264. https://doi.org/10.1177/0008417414539926

Section 504 of the Rehabilitation Act of 1973, as amended, 29 U.S.C. § 794 (2008).

Sodergren, S. C., Husson, O., Robinson, J., Rohde, G. E. Tomaszewska, I. M., Vivat, B., . . . Darlington, A-S. (2017). Systematic review of the health-related quality of life issues facing adolescents and young adults with cancer. *Quality of Life Research, 26,* 1659–1672. https://doi.org/10.1007/s11136-017-1520-x

Sparrow, J., Brennan, R., Mao, S., Ness, K. K., Rodriguez-Galindo, C., Wilson, M., & Qaddoumi, I. (2016). Participation in an occupational therapy referral program for children with retinoblastoma. *Journal of Pediatric Rehabilitation Medicine, 9*(2), 117–124. https://doi.org/10.3233/PROM-160372

Stinson, J. N., Sing, L., Gupta, A., White, M. E. Jibb, L. A., Dettmer, E., . . . Baker, N. (2012). Disease self-management needs of adolescents with cancer: Perspectives of adolescents with cancer and their parents and healthcare providers. *Journal of Cancer Survivorship, 6,* 278–286. https://doi.org/10.1007/s11764-012-0222-1

Strauser, D., Klosky, J. L., Brinkman, T. M., Wong, A. W. K., Chan, F., Lanctot, J., . . . Ness, K. K. (2015). Career readiness in adult survivors of childhood cancer: A report from the St. Jude Lifetime Cohort Study. *Journal of Cancer Survivorship, 9*(1), 20–29. https://doi.org/10.1007/s11764-014-0380-4

Swinth, Y. (2014). Education. In B. A. B. Schell, G. Gillen, & M. E. Scaffa (Eds.), *Willard & Spackman's occupational therapy* (12th ed., pp. 653–677). Baltimore: Lippincott Williams & Wilkins.

Upton, P., & Eiser, C. (2006). School experiences after treatment for a brain tumor. *Child: Care, Health and Development, 32*(1), 9–17. https://doi.org/10.1111/j.1365-2214.2006.00569.x

U.S. Department of Education. (2018). *Protecting students with disabilities.* Retrieved from https://www2.ed.gov/about/offices/list/ocr/504faq.html

U.S. Department of Education. (2020). *IDEA: Individuals with Disabilities Education Act.* Retrieved from https://sites.ed.gov/idea/regs/b/a/300.8/c/9

Weiner, L., & Sourkes, B. (2014). Communication. In R. I. Hoffman & S. E. Smith (Eds.), *A parent's guide for enhancing quality of life in children with cancer* (pp. 85-106). Beltsville, MD: American Childhood Cancer Organization.

Wilcock, A. A., & Hocking, C. (2015). Defining occupation in relation to health. In A. A. Wilcock & C. Hocking (Eds.), *An occupational perspective of health* (3rd ed., pp. 117–146). Thorofare, NJ: SLACK.

Willard, V. W., Cox, L. E., Russell, K. M., Kenney, A., Jurbergs, J., Molnar, A. E., & Harman, J. L. (2017). Cognitive and psychosocial functioning of preschool-aged children with cancer. *Journal of Developmental and Behavioral Pediatrics, 38,* 628–645. https://doi.org/10.1097/DBP.0000000000000512

Wilson, D. K., Hutson, S. P., Hall, J. M., & Anderson, K. M. (2016). Examining the digital story created by an adolescent with cancer: Insights and ideas from a case story. *Open Journal of Nursing, 6,* 426–434. https://doi.org/10.4236/ojn.2016.65044

World Health Organization. (1986). *Ottawa Charter for Health Promotion.* Geneva, Switzerland: Author. Retrieved from http://www.who.int/healthpromotion/conferences/previous/ottawa/en/

Work

25

Brent Braveman, OTR, PhD, FAOTA; Robin Newman, OTD, OT, OTR, CLT, FAOTA; Kathleen Lyons, ScD, OTR/L; and Mackenzi Pergolotti, PhD, OTR/L

LEARNING OBJECTIVES

After completing this chapter, readers should be able to
- Describe the development of work as an area of occupation across the lifespan;
- Identify and describe factors that influence the ability of cancer survivors to continue to work or to return to work;
- Describe components of an evidence-based approach to assist cancer survivors to continue to work or to return to work; and
- Identify resources on cancer and work for cancer survivors, employers, and health care providers.

KEY TERMS AND CONCEPTS

- Assessment of Work Performance
- Environment
- Financial toxicity
- Habituation
- Interests
- Model of Human Occupation
- Performance capacity
- Volition
- Work
- Work disability
- Work Environment Impact Scale
- Worker Role Interview
- Work values

INTRODUCTION

Work is an occupation that often begins in adolescence and then consumes much of adult life, extending into older adulthood for many. Cancer and its treatments can be disruptive to both the development of work skills in adolescents and young adults and to working in adults and older adults. According to the U.S. Bureau of Labor Statistics (BLS; 2019), the average American who is employed full-time works 44 hours per week, or 8.8 hours per day. A 2014 national Gallup Poll put the average number at 47 hours per week, or 9.4 hours per day, with many saying they work 50 hours per week (Ward, 2017). However, long work days are not unique to the United States—it ranks 17th out of 38 countries for average hours worked annually, at 1,786 (McPhillips, 2016; Organization for Economic Cooperation and Development [OECD], 2018). In contrast, Mexico, where the work week is limited to 48 hours by law, ranks first, at 2,148 (McPhillips, 2016; OECD, 2018).

Cancer and its treatments can have a dramatic impact on the ability of people to develop typical work habits and skills in childhood and adolescence, develop the worker role in adolescence and young adulthood, or enter work or continue working in adulthood or older adulthood. Although work issues for cancer survivors have recently received more attention, much opportunity exists for the development of and improvement in work-related services for these survivors (Newman et al., 2019). Occupational therapy practitioners can play a critical role in supporting cancer survivors by promoting participation and productivity in the occupation of work.

WORK AS OCCUPATION

Broadly, **work** as an occupation can include paid work and volunteer work (Braveman, 2012). In citing Christiansen and Townsend (2010), the *Occupational Therapy Practice Framework: Domain and Process* (3rd ed.; American Occupational Therapy Association, 2014) defines *work* as "labor or exertion; to make, construct, manufacture, form, fashion, or shape objects; to organize, plan, or evaluate services or processes of living or governing; committed occupations that are performed with or without financial reward" (Christiansen & Townsend, p. 423). *Work* can be conceptualized as a job, a career, or a "calling." It can be primarily either physical or cognitive in nature or involve a combination of the two, and it can be performed in a solitary manner or require occasional or frequent social interaction with others.

WORK ACROSS THE LIFESPAN

Developmental perspectives on careers recognize that vocational development constitutes a lifelong process from infancy through childhood, adolescence, adulthood, and old age that is affected by both personal and contextual factors (Hartung et al., 2005).

Children

From early childhood, children develop the basic skills to participate in social roles and to interact with others as they learn to navigate the various contexts and environments in which they take part. For young children, involvement in family activities (e.g., helping with meal preparation, grocery shopping, and household chores) not only prepares them to be responsible adults in general but also provides them an opportunity to develop basic work skills and habits (Braveman, 2012). Children also learn about work through observation of others, and they begin to understand the connection between work and identity, as illustrated in the simple question, "What do you want to be when you grow up?"

In middle and late childhood, children are exposed to the logistical issues of working, including schedules; work demands; and the basic nature of work expectations and social interactions with subordinates, peers, and bosses. This exposure happens as they watch parents, siblings, teachers and others involved in various jobs and forms of work. They are also exposed to work through television, social media, and clasroom activities. Fantasy about the exciting nature of occupations such as police officer, firefighter, or astronaut is tempered with the understanding that jobs require hard work, entail maintenance of a schedule, and involve demands that compete with other roles such as parent or spouse.

Adolescents

Adolescents begin to develop more advanced awareness and understanding of personal aptitudes, abilities, and interests and a more accurate sense of self-efficacy and personal agency (Braveman, 2012). Adolescence is typically a time of increasing responsibility and independence to explore the world. Exposure to positive or negative role models shapes adolescents' understanding of the world of work and can influence the assumptions that they have about working.

What is considered typical involvement in paid work during mid- and late adolescence varies greatly around the world. Whereas it is common in industrialized nations for adolescents to begin paid work in part-time jobs outside of the home, those in developing nations may struggle to attend school and be expected to contribute to family sustenance through farming or other activities. Youth from poor and working-class backgrounds are also more likely to take on greater household and financial responsibilities and have more adultlike interactions with adults than their more advantaged peers do (Benson & Elder, 2011). In the United States, late adolescence is often marked as a transition to full-time work or to continued education in a college or university or in a trade or technical school.

Young Adults

Young adulthood is typically the period when people transition to involvement in work as a primary means of supporting themselves, providing for their own housing and food, and meeting other needs. Schwartz et al. (2005) noted that young adult identity as a level of psychosocial maturation focuses on the psychological task of establishing a stable and viable identity through the capacity to adapt to changing demands, including the demands of work. Young adults begin to crystalize their identity as workers as they experience successes and failures and face firsthand the realities of working. Young adults also must learn how to balance work and other roles that are frequently assumed during young adulthood, including those of spouse or parent.

Stone et al. (2017) described how a life course perspective can be helpful in understanding cancer and work:

> A life course perspective on cancer can advance understanding of the unique ways cancer affects young adults. Cancer survivors encounter a variety of work experiences such as changes in responsibilities, decreased capacity to work, and perhaps job loss. Work ability is a complex concept that changes over time as a new balance between job demands and personal capacity is established. (p. 766)

Stone et al. also noted that working young adults with a cancer history may spend more years living with lasting effects of cancer or its treatment and experience different types of late effects than survivors diagnosed with cancer at older ages. The work-related issues for young adult cancer survivors during a career trajectory are complex, with physical and psychosocial implications. For example, these young adults may experience delays in obtaining education and employment as a result of their cancer diagnosis and treatment.

Middle Adulthood

During middle adulthood, work can consume much of people's focus and energy. In addition, people continue to face the challenges of balancing work with other occupations. Adults in their 30s, 40s, and 50s may feel the added pressure of caring for their parents in addition to their children. Midlife is a time when stresses involving multiple role demands or financial pressures may cluster and take a greater toll on physical health and psychosocial well-being (Aldwin & Levenson, 2001; Almeida & Horn, 2004; Lachman et al., 2014). Evidence also suggests that middle adulthood is commonly a point in the lifespan at which life satisfaction, including work satisfaction, may be at its lowest (Blanchflower & Oswald, 2008; Clark & Oswald, 2006; Stone et al., 2010; Ulloa et al., 2013).

Stressors felt during middle adulthood can be greatly amplified with the onset of disease, such as cancer, or disability. Some adults may reassess expectations regarding work and may choose to make career changes, whereas others may recommit to their current career or job. Some may perceive that they are stuck in work they find dissatisfying but have few options for change. Satisfaction with work has often been correlated with the likelihood of continuing to work during or returning to work after illness or injury (Heinesen et al., 2017; Islam et al., 2014).

Older Adults

The U.S. Census Bureau (2018) projects that by 2030 approximately 20% of the U.S. workforce will be older than age 65 years. According to the BLS (2017),

About 40 percent of people ages 55 and older were working or actively looking for work in 2014. That number, known as a labor force participation rate, is expected to increase fastest for the oldest segments of the population—most notably, people ages 65 to 74 and 75 and older—through 2024. In contrast, participation rates for most other age groups in the labor force aren't projected to change much over the 2014–24 decade. (p. 1)

Reasons for continued employment in older adulthood are varied but include financial necessity, a sense of enjoyment and fulfillment from work, and a desire to maintain social contact. The number of older adults who continue to work has increased more than at any time since the turn of the century, and according to the Pew Research Center (2016), they are spending more time on the job.

Health status and functional status vary widely in older adults, and functional status directly affects ability to work. The older population consists of an extremely heterogeneous group of people—the older the age group, the greater the variation found in cognition, physical and sensory function, and social engagement (Santoni et al., 2015). Colón-Emeric et al. (2013) noted the critical impact of comorbidities on functional status and disability in older adults:

> The severity of disability is determined by physical impairments caused by underlying medical conditions, and by external factors such as social support, financial support, and the environment. When multiple health conditions are present, they often result in greater disability than expected because the patient's ability to compensate for one problem may be affected by comorbid conditions. (p. 388)

Because cancer is a disease of aging to a large extent, we can expect that many older adult cancer survivors will be concerned about work in some capacity.

Meaning of Work

The meaning of work varies from person to person—some may see work primarily as a means of income, whereas others may derive great satisfaction and a strong sense of personal identity from their work. The centrality of work in people's lives can be heavily influenced by *work values*, and work values have been found to be stable across the lifespan. Kuron et al. (2015) cited a meta-analysis by Jin and Rounds (2012) that found that, except for the precareer school-to-work transition from ages 18 to 22, work values are "fairly stable" through the lifespan (p. 995). Overall, intrinsic work values (e.g., altruism, enjoyment) increased during the precareer stage and then slightly decreased, staying "relatively stable" through the lifespan (p. 995). However, extrinsic work values (e.g., economic reward, positive feedback) decreased during the precareer stage and then increased during entry to the workforce, staying "somewhat stable" through the lifespan (p. 995).

CANCER AND WORK

The significant impact that cancer and its treatments have on occupational performance and participation are documented throughout this book. Fatigue, cancer-related cognitive impairment, pain, chemotherapy-induced peripheral neuropathy, and the psychosocial effects of cancer can negatively affect the capacity for work. Moreover, as noted by Newman et al. (2019), "Reduced engagement in recreational activities, sexual activities, work, and daily activities can persist years after cancer treatment, even after physical impairments have resolved" (p. 1). Yet, many cancer survivors wish to continue to work either because of the meaning and satisfaction they find in this form of occupation or because of financial reasons. Cancer can cause severe financial strain, and many cancer survivors perceive the need to continue to work during their treatment or to return to work as quickly as possible. *Financial toxicity* is a term that describes the financial burdens of cancer survivors receiving treatment (Zafar & Abernethy, 2013). For example, cancer survivors are 2.65 times more likely to declare personal bankruptcy than people without a cancer diagnosis (Ramsey et al., 2013).

An increasing amount of evidence about the impact of cancer on the ability to continue to work or to return to work has been presented, with mixed results. Many studies that have investigated the negative effects of cancer on work have found that, in fact, the majority of cancer survivors return to work (Heisesen et al., 2018). Spelten et al. (2002) found in a review of the literature of factors that influence return to work (RTW) in cancer survivors that the rate of RTW varied from 30% to 93%, with a mean rate of 62%. However, other studies have confirmed that cancer is likely to reduce the probability of being employed, increase the probability of receiving a disability pension, and decrease earnings and wages (Dahl et al., 2019; Heinesen et al., 2018; Paltrinieri et al., 2018).

One reason for these mixed results may be because the impact of cancer and its treatments on work can be highly variable depending on the type of cancer and its staging. For example, Verdonck-de Leeuw et al. (2010) found that of 53 patients who were employed at the time of diagnosis of head and neck cancer, 44 returned to work (83%): 28 to the same work, 7 to adapted work, and 9 to other work. Median time for RTW was 6 months (range: 0–24 months), and 71% of the patients returned to work within 6 months after treatment. In this study, 32 patients (38%) with head and neck cancer were not working at the time of diagnosis, which was significantly associated with increased age and lower education level. Roelen et al. (2011) examined cancer survivors with breast, genital, gastrointestinal, lung, skin, or blood cancer selected from an occupational health register. Employees with lung cancer had the longest duration of sickness absence, with only 45% returning to work full-time 2 years after diagnosis compared with 88% of employees with genital cancer and 87% of employees with skin cancer.

Another reason for the mixed results may be that the variation in the severity of cancer and its treatment has variable effects on the identity of cancer patients (Rasmussen & Elverdam, 2008). As cancer affects a survivor's body, appearance, energy level, and ability to concentrate and causes a variety of symptoms such as fatigue or pain, survivors may be less likely to see themselves as workers. In addition, the everyday experience of work can provide structure, satisfaction, and contentment, contributing to a sense of identity. Cancer disrupts this everyday experience and can result in negative changes in identity (Rasmussen & Elverdam, 2008). Work is seen as a way to improve the quality of life (QoL) and as a source of social and emotional support in the face of illness such as cancer (Frazier et al., 2009). In addition, a metasynthesis of qualitative research suggested the need to focus on person-centered employment goals because goals vary across time and individuals (Wells et al., 2013).

There is no doubt that cancer can negatively affect the development of and participation in the occupation of work. However, although cancer is always a significant and life-altering event, not all cancers result in significant functional impairment. Even so, cancer survivors often struggle with multiple impairments. For example, a recent study of women with advanced breast cancer found that the average number of physical impairments was 3.2 (Lyons et al., 2019). Cancer can also cause great fear about the loss of health insurance if a cancer survivor is forced to stop working, and there is great variety in policies, depending on the workplace and health insurance (Nachreiner et al., 2011). Much of the research on cancer and work has been carried out in European countries. Because the intersection of health insurance policies, health care insurance, and public policies regarding work and income support greatly affects people who are injured or ill, more research on these issues is needed in the United States.

RETURN TO WORK

A large body of research literature describes the range of factors commonly shown to predict RTW after injury or illness, and most factors apply across multiple diseases and disabilities (Snippen et al., 2019; Steenstra et al., 2017; Stergiou-Kita et al., 2014; White et al., 2019). Factors commonly identified include those related to the person (e.g., identity, self-efficacy, work satisfaction, work capacity, motivation, perceived financial stress), the illness or the injury (e.g., symptom severity, type of disease or disability), the social environment (e.g., support or pressure from friends, families, and medical caregivers), and the work environment (e.g., relationships with supervisors and peers, type of work and work demands, flexibility and accommodations).

Most predictive models of RTW suggest that typically a combination of factors must be considered (McGirt et al., 2015; Schultz et al., 2004; Vooijs et al., 2015). Descriptions of effective and comprehensive work rehabilitation programs emphasize a multifactorial approach that addresses the full range of person factors, illness factors, and context and environmental factors (Cancelliere et al., 2016; Gupta et al., 2016; Kamper et al., 2015; McGill, 2015). Although predictive models can identify the combination of factors most likely to predict RTW at the population level, it is difficult to predict how they will influence an individual worker.

For example, income may predict an increased likelihood for RTW at the population level because concern about financial matters for those earning higher incomes makes them more likely to return to work (Giummarra et al., 2017). However, in individual cases, income can be mediated by other factors such as perceiving an opportunity to be a stay-at-home parent or to spend more time with children as highly desirable. Other factors, such as perceiving injustice or being treated unfairly such as the perception of being discriminated against due to a cancer diagnosis, might change individual outcomes. These variations highlight the importance of having a skilled, interprofessional team that provides a comprehensive and customized evaluation and intervention plan with each person. Occupational therapy practitioners are a critical member of this interprofessional team.

RTW INTERVENTIONS FOR CANCER SURVIVORS

The literature, including scoping reviews and comprehensive literature reviews, documenting work interventions for cancer survivors has slowly increased. Bilodeau et al. (2017) conducted a scoping review of RTW interventions for breast cancer survivors and found a wide variance in interventions to assist survivors to return to work. They noted that only one intervention referred to a theory linked to RTW. Forty-four percent of the interventions only provided educational information on RTW, such as an information booklet or individual or group sessions. Only 38% of the interventions were work-directed and offered other activities, such as coordination of services and information, as well as instructions for drawing up an RTW plan. Most of the interventions were provided by health care professionals. Interventions took place during the survivorship period (75%), at the hospital (44%), or an external rehabilitation center (38%).

De Boer et al. (2015) reported results of a Cochrane database search of randomized controlled trials of the effectiveness of psychoeducational, vocational, physical, medical, or multidisciplinary interventions that enhance RTW in patients with cancer. The primary outcome was RTW measured as either RTW rate or sick leave duration at a 12-month follow-up. The secondary outcome was QoL. They found that multidisciplinary interventions involving physical, psycho educational, or vocational components were more successful in promoting RTW in cancer patients than care as usual. QoL was similar. Psychoeducational, physical, and medical interventions were only equally successful in facilitating RTW as usual care.

OCCUPATIONAL THERAPY THEORETICAL PERSPECTIVES ON WORK AND OCCUPATIONAL DYSFUNCTION

The role of occupational therapy in addressing work, **work disability** (i.e., leaving the labor force or working at a lower level of function prior to becoming ill), RTW, and work as an occupation is well established. Occupational therapy's involvement in work-related practice can be traced to the roots of the profession and the *moral treatment era,* when harsh treatments such as regular bleeding and being placed in chains were replaced with involvement in occupations such as agriculture, tailoring, shoemaking, and sewing (Ross, 2007). Braveman (2019) noted that today occupational therapy practitioners provide work related interventions in a wide variety of settings across the globe. Examples of such settings include pre-employment screening, alternative employment for persons with developmental disabilities, transitional services for adolescents and young adults, supported employment in mental health, employer consultation for job and ergonomic analysis as well as compliance with the Americans with Disabilities Act (ADA; [P. L. 101-336]), onsite services in the workplace, vocational habilitation settings for persons who need to develop work skills and vocational rehabilitation programs in clinics and in the workplace to help persons return to work. (p. 411)

Some occupational therapy investigators have explored the use of occupational therapy conceptual practice models and the effectiveness of occupational therapy intervention to help people with various illnesses or disabilities continue working or to return to work. Although many of these efforts have focused on single diagnostic groups, were completed as requirements for a doctoral study, or had low participant numbers, it is a beginning. For example, Wisenthal (2015) used the Canadian Model of Occupational Performance and Engagement (CMOP–E; Townsend & Polatajko, 2013) to examine the theoretical underpinnings of a cognitive work hardening intervention. Fitzpatrick (2015) also used the CMOP–E to guide development of a RTW program for people with traumatic hand injury.

Desiron (2016) studied RTW in patients with breast cancer with the objective of developing an occupational therapy intervention to bridge the gap between health care and work. He found that three occupational therapy conceptual practice models met at least three of the following criteria:

- Is an occupational therapy model
- Is commonly used in adult rehabilitation
- Provides tools and instruments concerning RTW
- Addresses RTW in breast cancer survivors
- Has been validated in breast cancer.

These models were the **Model of Human Occupation** (MOHO; Kielhofner, 2008), the CMOP–E (Townsend & Polatajko, 2013), and the Person–Environment–Occupation–Performance Model (Law et al., 1996). He concluded that of these models, the MOHO was the most relevant, but adaptations were necessary to enhance its usability in RTW in breast cancer survivors.

The MOHO emphasizes that all occupational behavior (and in this case, work behavior) is always a result of the interaction of four elements, or constructs:

1. *Volition:* The pattern of thoughts and feelings about oneself as an actor in one's world that occur as one anticipates, chooses, experiences and interprets what one does.
2. *Habituation:* Internalized readiness to exhibit consistent patterns of behavior guided by habits and roles and fitted into the characteristic of routine temporal, physical, and social environments.
3. *Performance capacity:* The ability to do things provided by the status of underlying objective physical and mental components and corresponding subjective experience.
4. *Environment:* The physical and mental components and social features of the specific context in which one

performs an activity that impacts what one does and how it is done. (Braveman, 2012, p. 242)

A single factor alone usually does not sufficiently account for work failure or success. Consequently, the key to understanding how any person performs and experiences their work is to examine the intersection of that person's volition, habituation, and performance capacity with the physical and social environment.

Braveman (1999) conducted a review of research literature to determine whether empirical support existed for the theoretical arguments of the MOHO. This review involved 44 predictive studies in the area of work disability published over the previous 25 years. The review found that several predictive factors correspond with elements of the model, lending partial support for the theory. None of the factors most commonly cited as predictive of RTW or long-term disability were found to contradict the basic assertions of the model.

Exhibit 25.1 outlines the relationship between MOHO constructs and construct components to factors commonly identified as predictive of RTW. The MOHO was used as the theoretical model for two programs in Chicago designed to help people with HIV/AIDS return to work or other productive life roles with positive results. These programs are of interest because many people living with HIV/AIDS face many of the same challenges as cancer survivors, including fatigue, neuropathy, mild to severe cognitive impairment, pain, and issues around disclosure of their illness. The first program was vocational and was delivered at two outpatient locations. It evaluated the effectiveness of an occupational therapy intervention and found that the RTW rate for program completers was 66.7% (Kielhofner et al., 2004). The second program, Enabling Self-Determination for People Living With HIV/AIDS, was delivered at four assisted living facilities. Participants in the model intervention group showed significantly higher levels of productive participation, and an odds ratio of >3 reflected that participants were at least twice as likely to be productive at 3, 6, and 9 months post-intervention (Kielhofner et al., 2008).

Other efforts have explored applying MOHO to the problem of work dysfunction through assessments designed for workers with injuries or disabilities, including the Worker Role Interview (WRI; Braveman et al., 2005), the Work Environment Impact Scale (WEIS; Moore-Corner et al., 1998), and the Assessment of Work Performance (AWP; Sandqvist et al., 2010). The complexity of work disability cannot be overemphasized. Although assessment of each person is necessary, it is not sufficient to understand work dysfunction. Occupational therapy practitioners must recognize that structural factors beyond a client's immediate control and the environment shape occupational possibilities and occupational engagement (Gerlach et al., 2018).

FACTORS THAT MAY CONTRIBUTE TO OCCUPATIONAL DYSFUNCTION IN WORK

A wide range of factors have been shown to influence the capacity to work or return to work, including person factors, illness or injury factors, and contextual and

EXHIBIT 25.1.	The Relationship Between Model of Human Occupation Constructs and Construct Components to Factors Commonly Identified as Predictive of Return to Work	

MODEL CONSTRUCTS AND CONSTRUCT COMPONENTS	CONSTRUCT COMPONENTS	FACTORS COMMONLY IDENTIFIED AS PREDICTIVE OF RETURN TO WORK
Volition	Personal causation	<ul><li>Level of perceived disability</li><li>Perceived control over environment</li><li>Educational level</li><li>Perception of fault for injury</li><li>Age</li></ul>
	Values	<ul><li>Gender</li><li>Culture</li></ul>
	Interests	<ul><li>Job satisfaction before injury</li></ul>
Habituation	Roles	<ul><li>Work status (e.g., light duty vs. nonworking)</li></ul>
	Habits	<ul><li>Time at job before injury</li><li>Attendance record at work before injury</li></ul>
Performance capacity	Objective	<ul><li>Nature and severity of injury</li><li>Surgery history</li><li>Diagnosis</li></ul>
	Subjective	<ul><li>Perceived level of pain</li></ul>
Environment	Social groups	<ul><li>Supervisor interaction</li><li>Peer interaction</li><li>Work environment and work stress</li></ul>

environmental factors. For example, Cancelliere et al.'s (2016) extensive systematic review of studies and factors affecting RTW after injury or illness found that common factors associated with positive RTW outcomes were higher education and socioeconomic status, higher self-efficacy and optimistic expectations for recovery and RTW, lower severity of the injury or illness, RTW coordination, and multidisciplinary interventions that included the workplace and stakeholders. Common factors associated with negative RTW outcomes were older age, being female, higher pain or disability, depression, higher physical work demands, previous sick leave and unemployment, and activity limitations.

The literature that describes the factors that contribute to occupational dysfunction in work in cancer survivors is similar to literature for other illnesses and injuries such as back injury, cumulative trauma injuries, and HIV/AIDS. In their qualitative study of cancer survivors with various diagnoses, Duijts, van Egmond et al. (2017) provided a review of the multiple factors that must be considered in examining work and work dysfunction for RTW in cancer survivors:

- Physical (e.g., fatigue)
- Sociodemographic (e.g., age)
- Work-related (e.g., type of contract, flexibility, attitude of employer and colleagues, counseling from occupational physician)
- Psychosocial (e.g., concerns about prognosis, social network influences)
- Financial.

In addition, the participating cancer survivors considered employer accommodations, fatigue, and a positive attitude in life to be the most influential factors for RTW.

To appropriately understand cancer survivors who are experiencing work-related occupational dysfunction,

occupational therapy practitioners must assume a comprehensive approach that recognizes all of the factors at play. Raque-Bogdan et al. (2015) found in a study of young breast cancer survivors that cancer-related work challenges faced by these survivors fell into four major categories:

1. Deciding whether to continue working
2. Managing potential consequences of disclosure
3. Determining how cancer symptoms and side effects affect work
4. Managing workload and work schedule during treatment.

Client Factors

Research on RTW for people with a range of injuries and disabilities show that client factors play a significant role in the likelihood that they will continue to work or return to work (Donker-Cools et al., 2016; Schultz & Gatchel, 2016; Steenstra et al., 2017). Several nonmodifiable factors have been shown to negatively correlate with RTW for cancer survivors, including demographic factors (e.g., age), disease factors (e.g., cancer site), and medical factors (e.g., invasiveness of treatment; Courneya et al., 2007). Although these factors are nonmodifiable in themselves, occupational therapy practitioners can help cancer survivors moderate their impact on the work experience. For example, they can provide strategies to manage pain or other symptoms that occur in response to invasive treatments. They can also provide education and consultation on identifying reasonable accommodations under ADA that might support RTW.

Values and interests

The interaction of work values and injury or disability is very complex. At first it might appear that people who have a greater valuation of work will generally put forth more effort to return to work. Although true in many instances, other scenarios are possible. For example, people who strongly value work but are removed from work as a result of injury or acquired disability may experience great stress, devalue themselves, and be vulnerable to depression (Dorland et al., 2018; Isaksson et al., 2016).

Conversely, people with a very strong value of work may have a tendency to overlook limitations and be at greater risk to overexert and suffer injury or setbacks. People who strongly value a particular job or kind of work may have more difficulty coping with job modifications or a change in job tasks, position, or line of work. Alfano et al. (2017) noted that individuals experiencing distress are more likely to be unemployed or have adverse work outcomes and in return, unemployed patients report higher rates of psychosocial distress.

Sun et al. (2017) found in an investigation of RTW among breast cancer survivors that "for some, return to work may serve as a way to move forward, out of a 'sick role' and back into a sense of normalcy. Others may question whether the effort needed to return to work is worth it or search for the meaning of returning to work after experiencing a life-threatening illness" (p. 713). In addition, it is important to recognize that some cancer survivors will not perceive that continuing to work is a choice, regardless of the desire to work.

Interests refer to a person's attraction to different occupations and the factors that influence their preferences for one type of work over another. Vocational interests are important influences on what type of work many people choose. The enjoyment of physical labor, intellectual challenges, and interacting with people are examples of why people choose certain jobs and why they find them satisfying. Cancer and its treatments can affect the ability of people to pursue appropriate work-related interests, which can contribute to difficulties staying on the job or returning to the job. The ability to consider work-related interests may be limited by other factors such as limited education or more advanced age or by social factors such as being an undocumented immigrant.

Beliefs

People's beliefs, including personal causation, sense of self, perceived self-efficacy, and cultural beliefs, can influence decisions around working. As noted by Kielhofner et al. (1999), disability or an injury can strongly affect personal causation and may leave workers unsure of what they can and cannot do. It can be challenging for persons with a long-term disability to examine how their capacities can be used in different types of work and workers may under- or overestimate capacities. Underestimating one's capacity may lead to an unnecessarily pessimistic attitude about the ability to work and overestimating capacity may expose the worker to failure or injury. A worker's sense of efficacy may also be affected if the worker is unsure of how changes in capacity may influence work performance. The injured worker may be unsure about their performance at a previous job, what accommodations are needed and available to support job performance, or what new type of work is possible.

Ekbladh (2010) found that 5 of the 17 items in the WRI had a tentative predictive validity of RTW. The content area "personal causation" in the WRI had the best predictive validity. The results emphasized the importance of considering each client's unique beliefs and expectations of their effectiveness at work when assessing the client's ability to work and planning for further rehabilitation.

It must be recognized that individual beliefs and personal causation may not be sufficient to guarantee RTW or continued employment. Sociopolitical, economic, and policy issues may create challenges that result in cancer survivors wanting to work but being unable to do so. Laliberte Rudman and Aldrich (2016) described the situation of survivors who reported being "activated, but stuck," meaning that participants ultimately experienced their lives as "on hold," with feelings of "stuckness" heightened when engagement in policy-sanctioned activities repeatedly failed to result in secure, desired employment (p. 6).

Duijts, Bleiker, et al. (2017) found in a systematic literature search that applying behavior change models, such as the transtheoretical model of change or social cognitive theory, in the development of interventions for cancer survivors generally showed positive results. They found that the most frequently considered determinants of RTW were self-efficacy, social norms, workers' expectations toward work or recovery, attitude, motivation, and meaning of work. Although these models have been used extensively in RTW efforts with other populations, there is little documentation to date of their application in work-related programming specifically for cancer survivors.

Sun et al. (2017) noted that gender-based cultural views, such as attitudes toward the importance of women's careers, are more likely to be at play in breast cancer survivors and ultimately may affect the decision to return to work. People experiencing work-related disability seldom make decisions about work in isolation. In addition, supervisors and coworkers, friends, family members, and caregivers are likely to influence a cancer survivor's decisions about continuing to work or returning to work, and their gender-based assumptions can influence these decisions.

Body functions and body structures

The impact of impaired body functions—for example, cognitive function, vision, hearing, pain, musculoskeletal (e.g., power tone, endurance), cardiovascular, hematological, respiratory, voice and speech functions, and body structures (e.g., anatomical parts of the body including organs, limbs, and their components)—on work is clear. Common adverse consequences of cancer treatment can include fatigue, pain, lymphedema, neuropathies, balance problems, mobility issues, bladder and bowel problems, dysphonia and other communication difficulties, dysphagia, cardiopulmonary function declines, sexual dysfunction, cognitive and psychosocial problems, and so forth (Alfano et al., 2017).

The severity of symptoms can directly affect work outcomes. For example, the impact of lymphedema on work has been found to correlate with increased severity of lymphedema. In one study, the annual number of days off work for participants with subclinical or mild lymphedema was 1.4, versus 8.1 days for participants with moderate or severe lymphedema (Boyages et al., 2016). In addition, lower symptom interference was found to correlate with continued employment in a study of patients with metastatic cancer, and symptoms such as fatigue, drowsiness, memory problems, and neuropathy appeared to be most associated with a change to no longer working (Tevaarwerk et al., 2016).

Performance Skills

Impairments in physical functioning were consistently described as negatively affecting RTW and work ability in both quantitative and qualitative studies (Bijker et al., 2018). Performance skills are closely related to changes in body systems and body structures and can be influenced by both the underlying cancer and its treatments. Performance skills, including motor skills, process skills, and social interaction skills, are the typical focus of discrete assessment in occupational therapy services for cancer survivors and are explored in considerable depth in Section IV, "Sequelae of Cancer and Interventions Across the Lifespan," and Section V, "Cancer and Participation in Occupations Across the Lifespan," of this book.

Performance Patterns

Working can provide structure to cancer survivors' days, relieve feelings of boredom or isolation, distract from painful and difficult aspects of treatment, and promote a sense of belonging (Stergiou-Kita et al., 2014). RTW also provides a way for cancer survivors to leave behind the routines and activities of the "sick" or "patient" role and reassert their identity and role as a worker.

Perceived and real demands of other roles and responsibilities that are influenced by cultural expectations may influence the worker role. For example, Lee et al. (2017) found that Korean women who had children after cancer were less likely to return to work, noting that family cohesion and family-oriented values have strong traditions in Korean society and that women have important roles in maintaining these traditions. They posited that the breast cancer survivors in their study needed to negotiate the boundaries of work and family and that caring for their own health and their children took priority over working.

Context and Environment

Most research on and rehabilitation of workers with injuries and disabilities focus primarily on performance factors. Although the underlying capacity for performance is a necessary condition for doing a given job, it is not a sufficient condition for successfully adapting to work. Different perspectives within the field of work rehabilitation acknowledge that personal and environmental factors affect rehabilitation and the ability to return to work.

Support from others, including coworkers, supervisors, and family members, to continue or return to work has frequently been identified as an influential factor in individual outcomes. Support in the home, in the workplace, and from physicians can influence decision making by cancer survivors (Duijts, van Egmond et al., 2017).

As noted earlier, income and financial security can influence work-related outcomes. Some cancer survivors may perceive great pressure to continue to work to prevent income loss or return to work as quickly as possible to lessen income loss. Stergiou-Kita et al. (2014) reported in a systematic review of 39 studies that several studies discussed the negative impact that cancer and cancer-related treatment had on familial finances, future earning potential, and the related pressures that survivors felt to return to work.

Others may experience financial incentives (e.g., disability income) that make work less valuable as a sole source of income. These incentives, in turn, can lessen motivation to work toward treatment goals and improve function because a lesser functional status is necessary to secure the financial rewards. Some people with disability face a complex web of regulations governing income support systems and medical reimbursement that reduce or take away the value of work as a source of improving their life circumstance. For example, a person may find it more difficult to pay for housing or medical care if they return to work. Others fear that if they return to work but are unable to sustain a job, they will be unable to regain disability-related benefits. For them, there is a disincentive to even attempt to return to work because of the importance of not jeopardizing benefits.

OCCUPATIONAL THERAPY INTERVENTIONS FOR WORK

Occupational therapy interventions for work are becoming more frequently described in the literature, and interventions specific to cancer are an area ripe for development. Hunter et al. (2017) conducted a systematic review and found that three articles related to intervention for return to work met the criteria for the review, including one systematic review and one randomized controlled trial. There was moderate evidence indicating that high-intensity exercise (strength, interval, and home based) helped patients minimize the decrease in work ability after cancer and treatment (Thijs et al., 2012) and that multidisciplinary interventions that include physical and psychological aspects in addition to vocational support provided RTW benefits (de Boer et al., 2011). One Level III study provided limited evidence related to an occupational therapy intervention to help cancer patients return to work (Desiron, 2010).

Commonly Used Assessments for Work

It has been well established since the 1980s that addressing the full range of work-related problems faced by people with disabling conditions requires focusing beyond physical limitations for work (Frederickson et al., 1988; Waddell, 1987). It was recognized that the biomechanical approach overlooked aptitudes, interests, and vocationally relevant skills (Matheson et al., 1985; Waddell, 1987). A systematic review by de Boer et al. (2015) in the Cochrane database suggested that multidisciplinary rehabilitation interventions (i.e., a combination of psycho educational, physical, vocational, or medical components) lead to higher RTW outcomes compared with usual care.

Three previously mentioned assessments based on the MOHO—the WRI, WEIS, and AWP—have been

TABLE 25.1.   Sample of Assessments Used in Evaluating Return to Work Potential in Cancer Survivors

ASSESSMENT/AUTHOR	BRIEF DESCRIPTION
Worker Role Interview (Braveman et al., 2005)	Assesses psychosocial factors that influence workers with injuries or disabilities
Work Environment Impact Scale (Moore-Corner et al., 1998)	Assesses the impact of the work setting on a worker's performance, satisfaction, and well-being
Assessment of Work Performance (Sandqvist et al., 2010)	Assesses the impact of motor skills, process skills, and communication and interaction skills on work performance
Functional capacity evaluation	Evaluates a person's capacity to perform work activities related to their participation in employment (Soer et al., 2008); compares health status and body functions and structures to job demands and the work environment (Gerg et al., 2012)
Brief Fatigue Inventory (Mendoza et al., 1999)	Assesses the severity of fatigue experienced over the past 24 hours and its impact on function
Functional Assessment of Cancer Therapy–Cognitive (FACIT.org, 2016)	Assesses perceived cognitive function and impact on quality of life in cancer patients
Assessment of Motor and Process Skills (Fisher & Bray Jones, 2014)	Uses observations to assess ADL tasks in a natural, task-relevant environment, allowing scoring of the quality of the performance skills demonstrated
Assessment of Communication and Interaction Skills (Forsyth et al., 1998)	Uses observations to assess different aspects of communication and interaction skills according to three domains: physicality, information exchange, and relations
Occupational Performance History Interview (Kielhofner et al., 2005)	Measures past and current occupational functioning through life history narrative with a rating scale
Work Ability Index (Ilmarinen, 2007)	Uses a questionnaire during health examinations and workplace surveys to assess ability to work

Note. ADL = activities of daily living.

developed to supplement the biomechanical approach. The *WRI* is an assessment of the psychosocial factors that influence workers with injuries or disabilities; the *WEIS* is an assessment of the impact of the work setting on a worker's performance, satisfaction, and well-being; and the *AWP* is an assessment of the impact of motor skills, process skills, and communication and interaction skills on work performance (Braveman, 2019).

Note that effective RTW assessment and intervention must consider the full range of factors that can affect work performance. Table 25.1 provides a list of sample assessments specific to cancer that can be used by occupational therapy practitioners. Many of these assessments are noted in other chapters throughout this book. In addition, Case Example 25.1 provides a detailed account of occupational therapy assessments and interventions, including ones helpful for RTW, used for a women recently diagnosed with breast cancer.

Resources for Supporting Work

Increasingly, the needs of cancer survivors regarding working and RTW are being recognized, and some resources for them are available. For example, Cancer + Careers (www.cancerandcareers.org) is a free service offered by the Cosmetic Executive Women (New York) board of directors, and Cancer and Work (https://www.cancerandwork.ca) is offered by researchers at McGill University (Montreal) and the British Columbia Cancer Agency (Vancouver). These sites provide resources and tools for cancer survivors, employers, and health care providers. Examples include interactive tools such as a Return to Work Planner for Employers, a Cancer and Work Job Analysis, and a Cancer and Work (2019) Fatigue Tracking Tool. Springboard Beyond Cancer (https://survivorship.cancer.gov/) was developed by the National Cancer Institute (Bethesda, MD) and the American Cancer Society (Atlanta) and provides a

CASE EXAMPLE 25.1. ELLEN: WORKING POSTSURGERY FOR BREAST CANCER

Ellen is a 48-year-old woman who was diagnosed with right ductal carcinoma in situ of the right breast after a lump was found on a routine mammogram. A biopsy revealed Stage III breast cancer. Oncologic medical treatment involves chemotherapy, modified radical mastectomy, sentinel lymph node biopsy, breast tissue reconstruction, and 4 weeks of radiation therapy treatments

(5 days per week) targeting the right axilla and chest wall. Ellen underwent a modified radical mastectomy with sentinel lymph node biopsy and tissue reconstruction. She is currently in her last week of radiation treatment.

Ellen is the mother of two teenagers and is married to a woman who is deployed on active duty in the military. Before her diagnosis, Ellen worked full-time as an office

(Continued)

CASE EXAMPLE 25.1. ELLEN: WORKING POSTSURGERY FOR BREAST CANCER *(Cont.)*

manager for a law firm and was the sole at-home care-taker of her two children. She has support from family and friends, but no family members live in her town and they can visit only for a few days to a week every other month. Ellen's friends are supportive and frequently offer assistance, but Ellen is reticent to admit that she needs help and worries that her friends would perceive her as a burden. She also prides herself on being a strong and independent woman who "holds down the fort" while her wife is on active duty.

Ellen is being treated at a hospital that focuses on can-cer, and the oncologists are familiar with the rehabili-tation disciplines. Referrals to occupational therapy are typically for evaluation and treatment, and Ellen's oncol-ogist refers her to an occupational therapist. The occu-pational therapist completes a full evaluation, including developing an occupational therapy profile. She decides to focus on the following factors during the evaluation process:

- Obtaining baseline circumferential measurements of both upper extremities to assess for early lymph-edema and providing education on lymphedema prevention
- Assessing active and passive range of motion and providing education on stretching and strategies to maintain range of motion
- Screening for fatigue as part of comprehensive fatigue management
- Screening for signs of cancer-related cognitive impair-ment (CRCI) and providing intervention as appropriate

- Conducting an interview to assess ADLs and IADLs to understand any challenges that Ellen was expe-riencing and making recommendations for energy conservation and work simplification.

The screening and assessment tools used by the occu-pational therapist and a summary of Ellen's results are listed in Table 25.2.

During the initial assessment by the occupational therapist, Ellen voiced concern about her ability to con-tinue to work full-time because she was experiencing moderate levels of fatigue and mild cognitive impair-ment and was missing a lot of work because of multi-ple medical appointments, including occupational and physical therapy. Unfortunately, Ellen's commercial insurance does not reimburse for occupational therapy services related to work. However, the occupational therapist was familiar with issues involving cancer and working and therefore decided to administer the WRI to be able to provide some suggestions to Ellen. She used this assessment even though she would not include the results in her evaluation documentation.

Exhibit 25.2 shows the ratings for Ellen's WRI based on answers to questions asked during the initial assessment. Ellen has many factors that either support or strongly support her working in her current job. However, several factors may interfere with her work success:

- Ellen's expectation of limited job success because of her concern about balancing her parent role and her fatigue and CRCI

TABLE 25.2. Screening and Assessment Tools and Summary of Results for Ellen	
TOOL	**SUMMARY OF RESULTS**
Brief Fatigue Inventory (Mendoza et al., 1999)	Global average fatigue of 4 out of 10 over the last 24 hours. Ellen rates this fatigue as having minimal interference with her mood and relations with other people but significant interference with normal activities and with enjoyment of life.
Functional Assessment of Cancer Therapy–Cognitive Function (FACIT. org, 2016)	Scoring indicates that Ellen perceives difficulty with cognitive issues several times each week.
Circumferential measurements of upper extremities	Measurements indicate a small difference between the affected and nonaffected upper extremity, suggesting mild edema that has not yet progressed to Stage I lymphedema.
Interview regarding ADL/IADL performance	Ellen reports completing all basic ADLs independently but experiencing fatigue and occasionally feeling confused for a moment about what to do next, describing it as "a moment of fogginess." She is completing IADLs independently but reports moderate bouts of fatigue and that sometimes she has to stop in the middle of an activity such as folding laundry or meal preparation because she feels too fatigued to continue. She is extremely worried about being able to continue to independently care for her 2 children if her fatigue and cognitive symptoms continue to worsen.

Note. ADLs = activities of daily living; IADLs = instrumental activities of daily living.

(Continued)

CASE EXAMPLE 25.1. ELLEN: WORKING POSTSURGERY FOR BREAST CANCER *(Cont.)*

EXHIBIT 25.2.	Worker Role Interview Rating Form for Ellen

Purpose of Evaluation (circle one):   Initial Evaluation X   Discharge Evaluation

Name of client: Ellen   Name of therapist: Robin

Date of birth: 9-25-1972   Date of assessment: 1-19-2020

X Client is rated relative to his/her current job.   ☐ Client is rated relative to return to work in general.

Strongly Supports	Supports	Interferes	Strongly Interferes	Not Applicable
SS	S	I	SI	N/A
Strongly supports client returning to previous employment or finding and keeping work in general	Supports the client returning to previous employment or finding and keeping work in general	Interferes with the client returning to previous employment or finding and keeping work in general	Strongly interferes with the client returning to previous employment or finding and keeping work in general	Not applicable or not enough information to rate

Brief comments that support ratings

						Brief comments that support ratings
Personal Causation						
1. Assesses abilities and limitations	**SS**	S	I	SI	NA	Accurately describes fatigue and cognitive limitations
2. Expectation of job success	SS	S	**I**	SI	NA	Worried and stressed about success
3. Takes responsibility	**SS**	S	I	SI	NA	Accepts full responsibility
Values						
4. Commitment to work	**SS**	S	I	SI	NA	Highly committed due to children
5. Work-related goals	SS	**S**	I	SI	NA	Focused on success in current job
Interests						
6. Enjoys work	**SS**	S	I	SI	NA	Enjoys work and gains identity from work success
7. Pursues interests	**SS**	S	I	SI	NA	Pursues both work and nonwork-related interests
Roles						
8. Appraises work expectations	**SS**	S	I	SI	NA	Highly self-reflective and clarifies expectations
9. Influence of other roles	SS	S	**I**	SI	NA	Wife is deployed, and Ellen is stressed as only parent at home

(Continued)

CASE EXAMPLE 25.1. ELLEN: WORKING POSTSURGERY FOR BREAST CANCER (Cont.)

EXHIBIT 25.2. Worker Role Interview Rating Form for Ellen (Cont.)

Habits						
10. Work habits	**SS**	S	I	SI	NA	Strong habits, never misses work except for medical appointments
11. Daily routines	SS	S	**I**	SI	NA	Routines support working but some conflict with parenting and cancer symptoms
12. Adapts routines to minimize difficulties	SS	**S**	I	SI	NA	Using energy conservation and work simplification techniques
Environment						
13. Perception of work setting	SS	**S**	I	SI	NA	Generally perceived as supportive
14. Perception of family and peers	**SS**	S	I	SI	NA	Highly supportive, worries about being a burden
15. Perception of boss	SS	S	**I**	SI	NA	Unsure, has not disclosed her cancer to employer or supervisor
16. Perception of coworkers	**SS**	S	I	SI	NA	Highly supportive, has disclosed cancer to closest coworkers

- The stress of managing multiple life roles and being the only parent at home because her wife is deployed overseas
- Managing her daily routine including her parenting role given her treatment-related symptoms
- Not receiving support from her employer, who does not yet know about Ellen's cancer diagnosis.

Although the occupational therapist could not address Ellen's worker role directly in the goals that she and Ellen developed together, she could address Ellen's work issues throughout the intervention in the following ways:

- During education and training on fatigue management (including energy conservation and work simplification) and during sessions on management strategies for Ellen's CRCI, the occupational therapist helped Ellen problem solve by identifying strategies to participate in the occupations and scenarios that Ellen identified as most challenging for her, including ADLs, IADLs, work, and play.
- The occupational therapist provided Ellen with a variety of resources on cancer and work such as Cancer and Careers (https://www.cancerandcareers.org), Cancer and Work (https://www.cancerandwork.ca), and the job accommodations network (https://askjan.org).
- The occupational therapist referred Ellen to a breast cancer survivors' support group, where she could gain support and learn from the experience of other cancer survivors who struggled with cancer and work and balancing work with other occupational roles.

The occupational therapist referred Ellen to the Regional Americans With Disabilities (ADA) Center, which is part of a network of 10 resource centers nationwide. Ellen would be able to receive information on ADA and the process of disclosing her illness to her employer and requesting reasonable accommodations in the workplace.

As Ellen continued with occupational therapy sessions several times each week, she also actively explored the resources recommended by her occupational therapist. Through resources she found on the internet, recommendations from peers in her support group, and recommendations from a consultant at the ADA Center, Ellen developed a plan to manage her cancer symptoms while continuing to work and to perform her role as a parent.

As a result of her investigation, Ellen learned that she did not need to disclose to her employer the specific nature of her illness, so she decided to disclose that she had a health condition. She applied for intermittent family and medical leave and requested reasonable accommodations under the ADA (P. L. 101-336). These accommodations included

- An altered work schedule to accommodate medical appointments,
- Breaks throughout the day as necessary to help her manage her fatigue, and
- Access to written resource manuals from her orientation to serve as cues when necessary secondary to her CRCI.

At the urging of her new friends in a support group, Ellen had a conversation with several of her close friends

(Continued)

CASE EXAMPLE 25.1. ELLEN: WORKING POSTSURGERY FOR BREAST CANCER *(Cont.)*

and shared the challenges that she was facing, including symptoms from her cancer treatments and the stress she was feeling trying to manage both work and parenting. She shared that she could use their help but had worried about being perceived as a burden. Her friends responded by reassuring her and helping her develop a plan to ask for help whenever she was feeling overwhelmed. Ellen was also pleasantly surprised to find that her boss was supportive and made several suggestions

to aid Ellen that were above and beyond the reasonable accommodations that she had requested.

Ellen continued with occupational therapy for 4 weeks and actively used the strategies she learned to address her fatigue and cognitive impairment. She completed her home program and not only maintained but improved the active range of motion in her affected upper extremity. She also followed all recommendations to prevent the onset of lymphedema.

variety of resources about symptoms, emotions, and self-care for people with cancer. The Job Accomodations Network (https://askjan.org/) provides free guidance on work accomodations and disability employment issues.

SUMMARY

Many cancer survivors wish to continue to work during cancer treatment or to return to work after treatment. Reasons for this desire include maintaining the satisfaction gained through work; having a strong sense of self-efficacy and identity with being a worker; and continuing to earn an income, sometimes because of financial constraints. The impact that cancer and its treatments have on work capacity can range from mild to devastating. Work capacity can be influenced in complex ways through a combination of client factors, performance skills, performance patterns, and contextual and environmental factors.

Although there is an increasing amount of research on cancer and work, there is much to be learned. Research to date indicates that cancer is similar to other diseases or disabilities regarding work issues. Various factors interact in complex ways to influence the capacity for work or the likelihood to return to work, and effective work interventions must be multifaceted and address the full range of factors that affect work capacity. In addition, although resources are now available for cancer survivors, employers, and health care providers, there remains great opportunity for further resource development.

Occupational therapy practitioners can play a critical role in helping cancer survivors continue to work or return to work after their cancer diagnosis and treatment. Practitioners interested in this area of intervention can look to documented interventions with other populations for guidance in developing effective programming. In addition, a variety of occupational therapy–specific assessments are available that can be used with cancer survivors, and an increasing amount of research and literature is being produced by occupational therapy practitioners on cancer and work.

REFERENCES

Aldwin, C. M., & Levenson, M. R. (2001). Stress, coping, and health at mid-life: A developmental perspective. In M. E. Lachman (Ed.), *The handbook of midlife development* (pp. 188–214). New York: John Wiley & Sons.

Alfano, C. M., Kent, E. E., Padgett, L. S., Grimes, M., & de Moor, J. S. (2017). Making cancer rehabilitation services work for cancer patients: Recommendations for research and practice to improve employment outcomes. *PM&R, 9,* S398-S406.

Almeida, D. M., & Horn, M. C. (2004). Is daily life more stressful during middle adulthood? In O. G. Brim, C. R. Ryff, & R. C. Kessler (Eds.), *How healthy are we? A national study of well-being at mid-life* (pp. 425–451). Chicago: University of Chicago Press.

American Occupational Therapy Association. (2014). Occupational therapy practice framework: Domain and process (3rd ed.). *American Journal of Occupational Therapy, 68*(Suppl. 1), S1–S48. https://doi.org/10.5014/ajot.2014.682006

Americans With Disabilities Act of 1990, Pub. L. 101-336, 42 U.S.C. §§ 12101–12213 (2000).

Benson, J. E., & Elder, G. H., Jr. (2011). Young adult identities and their pathways: A developmental and life course model. *Developmental Psychology, 47,* 1646–1657. https://doi.org/10.1037/a0023833

Bijker, R., Duijts, S. F., Smith, S. N., de Wildt-Liesveld, R., Anema, J. R., & Regeer, B. J. (2018). Functional impairments and work-related outcomes in breast cancer survivors: A systematic review. *Journal of Occupational Rehabilitation, 28,* 429–451. https://doi.org/10.1007/s10926-017-9736-8

Bilodeau, K., Tremblay, D., & Durand, M. J. (2017). Exploration of return-to-work interventions for breast cancer patients: A scoping review. *Supportive Care in Cancer, 25,* 1993–2007. https://doi.org/10.1007/s00520-016-3526-2

Blanchflower, D. G., & Oswald, A. J. (2008). Is well-being U-shaped over the life cycle? *Social Science and Medicine, 66,* 1733–1749. https://doi.org/10.1016/j.socscimed.2008.01.030

Boyages, J., Kalfa, S., Xu, Y., Koelmeyer, L., Mackie, H., Viveros, H., . . . Gollan, P. (2016). Worse and worse off: The impact of lymphedema on work and career after breast cancer. *Springerplus, 5,* 657. https://doi.org/10.1186/s40064-016-2300-8

Braveman, B. (1999). The Model of Human Occupation and prediction of return to work: Related empirical research. *Work, 12,* 13–24.

Braveman, B. (2012). Volunteerism and play: Alternative paths to work participation. In B. Braveman & J. Page (Eds.), *Work: Promoting participation and productivity through occupational therapy* (pp. 221–244). Philadelphia: F. A. Davis.

Braveman, B. (2019). Work-related assessments: The Worker Role Interview, Work Environment Impact Scale, and Assessment of Work Performance. In, B. J. Hemphill-Pearson & C. Urish (Eds.), *Assessments in occupational therapy mental health: An integrative approach* (3rd ed., pp. 411–435). Thorofare, NJ: Slack.

Braveman, B., Robson, M., Velozo, C., Kielhofner, G., Fisher, G. S., Forsyth, K., & Kerschbaum, J. (2005). *The Worker Role Interview (Version 10).* Chicago: Model of Human Occupation Clearinghouse, Department of Occupational Therapy.

Cancelliere, C., Donovan, J., Stochkendahl, M. J., Biscardi, M., Ammendolia, C., Myburgh, C., & Cassidy, J. D. (2016). Factors affecting return to work after injury or illness: Best evidence synthesis of systematic reviews. *Chiropractic and Manual Therapies, 24,* 32. https://doi.org/10.1186/s12998-016-0113-z

Cancer and Work. (2019). *Interactive tools.* Retrieved from https://www.cancerandwork.ca/tools/

Clark, A. E., & Oswald, A. J. (2006). *The curved relationship between subjective well-being and age.* Retrieved from http://halshs.archives-ouvertes.fr/docs/00/59/04/04/PDF/wp200629.pdf

Colón-Emeric, C. S., Whitson, H. E., Pavon, J., & Hoenig, H. (2013). Functional decline in older adults. *American Family Physician, 88,* 388–394.

Courneya, K., Karvinen, K., & Vallance, J. (2007). Exercise motivation and behavior change. In M. Feuerstein (Ed.), *Handbook of cancer survivorship* (pp. 113–132). New York: Springer.

Dahl, A. A., Fosså, S. D., Lie, H. C., Loge, J. H., Reinertsen, K. V., Ruud, E., & Kiserud, C. E. (2019). Employment status and work ability in long-term young adult cancer survivors. *Journal of Adolescent and Young Adult Oncology, 8,* 304–311. https://doi.org/10.1089/jayao.2018.0109

de Boer, G., Taskila, T., Tamminga, S. J., Fings-Dresen, M. H., Feuerstein, M., & Verbeek, J. H. (2011). Interventions to enhance return-to-work for cancer patients. *Cochrane Database of Systematic Reviews, 2011,* CD007569. https://doi.org/10.1002/14651858.CD007569.pub2

de Boer, A. G. E. M., Taskila, T. K., Tamminga, S. J., Feuerstein, M., Frings-Dresen, M. H. W., Verbeek, J. H. (2015). Interventions to enhance return-to-work for cancer patients. *Cochrane Database of Systematic Reviews, 9,* CD007569. https://doi.org/10.1002/14651858.CD007569.pub3

Desiron, H. A. M. (2010). Occupational therapy and return to work for breast cancer survivors. *WFOT Bulletin, 61,* 45–51. https://doi.org/10.1179/otb.2010.61.1.013

Desiron, H. (2016). *Return to work in breast cancer patients* (Unpublished doctoral dissertation). Katholieke Universiteit Leuven, Leuven, Belgium.

Donker-Cools, B. H., Wind, H., & Frings-Dresen, M. H. (2016). Prognostic factors of return to work after traumatic or non-traumatic acquired brain injury. *Disability and Rehabilitation, 38,* 733–741. https://doi.org/10.3109/09638288.2015.1061608

Dorland, H. F., Abma, F. I., Van Zon, S. K. R., Stewart, R. E., Amick, B. C., Ranchor, A. V., . . . Bültmann, U. (2018). Fatigue and depressive symptoms improve but remain negatively related to work functioning over 18 months after return to work in cancer patients. *Journal of Cancer Survivorship, 12,* 371–378. https://doi.org/10.1007/s11764-018-0676-x

Duijts, S. F. A., Bleiker, E. M. A., Paalman, C. H., & van der Beek, A. J. (2017). A behavioural approach in the development of work-related interventions for cancer survivors: An exploratory review. *European Journal of Cancer Care, 26,* e12545. https://doi.org/10.1111/ecc.12545

Duijts, S. F., van Egmond, M. P., Gits, M., van der Beek, A. J., & Bleiker, E. M. (2017). Cancer survivors' perspectives and experiences regarding behavioral determinants of return to work and continuation of work. *Disability and Rehabilitation, 39,* 2164–2172. https://doi.org/10.1080/09638288.2016.1219924

Ekbladh, E. (2010). Return to work: The predictive value of the Worker Role Interview (WRI) over two years. *Work, 35*(2), 163–172.

FACIT.ORG. (2016). FACT—Cognitive Function (Version 3). Retrieved from https://www.facit.org/FACITOrg/Questionnaires

Fisher, A. G., & Bray Jones, K. (2014). *Assessment of Motor and Process Skills, Vol. 2: User manual* (8th ed.). Fort Collins, CO: Three Star Press.

Fitzpatrick, N. (2015). *An exploration of the return to work experiences of individuals who are managing a traumatic hand injury and the development of a return to work intervention* (Unpublished doctoral dissertation). London South Bank University, London, UK.

Forstyth, K., Salamy, M., Simon, S., & Kielhofner, G. (1998). *Assessment of Communication and Interactin Skills (ACIS).* Chicago: Model of Human Occupation Clearinghouse.

Frazier, L. M., Miller, V. A., Horbelt, D. V., Delmore, J. E., Miller, B. E., & Averett, E. P. (2009). Employment and quality of survivorship among women with cancer: Domains not captured by quality of life instruments. *Cancer Control, 16,* 57–65. https://doi.org/10.1177/107327480901600109

Fredrickson, B. E., Trief, P. M., VanBeveren, P., Yuan, H. A., & Baum, G. (1988). Rehabilitation of the patient with chronic back pain. A search for outcome predictors. *Spine, 13,* 351–353. https://doi.org/10.1097/00007632-198803000-00022

Gerg, M. J., Raptosh, D., Dorsey, J., Fick, F., & Kaskutas, V. (2012). *Occupational therapy's roles in functional capacity evaluation* [Fact sheet]. Retrieved from https://www.aota.org/~/media/Corporate/Files/AboutOT/Professionals/WhatIsOT/WI/Facts/Functional-Capacity.pdf

Gerlach, A. J., Teachman, G., Laliberte-Rudman, D., Aldrich, R. M., & Huot, S. (2018). Expanding beyond individualism: Engaging critical perspectives on occupation. *Scandinavian Journal of Occupational Therapy, 25,* 35–43. https://doi.org/10.1080/11038128.2017.1327616

Giummarra, M. J., Cameron, P. A., Ponsford, J., Ioannou, L., Gibson, S. J., Jennings, P. A., & Georgiou-Karistianis, N. (2017). Return to work after traumatic injury: Increased work-related disability in injured persons receiving financial compensation is mediated by perceived injustice. *Journal of occupational rehabilitation, 27*(2), 173–185.

Gupta, A. A., Papadakos, J. K., Jones, J. M., Amin, L., Chang, E. K., Korenblum, C., . . . Giuliani, M. E. (2016). Reimagining care for adolescent and young adult cancer programs: Moving with the times. *Cancer, 122,* 1038–1046. https://doi.org/10.1002/cncr.29834

Hartung, P. J., Porfeli, E. J., & Vondrick, F. W. (2005). Child vocational development: A review and reconsideration. *Journal of Vocational Behavior, 66,* 385–419. https://doi.org/10.1016/j.jvb.2004.05.006

Heinesen, E., Imai, S., & Maruyama, S. (2018). Employment, job skills and occupational mobility of cancer survivors. *Journal of Health Economics, 58,* 151–175. https://doi.org/10.1016/j.jhealeco.2018.01.006

Heinesen, E., Kolodziejczyk, C., Ladenburg, J., Andersen, I., & Thielen, K. (2017). Return to work after cancer and pre-cancer job dissatisfaction. *Applied Economics, 49,* 4982–4998. https://doi.org/10.1080/00036846.2017.1296555

Hunter, E. G., Gibson, R. W., Arbesman, M., & D'Amico, M. (2017). Systematic review of occupational therapy and adult cancer rehabilitation: Part 2. Impact of multidisciplinary rehabilitation and psychosocial, sexuality, and return-to-work interventions. *American Journal of Occupational Therapy, 71,* 7102100040. https://doi.org/10.5014/ajot.2017.023572

Ilmarinen, J. (2007). The Work Ability Index (WAI). *Occupational Medicine, 57*(2), 160. https://doi.org/10.1093/occmed/kqm008

Isaksson, J., Wilms, T., Laurell, G., Fransson, P., & Ehrsson, Y. T. (2016). Meaning of work and the process of returning after head and neck cancer. *Supportive Care in Cancer, 24,* 205–213. https://doi.org/10.1007/s00520-015-2769-7

Islam, T., Dahlui, M., Majid, H. A., Nahar, A. M., Taib, N. A. M., & Su, T. T. (2014). Factors associated with return to work of breast cancer survivors: A systematic review. *BMC Public Health, 14,* S8. https://doi.org/10.116/1471-2458-S3-S8

Kamper, S. J., Apeldoorn, A. T., Chiarotto, A., Smeets, R. J. E. M., Ostelo, R. W. J. G., Guzman, J., & Van Tulder, M. W. (2015). Multidisciplinary biopsychosocial rehabilitation for chronic low back pain: Cochrane systematic review and meta-analysis. *BMJ, 350,* h444. https://doi.org/10.1136/bmj.h444

Kielhofner, G. (2008). *Model of Human Occupation: Theory and application.* Philadelphia: F.A. Davis.

Kielhofner, G., Braveman, B., Baron, K., Fisher, G., Hammel, J., & Littleton, M. (1999). The Model of Human Occupation: Understanding the worker who is injured or disabled. *Work, 12,* 37–45.

Kielhofner, G., Braveman, B., Finlayson, M., Paul-Ward, A., Goldbaum, L., & Goldstein, K. (2004). Outcomes of a vocational program for persons with AIDS. *American Journal of Occupational Therapy, 58,* 64–72. https://doi.org/0.5014/ajot.58.1.64

Kielhofner, G., Braveman, B., Fogg, L., & Levin, M. (2008). A controlled study of services to enhance productive participation among people with HIV/AIDS. *American Journal of Occupational Therapy, 62,* 36–45. https://doi.org/10.5014/ajot.62.1.36

Kielhofner, G., Mallinson, T., Crawford, C., Nowak, M., Rigby, M., Henry, A., & Walens, D. (2005). *The occupational performance history interview (OPHI-II), version 2.1.* Chicago: Model of Human Occupational Clearinghouse.

Kuron, L. K., Lyons, S. T., Schweitzer, L., & Ng, E. S. (2015). Millennials' work values: Differences across the school to work transition. *Personnel Review, 44,* 991–1009. https://doi.org/10.1108/PR-01-2014-0024

Lachman, M. E., Teshale, S., & Agrigoroaei, S. (2014). Midlife as a pivotal period in the life course: Balancing growth and decline at the crossroads of youth and old age. *International Journal of Behavioral Development, 39,* 20–31. https://doi.org/10.1177/0165025414533223

Laliberte Rudman, D., & Aldrich, R. (2016). "Activated, but stuck": Applying a critical occupational lens to examine the negotiation of long-term unemployment in contemporary socio-political contexts. *Societies, 6,* 28. https://doi.org/10.3390/soc6030028

Law, M., Cooper, B., Strong, S., Stewart, D., Rigby, P., & Letts, L. (1996). The Person-Environment-Occupation model: A transactive approach to occupational performance. *Canadian Journal of Occupational Therapy, 63,* 9–23. https://doi.org/10.1177/000841749606300103

Lee, M. K., Kang, H. S., Lee, K. S., & Lee, E. S. (2017). Three-year prospective cohort study of factors associated with return to work after breast cancer diagnosis. *Journal of Occupational Rehabilitation, 27,* 547–558. https://doi.org/10.1007/s10926-016-9685-7

Lyons, K. D., Newman, R. M., Sullivan, M., Pergolotti, M., Braveman, B., & Cheville, A. L. (2019). Employment concerns and associated impairments of women living with advanced breast cancer. *Archives of Rehabilitation Research and Clinical Translation, 1,* 100004. https://doi.org/10.1016/j.arrct.2019.100004

Matheson, L. N., Ogden, L. D., Violette, K., & Schultz, K. (1985). Work hardening: Occupational therapy in industrial rehabilitation. *American Journal of Occupational Therapy, 39,* 314–321. https://doi.org/10.5014/ajot.39.5.314

McGill, S. M. (2015). *Low back disorders: Evidence-based prevention and rehabilitation.* Champaign, IL: Human Kinetics.

McGirt, M. J., Sivaganesan, A., Asher, A. L., & Devin, C. J. (2015). Prediction model for outcome after low-back surgery: Individualized likelihood of complication, hospital readmission, return to work, and 12-month improvement in functional disability. *Neurosurgical Focus, 39,* E13. https://doi.org/10.3171/2015.8.FOCUS15338

McPhillips, D. (2016). *The Labor Day weekend: A look at the hardest working countries.* Retrieved from https://www.usnews.com/news/best-countries/articles/2016-09-02/hardest-working-countries-ranked-by-hours-worked-per-year

Mendoza, T. R., Wang, X. S., Cleeland, C. S., Morrissey, M., Johnson, B. A., Wendt, J. K., & Huber, S. L. (1999). The rapid assessment of fatigue severity in cancer patients: use of the Brief Fatigue Inventory. *Cancer, 85,* 1186–1196. https://doi.org/10.1002/(sici)1097-0142(19990301)85:5<1186::aid-cncr24>3.0.co;2-n

Moore-Corner, R. A., Kielhofner, G., & Olson, L. (1998). *A user's manual for Work Environment Impact Scale (WEIS).* Chicago: Model of Human Occupation Clearinghouse, Department of Occupational Therapy.

Nachreiner, N. M., Ghebre, R. G., Virnig, B. A., & Shanley, R. (2011). Early work patterns for gynaecological cancer survivors in the USA. *Occupational Medicine, 62,* 23–28. https://doi.org/10.1093/occmed/kqr177

Newman, R. M., Alfano, C. M., Radomski, M. V., Pergolotti, M., Wolf, T. J., Sleight, A. G., . . . Daniels, E. (2019). Catalyzing research to optimize cancer survivors' participation in work and life roles. *OTJR: Occupation, Participation and Health, 39,* 189–196. https://doi.org/10.1177/1539449219844749

Organization for Economic Cooperation and Development. (2018). *Hours worked.* Retrieved from https://data.oecd.org/emp/hours-worked.htm

Paltrinieri, S., Fugazzaro, S., Bertozzi, L., Bassi, M. C., Pellegrini, M., Vicentini, M., . . . Costi, S. (2018). Return to work in European cancer survivors: A systematic review. *Supportive Care in Cancer, 26,* 2983–2994. https://doi.org/10.1007/s00520-018-4270-6

Pew Research Center. (2016). *More older Americans are working, and working more, than they used to.* Retrieved from https://www.pewresearch.org/fact-tank/2016/06/20/more-older-americans-are-working-and-working-more-than-they-used-to/.

Rasmussen, D. M., & Elverdam, B. (2008). The meaning of work and working life after cancer: An interview study. *Psycho-Oncology, 17,* 1232–1238. https://doi.org/10.1002/pon.1354

Raque-Bogdan, T. L., Hoffman, M. A., Ginter, A. C., Piontkowski, S., Schexnayder, K., & White, R. (2015). The work life and career development of young breast cancer survivors. *Journal of Counseling Psychology, 62*(4), 655–669. https://doi.org/10.1037/cou0000068

Roelen, C. A., Koopmans, P. C., Groothoff, J. W., van der Klink, J. J., & Bültmann, U. (2011). Sickness absence and full return to work after cancer: 2-year follow-up of register data for different cancer sites. *Psycho-Oncology, 20,* 1001–1006. https://doi.org/10.1002/pon.1820

Ross, J. (2007). *Occupational therapy and vocational rehabilitation.* Hoboken, NJ: Wiley.

Sandqvist, J., Lee, J., & Kielhofner, G. (2010). *A user's guide to the Assessment of Work Performance (AWP).* Chicago: Department of Occupational Therapy, University of Illinois at Chicago.

Santoni, G., Angleman, S., Welmer, A. K., Mangialasche, F., Marengoni, A., & Fratiglioni, L. (2015). Age-related variation in health status after age 60. *PloS One, 10,* e0120077. https://doi.org/10.1371/journal.pone.0120077.

Schultz, I. Z., Crook, J., Meloche, G. R., Berkowitz, J., Milner, R., Zuberbier, O. A., & Meloche, W. (2004). Psychosocial factors predictive of occupational low back disability: Towards development of a return-to-work model. *Pain, 107,* 77–85. https://doi.org/10.1016/j.pain.2003.09.019

Schultz, I. Z., & Gatchel, R. J. (2016). Where do we go from here in return to work research, policy, and practice?: A postscriptum. In I. Z. Schultz & R. J. Gatchel (Eds.), *Handbook of Return to Work* (pp. 695–703). New York: Springer-Verlag.

Schwartz, S. J., Côté, J. E., & Arnett, J. J. (2005). Identity and agency in emerging adulthood: Two developmental routes in the individualization process. *Youth and Society, 37,* 201–229. https://doi.org/10.1177/0044118X05275965

Snippen, N. C., de Vries, H. J., van der Burg-Vermeulen, S. J., Hagedoorn, M., & Brouwer, S. (2019). Influence of significant others on work participation of individuals with chronic diseases: A systematic review. *BMJ Open, 9,* e021742. https://doi.org/10.1136/bmjopen-2018-021742

Soer, R., van der Schans, C. P., Groothoff, J. W., Geertzen, J. H., & Reneman, M. F. (2008). Towards consensus in operational definitions in functional capacity evaluation: A Delphi survey. Journal of Occupational Rehabilitation, 18, 389–400. https://doi.org/10.1007/s10926-008-9155-y

Spelten, E. R., Sprangers, M. A., & Verbeek, J. H. (2002). Factors reported to influence the return to work of cancer survivors: A literature review. *Psycho-Oncology, 11*(2), 124–131. https://doi.org/10.1002/pon.585

Steenstra, I. A., Munhall, C., Irvin, E., Oranye, N., Passmore, S., Van Eerd, D., . . . Hogg-Johnson, S. (2017). Systematic review of prognostic factors for return to work in workers with sub-acute and chronic low back pain. *Journal of Occupational Rehabilitation, 27,* 369–381. https://doi.org/10.1007/s10926-016-9666-x

Stergiou-Kita, M., Grigorovich, A., Tseung, V., Milosevic, E., Hebert, D., Phan, S., & Jones, J. (2014). Qualitative meta-synthesis of survivors' work experiences and the development of strategies to facilitate return to work. *Journal of Cancer Survivorship, 8,* 657–670. https://doi.org/10.1007/s11764-014-0377-z

Stone, A. A., Schwartz, J. E., Broderick, J. E., & Deaton, A. (2010). A snapshot of the age distribution of psychological well-being in the United States. *Proceedings of the National Academy of Sciences, 107,* 9985–9990. https://doi.org/10.1073/pnas.1003744107

Stone, D. S., Ganz, P. A., Pavlish, C., & Robbins, W. A. (2017). Young adult cancer survivors and work: A systematic review. *Journal of Cancer Survivorship, 11,* 765–781. https://doi.org/10.1007/s11764-017-0614-3

Sun, Y., Shigaki, C. L., & Armer, J. M. (2017). Return to work among breast cancer survivors: A literature review. *Supportive Care in Cancer, 25,* 709–718. https://doi.org/10.1007/s00520-016-3446-1

Tevaarwerk, A. J., Lee, J. W., Terhaar, A., Sesto, M. E., Smith, M. L., Cleeland, C. S., & Fisch, M. J. (2016). Working after a metastatic cancer diagnosis: Factors affecting employment in the metastatic setting from ECOG-ACRIN's Symptom Outcomes and Practice Patterns study. *Cancer, 122,* 438–446. https://doi.org/10.1002/cncr.29656

Thijs, K. M., de Boer, A. G. E. M., Vreugdenhil, G., van de Wouw, A. J., Houterman, S., & Schep, G. (2012). Rehabilitation using high-intensity physical training and long-term return-to work in cancer survivors. *Journal of Occupational Rehabilitation, 22,* 220–229. https://doi.org/10.1007/s10926-011-9341-1

Townsend, E. A., & Polatajko, H. (2013). *Enabling occupation II: Advancing an occupational therapy vision for health, well-being, and justice through occupation* (2nd ed.). Ontario, Canada: Canadian Association of Occupational Therapists.

Ulloa, B. F. L., Møller, V., & Sousa-Poza, A. (2013). How does subjective well-being evolve with age? A literature review. *Journal of Population Aging, 6,* 227–246. https://doi.org/10.1007/s12062-013-9085-0.

U.S. Bureau of Labor Statistics. (2017). *Older workers: Labor force trends and career options.* Retrieved from https://www.bls.gov/careeroutlook/2017/article/older-workers.htm

U.S. Bureau of Labor Statistics. (2019). *Average hours employed people spent working on days worked by day of the week.* Retrieved from https://www.bls.gov/charts/american-time-use/emp-by-ftpt-job-edu-h.htm

U.S. Census Bureau. (2018). *What is ahead for the nation's aging workforce?* Retrieved from https://www.census.gov/library/stories/2018/04/aging-workforce.html

Verdonck-de Leeuw, I. M., van Bleek, W. J., Leemans, C. R., & de Bree, R. (2010). Employment and return to work in head and neck cancer survivors. *Oral Oncology, 46,* 56–60. https://doi.org/10.1016/j.oraloncology.2009.11.001

Vooijs, M., Leensen, M. C., Hoving, J. L., Daams, J. G., Wind, H., & Frings-Dresen, M. H. (2015). Disease-generic factors of work participation of workers with a chronic disease: A systematic review. *International Archives of Occupational and Environmental Health, 88,* 1015–1029. https://doi.org/10.1007/s00420-015-1025-2

Waddell, G. (1987). 1987 Volvo award in clinical sciences. A new clinical model for the treatment of low-back pain. *Spine, 12,* 632–644. https://doi.org/10.1097/00007632-198709000-00002

Ward, M. (2017). *A brief history of the 8-hour day, which changed how Americans work.* Retrieved from https://www.cnbc.com/2017/05/03/how-the-8-hour-workday-changed-how-americans-work.html

Wells, M., Williams, B., Firnigl, D., Lang, H., Coyle, J., Kroll, T., & MacGillivray, S. (2013). Supporting 'work-related goals' rather than 'return to work' after cancer? A systematic review and meta-synthesis of 25 qualitative studies. *Psycho-Oncology, 22,* 1208–1219. https://doi.org/10.1002/pon.3148

White, C., Green, R. A., Ferguson, S., Anderson, S. L., Howe, C., Sun, J., & Buys, N. (2019). The influence of social support and social integration factors on return to work outcomes for individuals with work-related injuries: A systematic review. *Journal of Occupational Rehabilitation, 29,* 636–659. https://doi.org/10.1007/s10926-018-09826-x

Wisenthal, A. (2015). *The effectiveness of cognitive work hardening in preparing people with depression to return to work* (Unpublished doctoral dissertation). Queens Univeristy, Kingston, Ontario.

Zafar, S. Y., & Abernethy, A. P. (2013). Financial toxicity, Part I: A new name for a growing problem. *Oncology, 27,* 80–81.

Social Participation

Mary Vining Radomski, PhD, OTR/L, FAOTA

26

LEARNING OBJECTIVES

After completing this chapter, readers should be able to
- Analyze how key social roles may be affected by cancer,
- Explain how social needs and priorities may change over the course of a client's cancer journey,
- Describe how social participation may be assessed as part of an occupational therapy evaluation, and
- Address social participation needs of cancer survivors through a variety of occupational therapy approaches.

KEY TERMS AND CONCEPTS

- Emotional support
- Social participation
- Social roles
- Social trajectory
- Support groups

INTRODUCTION

For many cancer survivors, social participation represents the "why" of their often arduous treatments and engagement in cancer rehabilitation. Maintaining or resuming **social roles** as parents, friends, spouses or partners, and coworkers is typically among cancer survivors' top concerns and priorities (Cubis et al., 2017). This is not surprising, given the importance of positive social relationships to overall health and psychological well-being (Ryff, 2014). Beyond its important contribution to quality of life (QoL), engagement in social roles can buffer the effects of stress and illness (Cubis et al., 2017). For all of these reasons, social participation for cancer survivors is of concern to occupational therapy practitioners.

This chapter explores cancer survivors' experience with social participation as relevant to the occupational therapy process. First, the construct of *social participation* is defined and examined in the context of cancer survivorship, which is followed by a summary of occupational therapy evaluation and intervention approaches. The goal of the chapter is to enable occupational therapy practitioners to appreciate the significance of their own roles in advancing social participation for cancer survivors, both as members of survivors' social support network and as experts whose services result in improvements that affect what matters most to cancer survivors.

SOCIAL PARTICIPATION AS OCCUPATION

The term **social participation** broadly refers to involvement in life situations that pertain to social roles valued by a person within their sociocultural context (Djurdjevic & Nikolic, 2009; McMullen et al., 2017; World Health Organization,

2001). The composition of these roles is unique to each person but may involve engaging and interacting with others as a family member, parent, spouse or partner, friend, coworker, and community member (McMullen et al., 2017). Successful social participation is the result of a person's ability to perform a wide array of occupations. For example, friendships are often maintained by sharing a meal at school or a restaurant, which is predicated on the cancer survivor's ability to swallow food and maintain their continence. Caring for one's young child may require sufficient stamina for meal preparation and cognitive proficiency to keep track of school activities.

Cancer has the potential to magnify the importance of social roles. Cancer and its treatments (as discussed in Chapter 2, "Cancer Treatment Approaches Across the Lifespan") may also cause physical and mental hardships that interfere with social participation priorities; side effects can include cancer-related fatigue (CRF), decreased sexual drive, cognitive inefficiency, chronic pain, incontinence, decreased range of motion, inability to eat or swallow, and lymphatic obstruction (Hwang et al., 2015). Occupational therapy practitioners can best address social participation by understanding the nature of typical concerns specific to various social roles and how social engagement needs change over time.

Examples of Cancer's Impact on Key Social Roles

Parenting relationships

Upon receiving a cancer diagnosis, most parents' primary concerns relate to the welfare of their children (Semple & McCance, 2010). In fact, parents with cancer tend to prioritize their children's needs over their own physical and emotional needs as patients (Tavares et al., 2017). Parents with new cancer diagnoses struggle with how to tell their children about cancer without worrying them (Houldin & Lewis, 2006). In addition to providing information tailored to a child's developmental stage, many parents prefer to tell their children about their illness after a treatment plan is in place (Semple & McCance, 2010). Cancer has the potential to significantly disrupt parenting activities and everyday family life. Therefore, many parents with cancer try to maintain their children's routines, which in turn reduces parental worry and guilt (Tavares et al., 2017). Having adolescent children may increase cancer survivors' stress and illness-related worry (Arès et al., 2014). Teenagers may be more distressed about cancer and experience more significant shifts in household and caretaking responsibilities than younger children (Arès et al., 2014).

Parenting dynamics may also shift when a child or adolescent has cancer. Parents typically become a critical source of support for their children, which can be both essential and complicated for adolescents who may also be struggling to gain independence from their families and develop identities within peer groups (Haluska et al., 2002). As their children emerge from the acute illness and treatment phase, some parents may struggle with a default toward overprotection (Ishibashi, 2001). See Chapter 5, "Special Considerations for Adolescents and Young Adults With Cancer," for more information.

Spouse or partner relationships

Cancer can take a significant toll on intimate relationships with spouses and partners (Fergus & Gray, 2009). There are many potential stressors on relationships, including renegotiation of family roles and responsibilities (Fergus & Gray, 2009). With activity and role shifts, some cancer survivors cope by trying to contribute in any way they can, including taking on new responsibilities that align with their abilities (Cubis et al., 2017). Even so, couples may experience relational frustrations when the cancer survivor remains overly directive and controlling regarding tasks that they are relinquishing to the spouse (Fergus & Gray, 2009).

Most couples experience significant losses related to sexual intimacy. Problems can be related to the cancer itself, the emotional consequences of cancer, and the side effects of cancer treatments (Djurdjevic & Nikolic, 2009). For example, some women with cancer are frightened by their own appearance (Holmberg et al., 2001) and experience early menopause as a result of cancer treatment as well as vaginal dryness and atrophy (Ferrell et al., 2003).

Some couples become less open in their communication in an effort to protect each other from fears and anxiety (Holmberg et al., 2001). Communication and reciprocal emotional support may be further compromised by differing expectations. For example, spouses may assume that the end of illness coincides with the end of treatment. Cancer survivors may experience this push to "return to normal" while struggling with renewed uncertainty and insecurity about their own health (Fergus & Gray, 2009).

Dating and romantic relationships

Many single cancer survivors worry about dating. Thinking about dating can be anxiety provoking, especially when considering how and when to disclose information about their diagnosis and altered physical appearance to a new partner (Holmberg et al., 2001). Unpartnered cancer survivors may have smaller social networks and thus may be vulnerable to problems with negative adjustment (Holmberg et al., 2001). Cancer may exaggerate many adolescents' worries about dating and their potential desirability to members of their peer group.

Friendships and extended family

Friends and members of the cancer survivor's extended family typically provide critical practical support (e.g., cooking, childcare, housework, transportation) and emotional support; this facilitates coping and hope (Cubis et al., 2017). Friendships may change over time and across the course of the disease: some deepen as other close friends withdraw to more distant relationships, which can be painful (Holmberg et al., 2001). Even as they appreciate the outpouring of generosity by members of their social network, many cancer survivors feel alone (Ferrell et al., 2003). This may be especially the case for children and adolescents with cancer, which may lead to physical and emotional isolation from friends (Haluska et al., 2002). Many children and adolescents with cancer fear losing friends who were previously close (Zebrack et al., 2014), in part because healthy friends do not know how to support them (Ishibashi, 2001).

Building new friendships with other cancer survivors can be important to long-term coping. **Support groups** expand the social network to include people with a shared cancer experience. These groups can help survivors rebuild self-confidence as they reintegrate back into the "normal" world (Arora et al., 2007). Children and adolescents whose social skills have been affected by the physical and cognitive impairments of cancer (e.g., brain tumor) can benefit from specialized group social skills interventions (Barrera et al., 2018).

Social Trajectory

In general, cancer survivors' social participation needs tend to change from the point of diagnosis through long-term survivorship (Cubis et al., 2017); this is called a **social trajectory**. Cubis et al. (2017) described three temporal themes in the social trajectory associated with a brain tumor, which have general applicability to other forms of cancer:

- *Life disrupted* reflects the shock of the unexpected diagnosis and rapid transition to treatments (Cubis et al., 2017). During this acute phase of decision making and treatment, cancer survivors primarily rely on emotional support and instrumental assistance from family and preexisting social networks (Cubis et al., 2017). Patients also rely heavily on health care providers for informational and decision-making support (Arora et al., 2007).
- *Navigating the new reality of life* reflects the period in which cancer treatment regimens become part of the patient and family's normal routine (Cubis et al., 2017). Because patients' days may be largely occupied with medical appointments, the information and emotional support provided by health care providers, including occupational therapy practitioners, becomes critical to patients' well-being (Cubis et al., 2017). During this

phase, previously performed social role activities associated with being a parent or spouse may be shifted to other family members, which may cause guilt and distress (Semple & McCance, 2010; Tavares et al., 2017). If this phase is protracted, family members may experience strain, and superficial acquaintances may disappear from the social network.

- *Social survivorship or separation* represents the cancer survivor's long-term social adaptation. With time, patients complete treatment and experience improved or stabilized function that allows for gradual social reengagement beyond immediate family and close friends (Cubis et al., 2017). Self-help groups may assume greater importance as a means of expanding social relationships that offer support as cancer survivors' resume normal life. Many cancer survivors want to reciprocate the support they've received from others (Cubis et al., 2017), which also contributes to their own coping and sense of purpose (Agarwal et al., 2010).

Cancer's Positive Impact on Social Relationships

Although cancer places new demands on social participation, for many cancer survivors it also contributes to a reinvigorated appreciation for relationships with family, children, and close friends (Cubis et al., 2017). For mothers and fathers, cancer often leads to reprioritizing of time devoted to being with children (O'Neill et al., 2016). Some couples report that although cancer contributed to interpersonal strain, it also brought about closeness and positive growth in the relationship (Ferrell et al., 2003). The reprioritization of family and social roles may prompt shifts upon return to work in favor of better work–life balance (O'Neill et al., 2016) and a focus on living in the moment and finding joy and meaning in spending time with others (Cubis et al., 2017). Even some adolescents find that the devastation of the cancer diagnosis and treatments prompts positive shifts in self-care, gratitude, and personal growth (Zebrack et al., 2014).

FACTORS THAT MAY CONTRIBUTE TO OCCUPATIONAL DYSFUNCTION IN SOCIAL PARTICIPATION

A wide range of factors may contribute to cancer-related occupational dysfunction in social participation. Client factors such as cancer type, cancer treatments and their side effects, illness chronicity and trajectory, and related impairments influence cancer survivors' proficiency with the activities that compose valued social roles.

For example, women with breast cancer–related lymphedema may have difficulty lifting their toddlers or experience fatigue during chemotherapy; these side effects may limit their ability to play with their children at the end of the day. A teenager with brain cancer may have cognitive impairments that contribute to decreased initiation of social activities or the appropriateness with which he interacts with peers at school. Therefore, occupational therapy practitioners appreciate that a client's social participation needs are driven by many factors, including personality type, premorbid socialization patterns and preferences,

cultural norms, composition of social network, and age and place in the lifespan.

Although this chapter outlines general themes related to social participation and cancer, developing a comprehensive occupational profile for each client allows occupational therapy practitioners to personalize the evaluation and intervention process in ways that defy preconceived ideas or stereotypes. See the following chapters for more information about age-related implications of cancer that may influence social participation: Chapter 4 (children), Chapter 5 (adolescents and young adults), Chapter 6 (adults), and Chapter 7 (older adults).

OCCUPATIONAL THERAPY EVALUATION OF SOCIAL PARTICIPATION

Even as cancer survivors may have profound challenges associated with social participation, rarely do these issues alone prompt referral to occupational therapy. Rather, cancer survivors are typically referred to occupational therapy for pain and musculoskeletal problems, deconditioning and endurance deficits, fatigue, lymphedema (Silver & Gilchrist, 2011), difficulty with ADLs and IADLs (Buckland & Mackenzie, 2017), and decreased cognitive functioning (Wolf et al., 2016). Practitioners must assess social participation as part of the occupational therapy evaluation for two reasons:

1. The aforementioned issues can interfere with social participation, and
2. Many cancer survivors are motivated to adhere to occupational therapy intervention when it advances their ability to participate in valued social roles.

When clients are referred to occupational therapy, occupational therapy practitioners try to understand who the client is and identify the areas of occupation that are both valued and difficult for the individual; they then determine what impairments or contextual or environmental factors interfere with occupational performance (American Occupational Therapy Association, 2014). Evaluating cancer survivors' social participation occurs within the context of identifying valued areas of occupation. Given the time and reimbursement limitations that are common in contemporary practice, engaging in informal, ongoing conversation with the client may be the best way to assure that the occupational therapy intervention remains relevant to the cancer survivor's most valued social roles. For example, occupational therapy practitioners might ask guiding questions such as:

- Tell me about the people in your life who are supporting you right now. In what ways are they providing assistance?
- During this part of your cancer journey, in what roles (such as parent, spouse, friend) do you most want to invest your time and energy? What, if anything, interferes with your ability to perform activities associated with these roles?
- How is your son dealing with your cancer treatment? Are there specific things we could address in therapy that might help you with your toddler (or teenager)?
- What routines are of particular importance to your family life? How are they going? Might it be helpful to explore new or modified routines?

- Have you been able to spend time with your friends or spouse to the degree you would like to in the past week or so? [If not] What seem to be the barriers to your doing so?

Informal interview questions for children with cancer should be somewhat more concrete such as, "Do you have a/Tell me about your best friend?" or "Tell me something about what you liked to do with your (friend, cousin, sibling) before you got sick." Parents should also be consulted to get their perspectives on what normal or optimal social participation looks like for their child. Conversations about an adolescent's social life may occur in increments as trust and comfort is established over the episode of care. For adolescents receiving inpatient care, occupational therapy practitioners should find out if they are experiencing any inadvertent barriers to socialization caused by the hospital policies or environment.

Beyond informal interview and conversation, formal assessment of social participation needs should occur within a comprehensive assessment of occupational performance needs. For example, use of the National Comprehensive Cancer Network (2018) Distress Thermometer and Problem List as part of the initial assessment gives occupational therapy practitioners a broad sense of where clients have concerns, including in the realm of social participation. Formal assessment methods specific to social participation should be reserved for situations in which practitioners need to quantify pre–post changes as a result of intervention for program evaluation or research; examples are summarized on Table 26.1. Note that both the Canadian Occupational Performance Measure (COPM; Law et al., 2019) and Reintegration to Normal Life Index (Wood-Dauphinee et al., 1988) may be used to inventory all of the client's occupational performance concerns, including social participation. The Patient-Reported Outcomes Measurement Information System (PROMIS) tools solely relate to satisfaction with social participation (National Institute of Health, 2014). The Child and Adolescent Scale of Participation may guide and quantify outcomes of therapy for younger clients (Bedell, 2004, 2009). Occupational therapy practitioners may also consider use of play and leisure or work-specific measures of social participation for some clients.

TABLE 26.1.   Examples of Formal Methods for Evaluating Social Participation in Cancer Survivors

DIMENSION	ASSESSMENT	DESCRIPTION
Self-identified priorities and self-reported status in areas of occupation	Canadian Occupational Performance Measure (COPM; Law et al., 2019)	The COPM (Law et al., 2019) is a well-established, reliable (Eyssen et al., 2005), and valid (Trombly et al., 1998) semistructured interview that helps the client inventory daily life performance concerns and identify the 5 performance areas that they would most like to address in therapy. Clients rate the top 5 problem areas on a scale of 1 to 10 as to how they perceive their ability to perform in each area (COPM–P) and how satisfied they are with their performance (COPM–S). The COPM has been used to identify problem–goal areas for hospitalized patients with cancer (Lindahl-Jacobsen et al., 2015) and men with metastatic prostate cancer (Huri et al., 2015).
Reintegration to normal social activities	Reintegration to Normal Living Index (RNL Index; Wood-Dauphinee et al., 1988)	The RNL Index is an 11-item self-report questionnaire that assesses global function and measures both clients' perceptions of their own capabilities and objective indicators of physical, social, and psychologic performance (Wood-Dauphinee et al., 1988). It may help identify cancer survivors at risk for physical performance limitations and for reduced capacity to participate in their desired family and societal roles (Nagarajan et al., 2008).
Satisfaction with social roles and activities Satisfaction with ability to participate in discretionary social activities	Patient-Reported Outcomes Measurement Information System (PROMIS) Satisfaction with Participation in Social Roles (National Institutes of Health [NIH], 2015) PROMIS Satisfaction with Participation in Discretionary Social Activities (NIH, 2014)	PROMIS measures were developed as part of a larger NIH initiative to develop psychometrically robust, easily interpretable, calibrated item banks to serve as patient-reported outcomes in research and clinical practice. These specific measures were developed to capture social health. - The PROMIS Satisfaction with Participation in Social Roles is a self-report questionnaire that assesses satisfaction with performing one's usual social roles and activities (e.g., "I am satisfied with my ability to participate in family activities"). - The PROMIS Satisfaction with Participation in Discretionary Social Activities assesses self-reported contentment with leisure interests and relationships with friends. This is separate from social roles (work and family responsibilities). The PROMIS measures are designed to be universal and not disease specific. Analyses of these two measures from oncology populations suggested that the self-report ratings were consistent with clinical experiences (Hahn et al., 2010).
Participation of children and adolescents	The Child and Adolescent Scale of Participation (CASP; Bedell, 2004, 2009)	The CASP measures the extent to which children and adolescents participate in home, school, and community activities as compared with children of the same age as reported by parents or family members. This 23-item questionnaire takes approximately 10 minutes to administer; has been translated into Spanish, French, German, Hebrew, and Mandarin; and has been validated across numerous studies (Bedell, 2011).

As in routine occupational therapy evaluation, informal and formal assessments are used to identify a client's occupational needs, including their social role priorities. Then, within the context of a comprehensive occupational therapy evaluation, occupational therapy practitioners may administer additional assessments to identify the impairments and barriers that can be remediated during intervention to improve social role performance. For example, a woman with breast cancer wants to return to babysitting her granddaughter but is fearful that she may fall while carrying the baby; the occupational therapy practitioner will likely further evaluate the client's peripheral neuropathy. Fatigue may be the primary barrier to a teenager's goal of returning to her role on the student council, which would require further quantification of this issue as part of the occupational therapy evaluation. Methods for further specifying impairments and interfering client and contextual factors are discussed in detail in other chapters (e.g., fatigue [Chapter 15], pain [Chapter 16], cognition [Chapter 17], neuropathy [Chapter 19], psychosocial issues [Chapter 20]).

OCCUPATIONAL THERAPY INTERVENTION FOR SOCIAL PARTICIPATION

Approaches to Improving Social Participation

Clients' social participation needs and priorities will likely change throughout the cancer survivorship journey. As those needs and priorities shift, so does the occupational therapy intervention plan, factoring in reimbursement and payment realities within various contexts of care. Therefore, occupational therapy practitioners address social participation using multiple approaches and potentially in different ways and environments across the cancer survivorship experience.

Provide social and informational support

During the active treatment phase of survivorship, many cancer survivors rely on health care providers for information and **emotional support** (Holmberg et al., 2001). Occupational therapy practitioners provide validation that concerns about social participation are typical and normal by inviting conversations about social participation. By making an effort to build rapport through humor and kindness, practitioners provide hope and reassurance to their clients with cancer (Cubis et al., 2017). Provision of timely, honest information to adolescents with cancer is especially critical to building trust and rapport during intervention (Ishibashi, 2001).

Address specific barriers to participation in valued social roles

Cancer survivors may experience a wide array of impairments, inefficiencies, and contextual or environmental factors that interfere with social role performance. Occupational therapy practitioners address these barriers in four ways: (1) providing equipment or environmental modifications, (2) addressing impairment remediation and symptom management, (3) working with hospitals, and (4) addressing problems with roles.

Provide equipment or contextual or environmental modifications. Occupational therapy practitioners can provide equipment or make adjustments to the environment to promote social participation. For example, by helping a client with lung cancer-related deconditioning obtain a wheelchair, the practitioner facilitates lunching with a friend.

Remediate impairments and advance symptom management. Occupational therapy intervention may specifically address problems with CRF. Physical activity interventions (e.g., aerobic exercise, resistance training) have been demonstrated to reduce fatigue and contribute to social functioning, in addition to other mental health and QoL benefits (Lahart et al., 2018). Similarly, occupational therapy intervention for cancer-related cognitive impairment ("chemobrain") has been demonstrated to improve cognitive performance and satisfaction with participation in social roles (Wolf et al., 2016).

That said, interventions that target impairments or symptoms may not automatically translate into improved social participation. Occupational therapy practitioners must simultaneously focus the intervention on impairments or symptoms and social participation. For example, a breast cancer survivor is referred to occupational therapy because of cognitive problems. Maintaining her role as mother to two elementary school–age children is among her greatest priorities. In occupational therapy, the client learns an array of cognitive compensatory strategies. She practices using a memory aid (e.g., her smartphone) to keep track of her children's school activities; she implements newly learned planning strategies in the context of organizing a family party. Aware of the benefits of exercise to fatigue management, the occupational therapy practitioner helps the client initiate a walking regimen accompanied by her daughter on a bicycle.

Make sure that hospital policies align with clients' need to maintain social connections. Ensuring hospital policies do no impede social participation includes advocating for liberal visitation policies; supporting attendance at school events, when possible; providing places for private conversations with friends; and availing clients with Internet access (Haluska et al., 2002).

Directly address problems or vulnerabilities related to role-specific concerns. Occupational therapy practitioners can advance social participation by identifying roles of particular importance to clients and addressing related concerns as part of the occupational therapy intervention (see Table 26.2).

Refer clients, spouses or partners, and their children to specialized services

As occupational therapy practitioners actively maintain a trust-based therapeutic alliance, clients with cancer may

TABLE 26.2.   Examples of Role-Specific Occupational Therapy Intervention Components

ROLE EXAMPLES	POSSIBLE OCCUPATIONAL THERAPY INTERVENTIONS
Parent	<ul><li>Provide information about age-specific developmental capabilities as clients make decisions about how to talk about cancer with their children.</li><li>Support clients' desire to maintain home routines for their children (Houldin & Lewis, 2006). This might mean helping clients determine which routines to prioritize and which to let go. Occupational therapy practitioners might assist clients in establishing new routines to reduce the cognitive load of frequently performed sequences. This might include developing a checklist to assure that a consistent sequence of steps is repeated and proceduralized until it becomes automatic (Radomski & Giles, 2014).</li><li>Acknowledge how planning family activities gives some clients a sense of control (Semple & McCance, 2010). Contribute to interactive problem solving with clients about ways to create meaningful leisure experiences with their families that align with their current abilities (Tavares et al., 2017).</li><li>Affirm the importance of the client's self-care to their long-term parental aspirations to counteract some clients' discomfort in occasionally putting their own health needs ahead of their children's needs (Semple & McCance, 2010).</li></ul>
Spouse or partner	<ul><li>As shaped by the client's self-reported priorities, normalize the challenges to relationships associated with cancer and encourage the client (and their spouse or partner as appropriate) to identify proactive actions that might help the couple to grow together (Fergus & Gray, 2009).</li><li>Given that clients and spouses or partners may be shifting task responsibilities at home, help the client determine what responsibilities to let go of and in what ways they can continue to contribute (Cubis et al., 2017). Explore task or equipment adaptations to optimize clients' ability to share responsibilities with their spouses or partners.</li></ul>
Friend	<ul><li>Encourage clients to accept practical help from social networks so they can preserve energy for valued social roles, especially during the active treatment phase (Semple & McCance, 2010). For many, being willing to receive help from others is a way to maintain connections with friends, which advances support and coping.</li><li>Help clients adjust expectations (if need be) and problem solve so they can pursue alternative activities or strategies to connect with others in meaningful ways (Cubis et al., 2017). For example, a client might derive a beneficial social connection by watching his buddies in a bowling tournament even if he is unable to bowl.</li><li>Provide clients with information about cancer support networks. Support groups may also help clients build new friendships, which might be especially important for individuals who have lost friends and acquaintances over the course of their illness.</li><li>Recognize that, especially after the active treatment phase, many cancer survivors support their own coping and find meaning by helping others (Agarwal et al., 2010; Cubis et al., 2017). Some cancer survivors want to pay it forward via volunteer work, and others find meaning in reciprocating the kindness they've received from friends.</li><li>When working with children or adolescents with cancer (and with their permission), explore ways to involve friends or siblings in therapy sessions. For example, an occupational therapy session to improve strength and endurance could involve playing active games with friends.</li><li>Work with school personnel to incorporate schoolwork into the occupational therapy intervention plan as well as to coordinate the client's return to school.</li></ul>

disclose social participation needs that are outside the domain of occupational therapy. By keeping a current list of other professionals in their organization or in the community, practitioners may best advance clients' social participation by referring them to other members of the interdisciplinary team. For example, some couples may benefit from counseling from psycho-oncology professionals or assistance from specialists for issues related to sexual function. Children or adolescents with cancer may benefit from groups or camps that allow them to connect with others in the same situation.

Summary of Evidence for Occupational Therapy to Support Social Participation

Despite the importance of social participation to the performance of roles and QoL, there is relatively little evidence to specify evidence-based interventions for occupational therapy practice. Studies that examine impairment-related interventions typically evaluate social participation as a secondary rather than primary outcome of the intervention (e.g., Lahart et al., 2018; Wolf et al., 2016). A recent systematic review examined 52 studies pertaining to occupational therapy–relevant psychosocial, sexuality, and return-to-work interventions (Hunter et al., 2017). Seven studies measured specific social role outcomes (e.g., social functioning, sexual activity, sexual function, social support, loneliness), only one of which involved an intervention delivered by an occupational therapist (Hegel et al., 2011).

A series of occupation-oriented interventions shows promise. In the study mentioned above, Hegel et al. (2011) used a small, randomized controlled trial to evaluate the feasibility of a problem-solving intervention for rural breast cancer survivors. Participants were randomized to Problem Solving and Occupational Therapy (PST–OT; $n = 15$) or usual care ($n = 16$). PST–OT involved 6 weekly sessions of a structured problem-solving intervention (goal setting and implementation/action planning) delivered via telephone. The intervention was found to be feasible, and measures of functioning, QoL, and emotional state favored the PST–OT condition.

In a prospective, one-group pretest–posttest pilot study, Lyons et al. (2018) extended this approach by combining a problem-solving treatment with behavioral activation within the context of six home-based occupational therapy sessions. The goal of the intervention was to use "strategic goal-setting, problem solving, and action planning to close the gap between what the person wanted to be able to do and what he or she was currently doing" (p. 2). The participants, 24 older adult cancer survivors, set 63 6-week goals. Twenty-two of the goals pertained to some dimension of social participation (i.e., leisure, socializing, volunteering), 12 (54.5%) of which were met over the 6 sessions.

In another prospective one-group pretest-posttest study, Maher and Mendonca (2018) evaluated the impact of a 1-week activity program on health, QoL, and occupational performance. Seventy-one breast cancer survivors completed the Camp Discovery intervention, which was offered 8 times over a 3-year period. Camp Discovery consisted of a 5-day group (4 hours per day) that involved classes and activities with both social and cognitive components (e.g., dance and Tai Chi [physical], poetry and scrapbooking [emotional], meditation and yoga [spiritual]). There were no pre–post changes in overall measures of QoL, except in the social relationships domain. Participants also demonstrated statistically significant pre–post improvements in occupational performance as measured by the COPM (Law et al., 2019). These occupation-oriented approaches warrant further study in the hopes that positive results will inform routine occupational therapy practice in the future.

SUMMARY

Maintaining or resuming activities that support participation in social roles is among many cancer survivors' top priorities. Returning to familiar social roles within family and social groups fosters feelings of accomplishment that remind cancer survivors that they are overcoming their cancer (Ferrell et al., 2003). However, many cancer survivors find it more difficult to maintain social activities than their everyday activities (Nikolić et al., 2015), suggesting that proficiency with ADLs and IADLs is not synonymous with social participation.

Occupational therapy practitioners can advance social role participation by formally or informally evaluating this dimension of occupational performance, regardless of the reason for which the client was referred to occupational therapy. Support to advance social participation can and should be routinely incorporated into the occupational therapy intervention plan for all cancer survivors by addressing the impairments that interfere with social role performance and providing education, support, and referrals to directly address social role distress.

REFERENCES

Agarwal, M., Hamilton, J. B., Crandell, J. L., & Moore, C. E. (2010). Coping strategies of African American head and neck cancer survivors. *Journal of Psychosocial Oncology, 28,* 526–538. https://doi.org/10.1080/07347332.2010.498456

American Occupational Therapy Association. (2014). Occupational therapy practice framework: Domain and process (3rd edition). *American Journal of Occupational Therapy, 68*(Suppl. 1), S1–S4. https://doi.org/10.5014/ajot.2014.682006

Arès, I., Lebel, S., & Bielajew, C. (2014). The impact of motherhood on perceived stress, illness intrusiveness and fear of cancer recurrence in young breast cancer survivors over time. *Psychology & Health, 29,* 651–670. https://doi.org/10.1080/08870446.2014.881998

Arora, N. K., Finney Rutten, L. J., Gustafson, D. H., Moser, R., & Hawkins, R. P. (2007). Perceived helpfulness and impact of social support provided by family, friends, and health care providers to women newly diagnosed with breast cancer. *Psycho-Oncology, 16,* 474–486. https://doi.org/10.1002/pon.1084

Barrera, M., Atenafu, E. G., Sung, L., Bartels, U., Schulte, F., Chung, J., . . . McConnell, D. (2018). A randomized control intervention trial to improve social skills and quality of life in pediatric brain tumor survivors. *Psycho-Oncology, 27,* 91–98. https://doi.org/10.1002/pon.4385

Bedell, G. M. (2004). Developing a follow-up survey focused on participation of children and youth with acquired brain injuries after discharge from inpatient rehabilitation. *NeuroRehabilitation, 19,* 191–205.

Bedell, G. (2009). Further validation of the Child and Adolescent Scale of Participation (CASP). *Developmental Neurorehabilitation, 12,* 342–351. https://doi.org/10.3109/17518420903087277

Bedell, G. (2011). The Child and Adolescent Scale of Participation (CASP). Administration and scoring guidelines. Retrieved from: Buckland, N., & Mackenzie, L. (2017). Exploring the role of occupational therapy in caring for cancer survivors in Australia: A cross sectional study. *Australian Occupational Therapy Journal, 64,* 358–368. https://doi.org/10.1111/1440-1630.12386

Buckland, N., & Mackenzie, L. (2017). Exploring the role of occupational therapy in caring for cancer survivors in Australia: A cross sectional study. *Australian Occupational Therapy Journal, 64,* 358–368. https://doi.org/10.1111/1440-1630.12386

Cubis, C., Ownsworth, T., Pinkham, M. B., & Chambers, S. (2017). The social trajectory of brain tumor: A qualitative metasynthesis. *Disability and Rehabilitation, 40*(16), 1857–1869. https://doi.org/10.1080/09638288.2017.1315183

Djurdjevic, A., & Nikolic, S. (2009). Profile of handicap situations in cancer patients. *Journal of the Balkan Union of Oncology, 14,* 435–440.

Eyssen, I. C. J. M., Beelen, A., Dedding, C., Cardol, M., & Dekker, J. (2005). The reproducibility of the Canadian Occupational Performance Measure. *Clinical Rehabilitation, 19,* 888–894. https://doi.org/10.1191/0269215505cr883oa

Fergus, K. D., & Gray, R. E. (2009). Relationship vulnerabilities during breast cancer: Patient and partner perspectives. *Psycho-Oncology, 18,* 1311–1322. https://doi.org/10.1002/pon.1555

Ferrell, B. R., Smith, S. L., Ervin, K. S., Itano, J., & Melancon, C. (2003). A qualitative analysis of social concerns of women with ovarian cancer. *Psycho-Oncology, 12,* 647–663. https://doi.org/10.1002/pon.681

Hahn, E. A., Devellis, R. F., Bode, R. K., Garcia, S. F., Castel, L. D., Eisen, S. V., . . . Cella, D. (2010). Measuring social health in the Patient-Reported Outcomes Measurement Information System (PROMIS): Item bank development and testing. *Quality of Life Research, 19,* 1035–1044. https://doi.org/10.1007/s11136-010-9654-0

Haluska, H. B., Jessee, P. O., & Nagy, M. C. (2002). Sources of social support: Adolescents with cancer. *Oncology Nursing Forum, 29,* 1317–1324. https://doi.org/10.1188/02.ONF.1317-1324

Hegel, M. T., Lyons, K. D., Hull, J. G., Kaufman, P., Urquhart, L., Li, Z., & Ahles, T. A. (2011). Feasibility study of a randomized controlled trial of a telephone-delivered problem-solving occupational therapy intervention to reduce participation restrictions in rural breast cancer survivors undergoing chemotherapy. *Psycho-Oncology, 20,* 1092–1101. https://doi.org/10.1002/pon.1830

Holmberg, S. K., Scott, L. L., Alexy, W., & Fife, B. L. (2001). Relationship issues of women with breast cancer. *Cancer Nursing, 24,* 53–60. https://doi.org/10.1097/00002820-200102000-00009

Houldin, A., & Lewis, F. M. (2006). Salvaging their normal lives: A qualitative study of patients with recently diagnosed advanced colorectal cancer. *Oncology Nursing Forum, 33,* 719–725. https://doi.org/10.1188/06.ONF.719-725

Hunter, E. G., Gibson, R. W., Arbesan, M., & D'Amico, M. (2017). Centennial Topics—Systematic review of occupational therapy and cancer rehabilitation: Part 2. Impact of multidisciplinary rehabilitation and psychosocial, sexuality, and return-to-work interventions. *American Journal of Occupational Therapy, 71,* 710210040 https://doi.org/10.5014/ajot.2017.023572

Huri, M., Huri, E., Kayihan, H., & Altuntas, O. (2015). Effects of occupational therapy on quality of life of patients with metastatic prostate cancer: A randomized controlled study. *Saudi Medical Journal, 36,* 954–961. https://doi.org/10.15537/smj.2015.8.11461

Hwang, E. J., Lokietz, N. C., Lozano, R. L., & Parke, M. A. (2015). Functional deficits and quality of life among cancer survivors: Implications for occupational therapy in cancer survivorship care. *American Journal of Occupational Therapy, 69,* 6906290010. https://doi.org/10.5014/ajot.2015.015974

Ishibashi, A. (2001). The needs of children and adolescents with cancer for information and social support. *Cancer Nursing, 24,* 61–67. https://doi.org/10.1097/00002820-200102000-00010

Lahart, I. M., Metsios, G. S., Nevill, A. M., & Carmichael, A. R. (2018). Physical activity for women with breast cancer after adjuvant therapy. *Cochrane Database Systematic Review, 1,* CD011292. https://doi.org/10.1002/14651858.CD011292.pub2.

Law M., Baptiste, S., Carswell, A., McColl, M. A., Polatajko, H., & Pollock, N. (2019). *Canadian Occupational Performance Measure Manual,* (5th ed., rev.). Altona, Man., Canada: COPM, Inc.

Lindahl-Jacobsen, L., Hansen, D. G., Wæhrens, E. E., la Cour, K., & Søndergaard, J. (2015). Performance of activities of daily living among hospitalized cancer patients. *Scandinavian Journal of Occupational Therapy, 22,* 137–146. https://doi.org/10.3109/11038128.2014.985253

Lyons, K. D., Newman, R. M., Kaufman, P. A., Bruce, M. L., Stearns, D. M., Lansigan, F., . . . Hegel, M. T. (2018). Goal attainment and goal adjustment of older adults during person-directed cancer rehabilitation. *American Journal of Occupational Therapy, 72,* 7202205110. https://doi.org/10.5014/ajot.2018.023648

Maher, C., & Mendonca, R. J. (2018). Impact of an activity-based program on health, quality of life, and occupational performance of women diagnosed with cancer. *American Journal of Occupational Therapy, 72,* 7202205040. https://doi.org/10.5014/ajot.2018.023663

McMullen, C., Liu, L., Bulkley, J. E., Hornbrook, M. C., Wendel, C., Grant, M., . . . Herrinton, L. (2017). Participation in activities associated with quality of life for long-term survivors of rectal cancer. *Permanente Journal, 21,* 16–011. https://doi.org/10.7812/TPP/16-011

Nagarajan, R., Mogil, R., Neglia, J. P., Robison, L. L., & Ness, K. K. (2008). Self-reported global function among adult survivors of childhood lower-extremity bone tumors: A report from the Childhood Cancer Survivor Study (CCSS). *Journal of Cancer Survivorship: Research and Practice, 3,* 59–65. https://doi.org/10.1007/s11764-008-0073-y

National Comprehensive Cancer Network. (2018). *National Comprehensive Cancer Network Distress Thermometer and Problem List.* Retrieved from https://www.nccn.org/about/permissions/thermometer.aspx

National Institutes of Health. (2014). *PROMIS satisfaction with social roles and activities.* Retrieved from https://www.assessmentcenter.net/documents/PROMIS%20Satisfaction%20with%20Participation%20in%20Social%20Roles%20Scoring%20Manual.pdf

National Institutes of Health. (2015). *PROMIS Satisfaction with Participation in Discretionary Social Activities.* Retrieved from https://www.assessmentcenter.net/documents/PROMIS%20Satisfaction%20with%20Participation%20in%20Discretionary%20Social%20Activities%20Scoring%20Manual.pdf

Nikolić, S., Ilić-Stosović, D., Kolarević, I., Djurdjević, A., Ilić, S., & Djuricić, M. (2015). Social participation of women with breast cancer. *Vojnosanitetski Pregled, 72,* 148–154. https://doi.org/10.2298/VSP1502148N

O'Neill, C., McCaughan, E., Semple, C. J., & Ryan, A. (2016). Fathers' experiences of living with cancer: A phenomenological study. *European Journal of Cancer Care, 27,* e12492. https://doi.org/10.1111/ecc.12492

Radomski, M. V., & Giles, G. M. (2014). Optimizing cognitive performance. In M. V. Radomski & C. A. T. Latham (Eds.), *Occupational therapy for physical dysfunction* (7th ed., pp. 725–752). Philadelphia: Lippincott Williams & Wilkins.

Ryff, C. D. (2014). Psychological well-being revisited: Advances in the science and practice of eudaimonia. *Psychotherapy and Psychosomatics, 83,* 10–28. https://doi.org/10.1159/000353263

Semple, C. J., & McCance, T. (2010). Experience of parents with head and neck cancer who are caring for young children. *Journal of Advanced Nursing, 66,* 1280–1290. https://doi.org/10.1111/j.1365-2648.2010.05311.x

Silver, J. K., & Gilchrist, L. S. (2011). Cancer rehabilitation with a focus on evidence-based outpatient physical and occupational therapy interventions. *American Journal of Physical Medicine and Rehabilitation, 90*(Suppl. 1), S5–S15. https://doi.org/10.1097/PHM.0b013e31820be4ae

Tavares, R., Brandão, T., & Matos, P. M. (2017). Mothers with breast cancer: A mixed-method systematic review on the impact on the parent-child relationship. *Psycho-Oncology, 27,* 1–9. https://doi.org/10.1002/pon.4451

Trombly, C. A., Radomski, M. V., & Davis, E. S. (1998). Achievement of self-identified goals by adults with acquired brain injury: Phase I. *American Journal of Occupational Therapy, 52,* 810–818. https://doi.org/10.5014/ajot.52.10.810

Wolf, T. J., Doherty, M., Kallogjeri, D., Coalson, R. S., Nicklaus, J., Ma, C. X., . . . Piccirillo, J. (2016). The feasibility of using metacognitive strategy training to improve cognitive performance and neural connectivity in women with chemotherapy-induced cognitive impairment. *Oncology, 91,* 143–152. https://doi.org/10.1159/000447744

Wood-Dauphinee, S. L., Opzoomer, M. A., Williams, J. I., Marchand, B., & Spitzer, W. O. (1988). Assessment of global function: The Reintegration to Normal Living Index. *Archives of Physical Medicine and Rehabilitation, 69,* 583–590.

World Health Organization. (2001). *International Classification of Functioning, Disability and Health—Short Version.* Geneva: Author.

Zebrack, B., Kent, E. E., Keegan, T. H. M., Kato, I., Smith, A. W., & AYA HOPE Study Collaborative Group 1. (2014). "Cancer sucks," and other ponderings by adolescent and young adult cancer survivors. *Journal of Psychosocial Oncology, 32,* 1–15. https://doi.org/10.1080/07347332.2013.855959

Caregiving

Tish Williams, OTR

LEARNING OBJECTIVES

After completing this chapter, readers should be able to
- Explain why the caregiver role is essential to the success of cancer care;
- Discover how the occupation of caregiving supports both the practical and the emotional aspects of cancer care for cancer survivors;
- Predict factors that contribute to occupational dysfunction among caregivers;
- Understand why evaluating caregiver needs and contributing to a plan of care helps support sustained occupational performance in caregiving; and
- Relate how meaningful, targeted interventions facilitate successful occupational engagement for supporting caregiver health, well-being, and self-efficacy.

KEY TERMS AND CONCEPTS

- Advocate
- Cancer survivors
- Care coordinator
- Caregiver burden
- Caregiver identity
- Caregivers
- Caregiving
- Direct care provider
- Early survivorship
- Emotional support provider
- End-of-life care
- Financial manager
- Late effects
- Legacy work
- Palliative care
- Quality of life
- Remission and survivorship
- Role engulfment
- Self-efficacy
- Shared identity
- Skilled performance
- Survivorship
- Telehealth

INTRODUCTION

Cancer survivors are individuals with a cancer diagnosis that is not yet life limiting. These individuals are considered to be survivors upon diagnosis until the end of life and often depend on caregivers to support their continued health and well-being as they transition from care provided by health care professionals to care provided in the home. Therefore, the role of the caregiver is essential to the success of cancer care. *Caregivers* may be parents, partners, siblings, children, friends, or any persons who share uncompensated responsibility for another individual's health, safety, and well-being. They are sometimes also referred to as *family caregivers* or *informal caregivers*.

During cancer treatment and *survivorship,* which begins on the day of diagnosis and extends beyond treatment until the end of life, cancer survivors come to rely on a designated caregiver to assist with supportive care for complex symptom management and various functional deficits, in addition to their medical team. Caregivers are increasingly being recognized as beneficial to overall health care for their ability to

- Contribute to patient satisfaction;
- Improve continuity of care;
- Assist with adherence to and acceptance of treatment;
- Prevent adverse events and rehospitalizations; and
- Reduce overall health care costs by decreasing emergency department visits, hospitalizations, and rehospitalizations.

Currently, caregivers represent the largest source of long-term care in the country, and their role of caring for those with chronic illnesses, such as cancer, is projected to grow by an estimated 85% between 2000 and 2050 (Eifert et al., 2015). Health care changes in recent years have contributed to the expansion of the occupation of *caregiving* to include performing medical tasks in the home that were once carried out by licensed professionals or provided only in hospitals or other facilities. This expansion of responsibilities is in addition to the assistance caregivers have typically provided with ADLs, IADLs, emotional support, and spiritual support. Many caregivers assume these responsibilities with little to no preparation or support from health care professionals and are at risk for experiencing caregiver-related stress or burden, which is known to negatively affect both emotional well-being and physical health.

Occupational therapy, with its focus on enabling participation in roles, habits, and routines, helps shape one's identity, health, and sense of competence or *self-efficacy* through occupational engagement (Kniepmann, 2012). Caregivers have identified successful occupational engagement as a way of evaluating and monitoring well-being and satisfaction in the role and as an indicator of whether they are providing good care (Williams, 2016). Occupational therapy practitioners support caregiver well-being and the occupation of caregiving, or nurturing the well-being of another individual, through screening for early identification of risk factors known to contribute to the decline of well-being; assessing for and assisting with the development of skills caregivers need to successfully execute the role; and using individualized, targeted interventions to facilitate successful occupational engagement in the role.

CAREGIVING AS OCCUPATION

Caregivers provide support important to both the practical and the emotional aspects of cancer care. Common occupations caregivers perform that support cancer survivors with practical needs may include assistance with transportation, finances, personal care, and symptom management. Emotional support may include encouraging cancer survivors in their spiritual concerns in addition to providing encouragement for anxiety, depression, and coping related to cancer and its treatment. A positive correlation is known to exist between perceived social and emotional support from family and the well-being of cancer survivors (Saritas et al., 2017).

However, the occupational needs and demands of the caregiver role are diverse and often change through the course of the illness trajectory. Kim and Carver (2012) categorized role demands caregivers reported according to phases of the illness trajectory to help guide occupational therapy practitioners in knowing what needs to address first during a particular phase. These phases include the early survivorship phase, the remission and survivorship phase, and the palliative and end-of-life phase. Not all cancer survivors experience all three phases.

- *Early survivorship* occurs from diagnosis through the initial treatment course. Caregivers spend substantial time providing informational and medical support to cancer survivors. Caregivers may be employed, with a need to balance both working and providing care. Greater levels of psychological stress and poorer health-related quality of life (QoL) compared with age-appropriate norms are reported in this phase.
- *Remission and survivorship* occurs after treatment and when cancer survivors are undergoing maintenance treatment interventions, are in remission, or are considered to be cancer free. This phase, when effects of the illness or treatment continue to require the attention of a caregiver, may last for decades. Caregivers report uncertainty about the future and fear that the disease may return. The financial burden from extended treatment and disruption in social relationships are sources of distress in this phase. Although overall distress may be reduced compared with the early survivorship phase, caregivers still often report high levels of psychological distress in this phase. They also tend to report that their needs in managing this distress go unmet (Ferrell et al., 2013).

- *Palliative and end-of-life care* occurs when the disease becomes life limiting, either during recurrence or if remission is not achieved. Caregiving needs tend to escalate in this phase as the burden of illness increases. Caregivers report needing formal, consistent, and no-cost help managing their loved one's symptoms and their own personal care. They also report needing spiritual, physical, and psychological support after the caregiver role ends because of the strain or burden induced by the role.

Caregivers often manage multiple roles in the context of caregiving. For example, a caregiver may take on both the care coordinator role and the role of direct care provider. In the care coordinator role, the caregiver assumes responsibilities for tasks the cancer survivor might have performed in a different stage of the illness trajectory, such as scheduling medical appointments or influencing medical decision making over a treatment course. The caregiver may be relied on at the same time to provide direct care for the ADL tasks of bathing and dressing and for IADL tasks of transportation to appointments and grocery shopping.

Categorizing or dividing the caregiver role can be useful in the development of interventions to address individual

TABLE 27.1.   Caregiver Roles and Common Associated Occupations

CAREGIVER ROLES	COMMON ASSOCIATED OCCUPATIONS
Direct care provider	- Provides medical symptom management (e.g., dispensing medication, monitoring body and medical device systems) - Assists with ADLs (e.g., bathing, dressing, toileting, grooming, eating, shaving, bowel bladder management, sexuality) - Helps with IADLs (e.g., cooking, shopping, running errands, completing household tasks, cleaning, reorganizing home environment)
Emotional support provider	- Provides companionship - Encourages cancer survivor self-efficacy - Includes spiritual support
Care coordinator	- Manages care across settings and providers - Schedules appointments - Provides transportation - Helps make medical decisions - Facilitates cancer survivor's understanding of care - Manages medical emergencies
Advocate	- Receives important information - Facilitates provider understanding - Helps maintain social relationships - Facilitates cancer survivor's self-care tasks
Financial manager	- Handles finances and financial issues - Helps facilitate legal support and advance care directives - Gathers resources and support

Note. ADLs = activities of daily living; IADLs = instrumental activities of daily living.
Source. Roles from O'Sullivan (2015).

caregiver needs. O'Sullivan (2015) categorized the caregiver role into five main roles: (1) direct care provider, (2) emotional support provider, (3) care coordinator, (4) advocate, and (5) financial manager (see Table 27.1).

The home is the preferred place to receive long-term care for many cancer survivors and is associated with decreased hospital-related infections, decreased costs, improved appetite, and improved QoL (Applebaum et al., 2016). Traditionally, caregivers provided assistance with ADL and IADL tasks, whereas other licensed providers carried out what were considered medical and nursing tasks such as managing prescription medications, wound care, ventilators, and tube feeding systems (O'Sullivan, 2015). However, many of the tasks that licensed providers once carried out have now fallen within the responsibility of caregivers to manage in the home because of

- Dramatic growth in the number of people living with serious and chronic illnesses, such as cancer, who need long-term care;
- Earlier discharges from acute care hospitals;
- Increased hospital inpatient-care costs;
- Changes in reimbursement for health care services;
- An increase in the aging population; and
- Advances in cancer treatment leading to long cancer survivorships (Ferrell & Wittenberg, 2017).

Developing effective interventions to support caregivers and reduce the negative effects associated with caregiving requires occupational therapy practitioners to take into account that

- Occupational needs and demands of the role change over time,
- Caregivers often manage multiple roles in the context of caregiving, and
- The caregiver role is expanding to include more complex tasks.

FACTORS CONTRIBUTING TO OCCUPATIONAL DYSFUNCTION IN CAREGIVING

Caregiver burden describes the potential negative effects that providing care can have on a caregiver's health, emotional status, and QoL, which often also adversely affects occupational, social, and personal roles (Kaveney et al., 2016). The caregiver role can last for months or years. It can continue after cancer treatment ends, placing caregivers at risk for decline in their own physical health and emotional well-being. Longer cancer survivorships tend to yield more complex interactions and unforeseen situations and challenges between caregivers and cancer survivors. This, along with the added financial strain, disruption of social roles, and decrease in QoL often associated with the role, can threaten the ability of caregivers to continue providing care (Lund et al., 2015). Poor QoL with a higher caregiver burden has been associated with

- Increased health care utilization and costs,
- Increased risk of care-recipient institutionalization,
- Increased risk of mortality for the caregiver, and
- Decreased overall utilization of resources and services for assistance (Sleight & Duker, 2016).

A reduction or cessation in valued occupations along with role changes often indicates that a caregiver is experiencing strain or a decline in well-being. Recognizing major risk factors that contribute to decline is important for effectively supporting caregivers and anticipating support they may need to reduce burden or strain. Major risk factors known to affect caregiver well-being are listed in Exhibit 27.1.

Drabe et al. (2015) found that the most important risk factors for the development of psychological stress among caregivers were being female and having past episodes of depression, followed by illness progression and physical burden. Lifestyle and role disruptions, an avoidant coping style, and problems interacting with the medical team were also important factors. Kim and Carver (2012) found that the major issues caregivers reported needing assistance with across the illness trajectory were

- Managing the psychological concerns of cancer survivors as well as their own,
- Obtaining help with ADLs and daily tasks, and
- Managing medical and side-effect symptoms.

Other factors that contribute to higher levels of caregiver distress included the caregiver

- Having inadequate knowledge and skills to deliver proper care;
- Not asking for care for themselves;
- Taking on a range of unfamiliar tasks;
- Feeling unprepared to manage or having low self-efficacy for managing symptoms;
- Receiving too little guidance from health care professionals;
- Lacking resources needed for caregiving such as finances, adequate transportation, or access to respite care; and
- Experiencing poor integration into the health care delivery system because medical insurance providers focus on the cancer survivor or beneficiary (Badr et al., 2015).

Occupational Performance and Caregiver Well-Being

Occupational therapy practitioners assess caregiver well-being and the sustainability of occupational performance by simultaneously attending to the caregiver's "body functions and structures, skills, roles, habits, routines, and contexts" (American Occupational Therapy Association [AOTA], 2014, p. S4) during occupational engagement.

Client factors

Physical well-being includes sleep quality, fatigue, and health problems along with physical functioning. Negative physical and psychological symptoms caused by caregiving can lead to fatigue and sleep disturbance such as insomnia. Nearly half of all cancer caregivers report sleep disturbances, a level comparable to that of cancer survivors (Kim & Carver, 2012). Diminished overall health because of caregiver burden was also reported by more than half of cancer caregivers, who listed arthritis, hypertension, and heart problems as common health concerns (Glajchen, 2012). Cancer caregivers report higher rates of physical ailments compared with persons their age who are not caregivers and report lower levels of overall subjective well-being (O'Sullivan, 2015).

EXHIBIT 27.1.	Risk Factors Affecting Caregiver Well-Being

Age
- Younger caregivers often need to balance employment with the caregiver role and other roles.
- Younger caregivers and caregivers to younger patients report higher levels of interaction problems and unmet needs (Lund et al., 2015).
- Elderly caregivers report depression, poorer self-rated health, and difficulty sustaining care at home.

Gender
- Women exhibit higher levels of burden and are at greater risk for depression, anxiety, and drug use than men.
- Men often treat caregiving as a job in which they can achieve "mastery," compared with women, who focus on providing physical assistance and on relationship changes.

Personality
- Caregivers who worry more than others tend to show increased distress levels.
- Extroverted caregivers may recruit more support and maintain pleasurable activities.
- Conscientious caregivers report lower levels of depression.
- Organized caregivers report lower levels of stress.

Relationship dynamics
- Preexisting relationship difficulties with the cancer survivor place caregivers at risk for distress.
- Spousal caregivers may have more distress if the role is expected of them rather than freely chosen.

Caregiver health and mental status
- Older caregivers experiencing cognitive impairment often struggle with depression and difficulty sustaining care at home.
- Older caregivers are at risk for engaging in potentially harmful behaviors toward cancer survivors.
- Caregivers report that providing psychosocial support is stressful but that caring for a cancer survivor with communication difficulties is the most stressful.

Level of care required
- Increased risk of mortality and cancer survivor institutionalization are associated with cancer survivors who need large amounts of physical, cognitive, or behavioral support over a long period of time.
- Caregivers who assist with cancer survivors' ADLs often demonstrate poor preventive health behaviors and decreased participation in leisure activity.
- As the level of care increases, caregiver levels of depression, general forgetfulness, excessive worry, and feelings of inadequacy often increase.

Access to resources and respite
- Caregivers confined to their home can experience decreased well-being because of physical isolation and decreased social relationships.

Stress triggers for harmful behaviors
- Higher levels of physical care over longer periods of time, cognitive impairments related to the cancer survivor's condition, inadequate access to community resources, and caregiver decline are associated with triggering caregiver depression, anxiety, low self-esteem, and substance abuse.
- Stress triggers place caregivers at risk for exhibiting physically or psychologically harmful behaviors such as yelling, withholding food, threatening institutionalization, insulting, and rough handling.
- Harmful behaviors are precursors to neglect and abuse.

Note. ADLs = activities of daily living.
Source. Information from Williams (2016).

QoL includes physical, mental, social, and spiritual well-being. Caregivers consistently report experiencing higher levels of mental health problems, such as depression, anxiety, fear, helplessness, uncertainty, and guilt, compared with their peers who are not caregivers (O'Sullivan, 2015). Those who care for individuals with incurable cancer tend to demonstrate high levels of depression and anxiety; their levels of anxiety often exceed that of the care recipient (Nipp et al., 2016).

In one study, caregivers were found to maintain spiritual well-being by relying on religion or other aspects of spiritual support while examining the meaning and purpose of life, but they reported struggling at times to maintain hope (Ferrell & Wittenberg, 2017). Overall, caregivers tend to report greater mental health symptoms, such as distress and sadness across time, versus cancer survivors, who report greater physical symptoms of pain, fatigue, and sleep disturbance (Nipp et al., 2016).

Performance skills

The ability of caregivers to maintain well-being depends not only on their ability to maintain QoL along with physical,

mental, and spiritual health but also on their ability to sustain skilled performance. *Skilled performance* within the context of well-being allows a caregiver to

- Continue providing care,
- Organize the coordination of care,
- Respond to the cancer survivor's needs as well as other social relationships,
- Adjust care according to changes in needs and demands, and
- Navigate the health care system and the financial and legal responsibilities related to providing care.

Caregiving can change well-established patterns of interaction between the caregiver and cancer survivor, which can strain the relationship and create family tension. For example, a spouse ceases to just be a spouse when the role of caregiver is added, or a parent–child relationship may shift so that the child begins caring for the parent. A caregiver often has a *shared identity* with the cancer survivor, or an identity based on the relationship or being part of a couple (Eifert et al., 2015). The disruption of shared identity affects shared performance skills, such as joint decision making or co-occupations. Changes in shared identity and other social factors, such as coping styles between the caregiver and cancer survivor, can cause conflicts to emerge or become exaggerated and can add to caregiver distress (Goldsmith et al., 2016). This can create a sense of loss for the relationship as it once was and is one of the many kinds of losses caregivers may experience that can affect their ability to sustain the performance skills needed to carry out their role (Family Caregiver Alliance, 2013).

Performance patterns

Health, well-being, and participation also depend on whether the essential skills individuals need to perform for an occupation are "embedded in a productive set of engagement patterns" (AOTA, 2014, p. S8), such as a self-care or exercise routine or weekly participation in a leisure interest. When habituation or an individual's usual pattern of habits and roles within a certain environment is challenged, they may lose the familiarity, consistency, and relative ease of daily life (Taylor, 2017). Role change accompanies this shift and involves alterations to identity, one's relationship to others, tasks one must perform, and the organization of one's lifestyle (Taylor, 2017).

Changes in role functioning usually occur as an illness progresses, when greater assistance with ADLs is required. The need to manage the cancer survivor's behavioral problems or an abrupt transition into the caregiver role may cause the caregiver to experience role overload or engulfment (Bastawrous et al., 2015). *Role engulfment* includes losing one's sense of self and happens when the responsibilities of caregiving leave little time for other activities and behaviors that might have previously defined the caregiver (Eifert et al., 2015). Caregivers may find they lack time and energy for performing their own self-care and exercise routines, preparing nutritious meals, or seeing health providers for their own care.

Caregiver burden and stress are associated with having a greater number of social roles (Family Caregivers in Cancer, 2019). Cancer caregivers often carry out multiple social roles, such as being a parent, employee, or caregiver for an elderly parent, while caring for a cancer survivor. An imbalance of care demands relative to the caregiver's personal time, social roles, resources, and physical and emotional states can increase social problems for the caregiver, such as isolation (Applebaum et al., 2016).

Contexts and environments

Maintaining familiarity, consistency, and the relative ease of daily life depends not only on the performance patterns of occupation but also on the contexts and environments where those performance patterns are being carried out. Support for or barriers to engagement and participation in an occupation also exist within the contexts and environment where an occupation is performed. Home continues to be the preferred environment for cancer survivors to receive care, especially those who need long-term care or care during a life-limiting illness (Marston et al., 2015). In the home environment, the caregiver's role is central to the health and well-being of the cancer survivor. Home is often considered the ideal environment to address caregiver needs because

- Caregiver tasks can be addressed in the context in which they are naturally performed,
- ADLs and IADLs that are usually home-based routines can be adapted in the home rather than recreated in a clinic or hospital setting,
- Specific customized recommendations and adaptations unique to the caring situation can be made, and
- The burden of accessing health care outside the home may be reduced (O'Sullivan, 2015).

In contrast, the hospital environment can fail to integrate the caregiver into decision making and care management, which can lead to feelings of helplessness if the caregiver was used to being the cancer survivor's main caregiver before hospital admission (Robinson et al., 2014). The hospital environment is also known for being busy and noisy and lacking privacy, which can present challenges for well-being, especially for dying patients and their caregivers.

OCCUPATIONAL THERAPY EVALUATION OF CAREGIVING

Occupational therapy practitioners use the occupational profile and an analysis of occupational performance during caregiver evaluation to systematically gather information for the development of targeted, individualized interventions. Such interventions are based on

- The multiple roles the caregiver holds,
- Gaps in knowledge and skills the caregiver needs to provide care,
- The resources and type of assistance the caregiver finds useful and acceptable,
- The strengths the caregiver brings to the caregiving situation, and
- Barriers the caregiver may face in meeting the cancer survivor's needs.

Occupational Profile

The caregiver's occupational history and experience, patterns of daily living, interests, values, needs, access to support and resources, and caregiving environment give insight into their perspective and support network through the development of the occupational profile.

Caregiver identity

Caregiver identity, or whether people identify themselves as caregivers, is assessed through the occupational profile and is associated with effective role navigation. Caregiver identity develops in association with a life change that necessitates the restructuring of a person's roles to focus on the activities and responsibilities associated with caregiving. Identifying with the caregiver role gives caregivers a context for effective problem solving, decision making, and role navigation.

Caregivers who identify themselves as caregivers usually

- Assume the role willingly,
- Find satisfaction in the role,
- Feel the positive aspects of the role outweigh the negative, and
- Demonstrate a greater use of support services and resources.

Cancer survivors have also been shown to appreciate care assistance more from self-identified caregivers. Self-identified caregivers report they find improved well-being and satisfaction from the role, gain a greater appreciation for life, feel important and useful, have greater inner strength and confidence, and feel they have a closer personal connection with the cancer survivor (Williams, 2016).

Research suggests that addressing the "challenges individuals face in identifying themselves as caregivers is potentially more important for developing effective interventions to address their needs than focusing on simply reducing the strain or burden associated with this role" (Williams, 2016, p. CE-1). Caregivers often struggle to identify themselves as such when they feel forced into the role or when they see the role merely as an extension of their role as a partner or child. Caregivers who do not identify themselves as caregivers tend to underuse support services and resources and describe feeling a lack of appreciation for their efforts by the cancer survivor as well as other family members, those in their social circles, and health care professionals. Exhibit 27.2 provides a template for an occupational profile that includes assessing caregiver identity.

Analysis of Occupational Performance

Occupational therapy practitioners synthesize information gathered from the occupational profile along with information from assessment tools and observed occupational performance to identify specific occupations and contexts that need to be addressed for sustained occupational performance. Selecting and using specific assessment tools assists practitioners in discovering those assets, problems, and potential problems that most support and hinder occupational performance. Guiding questions during the analysis of occupational performance useful to practitioners can include:

- Was the caregiver's perspective considered?
- Was the caregiver's understanding of the role and care task requirements clarified?
- Were measurable outcomes for the caregiver identified?
- Was the need for other supportive services and referrals identified?
- Were the limitations on the caregiver's time and energy respected?
- Were the caregiver's values and preferences incorporated into the care plan?
- Were the caregiver's health, well-being, and potential consequences of caregiving considered?
- Were requirements for care and occupational demands needed for care determined?

Assessments commonly used for caregiving

Occupational therapy practitioners can assess objective and subjective reactions to the caregiving situation through ADLs and IADLs. They can also use specific assessment tools to give insight into whether caregiver problems are related to specific caregiving tasks, the cancer survivor's symptoms, or the general effect of caregiving itself. Some commonly used assessments for caregiving are described in Exhibit 27.3.

EVIDENCE-BASED OCCUPATIONAL THERAPY INTERVENTIONS THAT SUPPORT CAREGIVING

Interventions using daily occupations to facilitate successful occupational engagement contribute to the well-being of both the caregiver and the cancer survivor as well as foster the continuity of the caregiver–survivor relationship. Effective interventions for caregivers share the following common features:

- *Timing:* Successful interventions match current occupational needs and role demands when the caregiver is ready to receive the support. Both educational and support needs as well as needs within the caregiving context change throughout the disease trajectory. Therefore, providing a combination of resources specific to a caregiver's needs at a particular time can help to decrease negative health consequences.
- *Relevance:* Functional recovery has been shown to be enhanced during the transition between care settings when interventions are specific, meaningful occupations in the form of "real-life tasks" relevant to a care situation. Caregivers demonstrate a need for occupational therapy practitioners to provide interventions beyond simple solutions because caregivers have often already faced difficult situations that required them to try and reject many interventions on their own (Williams, 2016).

EXHIBIT 27.2.	Assessing Caregiver Identity Through the Occupational Profile

History and experiences
- Age, gender, personality, dynamics of relationship to care recipient, mental and physical health status
- Presence of stress triggers for harmful behaviors

Interests and values
- Supported by or changed by the caregiver role
- Ability and frequency of engagement in desired and leisure activities
- Cultural and spiritual factors

Performance patterns: Roles and daily living patterns
- Level of care provided to the care recipient
- Roles currently engaged in; does the individual identify with the caregiver role?
- Successes and barriers to carrying out care tasks
- Feelings of role competence versus role challenges

Needs and priorities
- Perception of needs being acknowledged and met
- Coping skills and style
- Frequency of engagement in health preventive behaviors

Environment
- Barriers to performing caring tasks: physical, emotional, financial
- Need for modifications or simplifications

Support
- Access to and eligibility for resources and respite
- Level of support perceived as adequate or lacking
- Comfort level and ability to recruit support

Note. Adapted from Williams (2016).

EXHIBIT 27.3. Commonly Used Caregiver Assessment Tools

Brief Assessment Scale for Caregivers (Glajchen et al., 2005)
- 14-item tool measuring distress or burden among caregivers of patients with chronic illness

Caregiver Oncology Quality of Life Questionnaire (Kaveney et al., 2016)
- 29-item cancer-specific questionnaire assessing psychological well-being, burden, relationship with health care, finances, coping, physical well-being, self-esteem, leisure time, and social support

Caregiver Quality of Life Index—Cancer Scale (Weitzner et al., 1999)
- 35-item cancer-specific instrument measuring caregiver quality of life and physical, emotional, and financial well-being and functioning

Caregiver Reaction Assessment (Given et al., 1992)
- 24-item, 5-subscale tool for assessing schedule, health, finances, family support, and esteem for caregivers of older adults and adults with cancer, physical impairment, and Alzheimer's disease

Caregiver Self-Assessment Questionnaire (Health in Aging Foundation, 2015)
- 18-item questionnaire measuring physical and emotional distress of caregivers and their behavior and health risks when caring for chronically ill or older adults

Rapid Caregiver Well-Being Scale (Tebb et al., 2013)
- 6-item tool used to look at caregiver well-being from a strengths-based perspective of caregiver basic human needs and satisfaction with ADLs

Life Balance Inventory (Matuska, 2012)
- Uses 8 sections representative of life; takes a systematic approach, looking at how a person spends time and energy in a day for each section and the satisfaction the person has with the time and energy spent in each section

Modified Caregiver Strain Index (Thornton & Travis, 2003)
- 13-item questionnaire for caregivers of chronically ill and older adults to assess financial, physical, psychological, social, and personal well-being

Occupational Self Assessment (Baron et al., 2006)
- 21-item questionnaire assessing sense of competence for performing everyday occupations; assigns importance to those occupations to help with prioritization

Occupational Self-Assessment Short Form (Popova et al., 2019)
- 12-item client-centered, self-report measure for occupational competence and value

Preparedness for Caregiving Scale (Henriksson et al., 2011)
- 8-item questionnaire to assess how well prepared caregivers feel for providing physical and emotional care as well as setting up in-home supportive services and dealing with stress

Rewards of Caregiving Scale (Henriksson et al., 2011)
- Revised to a 16-item unidimensional scale measuring positive consequences of caregiving demands, palliative coping, depression, and caregiver burden

Role Checklist (Oakley et al., 1986)
- A written inventory, requiring approximately 15 minutes to administer, for use with adolescents, adults, and older adults. Part 1 assesses the major occupational roles that organize an individual's daily life along a temporal continuum. Part 2 identifies the degree to which each occupational role is valued.

Sense of Competence Questionnaire (Vernooij-Dassen et al., 1999)
- 35-item questionnaire assessing caregiver satisfaction with caregiver performance and satisfaction with the care recipient

Note. ADLs = activities of daily living.

- *Collaboration:* Collaborating with caregivers provides practitioners a way to recognize the knowledge, skills, and experience a caregiver already possesses to help promote improved carryover of interventions that are individualized and meaningful to the caregiver. Learning caregiving skills with guidance from experienced professionals has been shown to improve QoL and decrease preventable injuries (Williams, 2016).
- *Communication:* Practitioners who establish collaborative reasoning with caregivers often more accurately frame problems within the caregiving context and situation to help with acceptance of and adherence to occupational therapy interventions. Establishing a supportive environment for learning that is meaningful from the viewpoint of the caregiver may mean that the practitioner does not always need to assume the expert role.

Interventions offering a combination of education, skills training, environmental modification, and access to supportive resources help promote safety, health, and well-being

for caregivers and cancer survivors. Occupational therapy interventions supportive to caregivers in specific settings are listed in Exhibit 27.4.

Caregivers report decreased burden and improved QoL when trained on ADLs (Williams, 2016). The ability of caregivers to participate in preferred leisure activities has been shown to have a great impact on their overall well-being (Pierce, 2012). In one study, caregivers identified that they had the greatest need for developing strategies for
- Keeping the cancer survivor safe at home,
- Managing their own stress,
- Engaging the cancer survivor in care tasks,
- Finding time for themselves,
- Managing challenging behaviors,
- Balancing work and other family responsibilities, and
- Safely moving or lifting the cancer survivor (O'Sullivan, 2015).

Barriers to providing adequate interventions for caregivers include:
- Caregivers may not recognize when they need support.

EXHIBIT 27.4.   Occupational Therapy Interventions Supportive to Caregivers in Specific Settings

Clinic-based interventions
- Education and training on assisting with ADLs, mobility, and communication needs of care recipient
- Emphasis on physical and cognitive impairment remediation and compensatory strategy training for care recipient
- Emphasis on dressing and bowel–bladder management to ease caregiver burden
- Emphasis on safety training
- Beginning behavior management training
- Beginning medication management training
- Beginning stress management and relaxation techniques
- Referral to other services, such as counseling and nutrition

Home health interventions
- Role balance education for caregivers; emphasis on work balance with younger caregivers and on balancing the caregiver role with other family roles
- Ability and frequency of engagement in desired and leisure activities
- Emphasis on medication management
- Development of efficient daily routines with simplification strategies
- Emphasis on addressing the need for environmental modifications and safety training
- Time management and organization training for coordinating follow-up medical care, transportation needs, and other role demands
- Stress management and relaxation techniques
- Behavior management techniques
- Skills training on telehealth and other supportive technology assistance
- Skills training to access community resources and recruit support for respite
- Energy conservation and fatigue management training
- Referrals to other services such as counseling, financial and legal management

Community-based interventions
- Role balance education for resuming social activities, travel, and sexuality
- Emphasis on addressing community accessibility
- Skills training to access community resources and to recruit support and respite care
- Skills training on telehealth and other supportive technology assistance
- Stress management and relaxation techniques
- Behavior management techniques
- Energy conservation training
- Referrals to other services such as counseling, financial and legal management

Note. ADLs = activities of daily living.

Source. From "Supporting Caregiver Identity," by T. Williams, 2016, *OT Practice, 21*(19), p. CE5. Copyright © 2016 by the American Occupational Therapy Association. Used with permission.

- Caregivers may not have access to supportive resources or may not know how to access and use resources.
- Third-party payers and providers view health care as time limited and focus on the cancer survivor rather than the caregiver.
- Health care professionals report they have limited time to talk to or train caregivers and may view caregivers as intrusive.
- Caregivers or health care professionals may lack adequate communication skills.

Underutilization of support services has been found with the following caregiver behaviors:
- Refusal to take a physical break from the role,
- Reluctance to leave the cancer survivor unattended for even short periods,
- Belief that others cannot assist the cancer survivor as well, and
- Uncertainty in identifying whether help is needed (Williams, 2016).

Addressing Caregivers of Children and Adolescents

Parental caregivers continue to be their child's protector and nurturer and to facilitate life skills training through child rearing while fulfilling the caregiver role. Parental distress can negatively affect children and adolescents with cancer and their siblings and is often elicited by the perceived suffering of their child, poor symptom control, and the process of mourning the loss of the healthy child, or the child the parent imagined having. Zhukovsky et al. (2015) found that parents who overestimate their child's emotional distress compared with what the child reports may have distress for years both if the child survives or after bereavement.

Children and adolescent cancer survivors often demonstrate a pattern of limited personal care skills, chores, social activities, and school pursuits because of the "late effects" or toxic effects of cancer treatments (Berg & Hayashi, 2013). *Late effects* include any side effect related to cancer treatment that does not resolve after treatment is completed and manifests at a later time during growth, development, or aging. Common late effects include but are not limited to chronic pain, depression, fatigue, chemotherapy-induced cognitive impairment, and body image distortion.

Late effects often interfere with opportunities for adolescent cancer survivors or young adults to seek higher education, employment, and romantic relationships and to transition into independent living. These missed opportunities can result in significant financial strain for the parental caregiver as well as emotional, physical, and social strain. Parents have reported that social–emotional, practical, and financial support are crucial to their ability to cope with the caregiver role (Rosenberg-Yunger et al., 2013). In Case Example 27.1, Ricardo discusses with his son Enrique's occupational therapist the emotional strain he's experiencing with Enrique not wanting to return to school or to family gatherings after cancer treatment. Problems in relationships and family life as well as social isolation, depression, anxiety, and loneliness were the main problems parental caregivers reported they face as a result of their role (Fuentes et al., 2014).

Evaluating parental caregivers should include assessing their sense of competence as parents and how they can meet their own needs while caring for other family members, in addition to the evaluation process already discussed in this chapter. Interventions may include training on child behavior management strategies, advocating for support services, supporting the child's development, nurturing parents' relationship with their child, and helping them communicate with their child about the child's disease process (Cohn & Henry, 2008).

Addressing Caregivers of Older Adults

Caring for older adults with cancer often involves additional challenges that place caregivers at high risk for burden. More than half of all cancers occur among older adults, or those age 65 years and older (Pergolotti et al., 2015). Comorbidities, frailty, and geriatric syndromes are more common among older adults with cancer and are associated with morbidity and poor outcomes (Hsu et al., 2014). Geriatric syndromes such as delirium, falls, incontinence, functional decline, and pressure ulcers are common health conditions for older adults. Risk factors for geriatric syndromes (e.g., older age, impaired mobility, functional impairment, cognitive impairment), along with the effects of treatment protocols such as chemotherapy, have been associated with poorer physical and mental health, which leads to unplanned hospital admissions, longer stays, and readmissions because of both difficulty with symptom control and caregiver burden (Geddie et al., 2016; Pergolotti et al., 2015).

The average age of caregivers for older adults is age 63 years, with one-third of those caregivers reporting fair to poor health themselves (O'Sullivan, 2015). Although it is

CASE EXAMPLE 27.1. RICARDO: CAREGIVER TO AN ADOLESCENT

Ricardo is 47 years old and the father of 16-year-old **Enrique,** who has limited left upper-extremity and hand function after osteosarcoma to his cervical spine. Ricardo expressed that although he was pleased with Enrique's progress in the ability to use his arm, he was frustrated with Enrique's lack of desire to return to school and even more so with Enrique's disinterest in participating in family gatherings. Regularly meeting with their extended family and being close to them was important to Ricardo as part of passing on their family's culture to Enrique and his siblings.

Enrique openly shared with the occupational therapist that he did not plan to return to school or to attend family gatherings until his left arm looked and functioned normally. He said he was tired of his family feeling sorry for him for not being able to do things he used to do, and he did not want to be asked about his cancer and therapy every week. Ricardo told Enrique he was being disrespectful to the people who love him.

"See, this is why none of his kids want to spend time with him. You can't be human around this guy," Enrique said before walking out of the therapy session.

After a few moments of silence, Ricardo volunteered that there was no need to refer Enrique to counseling because he would not go.

Occupational therapy interventions used to support Ricardo included training on behavior management strategies. The occupational therapist asked whether Enrique kept in contact with any family members outside of the family gatherings. Ricardo replied that Enrique did keep in touch with one cousin a year younger and an uncle who was 5 years older. Ricardo agreed that

providing opportunities for Enrique to spend more time with his cousin and uncle would offer some interaction with their extended family until Enrique felt he could go to bigger gatherings.

The occupational therapist educated both Ricardo and Enrique on body image and the effects of body image disruption among adolescents going through changes from cancer and treatment. This assisted Ricardo in understanding the scope of the effects of his son's disease process. Ricardo said he knew Enrique was having difficulty with body image but did not know what to call it or what to do about it.

Ricardo shared that he had been hard on Enrique because he wanted the best for his son and often did not give him much of a break from working on his left arm at home or insisting he visit family. The occupational therapist asked Ricardo to recall things he enjoyed doing with Enrique that nurtured their relationship before Enrique's cancer diagnosis that did not involve Enrique working to improve himself. Ricardo said they used to listen to mariachi band music together but had not done that for some time.

Enrique's uncle brought him to his next therapy session, and Enrique wore workout gloves with the tips of his fingers exposed. He said his father had purchased them for him. Enrique liked that they made him look like he was getting ready to go to the gym. They hid the intrinsic muscle wasting and mild deformity of his left hand. When asked whether he had listened to any mariachi band music with his dad, Enrique said his father had asked him whether he wanted to, but they had not done so yet. Enrique said he might next time his father asked.

generally recognized that caregivers for older adults provide care that is high quality and in alignment with the care recipient's preferences, complex caregiving situations arise in caregiving for older adults that contribute to mental, emotional, and physical health problems for caregivers. When older caregivers who have their own health limitations experience burden, they may have difficulty sustaining care in the home and are known to have a greater mortality risk (Williams, 2016).

Older caregivers are more likely to care for someone with a need for greater ADL and IADL assistance. This, along with the caregiver's advanced age and health limitations, places the caregiver at a higher risk for depression. Older spousal caregivers may be at a higher risk for depression than the cancer survivor they are caring for (Jayani & Hurria, 2012). Caregivers who demonstrate high symptoms of depression and anxiety tend not to use formal support services, despite expressing an interest in those services (Dionne-Odom et al., 2018). Cognitive decline among caregivers places them at a greater risk for both depression and engaging in harmful behaviors such as rough handling, yelling, neglect, threats of institutionalization, and abuse (Williams, 2016). However, older caregiver age has also been associated with better adjustment during bereavement (Jayani & Hurria, 2012).

In Case Example 27.2, Karen shares with her sister Sarah's occupational therapist how overwhelmed she feels by not having adequate support or support services while caring for her sister. Evaluation for caregivers of older adults includes assessing for cognitive decline as well as other health-limitation barriers, access to support services, and the presence of risk factors for harmful behaviors and depression. Additional occupational therapy interventions may include training on managing mobility, ADL and IADL performance, cognitive decline, role balance (with attention paid to burden of care), and environmental modification for task simplification.

Addressing Caregivers at End of Life

Caregivers provide the majority of care at end of life and thus play an important role in the emotional and practical aspects of care along with end-of-life decision making. *End-of-life care* can be thought of as a continuum of palliative care that describes care when death is imminent, whereas *palliative care* itself focuses on effectively controlling symptoms and maintaining QoL at any stage of a life-limiting illness (Hammill et al., 2014; see Chapter 13, "Palliative Care and Hospice," for more information). QoL during end of life is a "dynamic process that is negotiated and renegotiated" (Mori et al., 2012, p. 666) among the caregiver, care recipient, and health care professionals. When physical symptoms are managed, QoL may be improved through opportunities for end-of-life preparation; remembrances; resolution

---

CASE EXAMPLE 27.2. KAREN: CAREGIVER TO AN OLDER ADULT

Karen is age 61 years and the caregiver for her sister **Sarah,** who is age 84 years and in remission for metastatic breast cancer, with an unknown cause of motoric slowing and executive function decline. Sarah was diagnosed with depression after her husband died 2 years earlier and has regular visits with her psychiatrist.

Karen moved Sarah into a senior living apartment after finding out that Sarah's home had a large hole in the roof and had not been cleaned in the 2 years since her husband's death. Sarah remains angry with Karen for this. She expects both transportation and emotional support from Karen but often says unkind things to her. Sarah refuses to meet anyone at her senior apartments and refuses to use their transportation services.

Karen is a business executive with a heavy work schedule. She enjoys her job and worked hard to obtain the position she holds. She identified herself as the caregiver for her husband, who has Parkinson's disease. Although Karen is the only person in Sarah's life who provides assistance for her or contacts her regularly, when she brought Sarah to one of her occupational therapy sessions, she did not identify herself as Sarah's caregiver. Each time the term *caregiver* was mentioned to her in reference to Sarah, Karen said, "She can't come live with me."

Karen shared she was already struggling with balancing her work projects with her husband's care. She resented Sarah's anger over being moved into a safer home environment and Sarah's lack of appreciation for Karen's help. Karen also felt their large age difference was a problem, with Sarah frequently getting upset because she perceived that her younger sister was telling her what to do. Karen admitted to engaging in the harmful behaviors of yelling, threatening to withhold visiting Sarah, and threatening at times to place Sarah in a nursing home.

After listening to both Karen and Sarah's needs as caregiver and cancer survivor, occupational therapy interventions used to support Karen included training Sarah in accessing community resources and getting her signed up with a medical transportation service to take her to doctor appointments. The occupational therapy practitioner provided stress management training and role prioritization using the Role Checklist (Oakley et al., 1986) and educated Karen that being Sarah's caregiver did not mean Sarah had to live with her.

Karen, the occupational therapy practitioner, and Sarah's psychiatrist used a telehealth intervention through weekly group emails for a consistent line of support from health care professionals. Karen later provided the most positive feedback for this intervention. Education and skills training for recruiting support and respite was also provided. Karen hired a personal care assistant for Sarah to assist her with errands and cooking. She also recruited Sarah's estranged, adopted son to spend one night per week addressing Sarah's needs to give Karen respite. Karen began identifying herself as Sarah's caregiver, and Sarah started attending an art group at her apartments.

of unfinished business; and *legacy work,* or purposefully leaving behind a sense or part of oneself through action or artifact (e.g., photo album, favorite family recipe, letters for children to open as they reach milestones in their lives).

Personal and health needs of caregivers often become overshadowed as the amount of physical and emotional support they provide increases alongside the complexity and urgency of the care recipient's medical and emotional needs. Many caregivers try to retain a sense of normalcy by focusing on continuing normal rituals and routines that involve the care recipient (Ugalde et al., 2012). Thus, facilitating shared family occupations around religious and spiritual practices as well as other usual family routines can help create a sense of health and normalcy for the caregiver (Pickens & Long, 2016). However, during end of life, care recipients often adopt and find new meaning in occupations that differ from familiar family rituals and routines, and caregivers may need assistance in accepting this "new normalcy." In Case Example 27.3, Darrell becomes aware that his wife Tameka will no longer be able to continue their morning routine and is educated by Tameka's occupational therapist about the need to adapt to new normalcy.

Evaluation during end-of-life care should include assessing the caregiver's knowledge of the care recipient's proximity to death, the symptoms of the dying process and possible disruptive behaviors that can occur, the caregiver's view of life and expectations of dying, and the cultural and spiritual expectations for the dying process. Occupational therapy interventions for caregivers may include training on

- Role balance, with attention to capacity to cope and burden of care;
- Environmental modifications to allow the caregiver and loved ones to be physically near each other and the care recipient;
- Time management and organization to coordinate taking care of financial, legal, and funeral needs;
- Facilitating both the practice of family rituals and routines and acceptance of "new normalcy;"
- Facilitating shared family occupations around religious and spiritual practices;
- Facilitating the caregiver role and providing assistance needed in legacy work; and
- Role transition and life restructuring for a new future without the care recipient.

CANCER CAREGIVERS AND TELECOMMUNICATION

A high prevalence of telecommunication or internet (74%) and social media use (39%) exists among caregivers of family members with cancer (Badr et al., 2015). The interest in having opportunities for both social engagement with cancer survivors and other caregivers and for coordination of care with health care professionals through telehealth interventions continues to grow. *Telehealth* is a mode of service delivery that connects the caregiver and the occupational therapy practitioner through some

---

CASE EXAMPLE 27.3. DARRELL: CAREGIVER DURING END-OF-LIFE CARE

Darrell is age 52 years and the husband of **Tameka,** who is age 48 years and has liver cell carcinoma with metastases to her lungs, multiple levels of her spine, and her right hip bone. She was told during this hospital stay that she is a candidate for hospice care and will likely need assistance with symptom management. Tameka has chosen to discharge home with hospice care.

Darrell does not know how he feels about Tameka dying at home because their twin young adult sons live with them while attending their first year of college. However, dying at home is Tameka's stated preference, and he wants to honor her wishes. Tameka says she wants to make a series of videos for her two sons for when they get married and start their own families. Darrell worries whether she will be able to do this because he reports she is exhausted after just getting up to go to the bathroom.

Occupational therapy interventions used to help support Darrell include environmental modification strategies and durable medical equipment (DME) recommendations. Although hospice will assist with getting the DME Tameka needs, the occupational therapist reviewed with Darrell recommendations for how to modify their home environment to make best use of the DME.

Tameka prefers to be upstairs in her room to sleep, and the only bath with a walk-in shower is upstairs, in

Tameka's preferred bathroom. She is currently able to go up and down stairs safely, despite her limp. In the environmental modification, the occupational therapist emphasized the importance of having areas both upstairs and downstairs where Tameka can rest to achieve positioning to decrease her pain and suggested areas where Darrell and her sons can be physically close to Tameka. Energy conservation and fatigue management training was provided for Darrell to help Tameka reserve the energy to complete her legacy work, help get her legal affairs in order, and spend quality time with her sons. Strategies on adapting and simplifying legacy work were also included because of the extensive project Tameka had chosen.

Education on adapting to new normalcy where new routines may be adopted in place of prior familiar routines was provided for Darrell after Tameka said she was not looking forward to continuing their morning routine of having breakfast and going for a walk, despite having been told walking would help with her strength and energy level. She reported she did not want to be seen by their neighbors and that eggs currently nauseated her. Instead, Tameka reported she thought she could drink a protein shake and walk with her husband in their backyard.

combination of visual and auditory real-time interactive communications technologies (Texas Board of Occupational Therapy Examiners, 2019). Integrating telehealth interventions into workflow systems

- Provides an opportunity to evaluate, consult with, and monitor caregivers who might not otherwise have frequent access to the occupational therapy practitioner;
- Eliminates the wait time for responses from a series of phone calls or emails when face-to-face video communication is used;
- Increases overall efficiency of care by providing caregivers information when they need it;
- Affects adherence to and the success of behavioral interventions when provided at the time the caregiver can use them; and
- Augments information from the occupational therapy practitioner by providing practical tips for managing the day-to-day aspects of cancer and cancer treatments (Long et al., 2015; Ugalde et al., 2012).

TABLE 27.2.   Resources for Caregiver Support

RESOURCE	URL
American Cancer Society ■ Caregiver support, coping information	cancer.org
CancerCare ■ Support groups, education, workshops, counseling services, financial assistance	cancercare.org
Cancer Support Community ■ Support groups, education, health and wellness programs, resources for children and teens	cancersupportcommunity.org
Caregiver Action Network ■ Education and support	caregiveraction.org/
CaringBridge ■ Site to share health news and coordinate care with family and friends	caringbridge.org
Family Career Alliance ■ Information, education, advocacy, research, and links to services	caregiver.org
National Alliance for Caregiving ■ Education, webcasts and conferences, research	caregiving.org
National Cancer Institute ■ Support, resources for children and teens	cancer.gov
National Caregiving Foundation ■ Caregiver support kit, links to resources	caregivingfoundation.org
Palliative Care Research Cooperative/ Family Caregiver Core ■ Research, family caregiver tools	palliativecareresearch.org

Source. From Bevans & Sternberg (2012) and Ferrell & Wittenberg (2017).

SUMMARY

Caregivers make up the largest source of long-term care in the country, and their role is projected to continue to grow. Advances in cancer treatment leading to increased survivorship, earlier discharges from acute care hospitals, and ongoing changes in health care reimbursement have contributed to a shift in the burden of care from health care professionals to caregivers. Increased survivorship has led to the extension of the demands of caregiving potentially for months or even years. Both the shift in burden of care and the extension of caregiver demands make caregivers more likely to experience caregiver burden, with declining physical and mental health and well-being, and ultimately may increase their risk for mortality. As caregiver burden increases, caregivers often give up their own desired occupations and develop health care needs that can compromise their ability to sustain care responsibilities.

Occupational therapy practitioners contribute to a plan of care of supportive services to both reduce the negative effects of caregiving and support the sustainability of occupational performance. Practitioners develop meaningful, targeted interventions that take into account the complexity of the role and its changing needs and demands to facilitate successful occupational engagement for the promotion of caregiver health, well-being, and self-efficacy. Table 27.2 provides other sources of caregiver support and their links.

REFERENCES

American Occupational Therapy Association. (2014). Occupational therapy practice framework: Domain and process (3rd ed.). *American Journal of Occupational Therapy, 68,* S1–S48. https://doi.org/10.5014/ajot.2014.682006

Applebaum, A., Bevans, M., Son, T., Evans, K., Hernandez, M., Giralt, S., & DuHamel, K. (2016). A scoping review of caregiver burden during allogeneic HSCT: Lessons learned and future directions. *Bone Marrow Transplant, 51,* 1416–1422. https://doi.org/10.1038/bmt.2016.164

Badr, H., Carmack, C., & Diefenbach, M. (2015). Psychosocial interventions for patients and caregivers in the age of new communication technologies: Opportunities and challenges in cancer care. *Journal of Health Communications, 20,* 328–342. https://doi.org/10.1080/10810730.2014.965369

Baron, K., Kiehofner, G., Iyenger, A., Goldhammer, V., & Wolenski, J. (2006). *The Occupational Self Assessment (OSA) Version 2.2.* Chicago: University of Illinois of Chicago, College of Applied Health Sciences, Department of Occupational Therapy.

Bastawrous, M., Gignac, M. A., Kapral, M. K., & Cameron, J. I. (2015). Adult daughters providing post-stroke care to a parent: A qualitative study of the impact that role overload has on lifestyle, participation and family relationships. *Clinical Rehabilitation, 29,* 592–600. https://doi.org/10.1177/0269215514552035

Berg, C., & Hayahi, R. J. (2013). Participation and self-management strategies of young adult childhood cancer survivors. *Occupational Therapy Journal of Research, 33,* 21–30. https://doi.org/10.3928/15394492-20120607-01

Bevans, M., & Sternberg, E. M. (2012). Caregiving burden, stress, and health effects among family caregivers of adult cancer patients. *Journal of the American Medical Association, 307,* 398–403. https://doi.org/10.1001/jama.2012.29

Cohn, E. S., & Henry, A. D. (2008). Caregiving and childrearing. In E. B. Crepeau, E. S. Cohn, & B. A. B. Schell (Eds.), *Willard & Spackman's occupational therapy* (11th ed., pp. 579–589). Philadelphia: Wolters Kluwer.

Dionne-Odom, J. N., Applebaum, A. J., Ornstein, K. A., Azuero, A., Warren, P. P., Taylor, R. A., . . . Bakitas, M. A. (2018). Participation and interest in support services among family caregivers of older adults with cancer. *Psycho-Oncology, 27,* 969–976. https://doi.org/10.1002/pon.4603

Drabe, N., Klaghofer, R., Weidt, S., Zwahlen, D., Buchi, S., & Jenewein, J. (2015). Mutual associations between patients' and partners' depression and quality of life with respect to relationship quality, physical complaints, and sense of coherence in couples coping with cancer. *Pyscho-Oncology, 24,* 442–450. https://doi.org/10.1002/pon.3662

Eifert, E. K., Adams, R., Dudley, W., & Perko, M. (2015). Family caregiver identity: A literature review. *American Journal of Health Education, 46,* 357–367. https://doi.org/10.1080/19325037.2015.1099482

Family Caregiver Alliance. (2013). *Grief and loss.* Retrieved from https://www.caregiver.org/grief-and-loss

Ferrell, B., Hanson, J., & Grant, M. (2013). An overview and evaluation of the Oncology Family Caregiver Project: Improving quality of life and quality of care for oncology family caregivers. *Psycho-Oncology, 22,* 1645–1652. https://doi.org/10.1002/pon.3198

Ferrell, B., & Wittenberg, E. (2017). A review of family caregiving intervention trials in oncology. *CA: A Cancer Journal for Clinicians, 67,* 318–325. https://doi.org/10.3322/caac.21396

Fuentes, C., Hernandez, C., Escobedo, L., Herskovic, V., & Tentori, M. (2014). Promoting self-reflection of social isolation through persuasive mobile technologies: The case of mother caregivers of children with cancer. *International Journal of Human–Computer Interaction, 30,* 802–814. https://doi.org/10.1080/10447318.2014.927279

Geddie, P. I., Loerzel, V. W., & Norris, A. E. (2016). Family caregiver knowledge, patient illness characteristics, and unplanned hospital admissions in older adults with cancer. *Oncology Nursing Forum, 43,* 453–463. https://doi.org/10.1188/16.ONF.453-463

Given, C. W., Given, B., Stommel, M., Collins, C., King, S., & Franklin, S. (1992). The Caregiver Reaction Assessment (CRA) for caregivers to persons with chronic physical and mental impairments. *Research in Nursing and Health, 15*(40), 271–283. https://doi.org/10.1002/nur.4770150406

Glajchen, M. (2012). Physical well-being of oncology caregivers: An important quality-of-life domain. *Seminars of Oncology Nursing, 28,* 226–235. https://doi.org/10.1016/j.soncn.2012.09.005

Glajchen, M., Kornblith, A., Homel, P., Fraidin, L., Mauskop, A., & Portenoy, R. K. (2005). Development of a Brief Assessment Scale for Cargivers of the medically ill. *Journal of Pain and Symptom Management, 29*(3), 245–254. https://doi.org/10.1016/j.jpainsymman.2004.06.017

Goldsmith, J., Wittenberg, E., Small-Platt, C., Iannarino, N. T., & Reno, J. (2016). Family caregiver communication in oncology: Advancing a typology. *Pyscho-Oncology, 25,* 463–470. https://doi.org/10.1002/pon.3862

Hammill, K., Bye, R., & Cook, C. (2014). Occupational therapy for people living with a life-limiting illness: A thematic review. *British Journal of Occupational Therapy, 77,* 582–589. https://doi.org/10.4276/030802214X14151078348594

Health in Aging Foundation. (2015). *Caregiver Self Assessment Questionnaire.* Retrieved from https://www.healthinaging.org/resources/resource:caregiver-self-assessment/

Henriksson, A., Andershed, B., Benzein, E., & Arestedt, K. (2011). Adaptation and psychometric evaluation of the Preparedness for Caregiving Scale, Caregiver Competence Scale, and Rewards of Caregiving Scale in a sample of Swedish family members of patients with life-threatening illness. *Palliative Medicine, 26,* 930–938. https://doi.org/10.1177/0269216311419987

Hsu, T., Loscalzo, M., Ramani, R., Forman, S., Popplewell, L., Clark, K., . . . Hurria, A. (2014). Factors associated with high burden in caregivers of older adults with cancer. *Cancer, 120,* 2927–2935. https://doi.org/10.1002/cncr.28765

Jayani, R., & Hurria, A. (2012). Caregiver of older adults with cancer. *Seminars in Oncology Nursing, 28,* 221–225. https://doi.org/10.1016/j.soncn.2012.09.004

Kaveney, S. C., Baumstarck, K., Minaya-Flores, P., Shannon, T., Symes, P., Loundou, A., & Auquier, P. (2016). Validation of the American version of the Caregiver Oncology Quality of Life (CarGOQol) Questionnaire. *Health and Quality of Life Outcomes, 14,* 82. https://doi.org/10.1186/s12955-016-0487-6

Kim, Y., & Carver, C. (2012). Recognizing the value and needs of the caregiver in oncology. *Current Opinion in Supportive and Palliative Care, 6,* 280–288. https://doi.org/10.1097/SPC.0b013e3283526999

Kniepmann, K. (2012). Female family carers for survivors of stroke: Occupational loss and quality of life. *British Journal of Occupational Therapy, 75,* 208–216. https://doi.org/10.4276/030802212X13361458480207

Long, J. T., Kovacs, C. J., Hoobler, A. J., Fritts, E. K., Cunningham, B. E., & Caldwell, C. M. (2015). Integrating telehealth: Experiences in incorporating telehealth tools and principles into a pediatric therapeutic environment. *OT Practice, 20*(7), CE-1–CE-8.

Lund, L., Ross, L., Peterson, M. A., & Groenvold, M. (2015). The interaction between informal caregivers and health care professionals: A survey of caregivers' experiences of problems and unmet needs. *Support Cancer Care, 23,* 1719–1733. https://doi.org/10.1007/s00520-014-2529-0

Marston, C., Agar, M., & Brown, T. (2015). Patients' and caregivers' perceptions of occupational therapy and adapting to discharge home from an inpatient palliative care setting. *British Journal of Occupational Therapy, 78,* 688–696. https://doi.org/10.1177/0308022615586417

Matuska, K. (2012). Validity evidence of a model and measure of life balance. *OTJR: Occupation, Participation and Health, 32,* 229–237. https://doi.org/10.3928/15394492-20110610-02

Mori, H., Fukuda, R., Hayashi, A., Yamamoto, K., Misago, C., & Nakayama, T. (2012). Characteristics of caregiver perceptions of end-of-life caregiving experiences in cancer survivorship: In-depth interview study. *Psycho-Oncology, 21,* 666–674. https://doi.org/10.1002/pon.1964

Nipp, R. D., El-Jawahri, A., Fishbein, J. N., Gallagher, E. R., Stagl, J. M., Park, E. R., . . . Temel, J. S. (2016). Factors associated with depression and anxiety symptoms in family caregivers of patients with incurable cancer. *Annals of Oncology, 27,* 1607–1612. https://doi.org/10.1093/annonc/mdw205

Oakley, F., Kielhofner, G., Barris, R., & Reichler, R. K. (1986). The role checklist: Development and empirical assessment of reliability. *Occupational Therapy Journal of Research, 6*(3), 157–170.

PDQ® Supportive and Palliative Care Editorial Board. PDQ Family Caregivers in Cancer. (2019). *Family Caregivers in Cancer (PDQ)—Patient Version*. Retrieved from https://www.cancer.gov/about-cancer/coping/family-friends/family-caregivers-pdq

Pergolotti, M., Deal, A. M., Lavery, J., Reeve, B. B., & Muss, H. B. (2015). The prevalence of potentially modifiable functional deficits and the subsequent use of occupational and physical therapy by older adults with cancer. *Journal of Geriatric Oncology, 6*, 194–201. https://doi.org/10.1016/j.jgo.2015.01.004

Pickens, N. D., & Long, T. (2016). Occupational therapy practitioners working with caregivers in adult palliative care and end-of-life care. *OT Practice, 21*(3), CE-1–CE-8.

Pierce, C. (2012). Profiling the caregiver. *Gerontology Special Interest Section Quarterly, 35*(4), 1–4.

Popova, E. S., Ostrowski, R. K., Wescott, J. J., & Taylor, R. R. (2019). Development and validation of the Occupational Self-Assessement—Short form (OSA-SF). *American Journal of Occupational Therapy, 73*, 7303205020. https://doi.org/10.5014/ajot.2019.030288

O'Sullivan, A. (2015). Collaborating with family caregivers in the home setting. *OT Practice, 20*(11), CE-1–CE-8.

Robinson, J., Gott, M., & Ingleton, C. (2014). Patient and family experiences of palliative care in hospital: What do we know? An integrative review. *Palliative Medicine, 28*, 18–33. https://doi.org/10.1177/0269216313487568

Rosenberg-Yunger, Z., Granek, L., Sung, L., Klaassen, R., Dix, D., Cairney, J., & Klassen, A. F. (2013). Single-parent caregivers of children with cancer: Factors assisting with caregiving strains. *Journal of Pediatric Oncology Nursing, 30*, 45–55. https://doi.org/10.1177/1043454212471727

Saritas, S. C., Kavak, F., Aksoy, A., & Saritas, S. (2017). Examination of the care burden of caregivers of oncology patients and the perceived social support from family. *International Journal of Caring Sciences, 10*, 447–454.

Sleight, A. G., & Duker, L. I. (2016). Toward a broader role for occupational therapy in supportive oncology care. *American Journal of Occupational Therapy, 70*, 7004360030. https://doi.org/10.5014/ajot.2016.018101

Taylor, R. R. (2017). Habituation: Patterns of daily occupation. In R. R. Taylor (Ed.), *Kielhofner's Model of Human Occupation: Theory and application* (5th ed., pp. 65–69). Philadelphia: Wolters Kluwer.

Tebb, S. S., Berg-Weger, M., & Rubio, D. M. (2013). The Caregiver Well-Being Scale: Developing a short-form rapid assessment instrument. *Health and Social Work, 38*(4), 222–230. https://doi.org/10.1093/hsw/hlt019

Texas Board of Occupational Therapy Examiners. (2019). *Occupational therapy rules: December, 2019*. Retrieved from https://www.ptot.texas.gov/idl/D4241942-233A-C3A1-8353-137E9423412E

Thornton, M., & Travis, S. S. (2003). Analysis of the reliability of the Modified Caregiver Strain Index. *Journal of Gerontology, 58*(2), S127–S132.

Ugalde, A., Krishnasamy, M., & Scofield, P. (2012). Role recognition and changes to self-identity in family caregivers of people with advanced cancer: A qualitative study. *Supportive Care in Cancer, 20*, 1175–1181. https://doi.org/10.1007/s00520-011-1194-9

Vernooij-Dassen, A., Felling, E., Brummelkamp, M., Dautzenber, G., van den Bosch, R. (1999). Assessment of caregiver's competence in dealing with the burden of caregiving for a dementia patient: A Short Sense of Competence Questionnaire (SSCQ) suitable for clinical practice. *Journal of American Geriatric Society, 47*, 256–257. https://doi.org/10.1111/j.1532-5415.1999.tb04588.x

Weitzner, M. A., Jacobsen, P. B., Wagner, H., Friedland, J., & Cox, C. (1999). The Caregiver Quality of Life Index-Cancer (CQOLC) Scale: Development and validation of an instrument to measure quality of life of the family caregiver of patients with cancer. *Quality of Life Research, 8*, 55–63. https://doi.org/10.1023/a:1026407010614

Williams, T. (2016). Supporting caregiver identity. *OT Practice, 21*(19), CE-1–CE-8.

Zhukovsky, D. S., Rozmus, C. L., Robert, R. S., Bruera, E., Wells, R. J., Chisholm, G. B., . . . Cohen, M. Z. (2015). Symptom profiles in children with advanced cancer: Parent, family caregiver, and oncologist ratings. *Cancer, 121*, 4080–4087. https://doi.org/10.1002/cncr.29597

Index

Note: Page numbers in *italic* indicate exhibits, figures, and tables.